National Key Book Publishing Planning Project of the 13th Five-Year Plan
"十三五" 国家重点图书出版规划项目
International Clinical Medicine Series Based on the Belt and Road Initiative
"一带一路" 背景下国际化临床医学丛书

国家出版基金项目
NATIONAL PUBLICATION FOUNDATION

Medical Microbiology

医学微生物学

Chief Editor   Jin Chengyun   Jin Qing   Cao Hong
主编   金成允   金清   曹虹

U0339675

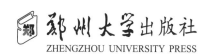
郑州大学出版社
ZHENGZHOU UNIVERSITY PRESS

图书在版编目(CIP)数据

医学微生物学 = Medical Microbiology：英文/金成允，金清，曹虹主编. — 郑州：
郑州大学出版社，2020.12
("一带一路"背景下国际化临床医学丛书)
ISBN 978-7-5645-7240-2

Ⅰ. ①医… Ⅱ. ①金…②金…③曹… Ⅲ. ①医学微生物学 – 英文 Ⅳ. ①R37

中国版本图书馆 CIP 数据核字(2020)第 161458 号

医学微生物学 = Medical Microbiology：英文

项目负责人	孙保营　杨秦予		策 划 编 辑	杨秦予
责 任 编 辑	刘宇洋		装 帧 设 计	苏永生
责 任 校 对	张锦森		责 任 监 制	凌　青　李瑞卿

出版发行	郑州大学出版社有限公司		地　　址	郑州市大学路 40 号(450052)
出 版 人	孙保营		网　　址	http://www.zzup.cn
经　　销	全国新华书店		发行电话	0371-66966070
印　　刷	河南文华印务有限公司			
开　　本	850 mm×1 168 mm　1 / 16			
印　　张	32.75		字　　数	1 258 千字
版　　次	2020 年 12 月第 1 版		印　　次	2020 年 12 月第 1 次印刷

书　　号	ISBN 978-7-5645-7240-2		定　　价	149.00 元

Staff of Expert Steering Committee

Chairmen

Zhong Shizhen   Li Sijin   Lü Chuanzhu

Vice Chairmen

Bai Yuting   Chen Xu   Cui Wen   Huang Gang   Huang Yuanhua
Jiang Zhisheng   Li Yumin   Liu Zhangsuo   Luo Baojun   Lü Yi
Tang Shiying

Committee Member

An Dongping   Bai Xiaochun   Cao Shanying   Chen Jun   Chen Yijiu
Chen Zhesheng   Chen Zhihong   Chen Zhiqiao   Ding Yueming   Du Hua
Duan Zhongping   Guan Chengnong Huang Xufeng   Jian Jie   Jiang Yaochuan
Jiao Xiaomin   Li Cairui   Li Guoxin   Li Guoming   Li Jiabin
Li Ling   Li Zhijie   Liu Hongmin   Liu Huifan   Liu Kangdong
Song Weiqun   Tang Chunzhi   Wang Huamin   Wang Huixin   Wang Jiahong
Wang Jiangang   Wang Wenjun   Wang Yuan   Wei Jia   Wen Xiaojun
Wu Jun   Wu Weidong   Wu Xuedong   Xie Xieju   Xue Qing
Yan Wenhai   Yan Xinming   Yang Donghua   Yu Feng   Yu Xiyong
Zhang Lirong   Zhang Mao   Zhang Ming   Zhang Yu'an   Zhang Junjian
Zhao Song   Zhao Yumin   Zheng Weiyang   Zhu Lin

专家指导委员会

Staff of Editor Steering Committee

Chairmen

Cao Xuetao   Liang Guiyou   Wu Jiliang

Vice Chairmen

Chen Pingyan   Chen Yuguo   Huang Wenhua   Li Yaming   Wang Heng

Xu Zuojun   Yao Ke   Yao Libo   Yu Xuezhong   Zhao Xiaodong

Committee Member

Cao Hong   Chen Guangjie   Chen Kuisheng   Chen Xiaolan   Dong Hongmei

Du Jian   Du Ying   Fei Xiaowen   Gao Jianbo   Gao Yu

Guan Ying   Guo Xiuhua   Han Liping   Han Xingmin   He Fanggang

He Wei   Huang Yan   Huang Yong   Jiang Haishan   Jin Chengyun

Jin Qing   Jin Runming   Li Lin   Li Ling   Li Mincai

Li Naichang   Li Qiuming   Li Wei   Li Xiaodan   Li Youhui

Liang Li   Lin Jun   Liu Fen   Liu Hong   Liu Hui

Lu Jing   Lü Bin   Lü Quanjun   Ma Qingyong   Ma Wang

Mei Wuxuan   Nie Dongfeng   Peng Biwen   Peng Hongjuan   Qiu Xinguang

Song Chuanjun   Tan Dongfeng   Tu Jiancheng   Wang Lin   Wang Huijun

Wang Peng   Wang Rongfu   Wang Shusen   Wang Chongjian   Xia Chaoming

Xiao Zheman   Xie Xiaodong   Xu Falin   Xu Xia   Xu Jitian

Xue Fuzhong   Yang Aimin   Yang Xuesong   Yi Lan   Yin Kai

Yu Zujiang   Yu Hong   Yue Baohong   Zeng Qingbing   Zhang Hui

Zhang Lin   Zhang Lu   Zhang Yanru   Zhao Dong   Zhao Hongshan

Zhao Wen   Zheng Yanfang   Zhou Huaiyu   Zhu Changju   Zhu Lifang

编审委员会

Editorial Staff

Reviewers

    Chen Zhesheng   St. John's University

    Yang Donghua   St. John's University

Honorary Chief Editor

    Li Jinfeng   The First Affiliated Hospital of Zhengzhou University

Chief Editors

    Jin Chengyun   Zhengzhou University

    Jin Qing   Yanbian University

    Cao Hong   Southern Medical University

Vice Chief Editors

    Zhu Bingdong   Lanzhou University

    Yu Haiyang   Tianjin University of Traditional Chinese Medicine

    Wu Wenlan   Henan University of Science and Technology

    Deng Maozi   Hubei University of Science and Technology

    Li Chunying   Henan Agricultural University

Editorial Staffs

    Dong Jianshu   Zhengzhou University

    Fu Xiangjing   Zhengzhou University(And Secretary)

    Jin Yingshan   Yangzhou University

    Ma Licai   China Agricultural University

    Li Jun   Chinese Academy of Medical Sciences

    Liu Rongzeng   Henan University of Science and Technology

    Qin Shangshang   Zhengzhou University

    Qiu Yuling   Tianjin Medical University

    Gong Yixia   Jiamusi University

    Sun Ruiqin   Henan University of Chinese Medicine

    Wang Qing   Henan Institute of Science and Technology

Wang Xiangpeng	Xinxiang Medical University
Wang Zhenya	Zhengzhou University
Yao Lan	Xinjiang Medical University
Zang Wenqiao	Zhengzhou University
Zhang Hao	Henan Normal University
Zhu Lingjuan	Shenyang Pharmaceutical University

作者名单

主　审
　　陈哲生　　圣约翰大学
　　杨冬华　　圣约翰大学

名誉主编
　　李金峰　　郑州大学第一附属医院

主　编
　　金成允　　郑州大学
　　金　清　　延边大学
　　曹　虹　　南方医科大学

副主编
　　祝秉东　　兰州大学
　　于海洋　　天津中医药大学
　　吴文澜　　河南科技大学
　　邓毛子　　湖北科技学院
　　李春英　　河南农业大学

编　委　（以姓氏汉语拼音为序）
　　董建树　　郑州大学
　　付向晶　　郑州大学（兼秘书）
　　金英善　　扬州大学
　　马立才　　中国农业大学
　　李　君　　中国医学科学院
　　刘熔增　　河南科技大学
　　秦上尚　　郑州大学
　　邱玉玲　　天津医科大学
　　宫益霞　　佳木斯大学
　　孙瑞芹　　河南中医药大学
　　王　青　　河南科技学院

王向鹏　　新乡医学院
王振亚　　郑州大学
姚　蓝　　新疆医科大学
臧文巧　　郑州大学
张　昊　　河南师范大学
朱玲娟　　沈阳药科大学

Preface

At the Second Belt and Road Summit Forum on International Cooperation in 2019 and the Seventy-third World Health Assembly in 2020, General Secretary Xi Jinping stated the importance for promoting the construction of the "Belt and Road" and jointly build a community for human health. Countries and regions along the "Belt and Road" have a large number of overseas Chinese communities, and shared close geographic proximity, similarities in culture, disease profiles and medical habits. They also shared a profound mass base with ample space for cooperation and exchange in Clinical Medicine. The publication of the International Clinical Medicine series for clinical researchers, medical teachers and students in countries along the "Belt and Road" is a concrete measure to promote the exchange of Chinese and foreign medical science and technology with mutual appreciation and reciprocity.

Zhengzhou University Press coordinated more than 600 medical experts from over 160 renowned medical research institutes, medical schools and clinical hospitals across China. It produced this set of medical tools in English to serve the needs for the construction of the "Belt and Road". It comprehensively coversaspects in the theoretical framework and clinical practicesin Clinical Medicine, including basic science, multiple clinical specialities and social medicine. It reflects the latest academic and technological developments, and the international frontiers of academic advancements in Clinical Medicine. It shared with the world China's latest diagnosis and therapeutic approaches, clinical techniques, and experiences in prescription and medication. It has an important role in disseminating contemporary Chinese medical science and technology innovations, demonstrating the achievements of modern China's economic and social development, and promoting the unique charm of Chinese culture to the world.

The series is the first set of medical tools written in English by Chinese medical experts to serve the needs of the "Belt and Road" construction. It systematically and comprehensively reflects the Chinese characteristics in Clinical Medicine. Also, it presents a landmark achievement in the implementation of the "Belt and Road" initiative in promoting exchanges in medical science and technology. This series is theoretical in nature, with each volume built on the mainlines in traditional disciplines but at the same time introducing contemporary theories that guide clinical practices, diagnosis and treatment methods, echoing the latest research findings in Clinical Medicine.

As the disciplines in Clinical Medicine rapidly advances, different views on knowledge, inclusiveness, and medical ethics may arise. We hope this work will facilitate the exchange of ideas, build common ground while allowing differences, and contribute to the building of a community for human health in a broad spectrum of disciplines and research focuses.

Nick Lemoine

Foreign Academician of the Chinese Academy of Engineering
Dean, Academy of Medical Sciences of Zhengzhou University
Director, Barts Cancer Institute, London, UK
6th August, 2020

Foreword

In accordance with the requirements of the National Ministry of Education with the goal of promoting international communication, improving English proficiency, and meeting the demands of bilingual teaching in China, we present this textbook "Medical Microbiology". We hope this book will better fit the needs of medical students in China. This textbook includes sections on introduction of microbiology, Bacteriology, Virology, Mycology, and Biosafety designed to improve the ease of study through well-defined sections from microbial structures to diagnosis. Information that is not pertinent for the understanding of this subject has been omitted to create a more useful reference.

All of the authors come from the forefront of teaching and research communities around China. They offer a variety of rich experiences in Medical Microbiology. The editor would like to acknowledge their contributions as well as extend thanks to the Zhengzhou University Publishing House who has helped this project reach its publishable goal.

In conclusion, we hope that our textbook can help the students, teachers, and clinicians whereas their nationalities throughout China. Although we have done our best to compile a comprehensive text, we realize some errors may be present due to the language barriers. We welcome any potential revisions or suggestions our readers might make.

Authors

Contents

Chapter 1

Microorganisms and Microbiology

1.1 Microorganism

1.1.1 Microorganism Development

Microorganism (microbe) is a group of microscopic organisms (less than 0.1 mm) with a simple structure and has to be visualized by an optical microscope or an electron microscope to magnify hundreds or tens of thousands of times instead of naked eyes.

Before people visualized microbes, some researchers had suspected their existence and considered them as the cause of diseases. The Roman philosopher Lucretius (about 98—55 B. C.) and the physician Girolamo Fracastoro (1478—1553) proposed that the disease was caused by invisible living organisms. Between 1625 and 1630, the Italian, Francesco Stelluti, performed microscopic observations on Bee and Weevil. Antony van Leeuwenhoek (1632—1723) from Netherlands created the microscope using polished lenses (Figure 1–1) and used it (from about 40 to 270 magnifications) to observe various forms of microorganisms from water, tartar and fecal matter. He also accurately described the morphology of organisms such as spheres, rods and spirals. This not only provides strong evidence for the existence of microorganisms, but also lays a foundation for microbial morphology.

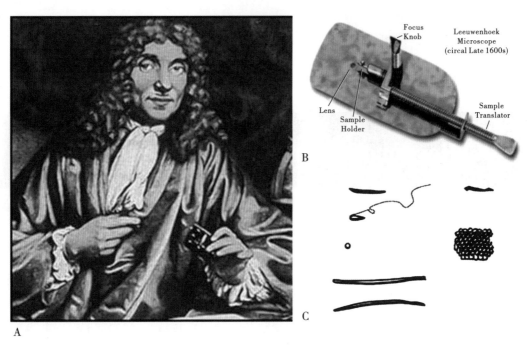

Figure 1-1   Antony van Leeuwenhoek(1632—1723)and microscope

A:Leeuwenhoek holds themicroscope;B:created the microscope;C:Bacteria in the human mouth observed by the microscope. From G. E. Dobell,Antony van Leeuwenhoek and his little animals(1932)

1.1.2   Spontaneous Generation

Once upon a time,people believed that living organisms could develop from non-living materials. Even the great Aristotle(384—322 B. C.)believed that some simple invertebrates could naturally arise. This opinion was first challenged by the Italian doctor Francesco Redi(1626—1697)who conducted a series of experiments testing the abiogenesis of maggots from carrion. He put the meat in three containers:the first was uncapped,the second was covered with paper and the third was covered with a fine gauze to keep files out. Eggs were laid on uncovered meat with maggots found. At the same time,no maggots were detected abiogenetically on the other two pieces of meat. However,files were attracted to the containers covered with gauze with eggs laid and maggots found. Therefore,maggots on carrion were from fly's eggs,but not from abiogenesis as people previously believed. Similar experiments conducted by others on larger organism also questioned the theory of abiogenesis.

Leeuwenhoek discovered the microbes and restored this controversy. Some people suggested that even though larger organisms were not abiogenetic,microbes were. They pointed out that microorganisms were detected in the extraction of hay or meat after a short while. In 1748,the British pastor John Needham(1713—1781)reported on his own experimental results on abiogenesis. Needham boiled mutton soup and plugged the flask. Finally,the soup in many flasks became turbid and contained microorganisms. He thought that the organic matter had vitality to make non-living materials living. Some years later,Italian priest and naturalist Lazzaro Spallanzani(1729—1799)improved Needham's experimental design by first sealing the glass flask with water and seeds. If the sealed flask had been boiled for 3/4 h,as long as the flask remained sealed,it contained no growth. He proposed that the air carried microorganism into the medium,but he also suggested that the outside air might be necessary for the growth of organisms already in the medium. So supporters of abiogenesis insisted that the sealed heating destroyed the ability of the air in the flask to sustain life.

Several researchers tried to overturn this argument. Theodore Schwann (1810—1882) lead the air to pass through a burning tube into a flask containing sterile nutrient solution. The flask remained sterile. Georg Friedrich Schroder and Theodor von Dasch then lead the air to pass through a sterile lint into a flask containing a heat-sterilized medium. Although the air was not heated, there was no growth in this medium. Although these experiments confirmed that the abiogenesis theory was wrong, in 1859, the French naturalist Felix Pouchet claimed that his experiment showed that microorganisms grew without air pollution. Louis Pasteur (1822—1895) decided to clarify this. First, Pasteur filtered the air through cotton cloth and captured plant spore-like objects. If a piece of air-filtered cotton cloth was placed in a sterile medium, microbial growth occurred. He then put the nutrient solution in the flask, heated its bottleneck over the flame and stretched the bottleneck into various patterns of bending with its end open and exposed to the atmosphere (Figure 1–2). He boiled the solution for a few minutes and let it cool down. Although the nutrient solution in flask was exposed to the air, no growth occurred. Pasteur pointed out that since dust and microorganisms were trapped on the wall of the bending bottleneck, no growth occurred. If the bottleneck was broken, growth would occur immediately. In 1861, Pasteur clarified that relationship between microbes and the fermentation, negated the abiogenesis, confirmed the microbiological etiology of infectious diseases and advocated vaccination, thus making an outstanding contribution to the development of microbiology.

In 1877, British physicist John Tyndall (1820—1893) confirmed that dust did carry microorganisms. If there was no dust and kept the broth sterile, no growth occurred even though it was exposed directly to the air. This gave the abiogenesis a deadly blow. In his research, Tyndall proved the presence of abnormally heat-resistant bacteria. The German botanist Ferdinand Cohn (1828—1898) also found the presence of endophytic spores of heat-resistant bacteria in his work.

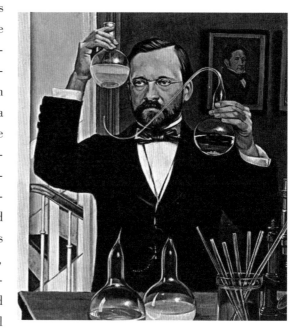

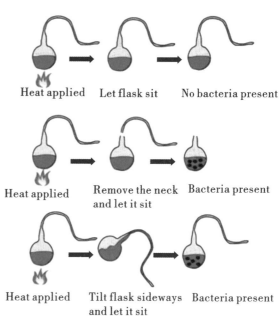

Heat applied　　Let flask sit　　No bacteria present

Heat applied　　Remove the neck　Bacteria present
　　　　　　　and let it sit

Heat applied　　Tilt flask sideways　Bacteria present
　　　　　　　and let it sit

Figure 1–2　Louis Pasteur(1822—1895) and his retorts

Left: Pasteur(1822—1895) is working in his laboratory for Autogenetic theory; Right: used in the experiment for microorganism autogenic theory Retorts. From Annales Sciences Naturelle, 4th Series, Vol. 16, pp. 1–98, Pasteur, L., 1861, "Mémoiresur les Corpuscules Organise's Qui Existent DansL' Atmosphère: Examen de la Doctrine des Générations Spontanées."

1.1.3 Microbial Role in Disease

1.1.3.1 Relationship Between Microbes and Diseases

The relationship between microorganisms and diseases was confirmed and known after many researches and years. It depends largely on the development of new technologies in microbiology. Once the disease caused by microbial infections are understood, microbiologists start to study the mechanisms of anti-microbial protection in hosts and explore how to prevent the disease. This gave rise to the immunology.

Regarding the occurrence and epidemic of infectious diseases, back to the early 11 th century, Liu Zhenren proposed that the tuberculosis was caused by insects in the late years of the Northern Song Dynasty. Plenciz (1705—1786) in Austria believed that the cause of infectious diseases was due to living objects. Italian Fracastoro (1483—1553) believed that infectious diseases might spread through direct contact, indirect contact and air. In preventive healthcare, Li Shizhen of the Ming Dynasty pointed out in the "Compendium of Materia Medica" that steamed cloths of the patient would not be contagious. In the Ming Dynasty (1567—1572), people used smallpox to prevent smallpox. But since the days of the Greek physician Galen (129—199), it had been widely accepted that disease was caused by an imbalance among four liquids (blood, mucus, yellow bile "rage" and black bile "melancholia"). In the early 19th century, pathogenic theory became polular. When Agostino Bassi (1773—1856) confirmed that Flacherie was caused by a fungal infection in 1835, he first pointed out that microorganisms was able to cause disease and proposed that many diseases were caused by microbial infections. In 1845, M. J. Berkeley proved that the serious potato disease in Ireland was caused by fungus. With the success of Pasteur's fermentation research, the French government asked him to investigate silkworm particles that damaged the silk industry. After a few years of work, Pasteur pointed out that the disease was caused by a parasitic protozoon which could be controlled by improving the ratio of larvae formed from eggs produced by healthy silkworm moths.

Indirect evidence of that microbes are human pathogenic factors came from the British surgeon Joseph Lister (1827—1912) who prevented the wound infections. He was inspired by Pasteur's findings on the involvement of microorganisms in fermentation and putrefaction and established an antiseptic surgical system preventing the entry of microorganisms into the window, such as: heating and sterilizing surgical instruments, disinfecting dressings with carbolic acid and spraying carbolic acid to disinfect the operating room. He applied his knowledge in microbiology in medical practice and laid the foundation for surgical aseptic surgery. Since the bacteria-killing carbolic acid also prevents wound infections, it also provided strong indirect evidence for the role of microorganism in diseases.

The first direct evidence for that bacteria cause disease came from the study of Anthrax by the German doctor Robert Koch (1843—1910) (Figure 1-3). Koch used the guidelines proposed by his teacher, Jacob Henle (1809—1885), to create a bacterial isolation culture method, established the relationship between Bacillus anthracis and Anthrax and published his findings in 1876. Koch injected healthy mice with substances from diseased animals and found all of these mice developed symptoms. After inoculating 20 mice to transfer anthrax, he incubated a piece of Spleen containing *Bacillus anthracis* in bovine serum. This Bacillus anthracis grew, reproduced and produced spores. When mice were inoculated with isolated bacilli or spores, Anthrax occurred. This thus proved a causal relationship between a microorganism and a specific disease, known as Koch's postulates. The law is summarized as follows: ①Pathogenic bacteria must exist in all affected individuals, but does not exist in healthy individuals; ②The pathogen must be isolated and cultivated to obtain pure breeds; ③When the pure-bred pathogen is inoculated into a healthy host, it must cause the same disease; ④The pathogenic microorganism must be separated again from this artificially infected and diseased host. This law plays an important role in the identification of pathogens. Subsequently, most of the pathogens of bacterial infectious diseases were discovered and successfully isolated and cultured.

Pasteur and his colleagues also used their work to confirm Koch's thesis that the Anthrax was caused by *Bacillus anthracis*. They discovered that after the dead animals were buried, the spores of anthrax were still alive and carried by the earthworms. When these spores were ingested by healthy animals, the animals would get infected.

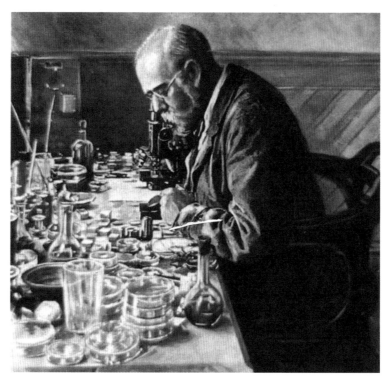

Figure 1–3   Robert Koch(1843—1910)working in his laboratory

1.1.3.2 Development of Microbial Pathogens Research Technology

When Koch studied bacterial diseases, in order to better isolate suspected bacterial pathogens, a solid medium using gelatin as a coagulant was created. Although gelatin has its advantages, it is not a good coagulant because many bacteria can digest it and it melts when the temperature rises to about 25 ℃. Fannie Eilshemius Hesse provided a better substitute. She was one of Koch's assistants and the wife of Walther Hesse (Figure 1–4). She suggested using agar as a coagulant and had been using agar to successfully make jelly for a while. Agar cannot be used by most bacteria and won't melt until the temperature reaches 100 ℃. One of Koch's assistants, Richard Petri, developed the Petri dish or plate, which holds the solid medium. These advances have not only made it possible to isolate pure cultures, but also directly promoted progress in all areas of bacteriology.

Fannie Hesse first suggested to use Agar in the medium.

Koch developed a medium suitable for the growth of bacteria isolated from the body. Since meat extracts and protein hydrolysates are similar to body fluids, they are used as the nutrient source and as a result, nutritive broths and nutrient agar culture medium which are still widely used today have been developed.

In 1882, Koch used these techniques to isolate bacilli that caused tuberculosis, followed by the isolation of most major pathogens (Table 1–1) over a period of 30–40 years.

In 1884, one of Pasteur's colleagues, Charles Chamberland (1851—1908), constructed a porcelain bacterial filter, which made it possible to discover the virus and its role in the disease. The first virus pathogen studied was the tobacco mosaic virus.

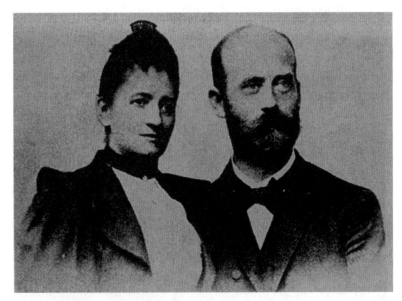

Figure 1-4　Fannie Eilshemius(1850—1934) and Walther Hesse(1846—1911)

Table 1-1　Important events in the development of microbiology

Date	Microbiological history
1546	Fracastoro proposes that Invisible organisms cause disease
1590—1608	Jansen develops the first useful composite microscope
1676	Antonie van Leeuwenhoek discovers "animalcules"
1786	Müller proposes the first bacterial classification
1838—1839	Schwann and Schleiden propose the cell theory
1857	Louis Pasteur shows that lactic acid fermentation is due to a microorganism
1861	Louis Pasteur shows that microorganisms do not arise by spontaneous generation
1867	Lister publishes his work on antiseptic surgery
1869	Miescher discovers nucleic acids
1876—1877	Robert Koch demonstrates that anthrax is caused by Bacillus anthracis
1880	Laveran discobers Plasmodium, the cause of malaria
1881	Louis Pasteur develops anthrax vaccine; Robert Koch cultures bacteria on gelatin
1884	Koch's postulates first published; Metchnikoff describes phagocytosis; High pressure sterilizer developed; Gram stain developed
1887	Richard Petri develops Petri dish (plate)
1921	Fleming discovers lysozyme

Continue to Table 1-1

Date	Microbiological history
1923	First edition of Bergey's Manual
1928	Griffith discovers bacterial transformation
1929	Fleming discovers penicillin
1933	Ruska develops first transmission electron microscope
1935	Stanley crystallizes the tobacco mosaic virus; Domagk discovers sulfonamide
1944	Avery shows that DNA carries information during transformation; Waksman discovers streptomycin
1953	Watson and Crick propose the double helix structure for DNA
1955	Jerne and Burnet propose theclonal selection theory
1973	Cohen, Boyer, Chang and Helling use plasmid vectors to clone genes in bacteria
1980	Development of the scanning tunneling microscope
1983—1984	Mullis develops the polymerase chain reaction
1990	First human gene-therapy testing begun
1997	Discovery of Thiomargaritanamibiensis, the largest known bacterium; Escherichia coli genome sequenced
2000	Discocery that Vibrio cholerae has two separate chromosomes

1.1.3.3　Immunology

During this period, advances had been made in determining how animals get resistant to diseases and establishing technologies to protect humans and livestock against pathogens. When Pasteur and Roux studied chicken cholera, they found that bacteria attenuated after a long time between transfer cultures. This indicated that bacteria had lost their ability to cause disease. If these cultures were used to vaccinate small chickens, they kept healthy and obtained resistance to this disease. To commemorate Edward Jenner, he called this attenuated culture Vaccin, because Jenner pioneered the usage of vaccinia to avoid smallpox many years ago. Shortly thereafter, Pasteur and Chamberland prepared the decayed anthrax vaccine in two ways: by treating the culture with Potassium dichromate and by culturing the bacteria at 42–43 ℃.

Pasteur later prepared a rabies vaccine in a different way. He cultured pathogens in a special host, the rabbit, to attenuated the pathogens. After the infected rabbits died, he extracted and dried the brains and spinal cords from the rabbit.

After the discovery of diphtheria-producing diphtheria, the German scholars Emil von Behring (1854—1917) and Shibasaburo Kitasato (1852—1931) inoculated rabbits with inactivated toxins to induce rabbits to produce antitoxins, a non-viable toxin in the bloodstream. It can resist diphtheria. Behring successfully treated a child with diphtheria in 1891 with diphtheria antitoxin-containing animal immune serum, when serology developed. Tetanus antitoxin was later produced and both antitoxins have been used in human treatment.

Antitoxin work proved that soluble substances in the blood caused immunity and it is now known as the antibody (humoral immunity). Elie Metchnikoff (1845—1916) discovered that some leukocytes in the blood were also important during the process of immunity (cellular immunity). He called these cells Phagocyte and this process Phagocytosis. The rise of immunology has opened the way for preventive medicine.

1.2 Microbiology

Microbiology is an important subject in the life sciences. It focuses on the basic structure, metabolism, inheritance and variation of microorganisms and the relationship between microorganisms and humans, other animals, plants and the natural world. As the scientist and writer Steven Jay Gould emphasized, we live in the era of bacteria. They are the first living organisms on our planet and they can effectively survive in any corner where other organisms live. The number of microorganisms is much more than any other species, possibly being the largest part of the total biological resources on earth. All ecosystems depend on their activities. They affect all aspects of the human society with a major impact on medicine, agronomy and food science, ecology, genetics, biochemistry and molecular biology. Therefore, modern microbiology is a major discipline with many different professional orientations. The microbiology focuses on general microbiology, microbial taxonomy, microbial physiology, microbial ecology, microbial genetics, molecular microbiology and genomics. According to the research object, microbiology can be divided into bacteriology, mycology and virology. According to the research and application fields, it can be divided into agricultural microbiology, industrial microbiology, medical microbiology, veterinary microbiology, food microbiology, marine microbiology and soil microbiology. The interdisciplinary, cellular microbiology, which is a fusion of microbiology and cell biology, focuses on the interaction between pathogenic microorganisms and host cells to explore the pathogenic mechanism of pathogenic microorganisms.

In recent decades, advances in biochemistry, genetics, cell biology and molecular biology and in electron microscopy, gas chromatography, liquid chromatography, immunological technology, monoclonal antibody technology and molecular biology technology have promoted the development of microbiology. At present, the genetic structure and function of pathogenic microorganisms, the material basis of pathogenicity and diagnostic methods are discussed at molecular level, which allows us to gain a deeper understanding of the metabolic laws of pathogenic microorganisms. Several new pathogenic microorganisms have been discovered, such as Legionella, Campylobacter, Lassa virus, Marburg virus, Human immunodeficiency virus and SARS coronavirus.

American plant virologists Diner et al. found that the pathogen of potato spindle tuber disease was an RNA virus without protein between 1967—1971. Such virulence factors are called viroid. Later, in the study of the viroid, a virusoid that causes diseases on plants such as clovers was found. In 1982, the cause of scrapie was a protein with a molecular mass of 27,000, which is known as prion.

In the diagnosis of infectious diseases, the rapid detection and diagnosis of pathogenic microorganisms has developed rapidly in the past decade, such as ELISA rapid detection of antigen and antibody technology, immunofluorescence technology, gene probes and PCR.

In the prevention of infectious diseases, corresponding vaccines have been developed and used as an artificial active immunity. Widespread vaccination has become the most effective and economical means to deal with many infectious diseases.

In the treatment of infectious diseases, new antibiotics have been continuously manufactured, effectively controlling the epidemic of bacterial infectious diseases. In contrast, the research progress of antiviral drugs is slow. In recent years, the use of cytokines (such as interleukin II and interferon, etc.) to treat certain viral diseases has achieved certain effects. In addition, the application of monoclonal antibodies and gene therapy in the treatment of viral diseases has become increasingly wider and deeper.

Now people have agreed that microbiology is a rapidly developing and the most dynamic frontier discipline in the life sciences. Some disciplines, including molecular biology, genetics and biomedical engineering, have achieved rapid development due to the use of microbial materials for research which cannot be achieved in other disciplines. Microbiology is not only closely related to and linked with biochemistry, pharmacology and genetics, but also has become an important pillar industry in many high technology areas including microbial engineering, cell engineering, enzyme engineering and genetic engineering. This suggests that microbiology plays an important role in promoting the sustainable development of the national economy. Microbiology will remain one of the leading disciplines in the 21st century.

Although people have made great achievements in the field of microbiology and the control of infectious diseases, the pathogens of some infectious diseases have not yet been fully understood and there is still no effective prevention and control method for certain diseases. Therefore, in the future, we should strengthen researches on the biological traits and pathogenicity of pathogenic microorganisms and establish a specific rapid and early diagnosis method. We need to strengthen the research on infection immunity, search for or artificially synthesize nonspecific and specific substances that can mobilize and improve the host defense, develop new vaccines and improve the existing vaccines to promote the efficacy of disease prevention and control. We must strengthen the study of genetic engineering, gene therapy used for some genetic diseases related to microbial infections to completely cure these diseases. We also must continue to strengthen links and collaborations of microbiology with immunology, biochemistry, genetics, cell biology, histology and pathology and adopt advanced technologies, especially molecular biology techniques. Only in this way can we accelerate the development of medical microbiology and contribute to the early control and elimination of various diseases that endanger human health.

Chapter 2

Microbial Molecular Biology

2.1 DNA as Genetic Material

Although it is now hard to imagine, it was once thought that DNA is too simple a molecule to store genetic information. It is composed of only four different nucleotides and it seemed that a molecule of much greater complexity must house the genetic information of a cell. It was argued that proteins, being composed of 20 different amino acids, were the better candidate for this important cellular function.

The early work of Fred Grifth in 1928 on the transfer of virulence in the pathogen *Streptococcus pneumoniae*, commonly called pneumococcus, sets the stage for research showing that DNA was indeed the genetic material. Grifth found that if he boiled virulent bacteria and injected them into mice, the mice were not affected and no pneumococci could be recovered from the animals. When he injected a combination of killed virulent bacteria and a living nonvirulent strain, the mice died; moreover, he could recover living virulent bacteria from the dead mice. Grifth called this change of nonvirulent bacteria into virulent pathogens transformation.

Oswald Avery and his colleagues then set out to discover which constituent in the heat-killed virulent pneumococci was responsible for transformation. These investigators used enzymes to selectively destroy DNA, RNA or protein in purified extracts of virulent pneumococci (S cells). They then exposed nonvirulent pneumococcal strains (R strains) to the treated extracts. Transformation of the nonvirulent bacteria was blocked only if the DNA was destroyed, suggesting that DNA was carrying the information required for transformation. The publication of these studies by Avery, C. M. MacLeod and M. J. McCarty in 1944 provided the first evidence that DNA carried genetic information.

Eight years later, Alfred Hershey and Martha Chase wanted to know if protein or DNA carried the genetic information of a bacterial virus called T2 bacteriophage. They performed experiments in which they made the virus's DNA radioactive with ^{32}P or they labeled its protein coat with ^{35}S. They mixed radioactive virions with Escherichia coli and incubated the mixture for a few minutes. This allowed the virions to attach to E. Coli and begin multiplying. The suspension was then agitated violently in a blender to shear off any adsorbed bacteriophage particles. After centrifugation, radioactivity in the supernatant (where the phage particles remained) versus the bacterial cells in the pellet was determined. They found that most radioactive protein was released into the supernatant, whereas 32P DNA remained within the bacteria. Since DNA entered the cells and T2 progeny were produced, the phage DNA must have been carrying the genetic information. Some luck was involved in their discovery, for the genetic material of many viruses is RNA and the researchers happened to select a DNA virus for their studies. Imagine the confusion if T2 had been an RNA virus! Te controversy surrounding the nature of genetic information might have lasted considerably longer than it did.

Subsequent studies on the genetics of viruses and bacteria were largely responsible for the rapid development of molecular genetics. Furthermore, much of the recombinant DNA technology has arisen from studies of bacterial and viral genetics. Research in microbial genetics has had a profound impact on biology as a science and on technology that affects everyday life.

2.2   Nucleic Acid and Protein Structure

DNA, RNA and proteins are often called informational molecules. The information exists as the sequence of monomers from which they are built. Here we describe the monomers and how they are linked together to form these important macromolecules.

2.2.1   Deoxribonucleic Acid Structure

Deoxribonucleic acid (DNA) is a polymer of deoxyribonucleotides linked together by phosphodiester bonds. It contains the bases adenine, guanine, cytosine and thymine. DNA molecules are very large and are usually composed of two polynucleotide chains coiled together to form a double helix 2.0 nm in diameter. The monomers of DNA are called deoxyribonucleotides because the sugar found in them is deoxyribose. The bond that links the monomers together to form the polymer is called a phosphodiester bond because it consists of a phosphate that forms a bridge between the 3′-hydroxyl of one sugar and the 5′-hydroxyl of an adjacent sugar. Purine and pyrimidine bases are attached to the 1′-carbon of the deoxyribose sugars and the bases extend toward the middle of the cylinder formed by the two chains. (The numbers designating the carbons in the sugars are given a prime to distinguish them from the numbers designating the carbons and nitrogens in the nitrogenous bases.) The bases from each strand interact with those of the other strand, forming base pairs. The base pairs are stacked on top of each other in the center, one base pair every 0.34 nm. The purine adenine (A) of one strand is always paired with the pyrimidine thymine (T) of the opposite strand by two hydrogen bonds. The purine guanine (G) pairs with cytosine (C) by three hydrogen bonds. This AT and GC base pairing means that the two strands in a DNA double helix are complementary. In other words, the bases in one strand match up with those of the other according to specific base-pairing rules. Because the sequences of bases in these strands encode genetic information, considerable effort has been devoted to determining the base sequences of DNA and RNA from many organisms, including hundreds of microbes.

The two polynucleotide strands of DNA ft together much like the pieces in a jigsaw puzzle. The two strands are not positioned directly opposite one another. Therefore when the strands twist about one another, a wide major groove and narrower minor groove are formed by the backbone. There are 10.5 base pairs per turn of the helix and each turn of the helix has a vertical length of 3.4 A. The helix is right-handed; that is, the chains turn counterclockwise as they approach a viewer looking down the longitudinal axis. The two backbones are antiparallel, which means they run in opposite directions with respect to the orientation of their sugars. One end of each strand has an exposed 5′-hydroxyl group, often with phosphates attached, whereas the other end has a free 3'-hydroxyl group. In a given direction, one strand is oriented 5' to 3' and the other, 3' to 5'.

The structure of DNA just described is that of the B form, the most common form in cells. Two other forms of DNA have been identified. The A form primarily differs from the B form in that it has 11 base pairs per helical turn, rather than 10. 5 and a vertical length of 2. 6 A, rather than 3. 4. Thus it is wider than the B form. The Z form is dramatically different, having a left-handed helical structure, rather than right-handed as seen in the B and A forms. The Z form has 12 base pairs per helical turn and a vertical rise of 3. 7 A. Thus it is more slender than the B form. At this time, it is unclear whether the A form is found in cells. However, evidence exists that small portions of chromosomes can be in the Z form. The role, if any, for these stretches of Z DNA is unknown.

There is another property of DNA that needs to be addressed: supercoiling. DNA is helical; that is, it is a coil. Whenever the rotation of a coil is restrained in some way, it causes the coil to coil on itself. The coiling of a coil is supercoiling. Recall that most bacterial chromosomes are closed, circular double-stranded DNA molecules. In this state, the two strands are unable to rotate freely relative to each other and the molecule is said to be strained. The strain is relieved by supercoiling. There are two types of supercoiling: positive and negative. For DNA, these are defined by the change in number of base pairs per turn in the double helix. As just discussed, the B form of DNA has 10. 5 base pairs per turn of the helix. Supercoiling that decreases the number of base pairs per turn is said to be negative supercoiling. Likewise, supercoiling that increases the number of base pairs per turn is called positive supercoiling. Bacterial chromosomes are generally negatively supercoiled.

What is the importance of supercoiling? Supercoiling helps compact DNA so that it fts into the cell. Importantly for this chapter, supercoiling also "loosens" up the DNA, making it easier to separate the two strands from each other. Separation of the two strands is an important early step in both DNA replication and transcription. Furthermore, positive supercoiling is often introduced into DNA during DNA replication. This can interfere with DNA replication and must be removed.

2. 2. 2　Ribonucleiz Acid Structure

Ribonucleic acid (RNA) is a polymer of ribonucleotides that contains the sugar ribose and the bases adenine, guanine, cytosine and uracil (instead of thymine). The nucleotides are joined by a phosphodiester bond, just as they are in DNA. Most RNA molecules are single stranded. However, an RNA strand can coil back on itself to form secondary structures such as hairpins with complementary base pairing and helical organization. The formation of double-stranded regions in RNA is often critical to its function.

2. 2. 3　Protein Structure

Proteins are polymers of amino acids linked by peptide bonds; thus they are also called polypeptides. An amino acid is defined by the presence of a central carbon (the a carbon) to which are attached a carboxyl group, an amino group and a side chain. Twenty amino acids are normally used to form proteins. However, two unusual amino acids have recently been discovered in some proteins. Amino acids differ in terms of their side chains. Depending on the structure of the side chain, the amino acid can be described as nonpolar, polar or charged. The peptide bonds linking the amino acids together are formed by a reaction between the carboxyl group of one amino acid and the amino group of the next amino acid in the protein. A polypeptide has polarity just as DNA and RNA do. At one end of the chain is an amino group and at the other end is a carboxyl group. Thus a polypeptide has an amino or N terminus and a carboxyl or C terminus.

Proteins do not typically exist as extended chains of amino acids. Rather, they fold back on themselves to form threedimensional structures, often more or less spherical in shape. The final shape is determined to a large extent by the sequence of amino acids in the polypeptide. This sequence is called the primary structure. Secondary and tertiary structures result from the folding of the chain. Finally, two or more polypeptide strands can interact to form the final, functional protein. This level of structure is called quaternary structure. These higher levels of structure are stabilized by intra-(and inter-) chain bonds.

2.3　DNA Replication in Bacteria

DNA replication is an extraordinarily important and complex process upon which all life depends. During DNA replication, the two strands of the double helix are separated; each then serves as a template for the synthesis of a complementary strand according to the base-pairing rules. Each of the two progeny DNA molecules consists of one new strand and one old strand and DNA replication is said to be semi-conservative. DNA replication is also extremely accurate; E. coli makes errors with a frequency of only 10^{-9} or 10^{-10} per base pair replicated [or about one in a million (10^{-6}) per gene per generation]. Despite its complexity and accuracy, replication is very rapid. In bacteria, replication rates approach 750 to 1,000 base pairs per second. Most of our discussion in this section is based on studies of chromosomal DNA replication in E. Coli.

2.3.1　Bacterial DNA Replication Initiates from a Single Origin of Replication

The replication of chromosomal DNA begins at a single point, the origin of replication. Synthesis of DNA occurs at the replication fork, the place at which the DNA helix is unwound and individual strands are replicated. Two replication forks move outward from the origin until they have copied the whole replicon-the portion of the genome that contains an origin that is replicated as a unit. When the replication forks move around the circular chromosomes observed in most bacteria, a structure shaped like the Greek letter theta (8)is formed. Because the bacterial chromosome is a single replicon, the forks meet on the other side and two separate chromosomes are released. Less is known about the replication of linear bacterial chromosomes. One well-studied organism with linear chromosomes belongs to the spirochete genus Borrelia. The replication of its chromosomes is considered on p. 300.

2.3.2　Replication Machinery

DNA replication is essential to organisms and a great deal of effort has been devoted to understanding its mechanism. The replication of E. coli DNA requires at least 30 proteins. Many of the archaeal and eukaryotic replication enzymes and proteins differ from those used by bacterial cells. In general, the archaeal replication machinery is more similar to the eukaryotic machinery than it is to the bacterial system. Despite these differences, the overall process of DNA replication is similar in all organisms.

Enzymes called DNA polymerases catalyze DNA synthesis. All known DNA polymerases catalyze the synthesis of DNA in the 5′ to 3′ direction and the nucleotide to be added is a deoxynucleoside triphosphate (dNTP). Deoxynucleotides are linked by phosphodiester bonds formed by a reaction between the hydroxyl group at the 3′ end of the growing DNA strand and the phosphate closest to the 5′ carbon (the a-phosphate)of the incoming deoxynucleotide. The energy needed to form the phosphodiester bond is provided by release of the terminal two phosphates as pyrophosphate (P Pi)from the nucleotide that is added. The P Pi is subsequently hydrolyzed to two separate phosphates (PJ Thus the deoxynucleoside triphosphates dATP, dTTP, dCTP and dGTP serve as DNA polymerase substrates while deoxynucleoside monophosphates (dNMPs; dAMP, dTMP, dCMP, dGMP) are incorporated into the growing chain. How Nucleotides Are Added in DNA Replication

For DNA polymerase to catalyze the synthesis of DNA, it needs three things. The first is a template, which is read in the 3′ to 5′ direction and is used to direct the synthesis of a complementary DNA strand. The second is a primer (e. g. , an RNA strand or a DNA strand) to provide a free 3′-hydroxyl group to which nucleotides can be added. The third is a set of dNTPs. E. coli has five different DNA polymerases (DNA polymerase I – V). DNA polymerase III plays the major role in replication, although it is assisted by DNA polymerase I.

DNA polymerase III holoenzyme is a multifunctional enzyme composed of 10 different proteins. Most evidence suggests that within the complex are found two core enzymes, although some evidence for three core polymerases exists. Each core enzyme binds one strand of DNA and is responsible for catalyzing DNA synthesis and proofreading the product to ensure fidelity of replication. Associated with each core enzyme is a subunit called the 1 clamp. The 1 clamp tethers a core enzyme to the DNA. At the center of the holoenzyme and represented by an octopus-like structure, is a complex of proteins called the clamp loader, which is responsible for loading the 1 clamp onto DNA. A dimer of another protein (tau) holds the holoenzyme together. Because there are two core enzymes, both strands of DNA are bound by a single DNA polymerase III holoenzyme.

DNA polymerase III holoenzyme is only one component of a huge complex of proteins called the replisome (Table 2–1). Other proteins found in the replisome include helicases, single-stranded DNA binding proteins and topoisomerases. Helicases are responsible for separating (unwinding) the DNA strands just ahead of the replication fork, using energy from ATP hydrolysis. Single-stranded DNA binding proteins (SSBs) keep the strands apart once they have been separated and topoisomerases relieve the tension generated by the rapid unwinding of the double helix (the replication fork may rotate as rapidly as 75 to 100 revolutions per second). This is important because rapid unwinding can lead to the formation of positive supercoils in the helix ahead of the replication fork and these can impede replication if not removed. Topoisomerases change the structure of DNA by transiently breaking one or two strands without altering the nucleotide sequence of the DNA (e. g. , a topoisomerase might tie or untie a knot in a DNA strand). DNA gyrase is an important topoisomerase in *E. coli*. It is not only important during DNA replication but also for introducing negative supercoiling in the bacterial chromosome that helps compact it.

Table 2–1 Component of the *E. coli* replication machinery

Protein	Function
DnaA	Initiation of replication; binds origin of replication
DnaB	Helicase (5′→3′); breaks hydrogen bonds holding two strands of double helix together; promotes DNA primase activity; involved in primosome assembly
DNA gyrase	Relieves supercoiling of DNA produced as DNA strands are separated by helicases; separates daughter molecules in final stages of replication
SSB proteins	Bind single-standed DNA after strands are separated by helicases
DnaC	Helicase loader; helps direct DnaB protein to DNA template
DNA primase	Synthesis of RNA primer; component of primosome

Continue to Table 2-1

Protein	Function
DNA polymerase Ⅲ holoenzyme	Complex of about 20 polypeptides; catalyzes most of the DNA synthesis that occurs during DNA replication; has 3'→5' exonuclease activity
DNA polymerase Ⅰ	Removes RNA primers; fills gaps in DNA formed by removal of RNA primer
Ribonuclease H	Removes RNA primers
DNA ligase	Seals nicked DNA, joining DNA fragments together
Tus	Termination of replication
Topoisomerase Ⅳ	Separation of chromosomes upon completion of DNA replication

Once the template is prepared, the primer needed by DNA polymerase Ⅲ can be synthesized. An enzyme called primase synthesizes a short RNA strand, usually around 10 nucleotides long and complementary to the DNA; this serves as the primer. RNA is used as the primer because unlike DNA polymerase, RNA polymerases (such as primase) can initiate RNA synthesis without an existing 3'-OH. It appears that primase requires the assistance of several other proteins and the complex of primase and its accessory proteins is called the primosome (Table 2-1). The primosome is another important component of the replisome.

As noted, DNA polymerase enzymes synthesize DNA in the 5' to 3' direction. Therefore only one of the strands, called the leading strand, can be synthesized continuously at its 3' end as the DNA unwinds. The other strand called the lagging strand, cannot be extended in the same direction as the movement of the replication fork because there is no free 3'-OH to which a nucleotide can be added. As a result, the lagging strand is synthesized discontinuously in the 5' to 3' direction (i. e. , in the direction opposite of the movement of the replication fork) and produces a series of fragments called Okazaki fragments, after their discoverer, Reiji Okazaki. Discontinuous synthesis occurs as primase makes many RNA primers along the template strand. DNA polymerase Ⅲ then extends these primers with DNA and eventually the Okazaki fragments are joined to form a complete strand. Thus while the leading strand requires only one RNA primer to initiate synthesis, the lagging strand has many RNA primers that must eventually be removed. Okazaki fragments are about 1,000 to 2,000 nucleotides long in bacteria and approximately 100 nucleotides long in eukaryotic cells.

2.3.3　Events at the Replication Fork

We present replication as a series of discrete steps, but in the cell these events occur quickly and simultaneously on both the leading and lagging strands. In *E. coli*, DNA replication is initiated at specific nucleotides called the oric locus (for origin of chromosomal replication). This site is AT rich. Recall that adenines pair with thymines using only two hydrogen bonds, so AT-rich segments of DNA become single stranded more readily than do GC-rich regions. This is important for initiation of replication.

1) The bacterial initiator protein DnaA is responsible for triggering DNA replication. DnaA proteins bind regions in oric throughout the cell cycle, but to initiate replication, DnaA proteins must bind a few particular oric sequences. The presence of DnaA at these sites recruits a helicase (usually DnaB helicase) to the origin.

2) The helicase unwinds the helix with the aid of topoisomerases such as DNA gyrase. The single strands are kept separate by SSBs.

3) Primase synthesizes RNA primers as needed. A single DNA polymerase Ⅲ holoenzyme catalyzes

both leading strand and lagging strand synthesis from the RNA primers. Lagging strand synthesis is particularly amazing because of the "gymnastic" feats performed by the holoenzyme. It must discard old 1 clamps, load new 1 clamps and tether the template to the core enzyme with each new round of Okazaki fragment synthesis. All of this occurs as DNA polymerase Ⅲ is synthesizing DNA.

4) Afer most of the lagging strand has been synthesized by the formation of Okazaki fragments, DNA polymerase Ⅰ removes the RNA primers. DNA polymerase Ⅰ does this because, unlike other DNA polymerases, it has the ability to snip off nucleotides one at a time starting at the 5′ end while moving toward the 3′ end of the RNA primer. This ability is referred to as 5′ to 3′ exonuclease activity. DNA polymerase Ⅰ begins its exonuclease activity at the free 5′ end of each RNA primer. With the removal of each ribonucleotide, the adjacent 3′-OH from the deoxynucleotide is used by DNA polymerase Ⅰ to fill the gap between Okazaki fragments.

5) Final the Okazaki fragments are joined by the enzyme DNA ligase, which forms a phosphodiester bond between the 3′-OH of the growing strand and the 5′-phosphate of an Okazaki fragment.

Amazingly, DNA polymerase Ⅲ, like all DNA polymerases (except DNA polymerases called reverse transcriptases), has an additional function that is critically important: proofreading. Proofreading is the removal of a mismatched base immediately after it has been added; its removal must occur before the next base is incorporated. One of the protein subunits of the DNA polymerase Ⅲ core enzyme (thee subunit) has 3′ to 5′ exonuclease activity. This activity enables the polymerase core enzyme to check each newly incorporated base to see that it forms stable hydrogen bonds. In this way, mismatched bases can be detected. If the wrong base has been mistakenly added, the exonuclease activity is used to remove it. A mismatched base can be removed only as long as it is still at the 3′ end of the growing strand. Once removed, holoenzyme backs up and adds the proper nucleotide in its place. DNA proofreading is not 100% efficient, the mismatch repair system is the cell's second line of defense against the potential harm caused by the incorporation of the incorrect nucleotide.

As we have seen, DNA polymerase Ⅲ is a remarkable multiprotein complex, with several enzymatic activities. In *E. coli*, the polymerase component is encoded by the dnaE gene. Bacillus subtilis, a Gram-positive bacterium that is another important experimental model, has a second polymerase gene called dnaEBs. Its protein product appears to be responsible for synthesizing the lagging strand. Thus while the overall mechanism by which DNA is replicated is highly conserved, there can be variations in replisome components.

2.3.4　Termination of Replication

In *E. coli*, DNA replication stops when the replisome reaches a termination site (ter) on the DNA. A protein called Tus binds to the ter sites and halts progression of the forks. In many other bacteria, replication stops spontaneously when the forks meet. Regardless of how fork movement is stopped, there are two problems that often must be solved by the replisome. One is the formation of interlocked chromosomes called catenanes. The other is a dimerized chromosome-two chromosomes joined together to form a single chromosome twice as long. Catenanes are produced when topoisomerases break and rejoin DNA strands to ease supercoiling ahead of the replication fork. The two daughter DNA molecules are separated by the action of other topoisomerases that break both strands of one molecule, pass the other DNA molecule through the break and then rejoin the strands. Dimerized chromosomes result from DNA recombination that sometimes occurs between two daughter molecules during DNA replication. Recombinase enzymes (e. g. , XerCD in *E. coli*) catalyze an intramolecular cross-over that separates the two chromosomes.

2.3.5 Replication of Linear Chromosomes

All eukaryotic chromosomes and some bacterial chromosomes are linear. In both cases, this poses a problem during replication because all DNA polymerases synthesize DNA in the 5′ to 3′ direction from a primer that provides a free 3′-OH. When the RNA primer for the Okazaki fragment at the 5′ end of the daughter strand is removed, the daughter molecule is shorter than the parent molecule. Over numerous rounds of DNA replication and cell division, this leads to a progressively shortened chromosome. Ultimately the chromosome loses critical genetic information, which is lethal to the cell. This problem is called the "end replication problem"; and a cell must solve it if it is to survive. Eukaryotic cells have solved the end replication problem with an enzyme called telomerase. Bacteria have taken a different approach.

Of those bacteria having linear chromosomes, the best understood mechanism for solving the end replication problem is that used by Borrelia burgdorferi. The approach B. Burgdorferi cells use is to disguise the ends so well that they are not really ends. How are the ends disguised? Consider a typical linear, double-stranded DNA molecule. At each terminus of the double helix is a strand having a 3′-OH and the complementary strand having a 5′-phosphate. B. burgdorferi chromosomes do not have these free ends. Rather, a phosphodiester bond links the two complementary strands together. This is made possible by inverted repeats at each terminus and the formation of a hairpin. The origin of replication is located between the hairpins. Interestingly, only leading strand synthesis occurs at each replication fork. When replication is complete, a circular molecule has been formed that is twice the length of the parent chromosome. Thus it is a dimerized chromosome. An enzyme called telomere resolvase (ResT) cuts the two chromosomes apart as it forms hairpin ends for each daughter molecule.

2.4　Bacterial Gene Structure

DNA replication allows genetic information to be passed from one generation to the next. But how is the information used? To answer that question, we must first look at how genetic information is organized. The basic unit of genetic information is the gene. Genes have been regarded in several ways. At first, it was thought that a gene contained information for the synthesis of one enzyme-the one gene-one enzyme hypothesis. This was modified to the one gene-one polypeptide hypothesis because of the existence of enzymes and other proteins composed of two or more different polypeptide chains (subunits) coded for by separate genes. A segment of DNA that encodes a single polypeptide is sometimes termed a cistron. However, not all genes encode proteins; some code instead for ribosomal RNA (rRNA) and transfer RNA (tRNA), both of which function in protein synthesis. In addition, it is now known that some eukaryotic genes encode more than one protein. Thus a gene might be defined as a polynucleotide sequence that codes for one or more functional products (i. e. , a polypeptide, tRNA or rRNA). In this section, we consider the structure of each of these three types of genes.

2.4.1 Protein-Coding Genes

Most of the genes found in bacterial genomes encode proteins. However, DNA does not serve directly as the template for protein synthesis. Rather, the genetic information in the gene is transcribed to give rise to a messenger RNA (mRNA), which is translated into a protein. For this to occur, protein-coding genes must contain signals that indicate where transcription should start and stop and signals in the resulting mRNA that indicate where translation should start and stop. During transcription only one strand of a gene directs mRNA synthesis. This strand is called the template strand and the complementary DNA strand is known as the coding strand because it is the same nucleotide sequence as the mRNA, except in DNA bases. Messenger RNA is synthesized from the 5′ to the 3′ end in a manner similar to DNA synthesis. Therefore the polarity of the DNA template strand is 3′ to 5′. In other words, the beginning of the gene is at the 3′ end of the template strand.

An important site called the promoter is located at the start of the gene. The promoter is the binding site for RNA polymerase, the enzyme that synthesizes RNA. The promoter is neither transcribed nor translated; it functions strictly to orient RNA polymerase so it is a specific distance from the first DNA nucleotide that will serve as a template for RNA synthesis. The promoter thus specifies which strand is to be transcribed and where transcription should begin. The sequences near the promoter often are very important in regulating when and at what rate a gene is transcribed.

The transcription start site represents the first nucleotide in the mRNA synthesized from the gene. However, the initially transcribed portion of the gene does not necessarily code for amino acids. Instead, it is a leader that is transcribed into mRNA but is not translated into amino acids. In bacteria, the leader includes a region called the Shine Dalgarno sequence, which is important in the initiation of translation. The leader sometimes is also involved in regulation of transcription and translation.

Immediately next to (and downstream of) the leader is the most important part of the gene, the coding region. The coding region typically begins with the template DNA sequence 3′-TAC-5′. This is transcribed into the start codon, 5′-AUG-3′, which codes for the first amino acid of the polypeptide encoded by the gene. The remainder of the coding region is transcribed into a sequence of codons that specifies the sequence of amino acids for the rest of the protein. The coding region ends with a sequence that, when transcribed, is a stop codon. I signals the end of the protein and stops the ribosome during translation. The stop codon is immediately followed by the trailer, which is transcribed but not translated. The trailer contains sequences that prepare the RNA polymerase for release from the template strand. Indeed, just beyond the trailer (and sometimes slightly overlapping it) is the terminator. The terminator is a sequence that signals the RNA polymerase to stop transcription.

In bacteria, the coding region is usually continuous, unlike the coding regions of eukaryotic genes, which are often interrupted by noncoding sequences called introns. Those rare bacterial genes that do contain introns are transcribed into an intron-containing mRNA. The introns are eventually removed but by a mechanism different than that used to remove introns from eukaryotic mRNAs.

2.4.2   tRNA and rRNA Genes

Actively growing cells need a ready supply of tRNA and rRNA molecules so that protein synthesis can occur. To ensure this, bacterial cells often have more than one gene for each of these molecules. Furthermore, it is important that the number of each tRNA or rRNA relative to other tRNAs or rRNAs be controlled. This is accomplished in part by having several tRNA or rRNA genes transcribed together, under the control of a single promoter.

In bacteria, genes for tRNA consist of a promoter, tRNA coding region, leader and trailer. When more than one tRNA is transcribed from the promoter, the coding regions are separated by short spacer sequences. Whether the gene encodes a single tRNA or multiple tRNAs, the initial transcript must be processed to remove the noncoding sequences (i. e. , leader, trailer and spacers, if present). This is called posttranscriptional modification and it is accomplished by ribonucleases-enzymes (and in some cases ribozymes)that cut RNA. In addition, many bacterial (and archaeal)tRNA genes contain introns that must be removed during tRNA maturation.

　Bacterial cells usually contain more than one rRNA gene. Each gene has a promoter, trailer and terminator and encodes all three types of rRNA. Thus, as seen for tRNA genes, the transcript from an rRNA gene is a single, large precursor molecule that is cut up by ribonucleases to yield the final rRNA products. Interestingly, in many bacteria, the trailer regions and the spacers often contain tRNA genes. Thus the precursor rRNA encodes for both tRNA and rRNA.

2.5　Transcription in Bacteria

　Synthesis of RNA under the direction of DNA is called transcription and the RNA product has a sequence complementary to the DNA template directing its synthesis. Although adenine directs the incorporation of thymine during DNA replication, it usually codes for uracil during RNA synthesis. Transcription generates three major kinds of RNA. Transfer RNA (tRNA)carries amino acids during protein synthesis and ribosomal RNA (rRNA)molecules are components of ribosomes. Messenger RNA (mRNA)bears the message for protein synthesis. Bacterial genes encoding proteins involved in a related process (e. g. , encoding enzymes for synthesis of an amino acid)are often located close to each other and are transcribed from a single promoter. Such a transcriptional unit is termed an operon. Transcription of an operon yields an mRNA consisting of a leader followed by one coding region, which is separated by a space from the second coding region and so on, with the final sequence of nucleotides being the trailer. Such mRNAs are said to be polycistronic mRNAs. Each coding region in the polycistronic mRNA is defined by a start and stop codon. Thus each coding region is translated separately to give rise to a single polypeptide. Many archaeal mRNAs are also polycistronic. However, polycistronic mRNAs are rare in eukaryotes. Instead, their mRNAs are usually monocistronic mRNAs, containing information of a single gene.

2.5.1　Bacterial RNA Polymerases

　RNA is synthesized by enzymes called RNA polymerases. In bacteria, a single RNA polymerase transcribes all genes. Most bacterial RNA polymerases contain five types of polypeptide chains: a, 1, 1', r and 0. The RNA polymerase core enzyme is composed of five polypeptides (two a subunits, 1, 1' and r) and catalyzes RNA synthesis. Interestingly, the subunits that form the core enzyme are conserved in archaeal and eukaryal RNA polymerases. However, their RNA polymerases consist of additional proteins and are larger and more complex than the bacterial enzyme. The sigma factor (c)has no catalytic activity but helps the core enzyme recognize the promoter. When sigma is bound to the core enzyme, the six-subunit complex is termed RNA polymerase holoenzyme. Only holoenzyme can begin transcription, but the core enzyme completes RNA synthesis once it has been initiated.

2.5.2　Stages of Transcription

　Transcription involves three separate processes: initiation, elongation and termination, which together are often referred to as the transcription cycle. Sigma factor is critical to the initiation process. It positions the RNA polymerase core enzyme at the promoter. Many bacterial promoters have two characteristic features: a sequence of six bases (often T TGACA)about 35 base pairs before (upstream) the transcription starting point and a TATAAT sequence called the Pribnow box, usually about 10 base pairs upstream of the transcriptional start site. These regions are called the-35 and-10 sites, respectively, because these are their distances in nucleotides upstream of the first nucleotide to be transcribed (i. e. , the +1 site). Sigma factor recognizes the-10 and-35 sequences and directs the RNA polymerase core enzyme to them.

At this point in our discussion, it is worth noting that bacterial cells produce more than one type of sigma factor. Each sigma factor preferentially directs the RNA polymerase to a distinct set of promoters. For instance, in *E. coli*, most genes have promoters recognized by a sigma factor called σ70. This sigma factor recognizes promoters having the-10 and-35 sequencesshown in Table 2−2. These sequences are the consensus sequences for σ70-recognized promoters. Promoters recognized by other sigma factors have different consensus sequences. The use of different sigma factors to initiate transcription is a common bacterial regulatory mechanism. Our focus here is on transcription of genes recognized by σ70.

Table 2–2   *E. coli* sigma factors and the sequences they recognize

Sigma factor	Consensus promoter sequences		Genes transcribed from promoter
σ70	TTGACAT	TATAAT	Most genes
σ54	CTGGNA	TTGCA	Genes for nitrogen metabolism
σ38	TTGACA	TCTATACTT	Genes for stationary phase and stress responses
σ32	TCTCNCCCTTGAA	CCCCATNTA	Genes for heat-shock response
σ28	CTAA	CCGATAT	Genes for chemotaxis and motility

Once bound to the promoter, RNA polymerase unwinds the DNA. The-10 site is rich in adenines and thymines, making it easier to break the hydrogen bonds that keep the DNA double stranded; when the DNA is unwound at this region, it is called an open complex. A region of unwound DNA equivalent to about 16 to 20 base pairs becomes the "transcription bubble"; which moves with the RNA polymerase as it synthesizes mRNA from the template DNA strand during elongation. Within the transcription bubble, a temporary RNA: DNA hybrid is formed. As RNA polymerase holoenzyme progresses along the DNA template, the sigma factor dissociates from the other subunits and can help another RNA polymerase core enzyme initiate transcription.

The reaction catalyzed by RNA polymerase is quite similar to that catalyzed by DNA polymerase. ATP, GTP, CTP and UTP are used to produce RNA complementary to the DNA template and pyrophosphate is produced as ribonucleoside monophosphates are incorporated into the growing RNA chain. Pyrophosphate is hydrolyzed to fuel the process. RNA synthesis also proceeds in a 5′ to 3′ direction with new nucleotides being added to the 3′ end of the growing chain, making the RNA complementary and antiparallel to the template DNA. As elongation of the mRNA continues, single-stranded mRNA is released and the two strands of DNA behind the transcription bubble resume their double helical structure. RNA polymerase is a remarkable enzyme capable of several activities, including unwinding the DNA, moving along the template and synthesizing RNA.

Termination of transcription occurs when the core RNA polymerase dissociates from the template DNA. This is brought about by the terminator. There are two kinds of terminators. The first type causes factor-independent termination. This terminator consists of an inverted repeat followed by an A-rich nucleotide sequence. RNA polymerase transcribes the inverted repeat, but it pauses within the A-rich region. This allows the inverted repeat to fold back on itself, forming a hairpin-shaped stem-loop structure. The A-U base pairs holding the DNA and RNA together in the transcription bubble are too weak to hold the RNA: DNA duplex together and RNA polymerase falls off.

The second kind of terminator is termed factor-dependent terminator because it requires the aid of a protein. The best-studied termination factor is rho factor (p). Rho factor can be involved in transcription termination of all types of genes, but its action is best studied for protein-coding genes. Current models propose that rho binds to mRNA at a site called rut for rho-utilization site. For rho to bind, rut must be free of ribosomes. Rho uses energy supplied by ATP hydrolysis to move along the mRNA, as it tries to catch up with RNA polymerase. However, rho's rate of movement is slower than that of RNA polymerase. Tus rho can only catch up with RNA polymerase if the polymerase pauses at a rho-dependent pause site. If this occurs, rho catches up with RNA polymerase and causes RNA polymerase to dissociate from DNA. How rho does this is not completely clear. However, it is known that rho factor has hybrid RNA:DNA helicase activity. This activity may cause unwinding of the mRNA-DNA complex.

2.6　The Genetic Code

The final step in the expression of protein-coding genes is translation. Protein synthesis is called translation because it is a decoding process. The information encoded in the language of nucleic acids must be rewritten in the language of proteins. During translation, the sequence of nucleotides is "read" in discrete sets of three nucleotides, each set being a codon. Each codon codes for a single amino acid. The sequence of codons is "read" in only one way-the reading frameto give rise to the amino acid sequence of a polypeptide. Deciphering the genetic code was one of the great achievements of the twentieth century. Here we examine the nature of the genetic code.

The genetic code, presented in RNA form. Close inspection of the code reveals several features that are related not only to the way cells use DNA to store information but also to why it is valuable for storing data. One feature is that the code words (codons) are three letters (bases) long; thus one small "word" conveys a significant amount of information. Each codon is recognized by an anticodon present on a tRNA molecule. Another feature is that the code has "punctuation": One codon, AUG, is almost always the first codon in the protein-coding portion of mRNA molecules. It is called the start codon because it serves as the start site for translation by coding for the initiator tRNA. Three other codons (UGA, UAG and UAA) are involved in termination of translation and are called stop or nonsense codons. These codons do not encode an amino acid and therefore do not have a tRNA bearing their anticodon. Thus only 61 of the 64 codons in the code, the sense codons, direct amino acid incorporation into protein. Finally, the genetic code exhibits code degeneracy; that is, there are up to six different codons for a given amino acid.

Despite the existence of 61 sense codons, there are fewer than 61 different tRNAs. It follows that not all codons have a corresponding tRNA. Cells can successfully translate mRNA using fewer tRNAs because loose pairing between the 5′ base in the anticodon and the 3′ base of the codon is tolerated. Thus as long as the first and second bases in the codon correctly base pair with an anticodon, the tRNA bearing the correct amino acid will bind to the mRNA during translation. This is evident on inspection of the code. Note that the codons for a particular amino acid most often differ at the third position. This somewhat loose base pairing is known as wobble and it relieves cells of the need to synthesize so many tRNAs. Wobble also decreases the effects of some mutations.

The description of the genetic code just provided is of the universal genetic code. However, there are exceptions to the code (Table 2-3). The first exceptions discovered were stop codons that encoded one of the 20 amino acids. For instance, some protists have a single stop codon (UGA); the other two stop codons are recognized by tRNAs bearing glutamine (Gln). More dramatic deviations from the code have also been discovered. Proteins from members of all three domains of life have been discovered to contain the amino acid selenocysteine, the twenty-first amino acid. Pyrrolysine, the twenty-second amino acid, can be found in the proteins of several methanogens and at least one bacterium. Genomic analysis indicates that pyrrolysine might also exist in many other bacteria and some eukaryotes. Selenocysteine is inserted at certain UGA codons, whereas pyrrolysine is inserted at UAG codons.

Table 2-3   Some exceptions to the universal genetic code

Codon	Amino acid inserted	Where observed
AGA and AGG	Stop	Mammalian mitochondria
AGA and AGG	Serine (Ser)	Invertebrate mitochondria
AUA	Methionine (Met)	Mammalian, invertebrate and yeast mitochondria
CUA	Threonine (Thr)	Yeast mitochondria
CUG	Serine	Some fungi
UAA and UAG	Glutamine (Gln)	Some protists
UAG	Pyrrolysine	Some methanogens and bacteria
UGA	Selenocysteine	Members of all three domains
UGA	Tryptophan (Trp)	Mammalian, invertebrate and yeast mitochondria
UGA	Glutamine	Mycoplasma bacteria

2.7   Translation in Bacteria

Translation involves decoding mRNA and covalently linking amino acids together to form a polypeptide; this occurs at the ribosome. Translation begins when a ribosome binds mRNA and is positioned properly so that translation will yield the correct amino acid sequence in the polypeptide chain. Transfer RNA molecules carry amino acids to the ribosome so that they can be added to the polyeptide chain as the ribosome moves down the mRNA molecule. Just as DNA and RNA synthesis proceeds in one direction, so too does protein synthesis. Polypeptide synthesis begins with the amino acid at the end of the chain with a free amino group (the N-terminal) and moves in the C-terminal direction. Thus translation is said to occur in the amino terminus to carboxyl terminus direction. Protein synthesis is accurate and very rapid. In E. coli, synthesis occurs at a rate of at least 900 amino acids added per minute; eukaryotic translation is slower, about 100 amino acids residues per minute.

Cells that grow quickly must use each mRNA with great efficiency to synthesize proteins at a sufficiently rapid rate. The two subunits of the ribosome (the 50S subunit and the 30S subunit in bacteria and archaea; 60S and 40S in eukaryotes) are free in the cytoplasm if protein is not being synthesized. They come together to form the complete ribosome complexed with mRNA only when translation occurs. Frequently mRNAs are simultaneously complexed with several ribosomes, each ribosome reading the mRNA message and synthesizing a polypeptide. At maximal rates of mRNA use, there may be a ribosome every 80 nucleotides along the mRNA or as many as 20 ribosomes simultaneously reading an mRNA that codes for a 50,000 dalton polypeptide. A complex of mRNA with several ribosomes is called a polyribosome or polysome. Polysomes are present in all organisms. Bacteria and archaea can further increase the efficiency of gene expression by coupling transcription and translation. While RNA polymerase is synthesizing an mRNA, ribosomes can already be attached to the mRNA so that transcription and translation occur simultaneously. Coupled transcription and translation is possible in bacterial and archaeal cells because a nuclear envelope does not separate the translation machinery from DNA, as it does in eukaryotes.

2.7.1   Transfer RNA and Amino Acid Activation

For translation to occur, a ready supply of tRNA molecules bearing the correct amino acid must be available. Thus a preparatory step for protein synthesis is amino acid activation, the process in which amino acids are attached to tRNA molecules. Before we discuss this process, we need to examine the structure of tRNA molecules.

Transfer RNA molecules are about 70 to 95 nucleotides long and possess several characteristic structural features. These features become apparent when the tRNA is folded so that base pairing within the tRNA strand is maximized. When represented two-dimensionally, this base pairing causes the tRNA to assume a cloverleaf conformation. However, the three-dimensional structure looks like the letter L. One important feature of tRNAs is the acceptor stem, which holds the activated amino acid. The 3′ end of all tRNAs has the same-C-C-A sequence and in all cases, the amino acid is attached to the terminal adenylic acid (A). Another important feature of the tRNA is the anticodon. The anticodon is complementary to the mRNA codon and is located on the anticodon arm.

Enzymes called aminoacyl-tRNA synthetases catalyze amino acid activation. As is true of DNA and RNA synthesis, the reaction is driven to completion when ATP is hydrolyzed to release pyrophosphate. The amino acid is attached to the 3′-hydroxyl of the terminal adenylic acid on the tRNA by a high-energy bond. The storage of energy in this bond provides the fuel needed to generate the peptide bond when the amino acid is added to the growing peptide chain.

There are at least 20 aminoacyl-tRNA synthetases, each specific for a single amino acid and its tRNAs (cognate tRNAs). It is critical that each tRNA attach the corresponding amino acid because if an incorrect amino acid is attached to a tRNA, it will be incorporated into a polypeptide in place of the correct amino acid. The protein synthetic machinery recognizes only the anticodon of the aminoacyl-tRNA and cannot tell whether the correct amino acid is attached. Some aminoacyl-tRNA synthetases proofread just like DNA polymerases do. If the wrong amino acid is attached to tRNA, the enzyme hydrolyzes the amino acid from the tRNA, rather than release the incorrect product.

2.7.2   Ribosome Structure

Protein synthesis takes place on ribosomes that serve as workbenches, with mRNA acting as the blueprint. Recall that ribosomes are formed from two subunits, the large subunit and the small subunit and each contains one or more rRNA molecules and numerous polypeptide chains. The region of the ribosome directly responsible for translation is called the translational domain. Both subunits contribute to this domain. The growing peptide chain emerges from the large subunit at the exit domain.

Ribosomal RNA is thought to have three roles. ①It contributes to ribosom structure. ②The 16S rRNA of the 30S subunit is needed for the initiation of protein synthesis because its 3′ end binds to a site on the leader of the mRNA called the Shine-Dalgarno sequence; thus the Shine-Dalgarno sequence is part of the ribosome-binding site (RBS). This helps position the mRNA on the ribosome. The 16S rRNA also binds a protein needed to initiate translation (initiation factor 3) and the 3' CCA end of amino-acyl-tRNA. ③The 23S rRNA is a ribozyme that catalyzes peptide bond formation.

2.7.3   Initiation of Protein Synthesis

Like transcription and DNA replication, protein synthesis is divided into three stages: initiation, elongation and termination. The initiation of protein synthesis is very elaborate. Apparently the complexity is necessary to ensure that the ribosome does not start synthesizing a polypeptide chain in the middle of a gene-a disastrous error.

Bacteria begin protein synthesis with a modified aminoacyl tRNA, N-formylmethionyl-tRNAfet (fet-tRNA), which is coded for by the start codon AUG. The amino acid of the initiator tRNA has a formyl group covalently bound to the amino group and can be used only for initiation because of the presence of the formyl group. When methionine is to be added to a growing polypeptide chain (i.e., at an AUG codon in the middle of the mRNA), a normal methionylt RNAMet is employed. Although bacteria start protein synthesis with N-formylmethionine, the formyl group is not retained but is hydrolytically removed. In fact, one to three amino acids may be removed from the amino terminal end of the polypeptide after synthesis.

The initiation stage is crucial for the translation of mRNA into the correct polypeptide. In bacteria, it begins when initiator fet-tRNA binds to a free 30S ribosomal subunit The 16S rRNA within the 30S subunit then binds the Shine Dalgarno sequence in the leader sequence of the mRNA. By aligning the Shine-Dalgarno sequence with the 16S rRNA, the initiator codon (AUG or some times GUG, though GUG is not as good an initiator) specifically binds with the fMet-tRNA anticodon. This ensures that the codon for the initiator fMet-tRNA will be translated first. When the 50S subunit of the ribosome binds to the 30S subunit-mRNA, an active ribosome mRNA complex is formed, with the fet-tRNA positioned at the peptidyl or P site (see description of the elongation cycle). This complex is referred to as the initiation complex. Three protein initiation factors (IF-1, IF-2 and IF-3) are required for formation of the initiation complex and GTP is hydrolyzed during the association of the 50S and 30S subunits. Eukaryotes and archaeal cells require more initiation factors.

2.7.4   Elongation of the Polypeptide Chain

Every addition of an amino acid to a growing polypeptide chain is the result of an elongation cycle composed of three phases: aminoacyl-tRNA binding, the transpeptidation reaction and translocation. The process is aided by proteins called elongation factors (EF). In each turn of the cycle, an amino acid corresponding to the proper mRNA codon is added to the C-terminal end of the polypeptide chain as the ribosome moves down the mRNA in the 5' to 3' direction.

The ribosome has three sites for binding tRNAs: ①the peptidyl or donor site (P site); ②the aminoacyl or acceptor site (A site); ③the exit site (E site). At the beginning of an elongation cycle, the P site is filled with either fMet-tRNA or a tRNA bearing a growing polypeptide chain (peptidyl-tRNA) and the A and E sites are empty. Messenger RNA is bound to the ribosome in such a way that the proper codon interacts with the P site tRNA (e.g., an AUG codon for fMet-tRNA). The next codon is located within the A site and is ready to accept an aminoacyl-tRNA.

The first phase of the elongation cycle is the aminoacylt RNA binding phase. The aminoacyl-tRNA corresponding to the codon in the A site is inserted so its anticodon is aligned with the codon on the mRNA. In bacterial cells, this is aided by two elongation factors and requires the expenditure of one GTP. Aminoacyl-tRNA binding to the A site initiates the second phase of the elongation cycle, the transpeptidation reaction. Transpeptidation is catalyzed by the peptidyl transferase activity of the 23S rRNA ribozyme, which is part of the 50S ribosomal subunit. In this reaction, the amino group of the A site amino acid reacts with the carboxyl group of the C-terminal amino acid on the P site tRNA. This results in the transfer of the peptide chain from the tRNA in the P site to the tRNA in the A site, as a peptide bond is formed between the peptide chain and the incoming amino acid. No extra energy source is required for peptide bond formation because the bond linking an amino acid to tRNA is high in energy.

The final phase in the elongation cycle is translocation. Three things happen simultaneously: ①the peptidyl-tRNA moves from the A site to the P site; ②the ribosome moves one codon along mRNA so that a new codon is positioned in the A site; ③the empty tRNA moves from the P site to the E site and subsequently leaves the ribosome. Translocation occurs by a ratcheting mechanism brought about by conformational changes in constituents of the ribosome and rotations of the 30S and 50S subunits relative to each other. This intricate process requires the participation of an elongation factor and GTP hydrolysis.

2.7.5　Insertion of Selenocysteine and Pyrrolysine

Insertion of the unusual amino acids selenocysteine and pyrrolysine during translation occurs by two distinctive mechanisms. Selenocysteine is synthesized from serine after it has been attached to certain tRNAs. The enzyme catalyzing the conversion is selenocysteine synthase. Once formed, the amino acid is recognized by a specific elongation factor and is incorporated when a UGA stop codon is encountered in association with nucleotide sequences called cis-acting selenocysteine insertion sequence elements (SECIS). In bacteria, SECIS are found immediately after the UGA stop codon. In archaea and eukaryotes, SECIS are located in the 3′ untranslated region of the mRNA.

Pyrrolysine insertion differs from that of selenocysteine in several ways. Pyrrolysine is synthesized from lysine before being attached to a tRNA. Organisms that use pyrrolysine make an unusual tRNA with a CUA anticodon; the pyrrolysine is attached by a specific aminoacyl-tRNA synthetase. Pyrrolysine is inserted at UAG stop codons located near a sequence element called pyrrolysine insertion sequence (PYLIS). Both SECIS and PYLIS form stem-loop structures that prevent cessation of translation.

2.7.6　Termination of Protein Synthesis

Protein synthesis stops when the ribosome reaches one of three stop codons: UAA, UAG and UGA. The stop codon is found on the mRNA immediately before the trailer. Three release factors (RF-1, RF-2 and RF-3) aid the ribosome in recognizing these codons. Because there is no cognate tRNA for a stop codon, the ribosome halts. Peptidyl transferase hydrolyzes the bond linking the polypeptide to the tRNA in the P site and the polypeptide and the empty tRNA are released. GTP hydrolysis occurs during this sequence of events. Next the ribosome dissociates from its mRNA and separates into 30S and 50S subunits. IF-3 binds the 30S subunit, which prepares it for the next round of protein synthesis. The termination of archaeal and eukaryotic protein synthesis is similar except that only one release factor appears to be active.

Protein synthesis is a very expensive process. Three GTP molecules probably are used during each elongation cycle and two ATP high-energy bonds are required for amino acid activation (ATP is converted to AMP, rather than to ADP). Therefore five high-energy bonds are required to add one amino acid to a growing polypeptide chain. GTP also is used in initiation and termination of protein synthesis. Presumably this large energy expenditure is required to ensure the fidelity of protein synthesis. Fidelity can be ensured both before and after formation of the peptide bond. When an aminoacyl-tRNA enters the A site, correct pairing of the anticodon and codon causes conformational changes in components of the ribosome such that the aminoacyl-tRNA is "locked into place" in a manner that facilitates peptide bond formation. On rare occasions, the incorrect aminoacyl-tRNA is selected and a peptide bond is formed between the growing polypeptide and the wrong amino acid. The ribosome is able to detect its error; how it does so is not clear. However, the presence of an incorrect amino acid is recognized by release factors. This leads to hydrolysis of the aberrant polypeptide from the tRNA, its release from the ribosome and termination of translation.

2.8   Protein Maturation and Secretion

As a polypeptide emerges from a ribosome, it is not yet ready to assume its cellular functions. Protein function depends on its three-dimensional shape. Proteins must be properly folded and in some cases associated with other protein subunits to generate a functional enzyme (e. g. ,DNA and RNA polymerases are multimeric proteins). In addition, proteins must be delivered to the proper subcellular or extracellular site. We now discuss these posttranslational events.

2.8.1   Protein Folding and Molecular Chaperones

Although the amino acid sequence of a polypeptide determines its final conformation, helper proteins aid the newly formed or nascent polypeptide in folding to its proper functional shape. These proteins, called molecular chaperones or simply chaperones, recognize only unfolded polypeptides or partly denatured proteins and do not bind to normal, functional proteins. Their role is essential because the cytoplasm is filled with new polypeptide chains. Under such conditions, it is possible for polypeptides to fold improperly and aggregate to form nonfunctional complexes. Molecular chaperones suppress incorrect folding and may reverse any incorrect folding that has already taken place. They are so important that chaperones are present in all cells.

Several chaperones and cooperating proteins aid proper protein folding in *E. coli*: chaperones DnaK, DnaJ, GroEL and GroES; and the stress protein GrpE. After a sufficient length of nascent polypeptide extends from the ribosome, a series of reactions involving DnaJ and DnaK fold the protein into its native conformation. This requires the expenditure of ATP. Sometimes the polypeptide does not reach its native conformation in one series of reactions and the folding process may be repeated.

Alternatively, the partially folded protein may be transferred to chaperones GroEL and GroES, which complete the folding. This chaperone system also expends ATP as it folds the protein into its proper conformation.

Chaperones were first discovered because they dramatically increase in concentration when cells are exposed to high temperatures, metabolic poisons and other stressful conditions that cause protein denaturation. Thus many chaperones are called heat-shock proteins. When an *E. coli* culture is switched from 30 ℃ to 42 ℃, the concentrations of some 20 different heatshock proteins increase greatly within about 5 minutes. If the cells are exposed to a lethal temperature, the heat-shock proteins are still synthesized but most other proteins are not. Thus chaperones protect the cell from thermal damage and other stresses as well as promote the proper folding of new polypeptides. For example, DnaK protects *E. coli* RNA polymerase from thermal inactivation in vitro. In addition, DnaK reactivates thermally inactivated RNA polymerase, especially if ATP, DnaJ and GrpE are present. GroEL and GroES also protect intracellular proteins from aggregation.

2.8.2   Protein Splicing

A further level of complexity in the formation of proteins has been discovered in microbes belonging to all three domains of life. Some microbial proteins are spliced after translation. In protein splicing, a part of the polypeptide is removed before the polypeptide folds into its final shape. Self-splicing proteins begin as larger precursor proteins composed of an internal intervening sequence called an intein (about 130 – 600 amino acids in length) flanked by external sequences called exteins. Inteins remove themselves from the precursor protein. When the splicing is completed, two proteins have been formed: the intein protein and the protein formed by splicing the two exteins together.

2.8.3   Protein Translocation and Secretion in Bacteria

It has been estimated that almost one-third of the proteins synthesized by cells leave the cytoplasm to reside in membranes, the periplasmic space of bacterial and archaeal cells or the external environment. It is not surprising then that over 15 different systems for moving proteins out of the cytoplasm have evolved. Some of these systems are found in all domains of life. Others are unique to bacterial cells and others are observed only in Gram-negative bacteria. When proteins are moved from the cytoplasm to the membrane or to the periplasmic space, the movement is called translocation. Protein secretion refers to the movement of proteins from the cytoplasm to the external environment. Many of the secretion pathways are designated with numbers (e. g. , type I secretion system, type II secretion system, etc.).

Why are so many proteins moved out of the cytoplasm? Many important proteins are located in membranes. These include transport proteins that bring needed materials into the cell and take wastes out of the cell. They also include proteins involved in electron transport. In Gram-negative bacteria, the periplasmic space is loaded with proteins such as chemotaxis proteins, enzymes involved in cell wall synthesis and periplasmic components of nutrient uptake systems. Many organisms secrete hydrolytic enzymes into the external environment. These enzymes break down macromolecules into monomers that are more easily brought into the cell. The protein subunits of external structures such as flagella and fimbriae must also be moved out of the cell and assembled on its external surface. Pathogenic microbes often release toxins that are important in the infection process.

Protein secretion poses different difficulties, depending on the structure of the cell envelope. For Gram-positive bacteria to secrete proteins, the proteins must be translocated across the plasma membrane. Once across the plasma membrane, the protein either passes through the relatively porous peptidoglycan into the external environment or becomes embedded in or attached to the peptidoglycan. Gram-negative bacteria have more hurdles to jump when they secrete proteins. They, too, must transport the proteins across the plasma membrane, but to complete secretion, the proteins must be transported across the outer membrane.

2.8.4   Common Translocation and Secretion Systems

The major pathway for translocating proteins across the plasma membrane is the secretion (Sec) pathway. In Gram-negative bacteria, proteins can be transported across the outer membrane by several different mechanisms, some of which bypass the Sec system, moving proteins directly from the cytoplasm to the outside of the cell. All protein translocation and secretion pathways described here require the expenditure of energy at some step in the process. The energy is usually supplied by the hydrolysis of high-energy molecules such as ATP and GTP. However, the proton motive force also sometimes plays a role.

The Sec system, sometimes called the general secretion pathway, is highly conserved, having been identified in all three domains of life. It translocates unfolded proteins across the plasma membrane or integrates them into the membrane itself. It does so either posttranslationally or cotranslationally. In posttranslational translocation, the protein is synthesized and released from the ribosome as a preprotein; the amino acid sequence at its amino terminus is called a signal peptide. The signal peptide is recognized and bound by chaperone proteins (e. g. , SecB). This helps delay protein folding, thereby helping the preprotein reach the Sec transport machinery in the conformation needed for transport. The chaperone protein "delivers" the preprotein to the Sec system. Certain Sec proteins (SecY, SecE and SecG) form a channel in the membrane through which the preprotein passes.

Another protein (SecA) binds to the SecYEG proteins and acts as a motor, using the energy released from ATP hydrolysis to translocate the preprotein. Recent studies suggest that two other proteins (SecDF) use the proton motive force to help fuel translocation through the plasma membrane. When the preprotein emerges from the plasma membrane, free from chaperones, an enzyme called signal peptidase removes the signal peptide. The protein then folds into the proper shape.

Cotranslational movement of proteins by the Sec system is mediated by a complex of RNA and protein called the signal recognition particle (SRP). It is thought that SRP binds a signal sequence (not the same as the signal peptide) in the protein as it leaves the ribosome and directs the protein together with the translating ribosome to SecYEG. As translation continues, the protein is threaded into the SecYEG channel and inserted into the plasma membrane, often with the aid of a protein called YidC. This process is similar to the cotranslational translocation that occurs in the eukaryotic Sec system that moves proteins across the membranes of the endoplasmic reticulum.

In bacteria and some archaea, another translocation system called the Tat system can move proteins across the plasma membrane. This system is distinguished from the Sec pathway by the nature of the protein transported. The Sec pathway translocates unfolded proteins; the Tat pathway translocates folded proteins. Furthermore, the Tat pathway only moves proteins that feature two or "twin", arginine residues in their signal sequence-in fact, Tat stands for twin arginine translocase. In Gram-negative bacteria, proteins translocated by the Tat pathway are delivered to a type II secretion system for transport across the outer membrane.

Type I secretion systems are ubiquitous in Gram-positive and Gram-negative bacteria, as well as in members of Archaea. Type I systems are members of a protein superfamily defined by the ABC transporters. In pathogenic Gram-negative bacteria, type I secretion systems are involved in the secretion of toxins (a-hemolysin), as well as proteases, lipases and specific peptides. Secreted proteins usually contain C-terminal secretion signals that help direct the newly synthesized protein to the type I machinery. In Gram-negative bacteria, the type I machinery spans the plasma membrane, the periplasmic space and the outer membrane. These systems move proteins in one step across both membranes, bypassing the Sec system.

Type IV secretion systems are unique in that they are used to secrete proteins as well as to transfer DNA from a donor bacterium to a recipient during a process called bacterial conjugation. These systems are observed in both Gram-positive and Gram-negative bacteria; however, in Gram-positive bacteria, they only function in DNA transfer. The type IV systems of Gram-negative bacteria are best studied. They are composed of many different proteins.

2.8.5 Protein Secretion in Gram-Negative Bacteria

Currently six protein secretion systems (types I to VI) have been identified in Gram-negative bacteria. Some of these systems have already been described as they are present in both Gram-negative and Gram-positive bacteria (type I and type IV secretion systems). All others are unique to Gram-negative bacteria.

Most are used to secrete virulence factors produced by plant and animal pathogens. Gram-negative bacteria use the type Ⅱ and type Ⅴ systems to transport proteins across the outer membrane after the protein has first been translocated across the plasma membrane by the Sec system. The type Ⅰ, type Ⅲ and type Ⅵ systems do not transport proteins with the help of the Sec system, so they are said to be Sec-independent. The type Ⅳ pathway sometimes is linked to the Sec pathway but usually functions on its own.

Three of the systems (Ⅲ, Ⅳ and Ⅵ) form a needlelike structure that extends beyond the outer membrane and can make contact with other cells. The type Ⅲ secretion system is best studied because it injects virulence factors directly into the plant and animal host cells that these pathogens attack. Its needle, called the injectisome, delivers virulence factors, including toxins, phagocytosis inhibitors, stimulators of cytoskeleton reorganization in the host cell and promoters of host cell suicide (apoptosis). Type Ⅲ systems also transport other proteins, including some of the proteins from which the system is built, proteins that regulate the secretion process and proteins that aid in the insertion of secreted proteins into target cells. In addition to *E. coli*, important examples of bacterial genera having members with type Ⅲ systems are Salmonella, Yersinia, Shigella, Bordetella, Pseudomonas and Erwinia.

Type Ⅴ and type Ⅵ secretion systems also warrant comment. Type Ⅴ systems employ proteins called autotransporters because after being translocated across the plasma membrane by the Sec pathway, the proteins are able to transport themselves across the outer membrane. Autotransporters have three domains. One is recognized by the Sec system and another forms a pore in the outer membrane through which the third domain (a virulence factor) is transported. Type Ⅵ systems are of interest because they are similar to the injection systems used by some bacteriophages to "push" their genomes into the cytoplasm of their bacterial hosts.

Chapter 3

Microbial Metabolism and Genetics

3.1 Metabolism：Important Principles and Concepts

It would be nice to think that microbes existed for the benefit of humans and that their metabolisms evolved for us to exploit, but of course this is not the case. Rather, they use their vast repertoire of chemical reactions to survive and reproduce, just as all organisms do. Thus metabolism is central to all life. The forces of evolution have shaped the metabolic process used by organisms for billions of years. Despite the diversity of chemical reactions that have evolved, there are several aspects of metabolism that are common to all organisms.

3.1.1 Cellular Work and Energy Transfers

Examine the common features of metabolism just described. It should be clear that cells must do work in order to survive and reproduce. Cells carry out three major types of work. Chemical work involves the synthesis of complex biological molecules from much simpler precursors (i. e. , anabolism) ; energy is needed to increase the molecular complexity of a cell. Transport work requires energy to take up nutrients, eliminate wastes and maintain ion balances. Energy input is needed because molecules and ions often must be transported across cell membranes against an electrochemical gradient. The third type of work is mechanical work. Energy is required for cell motility and the movement of structures within cells, such as partitioning chromosomes during cell division.

As just indicated, cells need energy to do work. Indeed, energy may be defined most simply as the capacity to do work. This is because all physical and chemical processes are the result of the application or movement of energy. Organisms obtain the energy they need from an energy source present in their environment. They convert the energy it provides into a useful form. The most commonly used form of cellular energy is the nucleoside triphosphate ATP. In addition, other nucleoside triphosphates and other high-energy molecules are required for specific processes.

To understand how energy is conserved in ATP and how ATP is used to do cellular work, some knowledge of the basic principles of thermodynamics is required. The science of thermodynamics analyzes energy changes in a collection of matter (e. g. , a cell or a plant) called a system. All other matter in the universe is called the surroundings. Thermodynamics focuses on the energy differences between the initial state and the final state of a system. It is not concerned with the rate of the process. For instance, if a pan of water is heated to boiling, only the condition of the water at the start and at boiling is important in thermodynamics, not how fast it is heated.

3.1.2   Laws of Thermodynamics

Two important laws of thermodynamics are critical to understanding energy transfers. The first law of thermodynamics says that energy can be neither created nor destroyed. The total energy in the universe remains constant, although it can be redistributed, as it is during the many energy exchanges that occur during chemical reactions. For example, heat is given off by exothermic reactions and absorbed during endothermic reactions. However, the first law alone cannot explain why heat is released by one chemical reaction and absorbed by another. Explanations for this require the second law of thermodynamics and a condition of matter called entropy. Entropy is a measure of the randomness or disorder of a system. The greater the disorder of a system, the greater its entropy. The second law states that physical and chemical processes proceed in such a way that the randomness or disorder of the universe (the system and its surroundings) increases. However, even though the entropy of the universe increases, the entropy of any given system within the universe can increase, decrease or remain unchanged.

Two types of energy units are employed to specify the amount of energy used in or evolving from a particular process. A calorie (cal) is the amount of heat energy needed to raise 1 gram of water from 14.5 ℃ to 15.5 ℃. The amount of energy also may be expressed in terms of joules (J), the units of work capable of being done. One cal of heat is equivalent to 4.1840 J of work. One thousand calories or a kilocalorie (kcal), is enough energy to boil 1.9 milliliters of water. A kilojoule is enough energy to boil about 0.44 milliliters of water or enable a person weighing 70 kilograms to climb 35 steps.

3.1.3   Free Energy and Chemical Reactions

The first and second laws of thermodynamics can be combined in a useful equation, relating the changes in energy that can occur in chemical reactions and other processes.

$$\Delta G = \Delta H - T\Delta S$$

ΔG is the change in free energy, ΔH is the change in enthalpy, T is the temperature in Kelvin (℃ + 273) and ΔS is the change in entropy occurring during the reaction. The change in enthalpy is the change in heat content. Cellular reactions occur under conditions of constant pressure and volume. Thus the change in enthalpy is about the same as the change in total energy during the reaction. The free energy change is the amount of energy in a system (or cell) available to do useful work at constant temperature and pressure. Therefore the change in entropy (ΔS) is a measure of the proportion of the total energy change that the system cannot use in performing work. Free energy and entropy changes do not depend on how the system gets from start to finish. A reaction will occur spontaneously-that is, without any external cause-if the free energy of the system decreases during the reaction or, in other words, if ΔG is negative. It follows from the equation that a reaction with a large positive change in entropy will normally tend to have a negative ΔG value and therefore occur spontaneously. A decrease in entropy will tend to make ΔG more positive and the reaction less favorable.

It is helpful to think of the relationship between entropy (ΔS) and change in free energy (ΔG) in terms that are more concrete. Consider the Greek myth of Sisyphus, king of Corinth. For his assorted crimes against the gods, he was condemned to roll a large boulder to the top of a steep hill for all eternity. This represents a very negative change in entropy-a boulder poised at the top of a hill is neither random nor disordered-and this activity (reaction) has a very positive ΔG. That is to say, Sisyphus had to put a lot of energy into the system. Unfortunately for Sisyphus, as soon as the boulder was at the top of the hill, it spontaneously rolled back down the hill. This represents a positive change in entropy and a negative ΔG. Sisyphus did not need to put energy into the system. He could simply stand at the top of the hill and watch the reaction proceed.

The change in free energy has a definite, concrete relationship to the direction of chemical reactions. Consider this simple reaction.

$$A+B \rightleftharpoons C+D$$

If molecules A and B are mixed, they will combine to form the products C and D. Eventually C and D will become concentrated enough to combine and produce A and B at the same rate as C and D are formed. The reaction is now at equilibrium; the rates in both directions are equal and no further net change occurs in the concentrations of reactants and products. This situation is described by the equilibrium constant (K_{eq}), relating the equilibrium concentrations of products and substrates to one another.

$$K_{eq} = \frac{[C][D]}{[A][B]}$$

If the equilibrium constant is greater than one, the products are in greater concentration than the reactants at equilibrium; that is, the reaction tends to go to completion as written.

The equilibrium constant of a reaction is directly related to its change in free energy. When the free energy change for a process is determined at carefully defined standard conditions of concentration, pressure, pH and temperature, it is called the standard free energy change (ΔG°). If the pH is set at 7.0 (which is close to the pH of living cells), the standard free energy change is indicated by the symbol $\Delta G^{\circ'}$. The change in standard free energy may be thought of as the maximum amount of energy available from the system for useful work under standard conditions. Using $\Delta G^{\circ'}$ values allows comparisons of reactions without considering variations in ΔG due to differences in environmental conditions. The relationship between $\Delta G^{\circ'}$ and K_{eq} is given by this equation.

$$\Delta G^{\circ'} = -2.303RT \cdot \log K_{eq}$$

R is the gas constant (1.9872 cal/mole-degree or 8.3145 J/mole-degree) and T is the absolute temperature. Inspection of this equation shows that when $\Delta G^{\circ'}$ is negative, the equilibrium constant is greater than one and the reaction goes to completion as written. It is said to be an exergonic reaction. In an endergonic reaction, $\Delta G^{\circ'}$ is positive and the equilibrium constant is less than one. That is, the reaction is not favorable and little product will be formed at equilibrium under standard conditions. Keep in mind that the $\Delta G^{\circ'}$ value shows only where the reaction lies at equilibrium, not how fast the reaction reaches equilibrium.

3.2   ATP: The Major Energy Currency of Cells

Energy is released from a cell's energy source in exergonic reactions (i.e., those reactions with a negative ΔG). Rather than wasting this energy, much of it is trapped in a practical form that allows its transfer to the cellular systems doing work. These systems carry out endergonic reactions (e.g., anabolism) and the energy captured by the cell is used to drive these reactions to completion. In living organisms, the most commonly used practical form of energy is adenosine 5′-triphosphate (ATP). In a sense, cells carry out certain processes so that they can "earn" ATP and carry out other processes in which they "spend" their ATP. Thus ATP is often referred to as the cell's energy currency. In the cell's economy, ATP serves as the link between exergonic reactions and endergonic reactions.

What makes ATP suited for its role as energy currency? ATP is a high-energy molecule. That is, it is hydrolyzed almost completely to the products adenosine diphosphate (ADP) and orthophosphate (P_i), with a strongly exergonic $\Delta G^{o'}$ of -7.3 kcal/mole (-30.5 kJ/mole).

$$ATP + H_2O \rightleftharpoons ADP + P_i + H^+$$

The energy released is used to power endergonic reactions.

The very negative $\Delta G^{o'}$ of hydrolysis of ATP is related to another important characteristic of ATP: its ability to transfer a phosphoryl group to another molecule. ATP is said to have a high phosphate transfer potential because it readily donates a phosphoryl group to other molecules. These molecules are generated during catabolism of organic molecules such as glucose. Some of these molecules have even higher phosphate transfer potentials than ATP. The fact that ATP does not have the highest phosphate transfer potential means that it can easily be made by cells from ADP, using molecules such as phosphoenolpyruvate (PEP) as the source of the phosphoryl group. This mechanism for making ATP is called substrate-level phosphorylation.

ATP, ADP and P; form an energy cycle. The energy released from an energy source is used to synthesize ATP from ADP and P;. When ATP is hydrolyzed, the energy released drives endergonic processes such as anabolism, transport and mechanical work.

ATP is the major energy currency for cells, but it is not the only energy currency. Other nucleoside triphosphates (NTP s) have major roles in metabolism. Guanosine 5′-triphosphate (GTP) supplies some of the energy used during protein synthesis. Cytidine 5′-triphosphate (CTP) is used during lipid synthesis and uridine 5′-triphosphate (UTP) is used for the synthesis of peptidoglycan and other polysaccharides.

3.3   Redox Reactions: Reactions of Central Importance in Metabolism

Free energy changes are related to the equilibria of all chemical reactions, including the equilibria of oxidation-reduction reactions. The release of energy from an energy source normally involves oxidation-reduction reactions. Oxidation-reduction (redox) reactions are those in which electrons move from an electron donor to an electron acceptor. 1 As electrons move from the donor to acceptor, the donor becomes less energy rich and the acceptor becomes more energy rich. Thus electrons can be thought of as packets of energy. The more electrons a molecule has and is able to donate in a redox reaction, the more energy rich the molecule is. This explains why molecules such as glucose, which can donate up to 24 electrons in redox reactions, are such excellent sources of energy.

Each redox reaction consists of two half reactions. One half reaction functions as the electron-donating half reaction (i. e. , an oxidation reaction) and the other functions as the electron-accepting half reaction (i. e. , the reduction). By convention, half reactions are written as reductions. Thus each half reaction consists of a molecule that can accept electrons (on the left side of the chemical equation), the number (n) of electrons (e^-) it accepts and the molecule it becomes after accepting the electrons. The latter is placed on the right side of the chemical equation and is referred to as a donor, because it has electrons it can give up. The acceptor and donor of a half reaction are referred to as a conjugate redox pair.

$$\text{Acceptor} + ne^- \rightleftharpoons \text{donor}$$

The equilibrium constant for a redox half reaction is called the standard reduction potential (E_0) and is a measure of the tendency of the donor of a half reaction to lose electrons. By convention, the standard reduction potentials for half reactionsare determined at pH 7 and are represented by E'_0. Standard reduction potentials are measured in volts, a unit of electrical potential or electromotive force. Therefore conjugate redox pairs are a potential source of energy.

The reduction potential has a concrete meaning. Conjugate redox pairs with more negative reduction potentials will spontaneously donate electrons to pairs with more positive potentials and greater affinity for electrons. Thus electrons tend to move from donors at the top of the list in Table 3-1 to acceptors at the bottom because the latter have more positive potentials. This may be expressed visually in the form of an electron tower in which the most negative reduction potentials are at the top. Electrons "fall down" the tower from donors higher in the tower (i. e. , those having more negative potentials) to acceptors lower in the tower (i. e. , those having more positive potentials).

Consider the case of the electron acceptor nicotinamide adenine dinucleotide (NAD$^+$). The NAD$^+$/NADH conjugate redox pair has a very negative E'_0. and NADH can therefore give electrons to many acceptors, including O_2.

$$NAD^+ + 2H^+ + 2e^- \rightleftharpoons NADH + H^+ \qquad E'_0 = -0.32 \text{ volts}$$

$$\frac{1}{2} O_2 + 2H^+ + 2e^- \rightleftharpoons H_2O \qquad E'_0 = +0.82 \text{ volts}$$

Because the reduction potential of NAD$^+$/NADH is more negative 1 than that of $\frac{1}{2} O_2/H_2O$, electrons flow from NADH (the donor) to O_2 (the acceptor). The redox reaction is shown here.

$$NADH + H^+ + \frac{1}{2} O_2 \rightarrow H_2O + NAD^+$$

The relatively negative E'_0 of the NAD+/NADH pair also means that the pair stores more potential energy than redox pairs with less negative (or more positive) E'_0 values. It follows that when electrons move from a donor to an acceptor with a more positive redox potential, free energy is released. The $\Delta G^{o'}$ of the reaction is directly related to the magnitude of the difference between the reduction potentials of the two couples ($\Delta E'_0$). The larger the $\Delta E'_0$, the greater the amount of free energy made available, as is evident from the equation

$$\Delta G^{o'} = -nF \cdot \Delta E'_0$$

in which n is the number of electrons transferred, F is the Faraday constant (23,062 cal/mole-volt; 96,480 J/mole-volt) and $\Delta E'_0$ is the E'_0 of the acceptor minus the E'_0 of the donor. For every 0. 1 volt change in $\Delta E'_0$, there is a corresponding 4. 6 kcal (19. 3 kJ) change in $\Delta G^{o'}$ when a two-electron transfer takes place. This is similar to the relationship of $\Delta G^{o'}$ and K_{eq} in other chemical reactions: the larger the equilibrium constant, the greater the $\Delta G^{o'}$. The difference in reduction potentials between NAD$^+$/NADH and $\frac{1}{2} O_2/H_2O$ is 1. 14 volts, a large $\Delta E'_0$ value. When electrons move from NADH to O_2, a large amount of free energy is made available and can be used to synthesize ATP and do other work.

Table 3-1　Selected biologically important half reactions

Half Reaction	E'_0(Volts)
$2H^+ + 2e^- \rightarrow H_2$	-0. 42
Ferredoxin (Fe^{3+}) + e$^-$ → ferredoxin (Fe^{2+})	-0. 42
NAD(P)$^+$ + H$^+$ + 2e$^-$ → NAD(P)H	-0. 32

Continue to Table 3-1

Half Reaction	E'_0(Volts)
$S + 2H^+ + 2e^- \rightarrow H_2S$	-0.27
$Acetaldehyde + 2H^+ + 2e^- \rightarrow ethanol$	-0.20
$Pyruvate^- + 2H^+ + 2e^- \rightarrow lactate^{2-}$	-0.19
$FAD + 2H^+ + 2e^- \rightarrow FADH_2$	-0.18
$Oxaloacetate2- + 2H^+ + 2e^- \rightarrow malate^{2-}$	-0.17
$Fumarate^{2-} + 2H^+ + 2e^- \rightarrow succinate^{2-}$	0.03
$Cytochrome\ b\ (Fe^{3+}) + e^- \rightarrow cytochrome\ b\ (Fe^{2+})$	0.08
$Ubiquinone + 2H^+ 2e^- \rightarrow ubiquinone\ H_2$	0.10
$Cytochrome\ c\ (Fe^{3+}) + e^- \rightarrow cytochrome\ c\ (Fe^{2+})$	0.25
$Cytochrome\ a\ (Fe^{3+}) + e^- \rightarrow cytochrome\ a\ (Fe^{2+})$	0.29
$Cytochrome\ a_3(Fe^{3+}) + e^- \rightarrow cytochrome\ a_3(Fe^{2+})$	0.35
$NO_3^- + 2H^+ + 2e^- \rightarrow NO_2^- + H_2O$	0.42
$NO_2^- + 8H^+ + 6e^- \rightarrow NH_4^+ + 2H_2O$	0.44
$Fe^{3+} + e^- \rightarrow Fe^{2+}$	0.77
$1/2O_2 + 2H^+ + 2e^- \rightarrow H_2O$	0.82

3.4 Electron Transport Chains: Sets of Sequential Redox Reactions

We have focused our attention on the reduction of O_2 by NADH because NADH plays a central role in the metabolism of many organisms. For instance, glucose is a common organic energy source. As glucose is catabolized, it is oxidized. Many of the electrons released from glucose are accepted by NAD^+, reducing it to NADH, which transfers the electrons to O_2. However, it does not do so directly. Instead, the electrons are transferred to O_2 via a series of electron carriers that are organized into a system called an electron transport chain (ETC). An ETC is similar to a bucket brigade. Each carrier represents a person receiving a pail of water (electrons) that are destined for the fire (terminal electron acceptor). The pail of water is passed down the line, just as electrons are passed from carrier to carrier. As soon as one person hands off a pail of water to the person after him in the line, he can receive a new bucket from the person before him in the line. Likewise, as electrons flow through the ETC, each carrier is sequentially reduced (given the pail full of water) and then reoxidized (passes the pail on to the next person in the brigade) and is ready to accept more electrons as catabolism continues.

The first electron carrier in an ETC has the most negative E'_0, each successive carrier is slightly less negative. Thus electrons are transferred spontaneously from one carrier to the next. The carriers direct the electrons to the terminal electron acceptor (in this case, O_2). This protects the cells from random, nonproductive reductions of other molecules in the cell. The use of several carriers in a chain also releases energy from an energy source such as glucose in a controlled manner so that more can be conserved and used to form ATP.

Electron transport chains are associated with or are in the plasma membranes and intracytoplasmic membranes of bacterial and archaeal cells. In eukaryotes they are localized to the internal membranes of mitochondria and chloroplasts. They are important to almost all types of energy conserving processes.

The electron carriers associated with ETCs differ in terms of their chemical nature and the way they carry electrons. NADH and its chemical relative nicotinamide adenine dinucleotide phosphate (NADPH), which donate electrons to ETCs, contain a nicotinamide ring. This ring accepts two electrons and one proton from a donor (e. g. , an intermediate formed during the catabolism of glucose) and a second proton is released. Flavin adenine dinucleotide (FAD) and flavin mononucleotide (FMN) bear two electrons and two protons on the complex ring system. P roteins bearing FAD and FMN are often called flavoproteins. Coenzyme Q (CoQ) or ubiquinone is a quinone that transports two electrons and two protons. Cytochromes and several other carriers use iron atoms to transport one electron at a time. In cytochromes, the iron atoms are part of a heme group or other similar ironporphyrin rings. There are several different cytochromes, each consisting of a protein and an iron-porphyrin ring.

Some iron-containing electron-carrying proteins lack a heme group and are called nonheme iron proteins. They are often referred to as iron-sulfur (Fe-S) proteins because the iron is associated with sulfur atoms. Ferredoxin is an Fe-S protein active in photosynthesis-related electron transport. Like cytochromes, Fe-S proteins carry only one electron at a time. The differences in the number of electrons and protons transported by electron carriers are of great importance to the operation of ETCs.

3. 5　Biochemical Pathways

Organisms carry out a myriad of chemical reactions and the products of these reactions are called metabolites. The reactions are organized into biochemical pathways, which can take various forms. Some are linear. In linear pathways, the first molecule in the pathway is often termed the starting molecule or the substrate of the pathway. The last molecule is called the end product. Those metabolites in between are pathway intermediates. Some linear pathways are branched and can yield more than one product. Biochemical pathways can also be cycles. In this case, all molecules in the pathway can be thought of as intermediates. For the cycle to continue running, there must be inputs into it. In both types of pathways, each reaction is represented by an arrow and is catalyzed by an enzyme or ribozyme.

Biochemical pathways are often illustrated as though they exist in isolation of each other. Unfortunately, this is very misleading (especially to students). In reality, biochemical pathways are connected and form a complex network. Thus, an intermediate of a pathway may be diverted from one pathway to another pathway. This is important to recognize because biochemical pathways are dynamic. As long as the starting molecules or inputs of the pathway are available and some end product is needed, these molecules will flow into and out of the many pathways that function in cells. Microbiologists are often concerned with metabolite flux. Metabolite flux is the rate of turnover of a metabolite; that is, the rate at which a metabolite is formed and then used. Metabolite flux can be used as a measure of pathway activity and to understand metabolic networks.

3.6 Enzymes and Ribozymes

An exergonic reaction is one with a negative L'. G0' and an equilibrium constant greater than one. An exergonic reaction proceeds to completion in the direction written (i. e. , toward the right of the equation). Nevertheless, reactants for an exergonic reaction often can be combined with no obvious result. For instance, if a polysaccharide such as starch is mixed in water, the hydrolysis of the starch into its component monosaccharides (glucose) is exergonic and will occur spontaneously; that is, it will occur on its own, given enough time. However, the time needed is very long. Even if an organic chemist carried out this reaction in 6 moles/liter (M) HCl and at 100 ℃, it would still take several hours to go to completion. A cell, on the other hand, can accomplish the same reaction at neutral pH, at a much lower temperature and in just fractions of a second. Cells can do this because they manufacture biological catalysts that speed up chemical reactions. Most of these catalysts are proteins called enzymes. Other catalysts are RNA molecules termed ribozymes. Enzymes and ribozymes are critically important to cells, since most biological reactions occur very slowly without them. Indeed, enzymes and ribozymes make life possible.

3.6.1 Enzyme Structure

Enzymes are protein catalysts that have great specificity for the reaction catalyzed, the molecules acted on and the products they yield. A catalyst is a substance that increases the rate of a chemical reaction without being permanently altered itself. The reacting molecules are called substrates and the substances formed are the products. Enzymes may be placed in one of six general classes and usually are named in terms of the substrates they act on and the type of reaction catalyzed (Table 3–2).

Table 3–2 Enzyme classification

Type of enzyme	Reaction catalyzed by enzyme	Example of reaction
Oxidoreductase	Oxidation reduction reactions	Lactate dehydrogenase: pyruvate + NADH + H$^+$ $\rightleftharpoons$ lactate+NAD$^+$
Transferase	Reactions involving the transfer of chemical groups between molecules	Aspartate carbamoyltransferase: Aspartate + carbamoylphosphate $\rightleftharpoons$ carbamoylaspartate+phosphate
Hydrolase	Hydrolysis of molecules	Glucose 6-phosphatase: glucose 6-phosphate + H_2O $\rightarrow$ glucose+P$_i$
Lyase	Breaking of C-C, C-O, C-N and other bonds by a means other than hydrolysis	Fumarase: L-malate $\rightleftharpoons$ fumarate+H_2O
Isomerase	Reactions involving isomerizations	Alanine racemase: L-alanine $\rightleftharpoons$ D-alanine
Ligase	Joining of two molecules using ATP (or the energy of other nucleoside triphosphates)	Glutamine synthetase: Glutamate + NH_3 + ATP $\rightarrow$ glutamine+ADP+P$_i$

Many enzymes are composed only of proteins. However, some are composed of two parts: a protein component called the apoenzyme and a nonprotein component called a cofactor. Cofactors include metal ions and a variety of organic molecules. The complete enzyme consisting of the apoenzyme and its cofactor is called the holoenzyme. If the cofactor is firmly attached to the apoenzyme, it is a prosthetic group. If the cofactor is loosely attached and can dissociate from the apoenzyme after products have been formed, it is called a coenzyme. Many vitamins required by humans serve as coenzymes or as their precursors (e. g. , riboflavin is incorporated into FAD). Coenzymes often carry one of the products of a chemical reaction to another enzyme or transfer chemical groups from one substrate to another.

3.6.2 How Enzymes Speed Up Reactions

It is important to keep in mind that enzymes increase the rates of reactions but do not alter their equilibrium constants. If a reaction is endergonic, the presence of an enzyme will not shift its equilibrium so that more products are formed. Enzymes simply speed up the rate at which a reaction proceeds toward its final equilibrium.

How do enzymes catalyze reactions? Some understanding of the mechanism can be gained by considering the course of a simple exergonic chemical reaction.

$$A + B \rightleftharpoons C + D$$

When molecules A and B approach each other to react, they form a transition-state complex, which resembles both the substrates and the products. Activation energy is required to bring the reacting molecules together in the correct way to reach the transition state. The transition-state complex can then resolve to yield the products C and D. The difference in free energy level between reactants and products is $\Delta G^{o'}$. Thus the equilibrium in our example lies toward the products because $\Delta G^{o'}$ is negative (i. e. , the products are at a lower energy level than the substrates).

A and B will not be converted to C and D if they are not supplied with an amount of energy equivalent to the activation energy. Enzymes accelerate reactions by lowering the activation energy; therefore more substrate molecules will have sufficient energy to come together and form products. Even though the equilibrium constant (or $\Delta G^{o'}$) is unchanged, equilibrium is reached more rapidly in the presence of an enzyme because of this decrease in activation energy.

Researchers have worked hard to discover how enzymes lower the activation energy of reactions. Enzymes bring substrates together at a specific location in the enzyme called the active or catalytic site to form an enzyme-substrate complex. How the enzyme and substrate interact still has not been fully elucidated. However, the induced fit model describes the interaction for many enzymes. In the induced fit model, the enzyme changes shape when it binds the substrate so that the active site surrounds and precisely fits the substrate. This mechanism is used by hexokinase. The formation of an enzyme-substrate complex can lower the activation energy in many ways. For example, by bringing the substrates together at the active site, the enzyme is, in effect, concentrating them and speeding up the reaction. An enzyme does not simply concentrate its substrates, however. It also binds them so that they are correctly oriented with respect to each other. Such an orientation lowers the amount of energy that the substrates require to reach the transition state. These and other catalytic site activities speed up a reaction by hundreds of thousands of times.

3.6.3 Substrate Concentration and Enzyme Activity

Enzyme activity varies in response to substrate concentration. At very low substrate concentrations, an enzyme makes product slowly because it seldom contacts a substrate molecule. If more substrate molecules are present, an enzyme binds substrate more often and the velocity of the reaction (usually expressed in terms of the rate of product formation) is greater than at a lower substrate concentration. Thus the rate of an enzymecatalyzed reaction increases with substrate concentration. Eventually further increases in substrate concentration do not result in a greater reaction velocity because the available enzyme molecules are binding substrate and converting it to product as rapidly as possible. That is, the enzyme is saturated with substrate and operating at maximal velocity (V_{max}). The resulting substrate concentration curve is a hyperbola.

The substrate concentrations in cells are often low. Therefore it is useful to know the substrate concentration an enzyme needs to function adequately. Usually the Michaelis constant (K_m), the substrate concentration required for the enzyme to achieve halfmaximal velocity, is used as a measure of the apparent affinity of an enzyme for its substrate. The lower the K_m value, the lower the substrate concentration at which an enzyme catalyzes its reaction. Enzymes with a low K_m value are said to have a high affinity for their substrates. Since the concentrations of substrates in cells are often low, enzymes with lower K_m values are able to function better.

3.6.4   Enzyme Denaturation

Enzyme activity is changed not only by substrate concentration but also by alterations in pH and temperature. Each enzyme functions most rapidly at a specific pH optimum. When the pH deviates too greatly from an enzyme's optimum, activity slows and the enzyme may be damaged. Enzymes likewise have temperature optima for maximum activity. If the temperature rises too much above the optimum, an enzyme's structure will be disrupted and its activity lost. This phenomenon is known as denaturation. The pH and temperature optima of a microorganism's enzymes often reflect the pH and temperature of its habitat. Not surprisingly, bacteria and archaea that grow best at high temperatures often have enzymes with high temperature optima and great heat stability.

3.6.5   Enzyme Inhibition

Microorganisms can be poisoned by a variety of chemicals (e. g. , cyanide) and many of the most potent poisons are enzyme inhibitors. A competitive inhibitor directly competes with the substrate at an enzyme's catalytic site and prevents the enzyme from forming product. Competitive inhibitors usually resemble normal substrates, but they cannot be converted to products.

Competitive inhibitors are important in the treatment of many microbial diseases. Sulfa drugs such as sulfanilamideresemble p-aminobenzoate (PABA), a molecule used in the formation of the coenzyme folic acid. Sulfa drugs compete with PABA for the catalytic site of an enzyme involved in folic acid synthesis. This blocks the production of folic acid and inhibits the growth of organisms that require its synthesis. Humans are not harmed because they do not synthesize folic acid but rather obtain it in their diet.

Noncompetitive inhibitors affect enzyme activity by binding to the enzyme at some location other than the active site. This alters the enzyme's shape, rendering it inactive or less active. These inhibitors are called noncompetitive because they do not directly compete with the substrate. Heavy metals such as mercury frequently are noncompetitive inhibitors of enzymes.

3.6.6   Ribozymes: Catalytic RNA Molecules

Biologists once thought that all cellular reactions were catalyzed by proteins. However, in the early 1980s Thomas Cech and Sidney Altman discovered that some RNA molecules also can catalyze reactions. Catalytic RNA molecules are called ribozymes. One important ribozyme is located in ribosomes and is responsible for catalyzing peptide bond formation between amino acid residues during protein synthesis. However, the best-studied ribozymes catalyze self-splicing, in which they cut themselves and then join segments of themselves back together (Table 3−3). Just as with enzymes, the shape of a ribozyme is essential to catalytic efficiency. Ribozymes even have Michaelis-Menten kinetics. One particularly interesting ribozyme is a self-splicing ribozyme produced by hepatitis delta virus. It is unusual in that it can fold into two shapes with quite different catalytic activities;the regular RNA cleavage activity and an RNA ligation reaction.

Table 3-3   Examples of self-splicing ribozymes

Function	Where observed
Splicing of pre-rRNA	Tetrahymena spp.
Splicing of mitochondrial rRNA and mRNA	Numerous fungi
Splicing of chloroplast tRNA,rRNA	Plants and algae
Splicing of viral mRNA	Viruses

3.7   Mutations

Perhaps the most obvious way genetic diversity can be created is by mutations (Latin mutare, to change). Several types of mutations exist. Some arise from the alteration of single pairs of nucleotides and from the addition or deletion of one nucleotide pair in the coding regions of a gene. Such small changes in DNA are called point mutations because they affect only one base pair in a given location. Larger mutations are less common. These include large insertions,deletions,inversions,duplications and translocations of nucleotide sequences.

Mutations occur in one of two ways. ①Spontaneous mutations arise occasionally in all cells and in the absence of any added agent. ②Induced mutations are the result of exposure to a mutagen,which can be either a physical or a chemical agent. Mutations are characterized according to either the kind of genotypic change that has occurred or their phenotypic consequences. In this section,the molecular basis of mutations and mutagenesis is first considered. Then the phenotypic effects of mutations are discussed.

3.7.1   Spontaneous Mutations

Spontaneous mutations result from errors in DNA replication,spontaneously occurring lesions in DNA or the action of mobile genetic elements such as transposons. A few of the more prevalent mechanisms are described here.

Replication errors can occur when the nitrogenous base of a nucleotide shifts to a different form (isomer)called a tautomeric form. Nitrogenous bases typically exist in the keto form but are in equilibrium with the rarer imino and enol forms. The shift from one form to another changes the hydrogen-bonding characteristics of the bases,allowing purine for purine or pyrimidine for pyrimidine substitutions that can eventually lead to a stable alteration of the nucleotide sequence. Such substitutions are known as transition mutations and are relatively common. On the other hand,transversion mutations-mutations where a purine is substituted for a pyrimidine or a pyrimidine for a purine-are rarer due to the steric problems of pairing purines with purines and pyrimidines with pyrimidines.

Replication errors can also result in the insertion and deletion of nucleotides. These mutations generally occur where there is a short stretch of repeated nucleotides. In such a location,the pairing of template and new strand can be displaced by the distance of the repeated sequence,leading to insertions or deletions of bases in the new strand.

　　Spontaneous mutations can originate from lesions in DNA as well as from replication errors. For example, it is possible for purine nucleotides to be depurinated; that is, to lose their base. This results in the formation of an apurinic site, which does not base pair normally and may cause a mutation after the next round of replication. Likewise, pyrimidines can be lost, forming an apyrimidinic site. Other lesions are caused by reactive forms of oxygen such as oxygen free radicals and peroxides produced during aerobic metabolism. For example, guanine can be converted to 8-oxo-7,8-dihydrodeoxyguanine, which often pairs with adenine, rather than cytosine, during replication.

3.7.2　Induced Mutations

　　Any agent that damages DNA, alters its chemistry or in some way interferes with its functioning will probably induce mutations. Mutagens can be conveniently classified according to their mode of action. Three common types of chemical mutagens are base analogues, DNA-modifying agents and intercalating agents. A number of physical agents (e. g. , radiation) are mutagens that damage DNA.

　　Base analogues are structurally similar to normal nitrogenous bases and can be incorporated into the growing polynucleotide chain during replication (Table 3-4). Once in place, these compounds typically exhibit base-pairing properties different from the bases they replace and can eventually cause a stable mutation. A widely used base analogue is 5-bromouracil, an analog of thymine. It undergoes a tautomeric shift from the normal keto form to an enol much more frequently than does a normal base. The enol tautomer forms hydrogen bonds like cytosine, pairing with guanine rather than adenine. The mechanism of action of other base analogues is similar to that of 5-bromouracil.

Table 3-4　Examples of Mutagens

Mutagen	Effects on DNA structure
Chemical	
5-Bromouracil	Base analogue
2-Aminopurine	Base analogue
Ethyl methanesulfonate	Alkylating agent
Hydroxylamine	Hydroxylates cytosine
Nitrogen mustard	Alkylating agent
Nitrous oxide	Deaminates bases
Proflavin	Intercalating agent
Acridine orange	Intercalating agent
Physical	
UV light	Promotes pyrimidine dimer formation
X rays	Cause base deletions, single strand nicks, cross linking and chromosomal breaks

　　There are many DNA-modifying agents-mutagens that change a base's structure and therefore alter its base-pairing specificity. Some of these mutagens are selective; they preferentially react with certain bases and produce a particular kind of DNA damage. For example, methyl-nitrosoguanidine is an alkylating agent that adds methyl groups to guanine, causing it to mispair with thymine. A subsequent round of replication can then result in a GC-AT transition. Hydroxylamine is another example of a DNA-modifying agent. It hydroxylates the nitrogen attached to the number 4 carbon (C-4) of cytosine, causing it to base pair like thymine.

Intercalating agents distort DNA to induce single nucleotide pair insertions and deletions. These mutagens are planar and insert themselves (intercalate) between the stacked bases of the helix. This results in a mutation, possibly through the formation of a loop in DNA. Intercalating agents include acridines such as proflavin and acridine orange.

Many mutagens and indeed many carcinogens, damage bases so severely that hydrogen bonding between base pairs is impaired or prevented and the damaged DNA can no longer act as a template for replication. For instance, ultraviolet (UV) radiation generates cyclobutane dimers, usually thymine dimers, between adjacent pyrimidines. Other examples are ionizing radiation and carcinogens such as the fungal toxin aflatoxin Bl and other benzo(a)pyrene derivatives.

3.7.3　Effects of Mutations

The effects of a mutation can be described at the protein level and in terms of observed phenotypes. In all cases, the impact is readily noticed only if it produces a change in phenotype. In general, the more prevalent form of a gene and its associated phenotype is called the wild type. A mutation from wild type to a mutant form is a forward mutation. The effect of a forward mutation can be reversed by a second mutation that restores the wild-type phenotype. The second mutation can occur at the same site as the original mutation or at another site. When the second mutation is at the same site as the original mutation (e. g. ,the same base pair in a codon), it is called a reversion mutation. Some reversion mutations re-establish the original wild-type sequence. Others create a new codon that codes for the same amino acid. Reversions can also restore the wild-type phenotype by creating a codon that specifies an amino acid that is similar to the amino acid found at that location in the wild-type protein (e. g. ,both amino acids are nonpolar). If the wild-type phenotype is restored by a second mutation at a different site than the original mutation, it is called a suppressor mutation. Suppressor mutations may be within the same gene (intragenic suppressor mutation) or in a different gene (extragenic suppressor mutation). Because point mutations are the most common types of mutations, their effects are the focus here.

3.7.4　Mutations in Protein-Coding Genes

Point mutations in protein-coding genes can affect protein structure in a variety of ways. Point mutations are named according to if and how they change the encoded protein. The most common types of point mutations are silent mutations, missense mutations, nonsense mutations and frameshift mutations.

Silent mutations change the nucleotide sequence of a codon but do not change the amino acid encoded by that codon. This is possible because the genetic code exhibits degeneracy. Therefore when there is more than one codon for a given amino acid, a single base substitution may result in the formation of a new codon for the same amino acid. For example, if the codon CGU were changed to CGC, it would still code for arginine, even though a mutation had occurred. When there is no change in the protein, there is no change in the phenotype of the organism.

Missense mutations involve a single base substitution that changes a codon for one amino acid into a codon for another. For example, the codon GAG, which specifies glutamic acid, could be changed to GUG, which codes for valine. The effects of missense mutations vary. They alter the primary structure of a protein, but the effect of this change may range from complete loss of activity to no change at all. This is because the effect of missense mutations on protein function depends on the type and location of the amino acid substitution. For instance, replacement of a nonpolar amino acid in the protein's interior with a polar amino acid can drastically alter the protein's threedimensional structure and therefore its function. Similarly the replacement of a critical amino acid at the active site of an enzyme often destroys its activity. However, the replacement of one polar amino acid with another at the protein surface may have little or no effect. Such mutations are called neutral mutations. Missense mutations play a very important role in providing new variability to drive evolution because they often are not lethal and therefore remain in the gene pool.

Nonsense mutations convert a sense codon (i. e. , one that codes for an amino acid) to a nonsense codon (i. e. , a stop codon; one that does not code for an amino acid). This causes the early termination of translation and therefore results in a shortened polypeptide. Depending on the location of the mutation in the gene, the phenotype may be more or less severely affected. Most proteins retain some function if they are shortened by only one or two amino acids; complete loss of normal function usually results if the mutation occurs closer to the beginning or middle of the gene.

Frameshift mutations arise from the insertion or deletion of base pairs within the coding region of the gene. Since the code consists of a precise sequence of triplet codons, the addition or deletion of fewer than three base pairs causes the reading frame to be shifted for all subsequent codons downstream. Frameshift mutations usually are very deleterious and yield mutant phenotypes resulting from the synthesis of nonfunctional proteins. In addition, frameshift mutations often produce a stop codon so that the peptide product is shorter as well as different in sequence. Of course, if the frameshift occurs near the end of the gene or if there is a second frameshift shortly downstream from the first that restores the reading frame, the phenotypic effect might not be as drastic. A second, nearby frameshift that restores the proper reading frame is an example of an intragenic suppressor mutation.

Changes in protein structure can alter the phenotype of an organism in many ways. Morphological mutations change the microorganism's colonial or cellular morphology. Lethal mutations, when expressed, result in the death of the microorganism. Because a microbe must be able to grow to be isolated and studied, lethal mutations are recovered only if they are conditional mutations. Conditional mutations are those that are expressed only under certain environmental conditions. For example, a conditional lethal mutation in Escherichia coli might not be expressed under permissive conditions such as low temperature but would be expressed under restrictive conditions such as high temperature. Thus the mutant would grow normally at cooler temperatures but would die at high temperatures.

Biochemical mutations are those causing a change in the biochemistry of the cell. Since these mutations often inactivate a biosynthetic pathway, they frequently eliminate the capacity of the mutant to make an essential molecule such as an amino acid or nucleotide. A strain bearing such a mutation has a conditional phenotype: it is unable to grow on medium lacking that molecule but grows when the molecule is provided. Such mutants are called auxotrophs and they are said to be auxotrophic for the molecule they cannot synthesize. If the wild-type strain from which the mutant arose is a chemoorganotroph able to grow on a minimal medium containing only salts (to supply needed elements such as nitrogen and phosphorus) and a carbon source, it is called a prototroph. Another type of biochemical mutant is the resistance mutant. These mutants have acquired resistance to some pathogen, chemical or antibiotic. Auxotrophic and resistance mutants are quite important in microbial genetics due to the ease of their detection and their relative abundance.

3.7.5   Mutations in Regulatory Sequences

Some of the most interesting and informative mutations studied by microbial geneticists are those that occur in the regulatory sequences responsible for controlling gene expression. Constitutive lactose operon mutants in E. coli are excellent examples. Many of these mutations map in the operator site and produce altered operator sequences that are not recognized by the repressor protein. There fore the operon is continuously transcribed and β-galactosidase is always synthesized. Mutations in promoters also have been identified. If the mutation renders the promoter sequence nonfunctional, the mutant will be unable to synthesize the product, even though the coding region of the structural gene is completely normal. Without a fully functional promoter, RNA polymerase rarely transcribes a gene as well as wild type.

3.7.6 Mutations in tRNA and rRNA Genes

Mutations in tRNA and rRNA alter the phenotype of an organism through disruption of protein synthesis. In fact, these mutants often are initially identified because of their slow growth. On the other hand, a suppressor mutation involving tRNA restores normal (or near normal) growth rates. In these mutations, a base substitution in the anticodon region of a tRNA allows the insertion of the correct amino acid at a mutant codon.

3.8 Detection and Isolation of Mutants

Mutations often arise spontaneously and provide genetic diversity, which enhances survival during changing environmental conditions; thus mutations are of value to microbes. Mutations are also of practical importance to microbial geneticists. Mutant strains have been used to reveal mechanisms of complex processes such as DNA replication, endospore formation and regulation of transcription. They are also useful as selective markers in recombinant DNA procedures.

To study microbial mutants, they must be readily detected, even when they are rare and then efficiently isolated from wild type organisms and other mutants that are not of interest. Microbial geneticists typically increase the likelihood of obtaining mutants by using mutagens to increase the rate of mutation. The rate can increase from the usual one mutant per 10^7 to 10^{11} cells to about one per 10^3 to 10^6 cells. Even at this rate, carefully devised means for detecting or selecting a desired mutation must be used. This section describes some techniques used in mutant detection, selection and isolation.

3.8.1 Mutant Detection

When collecting mutants of a particular organism, the wild type characteristics must be known so that an altered phenotype can be recognized. A suitable detection system for the mutant phenotype also is needed. The use of detection systems is called screening. Screening for mutant phenotypes in haploid organisms is straight forward because the effects of most mutations can be seen immediately. Some screening procedures require only examination of colony morphology. For instance, if albino mutants of a normally pigmented bacterium are being studied, detection simply requires visual observation of colony color.

Other screening methods are more complex. For example, the replica plating technique is used to screen for auxotrophic mutants. It distinguishes between mutants and the wild-type strain based on their ability to grow in the absence of a particular biosynthetic end product. A lysine auxotroph, for instance, grows on lysine-supplemented media but not on a medium lacking an adequate supply of lysine because it cannot synthesize this amino acid. Once a screening method is devised, mutants are collected. However, mutant collection can present practical problems. Consider a search for the albino mutants mentioned previously. If the mutation rate were around one in a million, on average a million or more organisms would have to be tested to find one albino mutant. This probably would require several thousand plates. The task of isolating auxotrophic mutants in this way would be even more taxing with the added labor of replica plating. Thus, if possible, it is more efficient to use a selection system employing some environmental factor to separate mutants from wild-type microorganisms.

3.8.2   Mutant Selection

An effective selection technique uses incubation conditions under which the mutant grows because of properties conferred by the mutation, whereas the wild type does not. Selection methods often involve reversion or suppressor mutations or the development of resistance to an environmental stress. For example, if the intent is to isolate revertants from a lysine auxotroph (Lys-), the approach is quite easy. A large population of lysine auxotrophs is plated on minimal medium lacking lysine, incubated and examined for colony formation. Only cells that have mutated to restore the ability to manufacture lysine will grow on minimal medium. Several million cells can be plated on a single Petri dish, but only the rare revertant cells will grow. Thus many cells can be tested for mutations by scanning a few Petri dishes for growth.

Methods for selecting mutants resistant to a particular environmental stress follow a similar approach. Often wild-type cells are susceptible to virus attack, antibiotic treatment or specific temperatures, so it is possible to grow the microbe in the presence of the stress and look for surviving organisms. Consider the example of a phage-sensitive wild-type bacterium. When it is cultured in medium lacking the virus and then plated on selective medium containing viruses, any colonies that form are resistant to virus attack and very likely are mutants in this regard.

Substrate utilization mutations also can be selected. Many bacteria use only a few primary carbon sources. With such bacteria, it is possible to select mutants by plating a culture on medium containing an alternate carbon source. Any colonies that appear can use the substrate and are probably mutants.

Mutant screening and selection methods are used for purposes other than understanding more about the nature of genes or the biochemistry of a particular microorganism. One very important role of mutant selection and screening techniques is in the study of carcinogens. Next we briefly describe one of the first and perhaps best known of the carcinogen testing systems.

3.8.3   Mutagens and Carcinogens

An increased understanding of the mechanisms of mutation and their role in cancer has stimulated efforts to identify environmental carcinogens-agents that cause cancer. The observation that many carcinogens also are mutagens was the basis for development of the Ames test by Bruce Ames in the 1970s. This test determines if a substance increases the rate of mutation; that is, if it is a mutagen. If the substance is a mutagen, then it is also likely to be carcinogenic if an animal is exposed to it at sufficient levels. Note that the test does not directly test for carcinogenicity. This is because it uses a bacterium as the test organism. Carcinogenicity can only be directly demonstrated with animals. Such testing is extremely expensive and takes much longer to complete than does the Ames test. Thus the Ames test serves as an inexpensive screening procedure to identify chemicals that may be carcinogenic and thus deserve further testing.

The Ames test is a mutational reversion assay employing several "tester" strains of Salmonella enterica serovar Typhimurium. Each tester strain has a different mutation in the histidine biosynthesis operon and therefore is a histidine auxotroph. The bacteria also have mutational alterations of their cell walls that make them more permeable to test substances. To further increase assay sensitivity, the strains are defective in their ability to repair DNA.

In the Ames test, tester strains of S. Typhimurium are plated with the substance being tested and the number of visible colonies that form are determined. To ensure that DNA replication can take place in the presence of the potential mutagen, the bacteria and test substance are mixed in dilute molten top agar to which a trace of histidine has been added. This molten mix is then poured on top of minimal agar plates and incubated for 2–3 days at 3rC. All of the histidine auxotrophs grow for the first few hours in the presence of the test compound until the histidine is depleted. This is necessary because replication is required for the development of a mutation. However, this initial growth does not produce a visible colony. Once the histidine supply is exhausted, only revertants that have mutationally regained the ability to synthesize histidine continue to grow and produce visible colonies. These colonies need only be counted and compared to controls to estimate the relative mutagenicity of the compound; the more colonies, the greater the mutagenicity.

Some chemicals tested may not be mutagenic unless they are transformed into another, more active form. In animals, such transformations occur in the liver. Indeed, many known carcinogens (e. g. , aflatoxins) are not actually carcinogenic until they are modified in the liver by enzymes that function to destroy toxins and other materials that may be circulating in the blood. However, in some cases, these enzymes transform chemicals into more dangerous forms. For this reason, a mammalian liver extract is often added to the molten top agar prior to plating the bacterial cells used in the Ames test. The extract converts potential mutagens into derivatives that readily react with DNA, mimicking the enzymatic transformations that occur in mammals. Carrying out the Ames test with and without the addition of the extract shows which compounds have intrinsic mutagenicity and which need activation after uptake. Despite the use of liver extracts, only about half of all potential carcinogens are detected by the Ames test.

3. 9   DNA Repair

If there is a microbial equivalent of an extreme sport, Deinococcus radiodurans's ability to repair its genome after it has been blasted apart by a high dose of radiation might be a contender. Surprisingly, this ability is primarily related to the resistance of D. radiodurans proteins and the structure of its genome, rather than to its DNA repair mechanisms. Its radiation-resistant proteins are able to begin repairing the genome quickly. Repair is aided by the genome consisting of two chromosomes, each having numerous areas of homology. This allows the DNA fragments to anneal to each other, facilitating the piecing together of the shattered genome. Other than this, D. radiodurans uses pretty much the same DNA repair mechanisms as other organisms. Obviously mutations can have disastrous effects. Therefore it is imperative that a microorganism be able to repair changes. Microbes have numerous repair mechanisms. Repair in *E. coli* is best understood and is briefly described in this section.

3. 9. 1   Proofreading: The First Line of Defense

Replicative DNA polymerases sometimes insert the incorrect nucleotide during DNA replication. However, these DNA polymerases have the ability to evaluate the hydrogen bonds formed between the newly added nucleotide and the template nucleotide and correct any errors immediately; that is, before the next nucleotide is added. This ability is called proofreading. When a DNA polymerase detects that a mistake has been made, it backs up, removing the incorrect nucleotide with its 3′ to 5′ exonuclease activity. It then restarts DNA replication, this time inserting the correct nucleotide. Proofreading is very efficient, but it does not always correct errors in replication. Furthermore, it is not useful for correcting induced mutations. *E. coli* uses other repair mechanisms to help ensure the stability of its genome.

3.9.2 Mismatch Repair

When proofreading by replicative DNA polymerases fails, mismatched bases are usually detected and repaired by the mismatch repair system. In *E. coli* the enzyme MutS scans the newly replicated DNA for mismatched pairs. Another enzyme, MutH, removes a stretch of newly synthesized DNA around the mismatch. A DNA polymerase then replaces the excised nucleotides and the resulting nick is sealed by DNA ligase. The MutS protein slides along the DNA until it finds a mismatch. Mutl binds MutS and the MutS/MutL complex binds to MutH, which is already bound to a hemimethylated sequence.

Successful mismatch repair depends on the ability of enzymes to distinguish between old and newly replicated DNA strands. This distinction is possible because newly replicated DNA strands lack methyl groups on their bases, whereas older DNA has methyl groups on the bases of both strands. DNA methylation is catalyzed by DNA methyltransferases and results in three different products: N6-methyladenine, 5-methylcytosine and N4-methylcytosine. After strand synthesis, the *E. coli* DNA adenine methyltransferase (DAM) methylates adenine bases in GATC sequences to form N6-methyladenine. For a short time after the replication fork has passed, the new strand lacks methyl groups while the template strand is methylated. In other words, the DNA is temporarily hemimethylated. The repair system cuts out the mismatch from the unmethylated strand.

3.9.3 Excision Repair

Excision repair corrects damage that causes distortions in the double helix. Two types of excision repair systems have been described: nucleotide excision repair and base excision repair. They both use the same approach to repair: Remove the damaged portion of a DNA strand and use the intact complementary strand as the template for synthesis of new DNA. They are distinguished by the enzymes used to correct DNA damage.

In nucleotide excision repair, an E. coli enzyme called UvrABC endonuclease removes damaged nucleotides and a few nucleotides on either side of the lesion. The resulting singlestranded gap is filled by DNA polymerase I and DNA ligase joins the fragments. This system can remove thymine dimers and repair almost any other injury that produces a detectable distortion in DNA.

Base excision repair employs enzymes called DNA glycosylases. These enzymes remove damaged or unnatural bases yielding apurinic or apyrimidinic (AP) sites. Enzymes called AP endonucleases recognize the damaged DNA and nick the backbone at the AP site. DNA polymerase I removes the damaged region, using its $5'$ to $3'$ exonuclease activity. It then fills in the gap and DNA ligase joins the DNA fragments.

3.9.4 Direct Repair

Thymine dimers and alkylated bases often are corrected by direct repair. For instance, photoreactivation repairs thymine dimers by splitting them apart with the help of visible light. This photochemical reaction is catalyzed by the enzyme photolyase. Methyl and some other alkyl groups that have been added to guanine can be removed with the help of an enzyme known as alkyl transferase or methylguanine methyltransferase. Thus damage to guanine from mutagens such as methyl-nitrosoguanidine can be repaired directly.

3.9.5 Recombinational Repair

Recombinational repair corrects damaged DNA in which both bases of a pair are missing or damaged or where there is a gap opposite a lesion. In this type of repair, a protein called RecA cuts a piece of template DNA from a sister molecule and puts it into the gap or uses it to replace a damaged strand. Although bacterial cells are haploid, another copy of the damaged segment often is available because either it has recently been replicated or the cell is growing rapidly and has more than one copy of its chromosome. Once the template is in place, the remaining damage can be corrected by another repair system.

3.9.6 SOS Response

Despite having multiple repair systems, sometimes the damage to an organism's DNA is so great that the normal repair mechanisms just described cannot repair all the damage. As a result, DNA synthesis stops completely. In such situations, a global control network called the SOS response is activated. In this response, over 40 genes are activated when a transcriptional repressor called LexA is destroyed. LexA negatively controls these genes and once it is destroyed, they are transcribed and the SOS response ensues.

The SOS response, like recombinational repair, depends on the activity of RecA. RecA binds to single- or double-stranded DNA breaks and gaps generated by cessation of DNA synthesis. RecA binding initiates recombinational repair. Simultaneously RecA takes on co protease function. It interacts with LexA, causing LexA to destroy itself (autoproteolysis). Destruction of LexA increases transcription of genes for excision repair and recombinational repair, in particular.

The first genes transcribed in the SOS response are those that encode the Uvr proteins needed for nucleotide excision repair. Then expression of genes involved in recombinational repair is further increased. To give the cell time to repair its DNA, the protein SfiA is produced; SfiA blocks cell division. Finally, if the DNA has not been fully repaired after about 40 minutes, a process called translesion DNA synthesis is triggered. In this process, DNA polymerase Ⅳ (also known as DinB; Din is short for damage inducible) and DNA polymerase Ⅴ (UmuCD; Umu is short for UV mutagenesis) synthesize DNA across gaps and other lesions (e. g. , thymine dimers) that had stopped DNA polymerase Ⅲ. However, because an intact template does not exist, these DNA polymerases often insert incorrect bases. Furthermore, they lack proofreading activity. Therefore even though DNA synthesis continues, it is highly error prone and results in the generation of numerous mutations.

The SOS response is so named because it is made in a life-or-death situation. The response increases the likelihood that some cells will survive by allowing DNA synthesis to continue. For the cell, the risk of dying because of failure to replicate DNA is greater than the risk posed by the mutations generated by this error-prone process.

Chapter 4

Evolutionary Microbiology and Microbial Diversity

4.1 Evolutionary Microbiology

The age of our planet is estimated to be about 4.6 billion years. The microbial cells were found in fossil remains from Stromatolites and Sedimentary rock that are approximately 3.5 – 3.8 billion years old (Figure 4 – 1) and in a carbonaceous meteorite, *Gloeodiniopsis*, from the Sakta Formation in the Ural Mountains that are approximately 1.5 billion years old. The fossil remains of a carbonaceous shale, *Palaeolyngbya*, from the Lakhanda Formation in the eastern Siberia region are about 950 million years old. Stromatolites are layered rocks, often domed, formed by the incorporation of mineral deposits into a microbial mat (Figure 4–2). Modern stromatolites are consist of cyanobacteria; it is estimated that at least some of the layered rock fossils were also formed in this way, indicating that prokaryotes appeared shortly after the earth cooled. The earliest bacteria may be anaerobic. Cyanobacteria and oxygen producing photosynthesis probably occurred between 2.5 billion to 3 billion years or earlier. As oxygen became richer, the microbial diversity increased greatly.

Left: Fossils of about 3.5 billion years from the ice-cut section of the ancient vein top in western Australia; Right: Gloeodiniopsis, about 1.5 billion years old, from the carbonaceous chert from the Sakta Formation in the southern Ural Mountains.

From Sha Yu Wan in Western Australia, modern stromatolites are spread out or layered rocks, made from the combination between calcium sulphate, calcium carbonate and other minerals with microbial mats. This microbial mat consists of cyanobacteria and other microorganisms.

In 1875, the German biologist Ferdinand J. Cohn (1828—1898) realized that bacteria can be classified by evolution when he first found bacteriology. However, due to the tiny structure of bacteria, it's impossible to study bacterial evolutionary in the way of studying living fossils in the Pacific era. Therefore, how to scientifically classify bacteria has always been a major challenge for microbiologists.

At the beginning of the 20th century, under the impetus of the American bacteriologist David Hendricks Bergey (1860—1937), a committee was established to develop a classification plan for all known bacteria. And, through this existing classification plan, all bacteria can be identified according to different criteria, such as Gram staining, morphology, colony and biochemical reactions. Bergey's Manual of Systematic Bacteriology was first published in 1923. The initial classification of bacteria was mainly based on the degree of similarity and has nothing to do with biological evolution. However, it cannot be denied that the classification method proposed by Bergey has made a great contribution to the development of bacteriology.

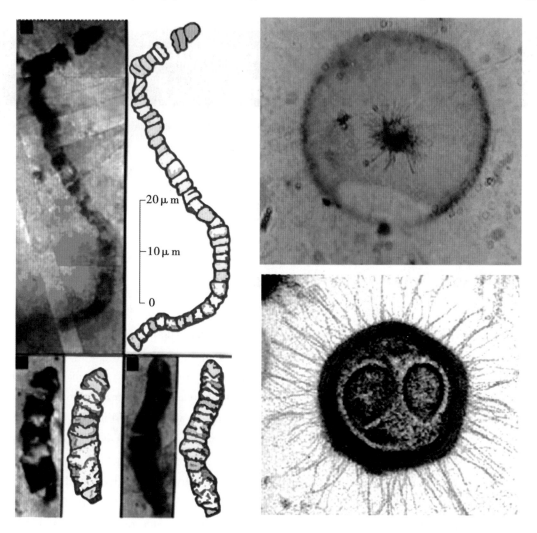

Figure 4-1　Microbial fossils

At the beginning of the 20th century, under the impetus of the American bacteriologist David Hendricks Bergey (1860—1937), a committee was established to develop a classification plan for all known bacteria. And, through this existing classification plan, all bacteria can be identified according to different criteria, such as Gram staining, morphology, colony and biochemical reactions. Bergey's Manual of Systematic Bacteriology was first published in 1923. The initial classification of bacteria was mainly based on the degree of similarity and has nothing to do with biological evolution. However, it cannot be denied that the classification method proposed by Bergey has made a great contribution to the development of bacteriology.

For much of the 20th century, prokaryotes were regarded as a single group of organisms and classified based on their biochemistry, morphology and metabolism. In a highly influential 1962 paper, Roger Stanier and C. B. van Niel first established the division of cellular organization into prokaryotes and eukaryotes, defining prokaryotes as those organisms lacking a cell nucleus. Adapted from Édouard Chatton's generalization, Stanier and Van Niel's concept was quickly accepted as the most important distinction among organisms; yet they were nevertheless skeptical of microbiologists' attempts to construct a natural phylogenetic classification of bacteria. However, it became generally assumed that all life shared a common prokaryotic ancestor.

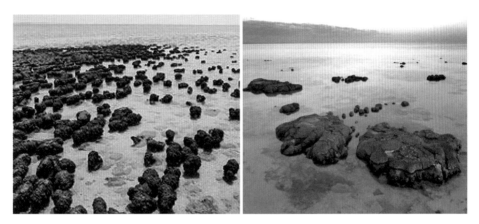

Figure 4-2   Stromatolites

Since the 1960s, the rapid development of molecular genetics and molecular biological technology has led bacterial taxonomy to enter an era of molecular biology. In the late 1960s, the American biologist and biophysicist, Carl Richard Woese (1928—2012), began to classify organisms using the oligonucleotide cataloging method of genetic material. He compared the signature sequences in ribosomal RNAs from various types of biological cells. It is believed that 16S rRNA is the most appropriate biochemical evolution clock. In 1977, Carl R. Woese and George E. Fox discovered the third form of life, Archaea, through analyzing the genetic sequence. Through the study of archaea, Woese further established a three-domain life theory and for the first time established a phylogenetic tree of all cellular organisms including bacteria based on evolutionary relationships. His three-domain system, based on phylogenetic relationships rather than obvious morphological similarities, divided life into 23 main divisions, incorporated within three domains: Bacteria, Archaea and Eucarya(Figure 4-3).

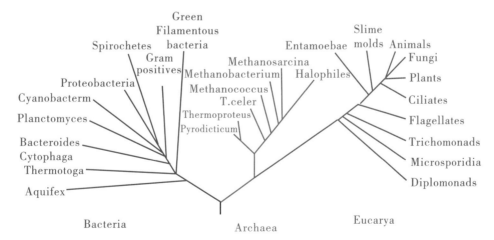

Figure 4-3   Phylogenetic tree based on Woese and Fox rRNA analysis

The vertical line at bottom represents the last universal common ancestor (LUCA).

As shown in the Figure, Archaea and Bacteria separate first and then Eucarya occurs. These three basic groups become domains and they are placed above the level of phylums and kingdoms (traditional kingdoms were distributed among these three domains). There are significant differences among domains. Eucanya, which mainly contains glyceryl diester lipid membrane and eukaryotic rRNAs, belongs to the eukaryotic domain. Organisms with diacyldiacyl glycerols predominantly lipid membranes and bacterial rRNAs belong to bacterial domains. A prokaryotic organism with isoprenoid diglyceride lipids in the bacertial membrane and Archaear RNA constitutes the third domain, the archaeal domain.

It seems that modern eukaryotic cells originated in prokaryotes 1.4 billion years ago. There are considerable speculations about how eukaryotes have developed from prokaryotic ancestors. Two hypotheses have been proposed. According to the first hypothesis, nuclei, mitochondria and chloroplasts are double-layer membrane structures formed from the invagination of the plasma membrane, which can further develop and differentiate. The similarity among chloroplasts, mitochondria and modern bacteria is due to the preservation of slowly-changing primitive prokaryotic characteristics of organelles; according to the more popular endosymbiotic hypothesis, the nucleus is initially formed in proto eukaryotic cells. The ancestors of eukaryotic cells may be formed by the fusion of ancient bacteria and archaea. It is possible that a gram-negative eubacterial host cell has lost its cell wall and engulfed archaea to form a symbiotic relationship. The archaea then lost its cell wall and plasma membrane and membrane folds formed in host eubacteria. Finally host genome was transferred to the original archaea to form nucleus and endoplasmic reticulum. The eubacteria and archaeal genes mgiht be lost when the eukaryotic genome was formed. It is worth emphasizing that many people believe that the genetic relationship between archaea and eukaryotes are closer than what suggested by the procedure of this hypothesis. They believe that eukaryotes differentiate directly from archaea and then form a nucleus that may come from the Golgi apparatus.

The discovery of an endosym biosiscyano bacteria supports the endosymbiotic hypothesis hypothesis. Cyanobacteria colonize and serve as the chloroplast of the bi-flagella protozoa β. This endosymbiont becomes a cyanelle similar to the detailed structure and being surrounded by a peptidoglycan layer of blue-green algae in the photosynthesis pigment system. Unlike blue-green algae, it lacks the lipopolysaccharide membrane of gram-negative bacteria. The cyanelle may be a recently-established endosymbiont and is evolving into a chloroplast. Further support comes from the rRNA tree, which determines the position of the chloroplast RNA in the blue-green algae.

Both hypotheses have supporters and perhaps new data will help answer this question. However, these hypotheses focus on the process that occurred in the distant past and cannot be observed directly. Therefore, a consensus that is completely consistent on this issue may never be reached.

4.2   Taxonomy of Microorganism

4.2.1   Classification Levels

Living organisms have puzzling diversity, so people expect to divide them into different groups based on their similarities among each other. Taxonomy is the science of naming and classifying organisms. In the widest sense, it consists of three separate but related parts: classification, nomenclature and identification. Classification classifies organisms as taxa based on their similarity or evolutionary relationship. Nomenclature is a branch of taxonomy that gives taxonomic units a name that matches the published rules. Identification is a practical aspect of taxonomy and is the process of determining whether a particular isolate belongs to a recognized taxon.

Taxonomy is important because: firstly, it allows people to organize a lot of knowledge about living things, because all members of a particular group have many common characteristics. In some sense, this provides a shortcut for information search in a huge file, like the flexible library directory. The finer the classification, the more informative and useful the system is. Secondly, taxonomy allows us to speculate and image in the further research based on the knowledge of similar organisms. If the relevant organisms have certain characteristics, the microorganisms under study may also have the same characteristics. Thirdly, taxonomy divides precisely named microbes into meaningful, useful taxa so microbiologists can use them for effective work and communication. Fourthly, in practical applications, taxonomy is necessary to the accurate identification of microorganisms.

The most commonly used levels (from high to low) in prokaryotic taxonomy include phylum, class order, family, genus and species. The nomenclature of each level of microbiota contains the suffix of that level (Table 4−1). Microbiologists often use informal names instead of official ones. For example, purple bacteria, spirochetes, methane oxidizing bacteria, reducing sulfur bacteria and lactic acid bacteria.

Table 4−1   classification levels and a sample

Level	Sample
Domain	Bacteria
Phylum	Proteobacteria
Class	ā-Proteobacteria
Order	Enterobacteriales
Family	Enterobacteriaceae
Genus	Shigella
Species	S. dysenteriae

The basic taxonomic group in microbial classification is species. Taxonomists who are working on higher organisms define the concept of species differently from microbiologists. Species of higher organisms are a group of natural populations reproducing by mating or potential hybrids that are separated from other groups by breeding. This is a good definition for organisms that can reproduce sexually, but not for microorganisms that do not reproduce sexually. The procaryotic species are defined by differences in phenotype and genotype. A procaryotic species is a collection of strains. These strains have many common stable characteristics and are significantly different from other strains. This definition is very subjective and can be interpreted in many ways. Some bacterial taxonomists propose a more precise definition. One species is a collection of strains having a similar G+C composition and 70% or greater similarity in DNA hybridization experiments. The ideal species should be distinguishable from other similar species on the phenotype. A strain is a biological group that is at least distinguishable from other populations in a particular taxonomy and is considered to be a single or pure culture microorganism. However, there are few differences among in species strains. Biovars are a variety of bacterial organisms that are biochemically or physiologically different. Morphovars are morphologically distinct and serovars have unique antigenic properties. A strain within a species is classified as a type strain. It is usually the strain that was first studied and its characteristics are better understood than other strains. However, it is not necessarily the most representative strain. The species specific strain is called a model species. It is a named model or has a species name. When the classification is rearranged, a named model is a marker guaranteeing the stability of names. For example, the model species must be within the genus of its naming pattern and only those strains that are quite similar to the model strain or model species are included in this species. Each species belongs to a genus, the next level of classification. A genus is a distinct group of one or more species that is significantly different from other genera. In fact, arranging species into one genus is quite subjective and taxonomists may not agree with the composition of the genus.

If an organism is assigned to another genus due to new information, the genus name can be changed. For example, according to rRNA analysis and other characteristics, *Streptococcus* has been divided into two new genera, *Enterococcus* and *Lactococcus*, so *Streptococcus faecalis* is now *Enterococcus faecalis*. Bacterial names are often abbreviated. At this time, the genus name is represented by a capital letter, such as *E. coli*. The list of approved bacterial names was published in the International Journal of Systems Science in 1980 and new valid names are regularly published. The Berger's System Bacteriology Handbook contains a contemporary, recognized prokaryotic taxonomy system.

4.2.2 Classification Systems

The classification system is established by two methods: organizing organisms together to form phenotypic systems based on overall similarity or establishing phylogenetic systems based on possible evolutionary relationships.

4.2.2.1 Phenetic Classification

Many taxonomists insist that the most natural classification is the classification with the largest amount of information or expected value. A good classification should order the biological diversity and define the morphological structure. For example, if certain microorganisms have both motility and flagella, the flagella may play a role in at least some types of movements. When considering in this way, the most natural classification system may be the phenetic system, which system based on the similarity of phenotypic characteristics between organisms. Although studies in phenotypic characteristics can show possible evolutionary relationships, they are not necessarily dependent on phylogenetic analysis. They compare many characteristics but do not consider that some features are more important than others in phylogeny, that is, non-significant characteristics are also included in analyzing statistical similarity. Obviously, the best characterization classification is the classification established by comparing as many traits as possible, classifying organisms with many common characteristics in a single taxa or taxon.

4.2.2.2 Numerical Taxonomy

The development of computers made quantitative methods possible, called numerical taxonomy. Peter H. A. Sneath and Robert Sokal defined numerical taxonomy as a method to group each taxonomic unit based on their characteristic conditions. Biological characteristics are converted into a table suitable for numerical analysis and then compared using computers. The final classification is based on the general similarity determined by the comparison of many characteristics, giving each characteristic equal importance. Because of the large number of calculations, this method is not feasible in the absence of a computer. This process first determines if there are characteristics in the taxa of the organism being studied. A feature is usually defined as an attribute that can be made into a separate table. In order to be precise and credible, many characteristics should be compared, at least 50, more appropriate hundreds and data of many different morphological, biochemical and physiological characteristics are preferably included.

After analyzing characteristics, the correlation coefficient is calculated for each pair of organisms in this taxon and this correlation coefficient can be used to measure the consistency of the characteristics from the two organisms. Simple matching coefficient is the most commonly used coefficient in bacteriology and it is the characteristic ratio, a distribution characteristic without considering if there is such attribute. The Jaccard coefficient is sometimes calculated without characteristics that does not exist in both organisms.

Numerical classification analysis results are often summarized in the dendrogram. In traditional classification terms, similarities between groups are used to define species, genus, etc. Sometimes groups are simply called phenons with a number indicating their similarity levels ahead (eg, a 70-phenons is a phenons with a similarity of 70% or greater between components). Phenones with 80% similarity are often equivalent to species.

It has been demonstrated that numerical classification is a powerful tool for microbial classification. Although it is only confirming existing classification plans, it sometimes still requires approved classifications. The numerical taxonomy can also be used to compare sequences of large molecules such as RNA and proteins.

4.2.2.3　Phylogenetic Classification

With the publication of the book Origin of Species by British naturalist Charles Robert Darwin (1809—1882) in 1859, biologists began to attempt to establish phylogenetic classification systems. These systems are based on evolutionary relationships rather than universal similarity [the term phylogeny (Greek phylon, race or variety, genesis, generation or origin) refers to the evolutionary development of a species]. Due to the lack of good fossil records, it is difficult to test in prokaryotes and other microorganisms, while direct comparison of genetic material and gene products such as RNA and proteins overcome many of these problems.

4.2.3　Major Characteristics Used in Taxonomy

Many characteristics are used for microbial classification and identification. These characteristics can be divided into two categories: classical characteristics and molecular characteristics.

4.2.3.1　Classical Characteristics

The classic method of taxonomy is the classification using morphological, physiological, biochemical and ecological and genetic characteristics. These characteristics have been used in microbial classification for many years. In routine identification, they are very useful and can provide phylogenetic information at the same time.

It is easy to observe and analyze morphology, especially in eukaryotic microorganisms and more complex prokaryotes. In addition, comparing morphology is also valuable because morphological characteristics are determined by the expression of many genes, which are generally genetically stable. Under normal circumstances (at least in prokaryotes), the morphology does not change significantly under environmental changes. Therefore, morphological similarity is often closely related to phylogenetic relationships.

Many different morphological characteristics are used for microbial classification and identification. Although fiber optics have always been a very important tool, a resolution of about 0. 2 μm has limited its use for viewing smaller microbes and structures. Transmission and scanning electron microscopy have greatly assisted the study of all microbial groups because of their higher resolution(Table 4−2).

Table 4-2   Some morphological characteristics used in classification and identification

Characteristics	Microbial groups
Cell shape	All major groups *
Cell size	All major groups
Colony morphology	All major groups
Ultrastructural characteristics	All major groups
Dyeing behavior	Bacteria, some fungus
Cilia and flagella	All major groups
Moving mechanism	Gliding bacteria, Spirochaeta
Endospore shape and position	Endospore bacteria
Spore shape and position	Bacteria, algae, fungus
Cell contents	All major groups
Color	All major groups

* At least used in the classification and identification of some bacteria, algae, fungus and protozoa.

Physiological and metabolic characteristics are directly related to the nature and activity of microbial enzymes and transporters, so they are very useful. Since proteins are the products of genes, analyzing these features provides indirect comparisons between microbial genomes. Most important characteristics associated with physiological and metabolic characteristics in microbial classification include: carbon and nitrogen sources, cell wall composition, energy sources, fermentation products, general nutrient types, optimal growth temperature and range, irradiance, energy conversion mechanisms, motility, permeation resistance, relationship with oxygen, optimum pH and growth range, photosynthetic pigments, salt requirement and tolerance, formation of secondary metabolites, sensitivity to metabolic inhibitors and antibiotics, storage inclusions, etc.

Ecological characteristics in nature influence the relationship between microorganisms and their environment. Because even microorganisms that are closely related to each other can be distinguished based on their ecological characteristics, these characteristics are useful in classification. Microorganisms living in different parts of the human body are different among each other and are also different from those living in freshwater, land and marine environments. Many characteristics such as life cycle types; natural symbiotic relationships; pathogenic capacity to specific hosts; habitat parameters such as temperature, pH, oxygen and osmotic concentration requirements, are also considered to be physiological characteristics.

Because most eukaryotes can reproduce sexually, genetic analysis in these taxa is quite useful. Although prokaryotes cannot reproduce sexually, it is sometimes useful to classify them by studying the chromosomal gene exchange occurred in transformation and integration.

Transformation can occur between different species of prokaryotes, but very rarely among genera. The occurrence of transformation between the two strains indicates that they are close related because no transformation can occur unless the bacterial genomes are quite similar. Transformation have been performed in several genera; Bacillus, Micrococcus, Haemophilus, Rhizobium and other genera. Although transformation is ineffective, the results of its transformation are sometimes difficult to interpret because transformation failures can be caused by other factors other than the major differences in DNA sequence.

Combined studies also provide useful data for classification, especially for gut bacteria. For example, Escherichelloa can be conjugated with Salmonella and Shigella but not with Proteus and Enterobacter. Analysis with other data suggests that relationship among the first three genera are closer than that between Proteus and Enterobacter.

Plasmids are undoubtedly important in taxonomy because most bacteria have plasmids. Many plasmids carry genes that encode phenotypic morphology. If the plasmid carries a gene encoding a major characteristic in the classification plan, the plasmid will have an important effect on the classification, however, it is best to classify it based on many characteristics. When classifying according to very few characteristics, if some of which are encoded by plasmid genes, erroneous results may be obtained. For example, hydrogen sulphide production and lactose fermentation are very important characteristics in gut bacterial classification. The genes encoding those characteristics can be either on the plasmid or on the bacterial chromosome. Care must be taken to avoid erroneous results caused by plasmid-carrying characteristics.

4.2.3.2   Molecular Characteristics

Some of the most powerful methods of taxonomy are through the study of proteins and nucleic acids. Because these substances are either direct gene products or their own, the comparison of proteins and nucleic acids will release important information about the true relevance. These new methods become more important in prokaryotic taxonomy.

The amino acid sequence of a protein is a direct reflection of the mRNA sequence, therefore, it is closely related to the structure of its coding gene. Because of this reason, comparing proteins from different microorganisms are very taxonomically useful. There are several ways to compare proteins. The most straightforward method is to sequence the amino acid of proteins with the same function. Protein sequences with different functions usually evolve at different rates; some sequences evolve quite rapidly, while others are very stable. However, if the protein sequences with the same function are similar, the organisms that possess them may be closely related. The protein sequences of cytochromes and other electron transport proteins, histones, heat shock proteins, transcription and translation proteins and various metabolic enzymes have been used in taxonomic studies. Because protein sequencing is slow and expensive, many indirect methods are often used in comparing proteins. The electrophoretic mobility of proteins is useful when studying phylogenetic relationships at both species and subspecies levels. Antibodies can be used to recognize very similar proteins and immunological techniques have been used to compare proteins from different microorganisms.

The physical, dynamic and regulatory properties of enzymes have been used for taxonomic studies. Because the enzyme behavior reflects the amino acid sequence, this method is useful when studying certain microbial groups. A specific group model of regulation has been found.

Microbe genomes can be directly compared and there are many ways to estimate the similarity of classification. The first technique may be the simplest and only measures DNA base composition. In double-stranded DNA, the $(G+C)/(A+T)$ ratio or $G+C$ content reflects the base sequence and changes with the base as follows:

The $G+C$ content of many microorganisms has been determined (Table 4-3). The $G+C$ content of eukaryotic and prokaryotic microorganisms varies greatly; Prokaryotic $G+C$ content is the most variable, ranging from approximately 25% to 80%. In addition to a wide range of variation, the $G+C$ content of a particular strain is stable. If the $G+C$ content of the two microorganisms differs by more than about 10%, their genomes have a greater difference in base sequence. On the other hand, there is no guarantee that organisms with very similar $G+C$ content will have similar DNA base sequences because DNA with very different base sequences can still have the same components with AT and GC base pairs. Only when the two microbial phenotypes are similar, it can be considered that their similar $G+C$ content indicates their close phylogenetic relationship.

Table 4-3   G+C contents of some bacterium

Bacteria	G+C(%)
Actinomyces	59–73
Bacillus	32–62
Bacteroides	28–61
Bdellovibrio	33–52
Caulobacter	63–67
Chlamydia	41–44
Fusiformis	21–54
Cellulus	33–42
Deinococcus	62–70
Escherichia	48–52
Micrococcus	64–75
Mycoplasma	23–40
Rickettsia	29–33
Salmonella	50–53
Spirillum	38
Staphylococcus	30–38
Spirochaeta	51–65

At least two aspects of G+C content data are useful in taxonomy. Firstly, in conjunction with other data, they can determine a general classification plan. If the biological G+C content in the same taxon differs too far, this taxon may need to be subdivided. Secondly, G+C content is useful in identifying bacterial genera, because even if the G+C content can vary greatly between genera, the content change within the same genus is often less than 10%. For example, the G+C content of *Staphylococcus* is between 30% and 38%, while the G+C content of Micrococcus DNA is between 64% and 75%. There are still many other characteristics of the two gram-positive cocci alike.

Comparing genomic similarities using nucleic acid hybridization is more directly. If the cooled single-stranded DNA mixture formed by heating the double strands can recombine with the complementary strand to form a double-stranded DNA at an incubation temperature of about 25 ℃ below *Tm*, the non-complementary chain will remain as single-stranded. Because the incompletely similar strain will form relatively stable double-stranded DNA hybrids at lower temperatures. It allows more single-stranded DNA to hybridize at 30–50 ℃ below Tm; only a nearly identical strain can hybridize at 10–15 ℃ below *Tm*.

In the most widely used hybridization technique, a nitrocellulose membrane with a non-radioactive DNA strand is incubated with a ^{32}P, ^{3}H or ^{14}C radiolabeled single-stranded DNA fragment at a suitable temperature. The radioactive fragment is bound to the membrane-bound single-stranded DNA. After hybridization, the membrane is rinsed to remove unhybridized single-stranded DNA and its radioactivity is measured. The amount of membrane bound radioactivity reflects the total amount of hybridization and therefore also reflects the similarity of the DNA sequence. The degree of similarity or homology is expressed as the comparison between the percentage of experimental DNA radioactivity on the membrane and the percentage of bound homologous DNA radioactivity under the same conditions. If the two strains are at least 70% related in DNA under optimum hybridization conditions and the difference of Tm value is less than 5%, they are considered to be members of the same species.

If DNA molecules differ greatly in sequence, they will not form stable, detectable hybrids, so DNA-DNA hybridization is only used to study closely related microorganisms. The relatively distant organisms are compared by DNA-RNA hybridization experiments using radioactive ribosomes or transfer RNA as materials because the rRNA and tRNA genes represent only a small part of the total DNA genome and do not evolve rapidly as most other microbial genes. This technique is similar to the technique used for DNA-DNA hybridization; membrane bound DNA is incubated with radioactive rRNA, rinsed and counted. A more accurate method of determining homology is to determine the temperature required to dissociate and remove half of the radioactive rRNA from the membrane; the higher the temperature is, the stronger the rRNA-DNA complex is and the more similar the sequences are.

In addition to G+C content assays and nucleic acid hybridization studies, genomic structure can be directly compared by sequencing DNA and RNA. Now there are techniques for rapid determination of DNA and RNA sequences; RNA sequences have so far been more widely used in microbial taxonomy.

More attention has been paid to the 5S and 16S rRNA sequences, which are isolated from the 50S and 30S subunits of prokaryotic ribosomes, respectively. These rRNAs are ideal materials for studying the evolution and interrelation of microorganisms because they are found to be essential to one of the major organelles of all microorganisms and their function in all ribosomes is the same. Therefore, their structure changes very slowly with time, probably because of their constant and necessary functions. Because rRNA contains variable and stable sequences, all closely related and very distant microorganisms can be compared. This is an important advantage. Just a small change in sequence can be used to study distantly related organisms.

The whole genome of some bacterial prokaryotes has been recently sequenced. Direct comparison of whole genome sequences in prokaryotes will undoubtedly be important.

4.3　Microbial Diversity

4.3.1　Biodiversity of Microorganisms

Biodiversity is a very important concept in ecology. It mainly refers to the overall diversity and variability of plants, animals, microbes and their systems. It consists of three levels: genetic diversity, species diversity and ecosystem diversity.

Species diversity is the core of biodiversity. It not only reflects the complex relationships between organisms and the environment, but also reflects the richness of biological resources. Species are the basic unit of taxonomy. In taxonomy, the identification of a species must take into account morphological, geographic and genetic characteristics. In other words, a species must meet the following requirements: ①It has a relatively stable and consistent morphological characteristic to distinguish with other species; ②It lives in a certain space in the form of population, occupies a certain geographical distribution area, survives and reproduces offspring in this region; ③Each species has a specific genetic gene database. Different individuals in the same species can be paired and reproduce offspring. There is reproductive isolation between different species of individuals; they cannot breed or produce progeny with reproductive ability after hybridization.

Species diversity refers to the abundance of animals, plants and microorganisms on the earth. Species diversity includes two aspects. One is the degree of species richness in a certain area, which can be called regional species diversity. The other is the degree of uniformity of species distribution in ecology, which can be called ecological diversity or community. Species diversity is an objective indicator to measure the abundance of biological resources in a certain area.

When describing the richness of the biodiversity in a county or area, the most commonly used indicator is the regional species diversity. There are three indicators for the measurement of regional species diversity: ①the total number of species, such as the number of species in a specific group within a specific area; ②the density of species which is the number of species in a specific group within a unit area; ③the percentage of endemic species referring as the proportion of the endemic species in a specific group in a given area to the total number of species in this area.

Genetic diversity is an important part of the biodiversity. The broad sense of genetic diversity refers to the sum of various genetic information carried by living things on earth. This genetic information is stored in the genes of individual organisms. Each species or individual organism holds a large number of genetic genes and, therefore, can be considered as a gene pool. The more abundant genes a species contains, the stronger adaptation to the environment it has. The diversity of genes is the basis for the evolution of life and the species differentiation.

The narrow sense of genetic diversity mainly refers to the changes of genes within biological species, including the genetic variation among different populations within the species and within the same population. In addition, genetic diversity can be reflected on multiple levels, such as molecular, cellular and individual levels. In nature, for the majority of sexually reproductive species, individuals within the population usually do not have exactly the same genotype. The population consists of these individuals with different genetic structures.

In the long-term evolution of organisms, genetic changes (or mutations) are the root of genetic diversity. There are two main types of mutations in genetic material: changes in the number and structure of chromosomes and changes in nucleotides within the gene locus. The former is called chromosome aberration and the latter is called gene mutation (or point mutation). In addition, genetic recombination can also lead to genetic variations in organisms.

The ecosystem is a natural complex consisting of various living things and their surrounding environment. All species are a part of the ecosystem. In the ecosystem, species not only depend on each other, but also restrict each other. Organisms also interact with various environmental factors. The ecosystem is mainly composed of producers, consumers and disintegrators. The function of the ecosystem is to circulate the various chemical elements on earth and maintain the normal flow of energy among the various components. The diversity of ecosystems mainly refers to the diversity of the composition and function of the ecosystem on the earth and the diversity of various ecological processes, including the diversity of habitats, biological communities, ecological processes and many other aspects. Among them, habitat diversity is the basis for the formation of ecosystem diversity. The diversity of biomes can reflect the diversity of ecosystem types.

Microbial diversity refers to the diversity of life forms of microorganisms, including the types of physiological metabolism, metabolites, genetic genes and ecological diversity. In modern biology, the microbiological community can be classified it into two categories, cellular and non-cellular organisms, depending on the cell structure (Figure 4-4). Cellular organisms can be divided into prokaryotes and eukaryotes according to the nuclear structure. The specific classifications are as follows:

In the study of microbial diversity, the basis for the classification of microorganisms emphasizes that the names of prokaryotes are continuously updated. The names of families and genera in the new system are established fairly well and stable (at least before new discoveries) ; in fact, the names of many families and genera in Bergey's Catalog of Systematic Bacteriology have not changed. Recently, many people think that Bergey's Catalog of Systematic Bacteriology is formal in some sense. The New Recommended names for the Effective Catalog in List of Approved Bacterial Names and International Journal of Systematic Bacteriology give a similar impression. However, it needs to be clarified that Bergey's Catalog of Systematic Bacteriology is not formal, but is the most consistent opinion at that time. Although people have invested great effort to obtain a viewpoint which is accep table to everyone, there is always a lack of data or confusion, resulting in different opinions and unstable classification. When Bergey's Catalog of Systematic Bacteriology was denied as a formal classification, many microbiologists might think that the building would overturn. In fact, many fields in taxonomy have been well established. Like all sciences, taxonomy still carries some subjective judgments and opinions. Before new information is obtained, different biologists can hold different opinions and shouldn't be forced to agree with any Formally Classify. It must be remembered that we still only know a small portion of bacterial species in nature. Technological advances also bring light to the relationship among bacteria. We therefore expect that the boundaries between populations will be reclassified in the future and many changes will occur in the coming decades, particularly in molecular biology.

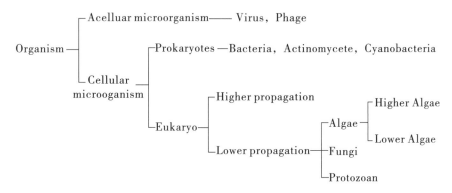

Figure 4-4   Classification of Microorganism

The status of Approved manual and Effective Catalog is quite similar. When bacteriologists agree to restart naming in bacteriology, they will face millions of names in past documents, the majority of which are ineffective because, apart from about 2,500 names, it is impossible to tell precisely what bacteria they refer to. These 2,500 names remained on the approved list. Only those names that are retained in the new bacteriological nomenclature are recognized with the rest are removed. When new bacterial names are proposed, the removed names will not be considered (although the name of the bacteria has sufficient reason to be recovered under special regulations).

It is required in the new international rules for bacterial nomenclature that all new names should be acknowledged by nomenclature through publication in a valid directory or publication in the "International Journal of Systematic Bacteriology" or elsewhere. The names on the valid directory only indicate that they are validly published (thus considering them in the bacterial nomenclature). It is not necessary to use names everywhere. Users do not need to use this name if they believe the new data is not scientific enough and the reasons for valid names are not sufficient. For example, the scientific community immediately accepted the use of Helicobacter pylori as *Campylobacter pylori*, but *Tatlockiamicdadei* instead of Legionella micdadei is not universally accepted. Taxonomy still requires scientific judgment and universal acceptance.

An excellent way to keep up with the latest style is through the use of the Bergey's Catalog of Systematic Bacteriology Trust website (www. cme. msu. edu/Bergeys/). This page contains information on changes in Bergey's Catalog of Systematic Bacteriology, basic microbial data and culture collections, as well as revisions of the Ribosomal basic data design phylogenetic tree (RDP) and validly named lists of prokaryotic species.

Chapter 5

General Bacteriology

5.1 The Shape and Structure of Bacteria

5.1.1 The Shape of Bacteria

Bacterial cells, as the fundamental units of bacteria, are one of the smallest living things in the world. There are various ways to distinguish bacteria from one another, such as morphology, antigenic, metabolic and staining characteristics. However, scientists usually divide bacteria based on their shape. The three most common shapes of bacteria are coccus, bacillus and spirillum, which depict the spherical bacterium, the rod-shaped bacterium and curved bacterium, respectively. Each bacterial shape is further subdivided according to the manner in which they arranged into multicellular organizations.

5.1.1.1 Coccus

Coccus usually has a spherical shape, resembling tiny balls. Most coccus is approximately 1 μm in diameter. The cocci arrange themselves into groups that are characteristic of a species. According to the arrangement of multicellular organization, coccus is subdivided into diplococcus, streptococcus, staphylococcus, tetrads and sarcina.

Diplococcus represents a diplo arrangement of coccus, such as *Neisseria*. *Neisseria* which is the most common causes of bacterial meningitis grows in pairs generally and has the ability of breaching the barrier.

Streptococcus whose progeny cells divide in the same plane and adhere to each other usually form long chains of cells. Although most streptococcal species are not pathogenic, some diseases, such as streptococcal pharyngitis, meningitis and bacterial pneumonia, are caused by streptococcus species. *Beta-hemolytic streptococcus* cause complete rupture of red blood cells.

Staphylococcus usually forms in grape-like clusters. The progeny cells of Staphylococcus divide in the different planes and are adherent in irregular clusters. Scientists have found that the staphylococcus genus includes at least 40 species and most are harmless. *Staphylococcus aureus* is one of the famous species of staphylococcus.

Cells of coccus that divide sequentially in two or three perpendicular planes form tetrads or sarcina, respectively. Tetradscells are adherent in square arrays of four, like *Gaffky's tetragena*. Sarcina cells are adherent in cubical arrays of eight, such as *Sarcine luted*.

5.1.1.2　Bacillus

Bacillus is shaped like a small rod with a rounded end or, sometimes, a tapered end. Bacillus comes in a wide variety of sizes. For example, the larger bacillus, such as *Bacillus anthracis*, is 1.0−1.2 μm wide by 3−10 μm long. While the smaller bacillus, such as *Brucella*, is 0.5−0.7 μm wide by 0.6−1.5 μm long. Some egg shaped bacillus are so short that they are called *coccobacillus*. The Bacillus species also arrange themselves into groups that are characteristic to other species. Cells forming long chains are called streptobacillus.

5.1.1.3　Spiral Bacteria

According to the number of twists per cell, cell flexibility and cell motility, spiral bacteria are subdivided into vibrio and spirillum. Vibrio is comma-shaped, such as *vibrio cholerae*, which is the pathogen of Asiatic cholera. Spirillum is S-shaped. The main pathogenic bacterial genus belonging to spirillum is *Spirillum minus*.

5.1.2　Bacterial Structure

Bacteria, belonging to the third kingdom proposed by Haeckel in 1886, constitute a large domain of prokaryotic microorganisms. It has been classified into prokaryotic cells because of their lack of a true nucleus. In fact, bacteria possess a much simpler structure than other organisms. It contains neither a nucleus nor a membrane-bound organelle. The bacterial structures are composed of essential structures and special structures in particular bacteria.

5.1.2.1　Essential Structures

Cell wall A bacterial cell has an internal osmotic pressure induced by the high concentrations of intercellular materials. Under this high osmotic pressure condition, the bacterial cell would not burst owing to the presence of the rigid cell wall. The major shape determinant of bacteria is the peptidoglycan cell wall which provides the bacterial cell with strength and rigidity against the high osmolarity. Besides the function of structural support, cell wall also serves as a filtering mechanism and protects the bacterial cells from outside environment. Cell wall lies outside the cytoplasmic membrane and mainly consists of the cross-linked polymer peptidoglycan. Peptidoglycan is also named mucopeptide, glycopeptide or murein. It is a mesh-like organic polymer composed of polysaccharide chains cross-linked byshortamino acidbridges. The composition of cell wall is complex and varies between species. According to the cell wall structure, bacteria can be divided into gram-positive bacteria and gram-negative bacteria. Either gram-positive or gram-negative bacteria, their glycan backbone formed by alternating N-acetylglucosamine and N-acetylmuramic acid peptidoglycan is same. While other components, such as tetrapeptide side chains and peptide cross-bridges, vary from species to species.

(1) Gram-positive Bacterial Cell Wall

Cell wall of gram-positive bacteria is thick and multilayered, usually 20−80 nm thick, 15−50 peptidoglycan layers. The main component of gram-positive bacterial cell wall, peptidoglycan, consists of glycan backbone, tetrapeptide side chains and peptide cross-bridges. Besides these, gram-positive bacterial cell wall also contains large amounts of teichoic acids which may comprise up to 50% of the dry weight of cell wall. There are two types of teichoic acids: wall teichoic acid and membrane teichoic acid (lipoteichoic acid), covalently linked to peptidoglycan and membrane glycolipid respectively. In addition, gram-positive wall may also include other components, such as lipoproteins and polysaccharide molecules. The wall of streptococci contains M protein, the staphylococci contain R protein in their cell walls. Teichoic acids are key factors in virulence. Lipoteichoic acids are the main factors launching host responses. These molecules confer major antigenic properties and they are the basis to distinguish bacterial serotypes.

(2) Gram-negative Bacterial Cell Wall

Gram-negative bacteria possess a thin cell wall, usually 10–15 nm thick, only one or two peptidoglycan layers. However, it is, structurally and chemically, more complex than gram-positive bacterial cell wall. The gram-negative wallis composed by an outer membrane, a peptidoglycan layer and a periplasmic space. The peptidoglycan of gram-negative bacterial wall consists of glycan backbone and tetrapeptide side chains. Teichoic acids are absent in the gram-negative bacterial cell wall.

Gram-negative wall also has its special components, such as outer membrane, comprising 80% of the dry weight of cell wall. Outer membrane locates in an area external to the peptidoglycan layer. Actually, outer membrane is covalently tied to the peptidoglycan by lipoprotein and is connected to the cytoplasm membrane at adhesion sites. It is an asymmetric bilayer structure composed by inner leaflet and outer leaflet. The inner leaflet is similar to the normal bacterial membrane containing phospholipids, while the outer leaflet contains a unique glycolipid, named lipopolysaccharide (LPS), which is different from any other biologic membrane. LPS is the endotoxin stimulating innate and immune responses. It can cause fever by activating leukocytes and monocytes. It can activate B cells to release interleukin-1, interleukin-6, tumor necrosis factor and other factors. LPS can also stimulate the complement cascade and clotting system, leading to local tissue damage and disseminated intravascular coagulation, respectively. Some gram-negative bacteria, such as *Neisseria* bacteria and *Haemophilus* bacteria contain lipooligosaccharide (LOS) as a stimulator of fever and other symptoms, which is similar to LPS.

Outer membrane also contains several proteins, although they are in a limited variety. Many of the proteins are transmembrane proteins as they traverse the entire lipid bilayer. Among these proteins, porins are one group being responsible for the diffusion of small hydrophilic molecules. However, for large or hydrophobic molecules, such as hydrophobic antibiotics and lysozyme, outer membrane serves as a permeability barrier protecting the cell from adverse environmental condition.

The area between the internal surface of the outer membrane and the external surface of the cytoplasmic membrane is called the periplasmic space. In fact, the periplasmic space plays essential roles in bacterial survival as it contains multiple enzymes that play important part in breakdown of large macromolecules by bacterial cells metabolism, such as phosphatases, lipases, proteases, nucleases and carbohydrate-degrading enzymes. In addition, the periplasmic space in some bacteria also contains hyaluronidases, β-lactamase, collagenases or various binding proteins.

Bacterial cell wall has several essential functions. ①Protecting bacteria from outside infections, mechanical stresses and pathogens. ②Enabling transport of substances and information in and out of the cell. ③Regulating osmolarity. ④Determining the bacterial shape.

Bacterial cell wall integrity is important to the bacterial viability. When the cell wall is weakened or ruptured, bacterial cell will become a protoplast or spheroplast and immediately occur lysis because of the high osmolarity. As a result, disruption of the cell wall by inhibiting its synthesis or cross-link has been considered to be a therapeutic method in antibacterial treatment. There are several enzyme that may cleave peptidoglycan and induce bacterial lysis, such as lysozymes, endopeptidases and amidases. Some antibiotics are also targeting at bacterial cell wall, such as penicillin.

Cytoplasmic membrane physically separates the intracellular materials from the extracellular environment and protects the bacterial cells from outside surroundings. Similar to the eukaryotic membrane, bacterial cytoplasmic membrane is a lipid bilayer structure embedded with multiple proteins. But different from eukaryotic membrane, bacterial cytoplasmic membrane does not consist steroids except for mycoplasmas. Besides these, cytoplasmic membrane also contains ion pumps and enzymes. As cytoplasmic membrane is the major structure that controls substance transportation and energy production, it is selectively permeable to ions and organic molecules. The transmembrane of substances is either passive or active transport. In addition, cytoplasmic membrane participates in a variety of cellular processes, including cell signaling and cell adhesion.

Cytoplasm Although the external structures of gram-positive and gram-negative bacteria are exactly different to each other, their internal structures, including the cytoplasm, are very similar. The cytoplasm of bacteria usually consists of proteins, ribosomes, DNA chromosome, mRNA, metabolites and ions. The cytoplasm is the main place where the bacteria metabolizes.

There are multiple cytoplasmic granules which are small particles consisting of insoluble substances in bacterial cytoplasm. Cytoplasmic granules, also called inclusion, is the place that bacteria store reserved materials, including starch, glycogen, lipid droplets and polymerized metaphosphate. Although the cytoplasmic granules are not always observed during a period of bacterial growth or they are different when the same bacteria grow in different environment, they play important roles in the survival of bacteria. For example, some bacteria convert carbon source materials pre-deposited in the granules to starch and glycogen when they are in a nitrogen source-absent condition. Some bacteria store polymerized metaphosphate in granules, also called volutin, assimilated from inorganic phosphate outside. Volutin can stain red with a blue dye and therefor be a characteristic of corynebacteria.

Bacterial ribosome is the place where bacterial proteins synthesize and suspends in the cytoplasm. Unlike eukaryotic 80S ribosome consisting of 40S and 60S subunits, bacterial ribosome is a 70S ribosome forming by 30S and 50S subunits. Bacterial ribosome is made up by RNA and proteins. It can bind to the bacterial mRNA to form polysome, which in turn facilitates the coupled transcription and translation. Antibacterial drugs mainly target on bacterial ribosome.

Bacterial plasmid is smaller, circular, extrachromosomal DNA suspended in cytoplasm. Although bacterial plasmid can replicate independently and is not essential for the survival of a bacterial cell, it often carries some genes, also called plasmid-borne genes, which may confer a selective advantage to the bacteria in specialized environments. That is to say, unlike the chromosome DNA which is bigger and contains genes essential for bacterial survival in normal conditions, plasmid is smaller and contains additional genes that may also be useful to the bacteria under particular conditions. For example, some characteristics of bacteria, such as antibiotic resistance, degradative metabolic pathways and host-to-host genetic material transfer, are controlled by bacterial plasmid.

Bacterial mesosome is a structure of the folded invagination of the plasma membrane. It is commonly observed in gram-positive bacteria. Scientists have found that mesosome may participate in chromosome replication, cell division and cell compartmentalisation. Furthermore, it may also play a role in cell respiration, which is analogous to the mitochondrion of eukaryotes. As this reason, the mesosome is also called chondroid of bacteria.

Nuclear material Nuclear material is also called nucleoid. It has been demonstrated that bacteria have a nucleoid instead of a nucleus which usually contains classic nuclear membrane and strands of DNA diploid genome in eukaryotes. The nucleoid of the bacteria can be observed under the light microscope and it is a discrete area in the center of a cell where DNA chromosome locates, mitotic apparatus and nuclear membrane absents. Bacterial nucleoid is Feulgen-positive because of the chromosome DNA. Bacterial chromosome DNA is haploid and exists as a single, double-stranded circle generally. Besides chromosome DNA, bacterial nucleoid also contains a small amount of RNA, RNA polymerase and proteins which might be the main composition of bacterial messenger RNA and transcription factor proteins.

5.1.2.2   Special Structures

Capsule & Slime layer Some bacteria are enveloped by a discrete covering layer, usually called capsule or slime layer, external to the cell wall. The former one refers to the polymers in a thickened gel appearance around each cell, while the latter refers to the polymers which are loosely adherent and easily washed off. Either capsule or slime layer is secreted extracellularly by bacteria. Capsule is usually composed by a large amounts of water and a small content of complex polysaccharides or proteins, but in some bacteria, such as *Bacillus anthracis*, the capsule contains water and polypeptide. The capsule is hard to observed microscopically. Until now, the method of negative staining in wet films with India ink is considered to be one of the most reliable methods to demonstrate the capsule.

The capsule and the slime also play important roles in bacterial cell survival, although they are not necessary during cell growth. The capsule is a major virulence determinant. The capsule can protect bacterial cells either from host ingestion or from attack of antibiotics. In addition, the capsule can also promote adherence of the bacteria to host tissue surfaces. For example, in *streptococcus mutans* the capsule composed by polymers of dextran and levan induces the bacteria to attach and adhere to the tooth enamel and finally causing dental caries. For *Bacillus anthracis*, the D-glutamic acid capsule is the mean by which the bacteria escape from antibiotics and host defenses.

Flagella Motile bacteria usually has flagella which are thread-like propellers and confer on bacteria motility. Flagella are found on almost all of the spiral bacteria and most bacilli. Flagellum is a long, hollow and thin filament and usually several times longer than the bacterial cell length. It anchors in the bacterial membrane and is extruded through the wall. The location and number of flagella vary between genera. Some bacteria having a single polar flagellum are called monotrichous, such as *Vibrio cholerae*. Some bacteria having two flagella and each flagellum locating at a pole are called amphitrichous, such as *Campylobacter jejuni*. For bacteria with multiple flagella, when the flagella locate at both poles of the cell, they are named lophotrichous, when the falgella are arranged around the entire cell, they are named peritrichous. For example, the flagella of *Spirillum* are clustered at both poles, *Pseudomonas* possesses 6 to 10 flagella which are peritrichous.

A flagellum mainly consists of a single kind of protein subunit, also known as flagellin. The most important function of flagella is its locomotive property. Interestingly, bacteria tend to swim toward localities with higher nutrient solutes (also called chemotaxis) and away from localities with higher disinfectant substances (also called negative chemotaxis). This motility is factually directed by the bacterial responses to the environmental nutrient solutes or poisons. Flagella provide bacteria with motility, allowing them to approach food and migrate to another direction. Moreover, flagella express antigenic and strain determinants. The power of bacterial active motility, to some extent, determines the pathogenicity. But notably, some non-motile pathogens are no less invasive than motile ones.

Fimbriae Fimbriae are filamentous appendages of bacteria, but they are different from the flagella. Fimbriae are thinner, more numerous than flagella and present in both motile and non-motile organisms. They are distributed peritrichously around the bacterial cell surface. Similar to flagella, fimbriae also consist of structured protein subunits, known as pilins.

Fimbriae are adhesion organs of bacteria. They provide firm adherence to surfaces of various kinds, such as cells of the host or other bacteria. For group A streptococci, fimbriae are responsible for the adherence of the bacteria to the hosts. As a result, fimbria is also an important virulence factor. Fimbriae are divided into two classes ordinary fimbriae and sex fimbriae. Ordinary fimbriae play important roles in adherence of symbiotic bacteria to host cells, while sex fimbriae play key roles in the attachment of donor and recipient cells in bacterial conjugation.

Endospore Some gram-positive bacteria, including those of the genera *Bacillus* and *Clostridium* can develop a structure, known as endospore, by which the organism can survive in harsh environment, such as nutrient scarcity. Such bacteria usually undergo a cycle of differentiation in response to survival condition. That process is named sporulation and germination. Sporulation happens as a response to nutrients depletion, including the loss of nitrogen, carbon and energy source or iron salt necessary to bacterial survival. Under these adverse conditions, the cell can form endospore that can be liberated immediately when the parent vegetative cell occurs autolysis. When returned to favorable condition, each endospore can be activated and give rise to a single vegetative cell. This process is germination. Endospore is considered to be the dormant state of bacteria dealing with adverse condition. When mature, endospore appears as a clear space in the stained cell protoplasm leaving itself not to be stained by simple stains.

Endospore is a dehydrated, multishelled structure, highly resistant to dry, heat and chemical agents. It is composed by an inner membrane, two peptidoglycan layers and a thin but tough outer coat. The inner membrane derives from the cytoplasmic membrane and wraps the spore protoplast. The two peptidoglycan layers, in which one layer is composed by thin, tightly cross-linked peptidoglycan and another is loose peptidoglycan layer, are also named cortex. The cortex is the thickest layer of the spore envelope and it gives the spore with impermeability. The outer coat which consists of a keratin-like protein with many intramolecular disulfide bonds confers on spores impermeability and relative resistance to antibacterial chemical agents. Inside of endospore is the spore protoplast, known as core. It contains a complete nucleus, large amounts of calcium dipicolinate and some essential proteins and ribosomes. All these characteristics of spore which is different from the vegetative cell make it to be high resistant.

5.2　The Growth and Metabolism of Bacteria

5.2.1　The Growth of Bacteria

5.2.1.1　The Nutritional Types of Bacteria

Due to the different enzyme system and metabolic activity of bacteria, different bacteria have different nutritional requirements. Based on this, bacteria are divided into two major types.

Autotrophic bacteria. This kind of bacteria survive with simple inorganic compounds as raw materials, such as CO_2, CO_3^{2-} as the carbon source and N_2, NH_3, NO_2^-, NO_3^- as nitrogen source. Inwhich, if the source of their required energy is mainly CO_2, H_2S, S or H_2 and other inorganic materials as hydrogen donor and they grow through photosynthesis, such bacteria are called photoautotrophic bacteria, such as green sulfur bacteria and blue Bacteria and so on. If the required energy source is mainly CO_2 or CO_3^{2-}, with H_2S, H_2, Fe^{2+} or NH_4^+ and other inorganic substances as hydrogen donor, they are called chemoautotrophic bacteria which using the chemical energy generated by the oxidation of inorganic substances to maintain the growth, such as nitrobacteriaand iron bacteria.

Heterotrophic bacteria. This kind of bacteria syntheses the body composition and obtains the energy with the organic materials such as protein, sugar and so on. Those using organic compounds as raw material and with the help of photosynthesis to grow are called photoheterotrophic bacteria and those using organic compounds as raw materials and the chemical energy produced by oxidation of organic matter to grow are called chemoheterotrophic bacteria. In nature, most bacteria are chemoheterotrophic bacteria. According to the different sources of organic materials, the chemoheterotrophic bacteria can be divided into saprophytic and parasitic bacteria. Saprophytic bacteria are a kind of chemoheterotrophic bacteria that use rotting, carcass or spoilage food of the soilas nutrients. Parasitic bacteria are a kind of chemoheterotrophic bacteria that parasitism in biological living organisms and use the organics nutrients of host. All pathogenic bacteria are heterotrophic bacteria and most of them belong to the parasitic bacteria.

5.2.1.2   The Nutrients of Bacteria

The nutrients needed for the growth of bacteria mainly include water, carbon source, nitrogen source, inorganic salt and growth factor.

Water is an essential substance to maintain the structure and survival of bacterial cells and plays an important role in the process of bacterial life. Water physiological functions are as follows: ①Water as a solvent involved in bacterial nutrient absorption and metabolic wastes excretion. ②Water is directly involved in biochemical reactions in bacterial metabolism, providing hydrogen and oxygen. ③Bound water is one of the components of bacterial cells. ④Water can transfer heat and regulate the temperature of cells.

Carbon source is the main element of bacterial synthesis, which provides energy for the growth of bacteria. All kinds of organic or inorganic substances containing carbon can be absorbed and utilized by bacteria. Inorganic carbon sources are mainly CO_2 or carbonates, such as CO_3^{2-}, HCO_3^-. Organic carbon source is rich in species, such as carbohydrates, lipids, alcohols, hydrocarbons and so on. Pathogens mostly use carbohydrate as their carbon source.

Nitrogen sources are mostly nitrogenous compounds that provide raw materials for the synthesis of bacterial strains, such as proteins, nucleic acids, enzymes and so on. The main nitrogen sources of bacteria are inorganic nitrogen sources and organic nitrogen sources. The common inorganic nitrogen sources include ammonium salt, nitrate and urea etc. Organic nitrogen sources mainly refer to animal or plant proteins and their degradation products, such as peptone, amino acid and so on. The pathogenic bacteria mainly obtain nitrogen from organic nitrogen compounds.

Inorganic salts provide the necessary metals and trace elements for the growth of bacteria. The elements require concentration of $10^{-3} - 10^{-4}$ mol/L as the common elements, including potassium, sodium, calcium, magnesium, sulfur, phosphorus, iron and so on. The elements that need a concentration of 10^{-6} to 10^{-8} mol/L are called trace elements, such as cobalt, manganese, copper, zinc, etc. The function of inorganic salts is mainly reflected in ①the formation of organic compounds involved in the formation of bacteria; ②as a component of the enzyme, maintaining enzyme activity; ③participating in energy storage and transport; ④regulating the osmotic pressure inside and outside the cell of the mycelium; ⑤some elements are closely related to the growth, reproduction and pathogenicity of bacteria. For example, the drug production of *Corynebacterium diphtheria* is closely related to the iron content in the bacterial living environment.

Growth factors refer to those the cell cannot synthesize or synthesis of insufficient, theymust rely on the outside world to provide trace amounts for bacteria to meet the growth and reproduction of organics, including vitamins, certain amino acids, purines and pyrimidine and so on. While, a few bacteria also require special growth factors. For example Haemophilus influenzae requires hemin (X) and Coenzyme Ⅰ or Coenzyme Ⅱ (V) factors. Bacteria require a very small amount of growth factors. Generally, vitamins are required at concentrations of 1 to 10 ng/mL and amino acids at concentrations of 20 to 50 μg/mL.

5.2.1.3 Conditions for the Growth of Bacteria

Sufficient nutrients, energy and suitable environment are the necessary conditions for the growth and reproduction of bacteria.

Nutrients provide necessary materials and energy for the metabolism, growth and reproduction of bacteria. Therefore, in a certain range, the concentration of nutrients is positively correlated with the growth rate of bacteria. Nutrients mainly include water, carbon source, nitrogen source, inorganic salt and growth factor.

The suitable environment for the growth of bacteria mainly refers to the suitable pH, temperature, osmotic pressure and gas environment.

The growth of bacteria is accomplished by various metabolic activities in the cell and every metabolic activity is dependent on the enzyme. And it is well known that enzymes need appropriate acidity and alkalinity to exert their biological activities. Hence, the growth of bacteria requires a suitable pH environment, that is, acidity and alkalinity. The most suitable growth pH of most bacteria ranges from 7.2 to 7.6. In this range, the bacteria have the strongest enzyme activity and the fastest growth rate. A few bacteria grow best in acid or alkaline environment, such as, the best pH range for *Vibrio cholerae* is 8.4 to 9.2 and the best pH range of *Mycobacterium tuberculosis* is 6.5 to 6.8. According to the optimum pH range of bacterial growth, the bacteria can be divided into three categories: neutrophilic bacteria (pH range 6.0–8.0), basophilic bacteria (pH range 8.0–10.5)and eosinophilic bacteria (pH range 3.0–6.0). As we know, most pathogens are neutrophilic bacteria.

The temperature has a great influence on the growth rate of bacteria. Different bacteria have different requirements for temperature. According to this, the bacteria are divided into three types: Psychrophiles, Mesophiles and Thermophiles. The overwhelming majority of pathogenic bacteria are Mesophiles and the optimum growth temperature is 37 ℃.

The gas related to the growth of bacteria is mainly oxygen and carbon dioxide. According to the need for oxygen or not in the process of bacterial growth, it is divided into four categories, obligate aerobic bacteria, microaerobes, facultative anaerobes and specific anaerobes. Obligate aerobic bacteria have perfect respiratory enzyme system, which must use molecular oxygen as hydrogen acceptor to complete aerobic respiration andthese bacteria can only grow in aerobic environment, such as *Mycobacterium tuberculosis*, *Vibrio cholerae*, etc. Microaerobic bacteria grow best in low oxygen environment, but higher oxygen concentration inhibits their growth, such as *Campylobacter jejuni* and *Helicobacter pylori* and so on. The facultative anaerobes can grow well in both aerobic and anaerobic environments and most of the pathogenic bacteria belong to this kind. Obligate anaerobes lack perfect respiratory enzyme system; they can only use other substances except oxygen molecules as hydrogen receptors and get energy through fermentation, such as Clostridium tetanus.

The salt concentration and osmotic pressure of the general medium are safe for most bacteria; however, a few bacteria, such as halophilic bacteria, require a higher salt concentration (3% NaCl).

5.2.1.4 Growth and Reproduction of Bacteria

Bacterial individuals reproduce asexual reproduction in a two split mode. Division of bacterial cells has three consecutive processes including nuclear DNA replicationand division, the formation of diaphragm and the progeny of cell division. After G$^+$ bacteria chromosome duplication is completed, the associated intermediaryis separated into two parts, the transversal mediators respectively pullthe replicated chromosomes to each sides of the cell, the middle of the cell membrane retracts to form the diaphragm and the cell wall grows inwards and cleaves the peptidoglycan covalent bond under the action of enzymes, eventually forming two descendant cells. G$^-$ bacterial chromosome is attached to the cell membrane, so the replication of the new chromosome also attached to the adjacent cell membrane, the new cell membrane formed between the two attachment points separates the respective chromosomes on both sides; finally, the cell wall invagination along the septumis divided into two and two descendant cells are formed. Under suitable conditions, most bacteria reproduce quickly. The time needed for multiplication of bacteria is called generation time. And the growth rate of bacteria is reflected by the time of generation.

In the laboratory process, take a certain number of bacteria inoculated in a suitable medium, continuously punctually sample to detect viable counts and choose the incubation time as the abscissa, the logarithmic number of cultured viable cells in the culture for the vertical axis, then draw a the growth curve of bacteria, founding that the growth and reproduction process of bacterial colony is divided into four stages as the lag phase, logarithmic phase, stationary phase and decline phase. Lag phase is the adaptation period of bacteria into the new environment, which shows the increase of the bacteria and the active metabolism, but with a slow propagation. The logarithmic growth period is also called exponential period; in this period, the growth of bacteria is rapid and the number of living bacteria increases with constant geometric progression and reaches the peak value directly. The logarithmic growth period of bacteria generally occurs at 8 to 18 h after culture, the morphology, chromosomes and physiological activities of bacteria are all typical, which are most sensitive to external environmental factors, thus they are mostly selected as research models. Due to the depletion of nutrients in the medium and the continuous accumulation of harmful metabolites, the reproduction rate of bacteria in the stationary phase slows down and the number of deaths slowly increases, both of which are in a state of equilibrium. At the declining stage, the bacterial propagation becomes more and more slow, the number of deaths increase significantly, the morphology of bacteria also changes obviously and the metabolic activity of the bacteria tended to stagnate. Especially, bacterial growth curve is of an important guiding significance in bacterial identification, research work and production practice.

5.2.2　Metabolism of Bacteria

The metabolism of bacteria is the sum of intracellular catabolism and anabolism. Catabolism is the process of substrate decomposition and energy generation. Anabolism is the process of bacteria using simple small molecular nutrients to synthesize cell bodies, cell structures and related metabolites. Catabolism provides raw materials and energy for anabolism, while anabolism provides a material basis for catabolism, both of which complement each other.

5.2.2.1　The Energy Metabolism of Bacteria

Bacterial energy metabolism mainly involves the conversion of ATP formal chemical energy; the basic biochemical reaction is biological oxidation, among which dehydrogenation or hydrogen transmission is the most common. Taking organic matter as a hydrogen carrier is called fermentation and using in organic matter as a hydrogen donor is called respiration. Utilizing molecular oxygen as a hydrogen carrier is aerobic respiration, while other inorganic substances, such as nitrate and sulphate, are anaerobic respiration. Aerobic respiration is carried out under aerobic conditions and anaerobic respiration and fermentation must be carried out under anaerobic conditions.

5.2.2.2　Bacterial Catabolism

The nutrients metabolism ofbacteria for polysaccharides, proteins, lipids and others large molecular, complex structure isnutrients is through the corresponding extracellular enzyme degradation and the simple structure of small molecule nutrients such as glucose and amino acids, is directly absorbed and utilized. The substrates for pathogen synthesizes cellular components and the energy are mainly sugars, which release energy through oxidative or glycolysis and store energy in the form of ADP, ATP with high-energy phosphate bonds. This section uses glucose as an example to briefly describe the energy metabolism of bacteria. Decomposition of glucose by bacteria is mainly through EMP pathway, pyruvate metabolic pathway and pentose phosphoric acid pathway.

The EMP pathway is the basic metabolic pathway for most bacteria and 1 molecule of glucose metabolized by EMP can produce 2 moleculesof pyruvic acid, 2 molecules of ATP and 2 molecules of NADH⁺H.

Pyruvate metabolic pathway: Under aerobic conditions, aerobic bacteria and facultative anaerobes oxidatively decarboxylate pyruvate to acetyl-CoA and then enter the tricarboxylic acid cycle to be completely oxidized to form CO_2 and H_2O, releasing a large amount of energy at the same time.

The pentose phosphate pathway is a branch of the EMP pathway that provides precursor and reductive energy for biosynthesis. One molecule of glucose-6-phosphate is metabolized by the pentose phosphate pathway to produce 1 molecule of glyceraldehyde-3-phosphate, 3 molecules of CO_2 and 6 molecules of NADH⁺ H.

5.2.2.3 Anabolic Products of Bacteria

Bacteria use the products and energy of catabolism to synthesize their own components, such as cell walls, proteins, nucleic acids and so on. At the same time, they can also synthesize some important metabolites in medicine. Some of them are related to the pathogenicity of bacteria, such as bacterial toxins. Some can be used for bacterial identification, such as bacterial pigments and others have important applications in medicine and pharmaceutical industry, such as antibiotics produced by Actinomyces.

5.3 Bacterial Genetics

Bacteria constitute a large domain of prokaryotic microorganisms. Just like other organisms, heredity and variation are common in bacteria. The bacterial morphological structure, physiological metabolism, pathogenicity, drug resistance, antigenicity and other biological traitsare determined by thegenetic material of bacteria. Heredity is the transmission of genetic characters from parents to their offspring, which are maintained relatively stable. Variation refers to the differences between a parent and offspring or between offsprings.

The properties of a bacterial cell at a particular time are referred to as the phenotype of the cell. These properties are determined not only by its genome (genotype), but also by its environment. Phenotypic variation occurs when the expression of gene is changed in response to the environment. The distinction is important: genotypic variation is heritable and maintained through changes in environmental conditions, whereas phenotypic variation is reversible, being dependent on environmental conditions and altering when these changes.

Continuous decoding of the bacterial genome and intensive research of the functional genome enhance the understanding of bacterial genetic variation. It promotes studies on the bacterial pathogenic mechanism, drug resistance mechanism, rapid diagnosis, vaccine development and new strategy of prevention and treatment.

5.3.1 Bacterial Variation

5.3.1.1 Morphological and Structure Variation

The shape, size and structure of bacteria may vary according to the change of external environment. When *Yersinia pestis* is cultured for a long time or on a culture medium with 30 g/L NaCl, the stick-shaped with bipolar staining bacterium may be changed into spherical, yeast-shaped, filamentous or polymorphous bacterium. Treated with β-lactam antibiotics, antibody, complement or lysozyme, normal bacteria become L forms because of interruption of cell wall synthesis. Some bacteria lose special structure after variation. For example, *Salmonella typhi* treated with some chemicals may lose flagella. This is called H-O variation, which means colony H (diffused growth on solid media with the motility of flagella) changes to colony O (single colony on solid media). The virulence of *Streptococcus pneumonia* attenuates after losing capsule. After being cultured at 42 ℃ for 10 to 20 days, *Bacillus anthracis* may lose its spore-forming ability and its virulence is also decreased.

5.3.1.2　Virulence Variation

Virulence variation includes the enhancement and attenuation of bacterial virulence. Infected by coryne bacteriophage, *Bacillus diphtheriae* acquires the ability of producing diphtheria toxin and becomes virulent strain. The virulence of *Mycobacterium tuberculosis* weakens after 230 times' passage on media with bile, glycerol and potato for 13 years. This is the process of the invention of Bacillus Calmette-Guerin, which is an effective vaccine for preventing tuberculosis.

5.3.1.3　Resistance Variation to Antimicrobial Agents

Bacteria become drug-resistance strains if they are tolerated with some antibacterial agents. Some bacteria, which are called multidrug resistant strains, show resistance to more than one drugs. From the extensive application of antibiotics, the constant increase of bacterial drug resistance has become a hot problem in the world. In addition, some bacteria are dependent on antibiotics after variation. The streptomycin-dependent attenuated strain of *Shigelladysenteriae*, for example, can be used for preventing dysentery.

5.3.1.4　Colony Shape Variation

Colony shape variation is often found in *Enterobacteriaceae*. S-R variation is the change from smooth (S) colony to rough (R) colony. This variation, which results from losing polysaccharide repeat units of LPS, are often followed with other characteristics alteration such as virulence, antigenicity and biochemical reaction.

5.3.1.5　Enzyme Activity Variation

Mutation may cause enzyme acticity variation. Some of these mutants called auxotrophs are unable to synthesize a certain kind of nutrient and require to be on midium with the nutrient that they cannot produce; or some mutants with enzyme activity variation lose the ability to ferment a particular carbohydrate and cannot grow on medium with certain carbohydrate as the only carbon source.

5.3.2　Bacterial Genes and Genome

Bacterial genetic information is encoded in DNA. Genome in bacteria is the totality of heritable information, include chromosomes, plasmids, bacteriophages and transposons.

5.3.2.1　Chromosome

Bacterial chromosomes, circular or linear, have no nuclear membrane. Most of bacteria have a single circular chromosome consisting of a double-stranded DNA (dsDNA) molecule (580−5,220 kb). A few bacterial chromosomes have two circular dsDNAs and the chromosome of *Borrella* contains a linear dsDNA. The chromosome of a typical bacterium *Escherichia coli* is $3×10^9$ Da (4,639 kilobase pairs) in size, an approximate length of 1.3 mm (i.e. nearly 1,000 times the diameter of the cell). Bacterial chromosome has a one-point replication origin and carries genetic information in the form of genes. Unlike eukaryotes, the genes in bacteria are often organized in operons and do not contain introns. The whole chromosome contains

4,000-5,000 genes and about 2,000 of them have been annotated. Genes are squences of nucleotides that have a biologic function; examples are protein-structural genes, ribosomal RNA genes and recognition and binds sites for other molecules (promoters and operators).

The main features of the bacterial genome are as follows: ①Non-coding sequences are relatively few, the number of genes and the size of genome are positively correlated; ②Most genes are single copies, but the rRNA gene is a multiple copy, which helps rapid synthesis of a large number of ribosomes to meet rapid growth and reproduction of the bacteria; ③Function-related genes are often arranged in clusters and their transcriptions are controlled by a common regulatory region orgene to form the operon; ④The structure of the bacterial gene does not have the intron and no splicing process is required after RNA transcription.

Different bacterial chromosomes have different G + C contents, which can be used to analyze bacterial species or the genetic origin. Genomic sequence analyses have revealed extensive genetic material exchanges within and between bacterial species. In the bacterial genome, exogenous DNA fragments (1-200 kb) can be observed, whose G+C percentage and codon usage bias are significantly different from those of the bacterial chromosome, both sides often contain repetitive sequences, insert sequences or tRNA, suggesting that these fragments are obtained by the lateral gene transfer. The carrying genes are associated with bacterial resistance, pathogenicity, virulence or some metabolisms, which are called resistant island, pathogenic island (PAI)/virulent island or metabolic island.

Bacterial chromosomes have various functional recognition sites, such as the origin of chromosomal replication (oriC), termination of chromosomal replication (TerC), transcription initiation site and termination site.

5.3.2.2 Plasmid

Plasmids are extrachromosomal genetic elements of closed, circular or linear, double stranded DNA in the cytoplasm. All natural plasmids contain an origin of replication (which controls the host range and copy number of the plasmid) and replicate independently of the chromosome and can exist in the cell as a unique copy or multiple copies. Genetic information carried in plasmids usually encode one or more biological traits to the host such as resistance to antibiotics or drugs, degradative functions and/or virulence, but usually do not include genes that are essential for cell growth or replication. Many plasmids contain mobile DNA sequences (transposons) that can move between plasmids and the chromosome.

Plasmids are classified into several types according to different criteria.

(1) Conjugative Plasmids and Non-conjugative Plasmids

Conjugative plasmids code for functions that promote transfer of the plasmid from the donor bacterium to other recipient bacteria, but non-conjugative plasmids do not. Large plasmids (>40 kb) are often conjugative. Non-conjugative plasmids are often less than 15 kb in size.

(2) Stringentplasmids and Relaxed Plasmids

The average number of molecules of a given plasmid per bacterial chromosome is called its copy number. Stringent plasmids have small copy numbers (1 to several per chromosome) and replicate only when the chromosome replicates. Relax plasmids have high copy numbers (typically 10-20 per chromosome) and replicate on their own.

(3) Compatible plasmids and Incompatible Plasmids

Closely related or identical plasmids demonstrate incompatibility; they cannot be stably maintained in the same bacterial host. The reason is that plasmids which are closely related to interfere with each other's replication. In contrast, compatibility means that unrelated plasmids can coexist stably in one cell.

(4) Classification Bygenetic Information

Many plasmids control medically important properties of pathogenic bacteria: ①Fertility plasmids (F plasmids) encode sex pili and promote transfer of the genetic elements from thedonor bacterium to other recipient bacteria; ②Resistance plasmids determine resistance toanti bacterial drugs. The conjugative resistanceplasmids are called R plasmids (R factors), whichare often found in gram-negative bacteria. Then on conjugative resistance plasmids are calledr plasmids, which can be transmitted between bacteria by transduction. ③Virulence plasmid sencode virulent factors associated with bacteria lpathogenicity. Representative toxins encoded by plasmids include heat-labile and heat-stable enterotoxins of *Escherichia coli*, exfoliative toxin of *Staphylococcus aureus* and tetanus toxin of *Closiridium tetani*.

5.3.2.3　Transposable Elements

Transposable elements are genetic units that can move from one site in a DNA molecule toother target sites in the same or a different DNA molecule. This transposition relies on their capacity to synthesize their own site-specific recombination enzymes, called transposases. Transposable elements are important genetic elements because they cause mutation mediate genomic rearrange ments or result in gene expression change adjacentto the insertion site.

(1) Insertion Sequence

Insertion sequences (IS) are short DNA segment of several hundred to 2,000 nucleotide pairs in length and only code for proteins implicated in the transposition activity. These proteins are usually the transposase which catalyses the enzymatic reaction allowing the IS to move and also one regulatory protein which either stimulates or inhibits the transposition activity. Insertion sequence is usually flanked by inverted repeats at their ends.

(2) Transposon

IS elements are components of tranposons and transposons are as much as 10-fold larger than IS elements. Except the genes responsible for transposition, transposons carry other genes that confer important properties on the bacteria carrying them. These often include drug resistance markers and other easily selectable genes. Transposons are classified into three types: ①Complex transposons contain insertion sequences at each end, usually as inverted repeats. The DNA between the terminal insertion sequences encodes specify resistance to one or more antibiotics. Complex transposons cause spread of drug resistance genes among bacteria. ②Tn3 family transposons have structures, which are similar to complex transposons. They possess terminal inverted repeats, but they lack terminal insertion sequences. ③Conjugative transposons are discovered in gram-positive bacteria, which have no terminal inverted repeats. These transposons are excised from the chromosome of the donor and transmitted by conjugation to the recipient.

(3) Bacteriophage Mu

Bacteriophage Mu is a phage, which hasbeen shown to cause genetictransposition. The entire phage genome inserts into host genes as a transposon. Prophage integration can occur at many different sites in the bacterial chromosome and often causes mutations. While Mu was specifically involved in several distinct areas of research (including *E. coli*, maize and HIV), the wider implications of transposition and insertion transformed the entire field of genetics.

5.3.2.4　Integron

Integrons are genetic elements that can capture and express genes from other sources.

An integron is minimally composed of three functional element. ①A gene encoding for integrase that catalyzes another type of site-specific recombination; ②A proximal recombination site, which is recognized by the integraseand at which gene cassettes may be inserted; ③a promoter that can express the newly integrated cassette-encoded genes.

Additionally, an integron will usually contain one or more gene cassettes that have been incorporated into it. The gene cassettes may encode genes for antibiotic resistance, although most genes in integrons are uncharacterized. Integrons have been found in a number of bacteria. They can occur in plasmids, transposons or on the chromosome to enhance the adaptability of bacteria.

5.3.2.5   Bacteriophages

Bacteriophages (phages) are viruses which infect bacteria, fungi, actinomycetes and spirochetes. They replicate as obligate intracellular parasites in host. Like all viruses, phages have common characteristics, such as small volume, consisting of either RNA or DNA but not both, containing no cytoplasm or cellular organelles, lack metabolic machinery of their own and are totally dependent on their host cell for replication, etc.

(1) Morphology and Structure

Extracellular phage particles are metabolically inert and consist principally of proteins plusnucleic acid (DNA or RNA, but not both). Theproteins of the phage particle form a protective shell(capsid) surrounding the tightly package dnucleic acid genome. Several morphologic allydistinct types of phage have been described, including polyhedral, filamentous and complex. Complex phages have polyhedral heads to whichtails and sometimes other appendages(tail plates, tail fibers, etc.)are attached (Figure 5-1).

(2) Classification

Phages are classified by the relationship between host and phages into two major groups: virulent and temperate. Virulent phages are which can only multiply in bacteria and kill thecell by lysis at the end of the life cycle. The lyticcycle is the multiply process of virulent phages which includes adsorption, penetration, biologicalsyn thesis, maturation and release.

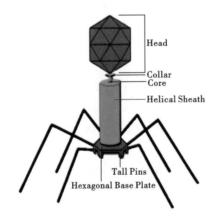

Figure 5-1   Structure of a complex phage

Temperate phages are those that can enter aquiescent state in the cell. In this quiescent statemost of the phage genes are not transcribed; the phage genome exists in a repressed state. Phage DNA in this repressed state is called a prophage because it is not a phage but it has the potentialto produce phage. In most cases the phage DNA actually integrates into the host chromo some and is replicated along with the host chromosome and passed onto the daughter cells. This process iscall lysogenic cycle.

The cell harboring a prophage is termed a lysogenic bacterium. The lysogenic state can be terminated by certain factors(e. g. exposure to UV or ionizing radiation). Prophages separate from the chromosome of the host and enter lytic cycleto generate new phages. Therefore, temperate bothlytic cycle and lysogenic cycle(Figure 5-2), but virulent phages only have lyticcycle.

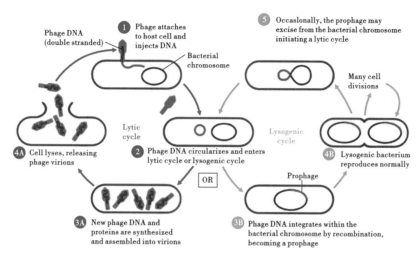

Figure 5-2   Lysogenic cycle and lytic cycle of a lysogenic bacterium

5.3.3   Mechanisms of Bacterialgenetic Variation

Genotypic variation is determined by the change of genic structure. Phenotypic variation occurs when the environmental conditions alter. The change of genic structure results from mutation and gene transfer and recombination.

5.3.3.1   Mutation

Mutation is heritable change in the base sequence of the nucleic acid genome of an organism, which will be passed on stably to subsequent generations. Both environmental and genetic factors affect mutation rates. Spontaneous mutations for a given gene generally occur with a frequency of $10^{-10}-10^{-6}$ in a population derived from a single bacterium. While the spontaneous rate of mutation is very low, many chemical, physical or biological agents can increase the mutation rate and are therefore said to induce mutations. The mutagenic agents are referred to as mutagens. Organisms selected as reference strains are called wild strains and their progeny with mutations are called mutant strains.

(1) Types of Mutation

Mutations can be classified into point and multisite mutations according to the effect on the structure of genes. Point mutations change only one or a few nucleotide, including substitution, insertion and deletion. Multisite mutations involve extensive chromosomal rearrangements such as deletion, duplication, inversion, insertion and translocation.

Mutations may cause different results. A missense mutation occurs when a change in base sequence converts a codon for oneamino acid to a codon for a different amino acid. Nonsensemutations occur when a codon for a specific amino acid isconverted to a chain-terminating codon. A synonymous mutation is a mutation that converts a codon for an amino acid to another codon that specifies the same amino acid; thus, it is likely that a synonymous mutation will affect the behavior of a cell. Frameshift mutations occur when a nucleotide is deleted or added to the coding portion of a gene. Frameshift mutations frequently jumble a large portion of the information encoded in a gene and can produce very defective protein products.

(2) Reversion and Suppression

Organisms selected as reference strains are called wild strains and their progeny with mutations are called mutant strains.

Mutations that convert the phenotype from wild-type to mutant are called forward mutations and mutations that change the phenotype from mutant back to wild-type are called reverse mutations. Reverse mutations that restore the exact nucleotide sequence of the wild type DNA are true reversions. Reverse mutations that do not restore the exact nucleotide sequence of the wild-type DNA are called suppressor mutations. Suppressormutations occurs at different site in the DNA and may cause restoration of wild type phenotype. Suppressormutations can be intragenic or extragenic. Intragenic suppressors are located in the same gene as the forward mutations that they suppress. Extragenic suppressors are located in different genes with from mutations whose effects they suppress.

5.3.3.2　Genetransfer and Recombination

A change in the genome of a bacterial cell may be caused either by a mutation in the DNA or result from gene transfer and recombination. Gene transfer termed recombination is an event of donate DNA from one bacterium to another bacterium. Bacterial genetic exchange is typified by transfer of relatively small fragments(e. g. , chromosome DNA fragments, plasmids or phage DNA) of a donor genome to a recipient cell. Because some types of transferred DNA do not contain an origin of replication, these genes will only be passed on to succeeding generations if the transferred DNA becomes incoporated into the recipient chromosome, which has an origin of replication. Plasmids contain their own origin of replication and can be maintained in a host through subsequent generations without being integrated into the chromosome. Genes can be transferred by three distinct mechanisms: transformation, conjugation and transduction.

(1) Transformation

Transformation is the process by which bacteria take up free DNA into a recipient cell and cause genetic change (Figure 5-3). The discovery of genetic transformation in bacteria was the one of outstanding events in biology and became keystone of molecular biology and modern genetics.

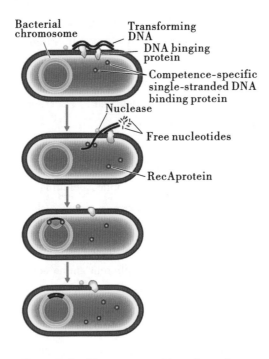

Figure 5-3　The process of transformation

Naturally transformable bacteria are found in several prokaryotes, including certain species of gram-nagative and gram-positive bacteria. The ability of bacteria to betransformed(called competence) depends on a physiologic state of the cell that allows extracellular DNA to cross cell membrane. Natural transformation is an active process demanding specific proteins produced by the recipient cell. In many species of bacteria, it is encoded by chromosomal genes that become active under certain environmental conditions. Many bacteria, unable to enter competent state, can be made permeable to DNA by treatment with agents that damage the cell envelope making an artificial transformation possible.

(2) Conjugation

Conjugation is a process by which bacteria transfer genetic information from donor to recipient cell via direct connection. The process requires the presence of a certain conjugative plasmid, such as F plasmid or R plasmid on donor cell, which makes DNA transfer.

1) F Plasmid: One of the well-characterized conjugative plasmids is F plasmid. It possess many *tra* genes encoding a sex pilus as well as the ability to form a conjugation bridge. A cell harboring F plasmid (F⁺ cell) function as donors, whereas strains that lack the F plasmid (F⁻ cell) behave as recipients. In matings between F⁺ and F⁻ bacteria, an intercellular cytoplasmic bridge is formed by sex pilus and one strand of the F plasmid DNA is transferred from donor to recipient. The transferred strand is converted to circular double-stranded F plasmid DNA in the recipient bacterium and a new strand is synthesized in the donor to replace the transferred strand. Both of the exconjugant bacteria are F⁺ (Figure 5-4).

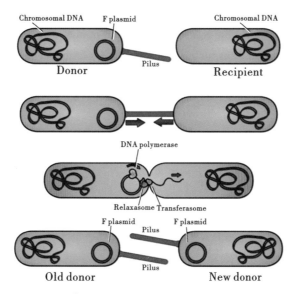

Figure 5-4   Schematic drawing of bacterial conjugation

Another important consequence of a tra region in F plasmid is can be integrated into the bacterial chromosome. In that case, donor strains with integrated F factors can transfer chromosomal DNA to recipients with high efficiency. These strains of bacteria that have a chromosome-integrated F plasmid are called Hfr (High frequency recombination). In matings between Hfr and F⁻ strains, transfer of single-stranded DNA from an Hfr donor to a recipient begins from the origin within the F plasmid. Transfer of this entire replicon, including the bacterial chromosome, requires approximately 100 minutes. Because the mating bacteria usually separate spontaneously before the entire chromosome is transferred, conjugation typically transfers only a fragment of the donor chromosome into the recipient. The segment of the F plasmid is transferred last, so conjugation between an Hfr and F⁻ cells leaves the recipient cell still F⁻.

Integrated F plasmids in Hfr strains can sometimes be excised from the bacterial chromosome and the possibility exists for the incoporation at that time of neighbouring chromosomal genes into the liberated F plasmid. Such F plasmid containing chromosomal genes are called F' plasmids.

2) R Plasmid: R plasmid is a conjugative plasmid in bacterial cells that promotes resistance to agents

such as antibiotics, metal ions, ultraviolet radiation and bacteriophage. R plasmid is composed of resistance transfer factor(RTF) and determinant (r-det). The functions of replication, conjugation and transfer are determined by RTF; r-det encode the genes of antibiotic resistance. R plasmid sare commonly shared between bacterial species, genera and even families through conjugation. Transfer of R plasmid can confer multiple resistance to antibiotics such as tetracycline, chloramphenicol and penicillin.

(3) Transduction

Transduction refers to transfer of genetic information from donor to recipient bacteria cell via a bacteriophage vector. Transduction can occur in two ways: generalized transduction and specialized transduction.

1) Generalized transduction: When bacteriophages multiply inside an infected bacterial cell, each phage head is normally filled with a copy of the replicated phage genome. However, with certain types of phage, a random fragment of bacterial chromosome DNA is accidentally encapsulated in a phage protein coat in place of the phage DNA at a frequency of $10^{-5} - 10^{-7}$. When such rare phage infects a recipient cell, the DNA fragment of donor cell can be transduced by the phage. Since phages of this type pick up any port the bacterial chromosome at random, they can transduce any chromosome genes at approximately the same frequency and are termed generalized transduction phages.

When a generalized transducing phage infects a recipient cell, expression of the transferred donor genes occurs. Abortive transduction refers to the transient expression of one or more donor genes without formation of recombinant progeny. In abortive transduction the donor DNA fragment does not replicate and among the progeny of the original transductant only one bacterium contains the donor DNA fragment. Complete transduction is characterized by production of stable recombinants that inherit donor genes and retain the ability to express them (Figure 5–5).

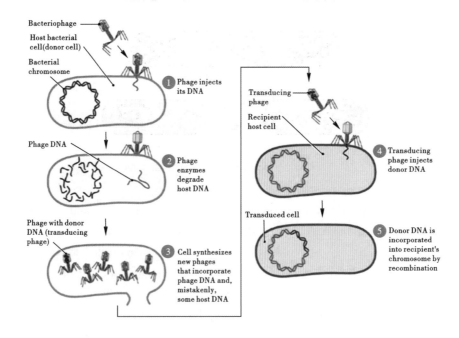

Figure 5–5   The process of generalized transduction

2) Specialized transduction: Specialized transduction is mediated by specific temperate phages. Phage DNA integrates into the host chromosome to form prophage. When a lysogen carrying such a prophage is induced to produce virions, excision of the viral genome from host chromosome occasionally occurs imprecise-

ly, carrying a small segment of host genes with it. A specialized tranducing phage particle contains both phage and bacterial DNA joined together as a single molecule. After infecting recipient cell, this joint molecule integrates into the recipient chromosome just as phage DNA normally does in the process of becoming a prophage. A few specific donor genes(usually those adjacent to their integration sites in the genome)can be transferred to recipient bacteria.

3)Lysogenic conversion: Lysogenic conversion is a change in the properties of host cell by the presence of a prophage. When the temperate phage DNA integrates into the host chromosome, the host cell becomes lysogenized. The genes carried by the phage are expressed and the characteristics of the host cell are changed. Loss of the prophage leads to the loss by the bacterium of the properties that originated during the lysogenic conversion. For example, *Corynebacterium diphtheria* produces diphtheria toxin only when it is infected by the β phage. In this case, the gene that codes for the toxin is carried by the β phage, not the bacteria. Erythrogenictoxin by group A hemolytic streptococci and botulinum toxin by *Clostridium botulinum* are also resulted from lysogenic conversion.

4)Protoplast fusion: Protoplasts are prepared by treating bacteria with a lytic enzyme such as lysozyme to remove the cell wall. As a result of this treatment the cell content would be enclosed only by a cell membrane and the protoplasts survive in osmotically protective media. During fusion, two or more protoplasts come in contact and adhere with one another either spontaneously or in the presence of fusion inducing agents such as polyethylene glycol. protoplasts are induced to fuse and form transient hybrids or diploids. During this hybrid state, the genomes may re-assort and genetic recombination can occur.

5.3.4　Application of Bacterial Heredity and Variation

5.3.4.1　Diagnosis, Treatment and Prophylaxis

(1)Variation in Morphology and Biological Characteristics and Bacteriological Diagnosis

Atypical characteristics of variants often bring about difficulties in bacterial identification. L form, for example, does not grow on regular media and must be cultivated on media with perosmosts. Therefore, it is essential to understand the law of bacterial variation for diagnosing diseases correctly.

Many rapid methods for identification of bacteria have developed on the basis of bacterial genetics. Polymerase chain reaction (PCR)is an effective diagnosis technique of high sensitivity and specificity for bacterial infections. PCR can be used to identify those bacteria, which are not easily cultivated such as *Bacillus tuberculosis* and *legionella pneumophila* through amplifying their conservative and specific DNA fractions.

(2)Variation in Bacterial Drug Resistance and Control

Due to variation in drug resistance and lateral transfer of drug resistance gene, combined with the clinical use of antibiotic screening, the number of drug-resistant bacteria continue to increase and a variety of drug-resistant strains appear. Variation and spread of bacterial drug resistance bring great difficulties to the clinical treatment. For example, among the isolated *Staphylococcus aureus*, more than 90% of strains are resistant to the drugs such as penicillin, sulfa, etc. In order to improve the efficacy of antibacterial drugs and prevent the spread of drug-resistant strains, the drug-sensitive test is used routinely to select sensitive antibiotics. In the clinical practice, for the reasonable selection and application of antibiotics, the drug resistance is monitored, the change in the drug-resistant spectrum is analyzed and the drug-resistant mechanism is studied to reduce the variation in drug resistance and prevent the spread of drug-resistant bacteria.

(3)Variation in the Bacterial Virulence and Disease Control

Bacterial variations includeen hancement and attenuation of the virulence. During bacterial identification, the bacterial virulence and expression of the virulence factors should be detected.

1) Variation in bacterial virulence and development of attenuated live vaccine: Vaccines were prepared for the prevention of bacterial diseases by screening strains with reduced virulence and retained immunogenicity. For example, the attenuated live vaccine of *Bacillus anthracis* has been used in the prevention of anthrax; Bacillus of Calmette Güerin (BCG) is used in the prevention of tuberculosis. With the advancement of genome-wide bacterial sequencing, the comparative genomics analysis will allow site-directed mutagenesis, induce targeted reduction of bacterial virulence when preserving its immunogenicity and avoid the possibility of reverse mutation of the virulence and enhance the development of more ideal effective vaccines.

2) Conditional lethal mutation strains and development of vaccines: When the genes necessary for bacterial growth are mutated, the gene products are only active under specific culture conditions and the mutants can survive under these conditions, which are called conditional lethal mutants. Temperature-sensitive mutants are common and valuable in the vaccine strain screening.

5.3.4.2　Screening Potential Carcinogen

Chemicals that are carcinogenic for animals are often mutagenic for bacteria. The substances inducing bacterial mutation are called potential carcinogens. Ames test is used as screening procedures to identify environmental agents that may be carcinogenic in humans. The test is based upon the reversion of mutations in the histidine (his) operon in the bacterium *Salmonella typhimurium*. The mutants are unable to grow without added histidine, whereas revertants that restore the His$^+$ phenotype can do. If the potential mutagen results in more colonies in medium without histidine than the control, thus it really is a mutagen and is a likely carcinogen.

5.3.4.3　Molecular Epidemiology

The use of molecular techniques makes the epidemiologic investigation precisely trace a specific strain of an infectious pathogen or gene. Molecular techniques include pulsed-field gel electrophoresis (PFGE), plasmid analysis, PCR-Restriction Fragment Length Polymorphism (RFLP), multiple Multilocus sequence typing (MLST) and nucleic acid sequence analysis, etc. These techniques help to determine the origin of the epidemic strains or genes or detect the spread of nosocomial drug-resistant plasmids in different bacteria and have emerged as revolutionary tools for epidemiological studies.

5.3.4.4　Molecular Biology and Genetic Engineering

Microbial genetics initiates from the study of bacteria. Many important theories of molecular biology and molecular genetics also originate from research to bacteria. Tool enzymes (e. g. , endonulease, ligase, polymerase, Taq enzyme), vectors, transposons and DNA recombination (e. g. , transformation, conjugation, transduction) were all first discovered in bacteria and they continue to be extensively applied up to now.

Genetic engineering refers to the development of microorganisms with genetic structure altered by biochemical manipulation. This kind of biochemical procedure is termed recombination DNA technology. This technology consists of isolating, purifying and identifying genetic material from one source, tailoring it for insertion into a new host; and isolating a colony of cells with the desired new genes.

Utilizing the characteristics of plasmids or phages, the target gene can be recombined with the vector and transferred into recipient bacteria to express the trait of the target gene. At present, many bioactive substances that are not readily available in large quantities from natural organisms, such as insulin, interleukin, interferon, growth hormone and clotting factors, can be mass-produced through genetic engineering. The development of genetically engineered vaccines has also made progress, which has played a positive role in the prevention and treatment of diseases.

5.4   Bacterial Infection and Immunity

5.4.1   Innate Immunity

5.4.1.1   Skin and Mucous Barriers

(1)The Skin and the Antimicrobial Substances

Intact skin provides a physical barrier against microorganism infection. Although the bacteria can enter sweat or sebaceous glands and hair follicles, fatty acid produced in sebaceous glands, lactic acid in perspiration and the acid pH of secretions, tend to eliminate pathogenic organisms. In the gastrointestinal tract, numerous hydrolytic enzymes in saliva inactivate bacteria and the acidity of the stomach kills many ingested bacteria. The bile in intestines inactivates many microbes too.

(2)Mucous Membranes

In the upper respiratory tract the mucosal epithelium is protected by mucus secretions and cilia and a film of mucus is constantly being driven upward. Bacteria tend to stick to this film and are continuously transported toward the mouth. Cigarette smoke or other pollutants can damage the ciliated epithelial cells.

(3)Normal Flora

Most mucous membranes of the body carry a constant normal microbial flora, which ensures competition for pathogens to which the skin is exposed. By this and other mechanisms, flora opposes establishment of pathogenic microorganisms.

5.4.1.2   Cellular Components of Innate Responses

(1)The Cellular Components and Their Activation

The cells involved in innate immunity include granulocytes (basophils, eosinophils and neutrophils), monocytes and macrophages, mast cells, natural killer cells, NKT cells and γ/δ T cells, etc. These cells express different combinations of pattern recognition receptors (PRRs)and danger and damage sensors for microbes and cell trauma. PRRs, like the Toll-like receptors(TLRs), bind repetitive structures of microbe that form pathogen-associated molecular patterns (PAMPs) including lipopolysaccharide (LPS), lipoteichoic acid, unmethylated cytosine-guanosine units of DNA [CpG oligodeoxynucleotides (ODNs)] and other molecules. Cytoplasmic sensors, nucleotide-binding oligomerization domain protein (NOD)-like receptors (NLRs) recognize bacterial peptidogly can and other components in cytoplasm. The interaction between PRRs and PAMPs leads to the activation of innate immunity. In addition, in response to PAMPs or tissue damage, a multiprotein complex inflammasome is assembled in myeloid cells. The inflammasome activates the caspase 1 protease, which then cleaves, activates and promotes the maturation of the release of inflammatory cytokines interleukin 1β (IL-1β)and interleukin 18 (IL-18).

Neutrophils play a major role in antibacterial protections. The neutrophil surface is decorated with receptors, such as lectins, scavenger receptors and Fc and C3b opsonin receptors. These receptors promote phagocytosis of the microbe. Neutrophils have many granules that contain antimicrobial proteins and substances, which contribute to the subsequent killing of phagocytosed bacteria. Neutrophils spend less than 3 days in the blood, rapidly die in tissue and become pus at the site of infection.

Macrophages represent a family of mononuclear leukocytes that are distributed throughout the body. Monocytes are small leukocytes that circulating in the blood and mature into macrophage in all tissues. Some macrophages are activated by IFN-γ which is produced by NK cells and T cells as part of the TH1 response. Activated macrophages are long lived and produce enzymes and other molecules to promote antimicrobial function and reinforce local inflammatory reactions by producing chemokines and acute-phase cytokines. Macrophages capture extra-and intracellular pathogens, eliminate invaders and deliver them to subcompartments of lymphoid organs. They also process and present antigens to activate T cells, although dendritic cells (DCs) are the main antigen presenting cells (APCs). In the case of an unresolved mycobacterial infection, continuous (chronic) stimulation of macrophages by T cells promotes fusion of the macrophages into multinucleated giant cells and large macrophages called epithelioid cells that surround the infection and form a granuloma.

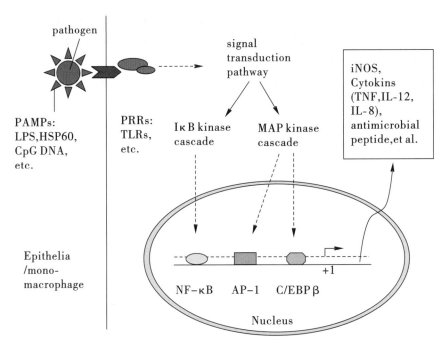

Figure 5-6   The interaction between PRRs and PAMPs leads to activation of innate immunity

NK cell sare innate lymphoid cells (ILCs) that provide an early cellular response to an infection, have antitumor activity and amplify inflammatory reactions after bacterial infection. NK cells are also responsible for antibody-dependent cellular cytotoxicity (ADCC), in which they bind and kill antibody-coated cells. NK cells are large granular lymphocytes (LGLs) that share many characteristics with T cells, except the mechanism for target cell recognition. NK cells do not express a T-cell receptor (TCR) or CD3 and cannot produce IL-2. They neither recognize a specific antigen nor require presentation of antigen by MHC molecules.

NKT cells and γ/δ T cells reside in tissue and in the blood and differ from other T cells because they have a limited repertoire of T-cell receptors. Unlike other T cells, NKT and γ/δ T cells can sense nonpeptide antigens, including bacterial glycolipids (mycobacteria) and phosphorylated amine metabolites from some bacteria (*Escherichia coli*, mycobacteria) but not others (streptococci, staphylococci). These T cells and NK cells produce IFN-γ, which activates macrophages and DCs to enforce a protective TH1 cycle of cytokines and local cellular inflammatory reactions. NKT cells also express NK-cell receptors.

(2) Phagocytosis

The process of phagocytosis includes chemotaxis, migration, ingestion and microbial killing. Migration is dependent on the release of chemoattractant signals produced by either host cells or pathogen. One chemoattractant is IL-8 which attracts neutrophils and other granulocytes. Neutrophils attach to the endothelial cell surface and migrate from the circulation through the endothelium into the tissues and to the site of infection. Neutrophils and macrophages are main cells that engulf and kill pathogens. The phagocyte recognizes, engulfs and internalizes the pathogen into an endocytic vesicle called phagosome. Then phagosome fuse with lysosomes to form mature phagolysosomes. The bacteria are killed and digested in phagolysosomes.

There are several mechanisms used by phagocytes to kill the pathogen, which can be fundamentally divided as oxygen-dependent killing and oxygen-independent killing. ①Oxygen-dependent killing is mediated by the generation of reactive oxygen species (ROS), which include reactive oxygen intermediate (ROI) and reactive nitrogen intermediate (RNI). The oxygen-dependent process, also referred to as the "respiratory burst", leads to the generation of O_2^-(superoxide anion). O_2^- is converted by superoxide dismutase into hydrogen peroxide, which is then metabolized into hypochlorous acid in the presence of myeloperoxidase and halogens. O_2^- can also reacts with nitric oxide, which is generated through activation of nitric oxide synthase, to form cytotoxic oxidant peroxynitrite. ②Oxygen-independent process consists of the following mechanism: ①Acidification within the phagosome. The phagosome pH is 3.5-4.0 that is bacteriostatic or bactericidal; ②The release of lysozyme. Lysozyme hydrolyses preferentially the β-1,4 glycosidic linkages between the N-acetylmuramic acid and N-acetylglucosamine that occur in the peptidoglycan cell wall structure of bacteria, particular Gram-positive bacteria; ③The generation of antimicrobial peptides, such as cathelicidin and defensins. These cationic peptides kill Gram-negative bacteria by disrupting their cell wall integrity.

(3) Outcome of Phagocytosis

The phagocytic cells may kill ingested microorganisms. But in some situation some bacteria can escape from killing and survive, even multiply in the phagocytic cells. The nature of the microorganism and function of the phagocytic cells determine the outcome of phagocytosis.

5.4.1.3　Humoral Components

(1) Complement

The complement system constitutes an alarmand serves as first lines of defense against microorganism. There are three activation pathways of complement: classic pathway, alternative pathway and lectin pathway. The complement system is activated by complexes of antibody and antigen (classical pathway). Moreover, the complement system is directly activated by microbial surfaces (alternative pathway) and by mannose-binding lectin (MBL) binding to mannose residues on the bacterial or fungal cell surface(lectin pathway) in the absence of antibody. In all three pathways, C3-convertase cleaves and activates components C3, creating C3a and C3b and causes a cascade of further cleavage and activation events. The complement peptides, C3a, C4a and C5a, have anaphylatoxin activity and have a wide variety of biological activities, contributing to amplification of inflammatory responses and C3b has most important opsonizing activity. At last C5b recruits and assembles C6, C7, C8 and multiple C9 molecules to assemble a membrane attack complex (MAC), (C5b,6,7,8)1(C9)n complex, on target cell membranes and drills a hole in the membrane, leading to osmotic lysis of the target cell. *Neisseria* bacteria are very sensitive to this manner of killing, whereas gram-positive bacteria with abundant peptidoglycan are relatively insensitive.

(2) Lysozyme

Lysozyme is abundant in secretions such as tears, saliva and mucus. It is also present in cytoplasmic granules of the macrophages and the polymorphonuclear neutrophils (PMNs). Lysozyme induces lysis of bacteria by catalyzing the hydrolysis of 1,4-beta-linkages between N-acetylglucosamine (GlcNAc) and N-acetylmuramic acid (MurNAc) residues in peptidoglycan of bacteria. Lysozyme is used to lyse gram negative bacteria. Its activity increases with increasing temperatures, up to 60 ℃, with a pH range of 6.0-7.0.

(3) Antimicrobial Peptides and Chelators

Antimicrobial peptides including defensins were produced by epithelial cells and other cells and found in secretions at mucosal surfaces (tears, mucus and saliva). Defensins are small (≈ 30 amino acids) cationic peptides that can form holes in bacterial cell walls and hence kill bacteria. The production of antimicrobial peptides may be constitutive or stimulated by microbial products (PAMPs) or cytokines (IL-8, etc.).

Living organisms produce some complex proteins, one kind of chelators that bind very tightly to metal ions. These metal ion-binding proteins bind iron (e. g., lactoferrin, transferrin, ferritin, siderocalin) or bind zinc (e. g., calprotectin), which are essential for bacteria and consequently prevent growth of bacteria and yeast. However, many pathogens such as *Mycobacterium tuberculosis* have developed alternate means for acquiring these ions.

5.4.1.4 Acquired Immunity

Acquired or adaptive immunity provided by T and B cells and antibody is highly antigen specific and has immunologic memory. It involves antibody-mediated and cell-mediated immunity. Following antigen stimulation, the immune response rapidly expands in strength and cell number along with specificity. The main differences between innate immunity and adaptive immunity are listed in the following Table 5-1.

Table 5-1　The comparison between innate immunity and adaptive immunity

	Innate immunity	Adaptive immunity
Host	Multicellular organism	Vertebrates
Ligand	PAMPs (pathogen-associated molecular patterns)	Particular epitope
Receptor	PRRs (pattern recognition receptors)	B-cell and T-cell receptors for antigen
Response	Immediate response	Slow (3–5 days) response
Effective agent	Antimicrobial peptides *et al.*	Specific B and T cells *et al.*

(1) Antigen and Antigen Presentation

There are a wide variety of features that determine the immunogenicity of antigen: ①Recognition of foreignness ("nonself"). ②Size: Proteins with a molecular weight less than 10,000 are weakly immunogenic. Some small molecular, called haptens, become immunogenic when linked to a carrier protein. ③Chemical and structural complexity. ④Dosage, route and timing of antigen administration.

On ingestion of bacteria, antigen-presenting cells (APCs) such as Langerhans cells and immature dendritic cells (iDCs) become mature and move to the lymph nodes to process and present their internalized antigen to naïve CD4$^+$ Th0 T cells, which are bound to class Ⅱ major histocompatibility complex (MHC) molecules. The activated APCs and Th0 cells produce IL-2, IFN-γ and IL-4. CD4$^+$ Th0 cells differentiate into Th1 and Th2 types, which contribute to setting up cell-mediated immunity and antibody-mediated immunity respectively. The intracellular bacteria can also activate CD8$^+$ T cells through MHC class Ⅰ molecules. Simultaneously, bacterial molecules with repetitive structures (e. g., capsular polysaccharide) interact with B cells expressing surface IgM and IgD specific for the antigen and activate the cell to grow and produce IgM. These are primary antigen-specific immune responses. During a secondary or memory response, B cells, macrophages and DCs can present antigen to initiate the response.

Some bacterial proteins are able to activate large numbers of T cells. These proteins are called superantigens, which are able to bind to MHC molecules outside the peptide-binding cleft and therefore can stimulate much larger numbers of T cells. Some bacterial toxins including staphylococcal enterotoxins, toxic shock syndrome toxin and group A streptococcal pyrogenic exotoxin A, are superantigens.

(2) Antibody-mediated Immunity

B lymphocyte recognizes antigen, then interacts with antigen-specific helper CD4 T cells and secreted cytokines, at last proliferate and differentiate into either antibody-producing plasma cells or memory B cells. Some bacterial antigens like LPS can directly stimulate antibody production and do not require T cell help to activate B cells, which induce B-cell responses with limited class switching and do not induce memory B cells.

There are several immunoglobulin classes: IgG, IgM, IgA, IgE and IgD. Initially, all B cells bound to an antigen carry IgM and produce antigen-specific IgM. Later, gene rearrangement generates the same antigen-specific antibodies of different immunoglobulin classes (IgG, IgA or IgE). When an individual encounters an antigen, the first antibodies are IgM (within 3 days), then following with IgG, IgA or both (approximately 8 days). IgM levels decline sooner than IgG levels. Re-exposure to an immunogen, a secondary response (also termed anamnestic response), induces a much more rapid production of antibody, which lasts longer and reaches a higher titer.

Antibodies recognize and bind to specific pathogen or toxin and produce resistance against bacteria through following mechanisms: ①Enhanced phagocytosis by opsonizing (coating) organisms; ②Neutralization of toxins and inactivate their harmful effects; ③Complement-mediated lysis by activating the complement system; ④Antibody-dependent cell cytotoxicity (ADCC) by a killer cell (NK, macrophage, neutrophil, eosinophil) that binds to the Fc proton of antibody; ⑤preventing adhesion of bacteria by secretory IgA at epithelial cell surfaces.

(3) Cell-mediated Immunity

$CD4^+$ helper T cell, $CD8^+$ killer T cell and NKT cell, etc. mediate immunity against microbes that survive in phagocytes and microbes that infect non-phagocytic cells, such as virus, intracellular bacteria, fungi and protozoans. Cell-mediated immunity (CMI) involves the activation of antigen specific T lymphocytes, release of various cytokines and activation of phagocytes in response to antigen. The effector $CD4^+$ T cells can develop into one of four main categories: Th1 cells, Th2 cell, Th17 cells or T regulatory (Treg) cells. Th1 cells produce IL-2 and IFN-γ and contribute to the activation of CMI. CD8 cells differentiate into effector cytotoxic cells. Following activation, the cytotoxic T lymphocytes (CTL) kill the infected cell through releasing cytotoxic granules containing perforin.

Besides differentiating to effector cells, CD4 and CD8 T cells develop into memory T cells (T_M) following antigen stimulation. Memory T cells can be divided into effector memory T cells (T_{EM}), central memory T cells (T_{CM}) and tissue-resident memory T cells (T_{RM}). The short-lived T_{EM} confers immediate protection for incoming pathogens, while T_{CM} survive for long periods and readily proliferate and differentiate to T_{EM} and effector cells upon re-stimulation with the same antigen. Upon chronic or nonsterile infection, the persistent antigen induces T_{EM} as well as effector cells constantly. Therefore, the nonsterile immunity, also called concomitant immunity, has been associated with enhanced protection by T cells. However, severe chronic infection could induce T cell exhaustion.

5.5   **Laboratory Diagnosis**

5.5.1   Sample Collection

Aspirates from unopened lesions, in sterile syringes or sterile containers, are preferred. Swabs in transport media are acceptable. Milk is collected into containers under sterile precautions. Blood and urine cultures are appropriate for staphylococcal isolation.

5.5.2　Direct Examination

Staphylococci appear as Gram-positive cocci in pairs, clusters or short chainsin Gram-stained films. They may be sparse in specimens from skin pustules.

5.5.3　Isolation and Identification

Bovine blood agar is best for the detection of beta toxin ("water stain" appearance), which is diagnostic for coagulase-positive staphylococci (*S. aureus*, *S. intermedius* and *S. schleiferi* ssp. *coagulan*). Colonial appearance is as described. Biochemical tests are used to identify staphylococcal isolates. Commercial kits are available.

5.6　Treatment and Control

Abscesses are drained pus. Topical application of mild antiseptics (hexachlorophene) may be adequate for the most superficial pyoderma.

Extensive, inaccessible and disseminated infections require systemic treatment. Staphylococci are commonly resistant to penicillin G, streptomycin and tetracycline. Usually effective antimicrobics include penicillinase-resistant penicillins, fluoroquinolones, chloramphenicol, cephalosporins (first generation), vancomycin, lincosamides (lincomycin and clindamycin), the macrolides (erythromycin, azithromycin, c1arithromydn) and trimethoprim-sulfas. Clavulanic acid inactivates the beta-lactamase produced by *S. aureus* and *S. intermedius*, therefore cell wall antibiotics containing this substance are protected (e. g. , clavulanic acid/amoxicillin). The penicillinase-resistant penicillin cloxacillin is effective in treating staphylococcal mastitis, especially ill dry rows.

For staphylococcal cystitis, penicillins remain ertecetse because of their high urinary concentrations. Cloxacillin is used topically and systemically on exudative epidermitis due to *S. hyicus*.

A controversial approach to prevention of staphylococcal infections in infants utilizes "bacterial interference": the implantation of a nonvirulent strain to preclude colonization by virulent staphylococci. The method shows promise for control of staphylococcosis in turkeys.

5.7　Bacterial Drug Resistance

5.7.1　Antimicrobial Agents

In 1942, the application of penicillin as a therapeutic agent opens up the era of antimicrobial chemotherapy and marks a key milestone in medicine. Many additional classes of antibiotics that involve an extensive range of chemical structures and targets, form the foundation of the current armory of antibiotics.

Selective toxicity is a significant character of an ideal antimicrobial agent, which means that the antibiotic is harmful to pathogens without being harmful to the host. The current antimicrobial agents used for treating bacterial infections can be divided into different classes on the basis of their chemical structure, mechanisms of action or spectrum of activity. Main antibiotic families and their mechanisms of action were summarized inTable 5-2. According to their chemical structure, the major categories of antibiotics include: ① β-lactam antibiotics (e. g. , penicillins, cephalosporins) ; ② macrolides (e. g. , erythromycin, azithromycin, clarithromycin) ; ③ chloromycetins (e. g. , chloromycetin, dextrosulfenidol) ; ④ tetracyclines (e. g. , tetracycline, doxycycline, lymecycline) ; ⑤ aminoglycosides (e. g. , gentamicin, amikacin) ; ⑥ fluoroquinolones (e. g. , norfloxacin, ciprofloxacin, ofloxacin) ; ⑦ sulphonamides (e. g. , trimoxazole, trimethoprim) ; ⑧ peptides (e. g. , bacitracin).

Table 5-2   Main antibiotic families and their mechanisms of action

Mechanism of action	Antibiotic families
Inhibition of cell wall synthesis	β-lactam antibiotics; daptomycin; glycopeptides
Inhibition of protein synthesis	Macrolides; tetracyclines; aminoglycosides; lincosamides
Inhibition of DNA synthesis	Fluoroquinolones
Competitive inhibition of folic acid synthesis	Sulfonamides; trimethoprim
Inhibition of RNA synthesis	Rifampin

5.7.2   What Causes Drug Resistance?

There are two main components considered to be responsible for the emergence of antimicrobial resistance problem. One is the antibiotic or antimicrobial agent, which inhibits susceptible bacteria and selects the resistant ones; and the other is the genetic resistance determinant in microorganisms selected by the antimicrobial agent. Drug resistance occurs only when the two components come together in an environment or host, which can pose a threat to clinical therapy. Under continued antimicrobial pressure, the selected resistance genes and their hosts spread and propagate, leading to amplify and extending the problem to other hosts and other geographic locations.

Antibiotic targets, generally conserved, are involved inessential physiological or metabolic functions of the bacterial cell whereas absent from or sufficiently different in eukaryotes. Unfortunately, none of the current antimicrobial agents has escaped from a resistance mechanism (Figure 5-7). But how do bacteria acquire drug resistance? Drug resistance is mobile the genes for resistance characteristic can be transferred among bacteria of various taxonomic and ecological groups with the aid of mobile genetic elements such as plasmids, naked DNA, bacteriophages or transposons.

5.7.3   Biological Mechanism of Antimicrobial Resistance

The basic mechanisms by which a microorganism can exhibit resistance to an antimicrobial agent are: prevention of access to target; changes in antibiotic targets; and direct modification of antibiotics. Furthermore, bacteria can possess one or all of described above mechanisms simultaneously (Figure 5-8).

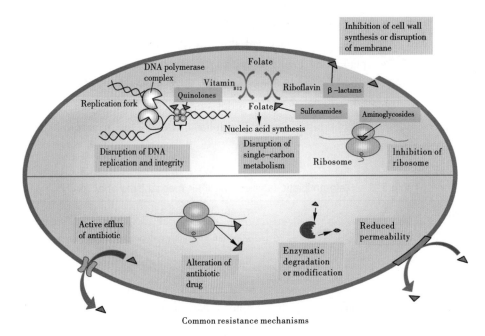

Figure 5-7　Common Mechanisms of Antibiotic Action and Antibiotic Resistance

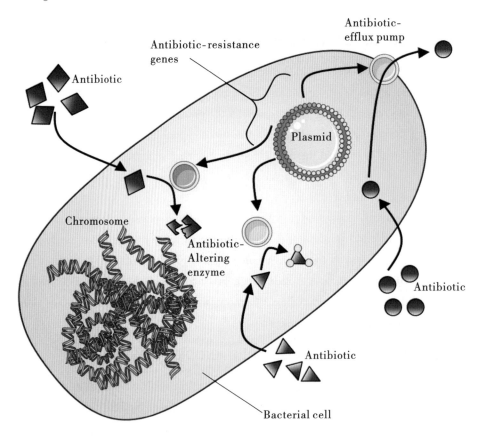

Figure 5-8　Biological Mechanisms of Resistance

5.7.3.1　Prevention of Access to Target

（1）Reduced Permeability

Gram-negative bacteria are intrinsically less permeable to many antibiotics because their outer membrane forms a permeability barrier when compared with Gram-positive species. These microorganisms have evolved porin proteins (e. g. ,*Omp*F in *E. coli* and *Opr*D in *P. aeruginosa*) that function as "nonspecific" entry and exit targets for drugs and other small molecule organic chemicals in order to circumvent this permeability barrier. Hydrophilic antibiotics across the outer membrane by diffusing through outer membrane porin proteins. As a consequence, reduction of porin gene expression can reduce the permeability of the outer membrane and restrict antibiotic entry into the bacterial cell, leading to clinical antimicrobial resistance.

(2)Increased Efflux

Efflux, a kind of mechanism of antibiotic resistance is nowwell-appreciated and commonly found. Bacterial efflux pumps actively transport structurally diverse antibiotics out of the cell. Furthermore, efflux pumps are mainly responsible for intrinsic resistance of Gram-negative bacteria to a variety of he drugs that can be used to treat Gram-positive bacterial infections.

Once overexpressed, efflux pumps can also confer high level resistance to previously described clinically useful antimicrobial agents. Some efflux pumps have narrow substrate specificity (e. g. ,the Tet pumps), while others can transport a broad range of structurally dissimilar substrates and are known as multidrug resistance (MDR) efflux pumps.

Most MDR efflux proteins belong to five different protein families: the resistance-nodulation-cell division (RND),major facilitator (MF),staphylococcal/small multidrug resistance (SMR),ATP-binding cassette (ABC) and multidrug and toxic compound extrusion (MATE) families. Efflux by proteins in the RND,SMR,MF and MATE families is driven by proton (and sodium) motive force and is therefore called secondary transport. ATP hydrolysis drives efflux in the primary (ABC) transporters. Members of the RND family of efflux pumps, identified in Gram-negative bacteria, are the best characterized of the clinically relevant MDR efflux transporters, which is the most important in mediating antibiotic resistance. RND family efflux pumps confer clinically increased levels of MDR and export an extremely broad range of substrates when overexpressed. Well-studied examples include the multidrug efflux pump AcrAB-TolC in *E. coli* and CmeABC in *Campylobacter jejuni*.

5.7.3.2   Changes in Antibiotic Targets

(1) Changes in Antibiotic Targets by Mutation

Most antibiotics bind to their targets specifically with high affinity, thus preventing the normal activity of the target. Changes to the target structure that prevent efficient antibiotic binding can confer resistance to antibiotics, however, it still enables the target to perform its normal function. eg. The penicillin-resistant *S. aureus* which expressed a β-lactamase conferring resistance to penicillin was first identified in the mid-1940s. Methicillin, a penicillin derivative, which is resistant to this β-lactamase was subsequently introduced to treat the penicillin-resistant isolates in 1959, but *S. aureus* with methicillin resistance were identified shortly there after. Here, the β-lactam resistance was attributed to the acquisition of a gene encoding an altered PBP named PBP2a.

(2) Modification (and Protection) of Targets

Modification of the target as a sort of protection mean can also result in antibiotic resistance that does not require a mutational change in the genes encoding the target molecules. For example, the erythromycin ribosome methylase (*erm*) family of genes methylate 16S rRNA and alter the drug-binding site, thus preventing the binding of macrolides, lincosamines and streptogramins and conferring bacteria resistant to these classes of antibiotics.

5.7.3.3   Direct Modification of Antibiotics

(1)Inactivation of Antibiotics by Hydrolysis

Since the first use of antibiotics, with the discovery of penicillinase (aβ-lactamase) in 1940, the major mechanism of antibiotic resistance is modification of antibiotics by enzyme catalysis. Thousands of enzymes have since been identified that can degrade and modify different classes of antibiotics, including β-lactams, aminoglycosides, phenicols and macrolides. e. g. The antibiotics of β-lactams all have a common element in their molecular structure: a four-atom ring known as a β-lactam, while β-lactamase can break this structures and provide antibiotic resistance. Through hydrolysis, the lactamase enzyme breaks the β-lactam ring and deactivates the molecule's antibacterial properties.

(2) Inactivation of Antibiotic by Transfer of a Chemical group

The addition of chemical groups tovulnerable sites on the antibiotic molecule catalyzed by bacterial enzymes confers antibiotic resistance, which prevents the antibiotic from binding to its target protein as a result of steric hindrance. Various different chemical groups can be transferred, including acyl, phosphate, nucleotide and ribitoyl groups and the enzymes that are responsible for a large and diverse family of antibiotic-resistance enzymes. e. g. There are three main classes of aminoglycoside-modifying enzymes: acetyltransferases, phospho transferases and nucleotidyl transferases, conferring high levels of resistance to the antibiotic (or antibiotics) that they modify. These classes described above are evolutionarily diverse and vary in the aminoglycosides that they can modify and in the part of the molecule that is modified.

5.7.4 The Genetic Basis of Drug Resistance

Antibiotic resistance is divided into intrinsic and acquired resistance according toa genetic basis. The natural insusceptibility of an organism is responsible for intrinsic resistance. In contrast, acquired resistance involves changes in the DNA content of a cell, so that the cell acquires an antibiotic resistant phenotype.

5.7.4.1 Intrinsic Resistance

The intrinsic resistance of a bacterial species to a particular antibiotic is the ability to resist the action of that antibiotic resulting from inherent structural or functional characteristics(Figure 1). In an individual species, the simplest example of intrinsic resistance is attributed to the absence of a susceptible target of a specific antibiotic.

5.7.4.2 Acquired Resistance

Bacteria acquire antimicrobial resistance as a consequence of chromosomal mutations or the horizontal exchange of genetic material among related or unrelated bacterial species.

(1) Chromosomal Mutation

In all bacterial populations, random spontaneous mutations occur continuously at a low frequency and some mutations may confer resistance to a particular antibiotic. The rate at which these mutations occur is not influenced by the antibiotic, however, the resistant mutations can survive, grow and eventually become the predominant only in the presence of the drug. For example, the ribosomal protein L4 and L22 on the 50S subunit are macrolide-binding site and bacteria may acquire macrolide resistance when the genes encoding L4 and L22 proteins sustain mutations that alter the drug binding site.

(2) Transferable Antibiotic Resistance

The horizontal transfer of resistance determinants carried on transposons, bacteriophages, plasmids and other mobile genetic material is responsible for the dissemination of antibiotic resistance among related or unrelated bacterial species. In general, this exchange is accomplished through the processes of transduction (via bacteriophages), conjugation (via plasmids and conjugative transposons) and transformation (via incorporation into the chromosome of chromosomal DNA, plasmids and other DNAs from dying organisms) (Figure 5-9). Another genetic element involved in resistance is integron, which was discovered in 1980s. Integron is a mobile DNA element that can capture and carry genes, particularly those leading to antibiotic resistance. Integron structure is composed of two conserved regions (5′ conserved region and 3′ conserved region) flanking a variable region (gene cassette), which includes one or more resistance genes. The 5′ region contents an integrase gene related to the integration and excision of the gene cassette and a promoter to drive transcription. Integrons can insert into transposons or conjugative plasmids conferring dissemination of antibiotics resistance among different species of bacteria.

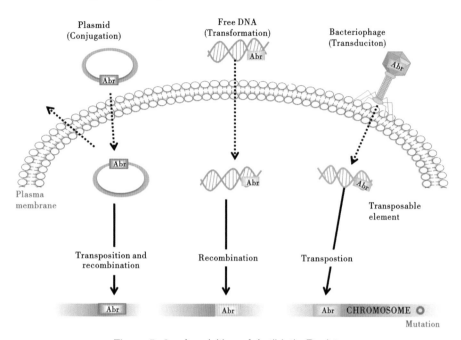

Figure 5-9   Acquisition of Antibiotic Resistance

5.7.5   Control of Resistance

A number of measures to control bacterial resistance include: ① controlling, reducing or cycling antibiotic usage; ② improving hygiene in hospital and hospital personnel to eliminate the dissemination of resistance organisms within hospitals; ③ discovering or developing new antibiotics; ④ developing inhibitors of antibiotic-modifying enzymes; ⑤ defining agents that would cure resistance plasmids.

5.8   Disinfection and Sterilization

Disinfection and sterilization are methods which are often used to decontaminate microbial and remove undesirable microorganisms. Disinfection means killing or removing of harmful vegetative microorganisms and sterilization means complete killing of all forms of microorganisms, including bacterial spores.

The object of disinfection and sterilization is to remove or destroy microorganisms which may cause contamination, infection and decay from materials or from areas. In many situations, such as surgery, food and drug manufacture, it is necessary to ensure safety from contaminating organisms by sterilization process. Sterilization methods include physical and chemical methods. In this section, physical methods of sterilization including heat, radiation and filtration for preventing microbial growth or to decontaminate areas or materials harboring microbes will be discussed. The followings are some definitions:

（1）Sterilization

Sterilization refers to complete destruction or elimination of all forms of microbial life present in a particular location or material. It can be accomplished through various means, including: incineration, nondestructive heat treatment, certain gases, exposure to ionizing radiation, some liquid chemicals, high pressure and filtration.

（2）Disinfection

Disinfection is to destruct or remove of all pathogenic microorganisms but does not necessarily kill all microorganisms, such as bacterial spores organisms with waxy coats（e. g. , mycobacteria）and some viruses, which are resistance to the common disinfectants; it fails to meet the criteria for sterilization.

（3）Antisepsis

Antisepsis means the inhibition of the growth of bacteria in wounds or living tissue to reduce the possibility of infection, sepsis or putrefaction. Antiseptics are some chemical disinfectant agents which are less toxic than environmental disinfectants but are usually less effective in killing vegetative organisms. They can act on normal flora and pathogenic contaminants on body surfaces such as the skin or vaginal tract.

（4）Sanitization

Sanitization which is used primarily inhouse-keeping and food preparation contexts aims to reduce microbial counts to safe public health levels and minimize the chances of disease transmission among patients. It has a little vague meaning somewhere between disinfection and cleanliness.

（5）Asepsis

Asepsis describes the state of being free from pathogenic microorganisms in a protected environment. It often refers to those practices used in the operating room, in the preparation of therapeutic agents, in technical manipulations and in the microbiology laboratory. The sterilization of all materials and equipment used is an essential part of aseptic techniques.

5.8.1 Physical Methods of Sterilization and Disinfection

Microbial decontamination can be achieved by physical methods, including heat, radiation and filtration, which are standard methods used to destroy or eliminate undesirable microorganisms.

The availability of reliable methods of sterilization and disinfection have contributed to not only the major developments in surgery and intrusive medical techniques that have helped to revolutionize medicine over the past century, but also the progress of many food preservation procedures. The following are the mechanisms of action and some practical examples that employ these methods to remove bacterial.

5.8.1.1 Sterilization by Heat

Heat which is the most reliable method of sterilization and disinfection should be the first choice unless contraindicated. It's a good way for materials that maybe damaged by heat to be sterilized at lower temperatures, for longer periods or by repeated cycles. There are some factors influencing sterilization by heat, involving properties of heat-dry heat or moist heat, exposure temperature and time, number of microorganisms present, characteristics of the organisms and so on.

The kinetics of heat sterilization is: departure from a microbe's temperature of adaptation suddenly is likely to have a detrimental effect on it. All microorganisms have a maximum temperature for growth, beyond which the microbicidal effects occur, because almost all macromolecules lose their structure and their ability to function at very high temperatures, which is known as denaturation. And it occurs more rapidly as the temperature rises and rate of death is proportional at any time to the concentration of organisms. These facts indicate that if we intend to sterilize a microbial population, lower temperatures need more time than at higher temperatures. So for each specific set of conditions, adjusting the time and temperature is vital to achieve sterilization. In addition, it is important to understand the nature of the heat: dry heat has worse penetrating power than moist heat which contributes to a faster reduction in the number of living organisms at a given temperature.

Vegetative cells and bacterial endospores from the same organism show distinctly different resistance to heat. Bacterial endospores are capable of surviving heat which would rapidly kill vegetative cells from the same species. The amount and state of water within the endospore mainlylead to heat resistance. During endospore formation, the accumulation of Ca^{2+}, *small acid-soluble spore proteins* (SASPs) and synthesis of dipicolinic acid lead to formation of a gel-like structure, reducing the protoplasm to a minimum volume. At this stage, around the protoplast core, there forms a thick cortex. Its contraction results in a shrunken, dehydrated protoplast, whose water content is only 10% –30% of a vegetative cell. The heat resistance of the spore is determined by water content of the protoplast coupled with the concentration of SASPs. Endospores with a low concentration of SASPs and high water content have low heat resistance; while endospores with a high concentration of SASPs and low water content have high heat resistance. Water moves freely in and out of spores, so it is the gel-like material in the spore protoplast rather than the impermeability of the spore coat that excludes water.

The killing of both vegetative cells and spores is also influenced by the nature of the medium in which heating takes place. Acidic foods such as tomatoes, fruits and pickles are much easier to sterilize than neutral pH foods such as corn and beans, which verifies that microbial death is more rapid at acidic pH. Besides, high concentrations of sugars, proteins and fats decrease heat penetration, usually increasing the resistance of organisms to heat, whereas it is depending on the organism that high salt concentrations may either increase or decrease heat resistance. In addition, dry cells (and spores) are more resistant to heat than moist ones; as a consequence, higher temperatures and longer times are required for heat sterilization of dry objects than moist objects.

(1)Sterilization by Dry Heat

Dry heat utilizes hot air that is either free from water vapor or has very little of it, while moisture plays a minimal or no role in the process of sterilization. Protein denaturation, oxidative damage and the toxic effect of elevated levels of electrolytes result in the killing effect of dry heat.

1)Hot air sterilizer: Materials which are likely to be affected by contacting with steam but can withstand high temperature for the length of time, such as empty glassware, forceps, scissors, porcelain, all-glass injection syringe, can be sterilized by hot air sterilizer. It is reliable to treat materials at 160–170 ℃ for 2 hours (Figure 5–10).

2)Incineration: Incineration is a waste treatment process involving the combustion of organic substances contained in waste materials. This is an excellent sterilization method which can safely destroy contaminated materials at a high temperature, especially for animal corpses or pathological waste materials before they are discarded with non-hazardous waste. Bacteria incinerators incinerate and kill off any microorganisms that may be on an inoculating loop or wire by using mini furnaces.

3)Flaming: The flaming sterilization includes exposure of inoculating loops and the necks of flasks in laboratory to a Bunsen flame until it glows red ensures that any infectious agent is inactivated. Besides, dipping inoculation loops and needles with infective material in methylated spirit and burning off the alcohol can be used to prevent spattering(Figure 5–11).

4)Microwaves: Microwaves are a form of electromagnetic radiation with wavelengths ranging from one meter to one millimeter; the heating effect in micro-wave-oven is not uniform and it is easy to isolate bacteria from the interior of recently used microwave oven. Therefore, sterilization process using microwaves is unreliable and presently unavailable for non-metal instrument, tableware and so on.

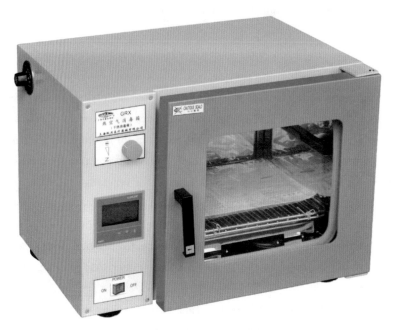

Figure 5-10   **Dry Heat Sterilizer**

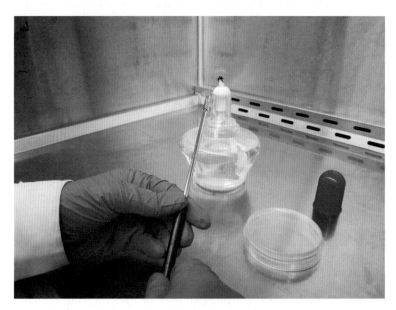

Figure 5-11   **Flaming Sterilization**

(2)Sterilization by Moist Heat

Moisture plays an important role in the moist heat sterilization which causes destruction of microorganisms by denaturation and coagulation of protein. Boiling a sample for 30 minutes or more will kill virtually all vegetative cells present except spores, which can germinate shortly thereafter and resume growth. Therefore, boiling is an insufficient method to achieve sterilization. Steam can raise the temperature of that surface by releasing the latent heat when it condenses on a cooler surface. In the case of the spore, steam can kill them by condensing on it, increasing its water content withthe ultimate hydrolysis and break down of the bacterial protein. Because bacteria, like many proteins, are more resistant to heat in a completely moisture-free atmosphere, they are killed due to oxidation of the cell constituents occurs, which requires much higher temperatures than that needed for coagulation of proteins.

1) Pasteurization: Pasteurization is a process that can inactivate important pathogenic organisms and reduce the number of viable pathogens in foods by using heat at a temperature sufficient tokill microbes but below that needed to ensure sterilization. It is named for French scientist Louis Pasteur during the nineteenth century. Pasteur discovered that heating beer and wine can kill most of the bacteria that caused spoilage, preventing these beverages from turning sour. Unlike sterilization, pasteurization is unable to kill all microorganisms in the food. Originally, pasteurization of milk was used to reduce the number of pathogenic bacteria, especially the microbial-induced tuberculosis, brucellosis, Q fever and typhoid fever and luckily the shelf life of milk was also improved at the same time. Besides, pasteurization prevents the spread of pathogens such as *Salmonella* species and *Escherichia coli* O157 ： H7 through common sources such as milk and juices in developed countries where these pathogens are no longer common in food. Pasteurization also acts on spoilage organisms, dramatically increases the shelf life of perishable liquids.

Passing the milk through a heat exchanger can achieve pasteurization of milk. Older pasteurization methods used temperatures (e. g. 63–66 ℃ for 30 minutes) below boiling to prevent micelles of the milk protein casein from aggregating irreversibly or curdle. However, they are less satisfactory because the milk heats and cools slowly and must be held at high temperatures for longer times. Newer methods use higher temperature, but shorten the time, such as *flash pasteurization*: the milk is fed through tubing which is connected to a heat source. The key steps are careful control of the milk flow rate, the size and temperature of the heat source to raise the temperature of the milk to 71 ℃ for 15 seconds then rapidly cooled it. The whole process is called *flash pasteurization* which alters the flavor less, kills heat-resistant organisms more effectively and is normally done on a continuous-flow basis. The flash pasteurization method which is more adaptable to large dairy operations, often with even shorter exposure times and higher temperatures is employed in modern dairies (Figure 5–12).

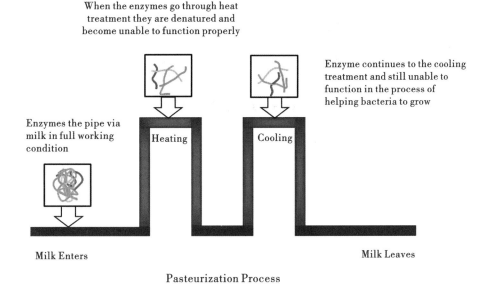

Figure 5–12　General Overview of the Pasteurization Process

2) Boiling water: Boiling water is intended to kill microbes that may be present, making it potable. Different microorganisms have different sensitivity to heat, but if water is held at 70 ℃ (158 °F) for ten mi-

nutes, many organisms are killed, but some are more resistant to heat. For example, vegetative bacteria are killed at 100 ℃ for 5 minutes, but spore bacteria require prolonged periods of boiling for 1-2 hours. Adding 2% sodium bicarbonate to the water can promote sterilization. Boiling which can't sterilize of instrument used for surgical procedures should be considered only as a mean of disinfection for tableware, instrument used for surgical procedures and glass syringe.

3) Steam under pressure sterilization: The autoclave whichplays a pivotal role in heat sterilization is a sealed pressure chamber that allows the entrance of steam is under pressure. It is common sensible that when water is heated to its boiling point, it will boil and produce steam; besides, the vapour pressure of water is equal to the pressure exerted on it by the surrounding atmosphere. The higher the pressure is, the higher the boiling point is. Heating at temperatures above boiling and the use of steam under pressure is essential to sterilize the heat resistant endospores. Note that it is the high temperature under the corresponding steam pressure rather than the pressure of the autoclave that kills the microorganisms. At sea-level, water boils at 100 ℃ under atmospheric pressure. Since liable sterilization with moist heat requires temperature above that of boiling water, pressure in an autoclave should be higher. At 103.4 kPa (1.05 kg/cm^2), the temperature may be up to 121.3 ℃ and all microorganisms including bacterial spores can be killed for 15-20 minutes, so it is widely used to sterilize ordinary medium, saline, operation dressing, intravenous equipment and all materials, which can withstand high temperature, moisture and pressure (Figure 5-13).

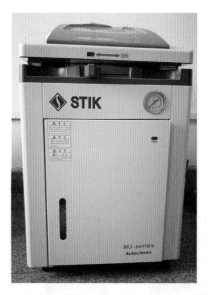

Figure 5-13   **High pressure steam sterilizer**

5.8.1.2   Sterilization by Radiation

However, each type of radiation is achieved through a specific mechanism. For example, microwaves act on the microorganisms through thermal effects. Antimicrobial effects of microwaves are due, at least in part, to thermal effects. Non-ionizing and ionizing are two types of radiation used for sterilization. The non-ionizing low energy type includes infrared and ultraviolet rays while the high energy ionizing type includes X-rays, γ-rays and high energy electrons, which is an effective way to sterilize or reduce the microbial burden in almost any substance.

(1) Non-ionizing Radiation

UV light is used to disinfect surfaces, air and other materials that do not absorb the UV waves, which cause breaks in DNA and lead to the death of the exposed organism. The 260 nm UV wavelength is the most effective for killing microbes and widely used to control microbes in air for disinfecting enclosed areas such as entryways, operation theatres and laboratories. However, there are some disadvantages about ultraviolet radiation. A major disadvantage of UV light as a disinfectant is that the radiation is not very penetrating. So if protected by solids and such coverings as paper, glass and textiles and not directly exposed to the rays, the organisms are not killed. Besides, UV light is harmful to human eyes and skin, if exposed for a long time, can cause burns and skin cancer in human by producing non-mutagenic effects.

(2) Ionizing Radiation

Ionizing radiation such as X-rays, γ-rays and cosmic rays is electromagnetic radiation of enough energy to liberate electrons from atoms or molecules, thereby ionizing them and producing electrons, e^-, hydroxyl radicals, OH · and hydride radicals, H · , which are capable of degrading and altering biopolymers such as deoxyribonucleic acid (DNA) and protein, leading to the death of irradiated cells. In addition, ionizing radiation can interact directly with DNA and cause breaks in the polymer. Unlike non-ionizing radiation, they have very high penetrative power. And the sterilizing effects of ionizing radiation are useful for cleaning medical instruments, food irradiation and so on.

Ionizing radiation has several sources, which include X-ray machines, cathode ray tubes and radioactive nuclides. Either X-rays or γ-rays they produce have sufficient energy and penetrating power which can effectively inhibit microbial growth in solid and liquid culture medium. The radioactive nuclides emitting γ-rays are supreme sources of commercially useful ionizing radiation. ^{60}Co and ^{137}Cs comparatively inexpensive secondary products of nuclear fission are the most generally used radioactive isotopes. At present, radiation is used for sterilization and decontamination in the medical supplies and food industries. However, because of fears of possible radioactive contamination, alteration in nutritional value, production of toxic or carcinogenic products and production of "off" tastes in irradiated food, the use of radiation is slow to gain acceptance in other purposes in many countries.

(3) Sterilization by Ultrasonic and Sonic Vibration

Ultrasonic and sonic waves are considered to be able to kill bacteria but microorganisms vary in their sensitivity to them and spores will remain on the objects after such treatment. Hence this method is normally followed by sterilization.

5.8.1.3 Sterilization by Filtration

In most situations, we tend to heat liquids for purpose of sterilization. But for some heat-sensitive liquids or gases, filtration should be used. Positive or negative pressure filtration can remove both live and dead microorganisms from liquid. A filter is a device with many pores, which is too small for the corridor of microorganisms but large enough to allow the liquid or gas to pass.

Now we have three major types of filters. The oldest type is the depth filter, in which the particles will pass tortuous paths. The main structure of depth filter is the fibrous sheet or mat that is made from the random array of overlapping paper, asbestos or glass fibers. Depth filters are often used as prefilters to remove larger particles from a solution in case of clogging in the final filter sterilization process, because they are rather porous.

Themembrane filters which are usually composed of cellulose esters (e. g. , cellulose acetate) whose pore sizes range from 0. 005 μm to 1 μm, are the most frequently used for sterilization in the field of microbiology, which contain a large number of tiny holes. Filters with a pore size of 0. 2 μm act not only mechanically but also by electrostatic adsorption of particles to their surface to remove bacteria. The size of those holes in the membrane (the size of the molecules passing through) can be accurately controlled by adjusting the polymerization conditions during manufacture. The membrane filter's function is more like a sieve, trapping many of the particles on the filter surface (Figure 5-14).

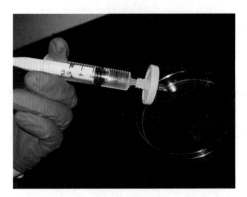

Figure 5-14 Sterilization by Filtration

The third type in common use is the nucleation track (Nucleopore) filter. These filters are produced by treating very thin polycarbonate films (10 μm in thickness) with nuclear radiation and then etching the film with a chemical. First, localized damage will be caused in the film by the radiation; then these damaged locations will be enlarged into holes by the etching chemical. We can accurately control the sizes of the holes by the strength of the etching solution and the etching time. There are very uniform holes arranged almost vertically through the thin film in a typical Nucleopore filter, which can remove an organism from liquid and concentrate it in a single plane on the top of the filter. Then we can observe this organism with the microscope readily.

As a sterilizer, the filter itself needs to be sterilized. At the time of filtration, the filter apparatus and the filter will be assembled into the apparatus aseptically after sterilized separately. For large-volume sterile filtration, the membrane filter material is arranged in a cartridge and placed in a stainless steel housing. And it is very common to see the large-volume filtration of heat-sensitive fluids in the pharmaceutical industry. Filtration forces the liquid through the filtration apparatus into a sterile collection vessel by using a syringe, pump or vacuum. Conversely, in most laboratories, presterilized membrane filter assemblies for sterilization of small to medium volumes are more routinely used.

Filtration sterilization is used to disinfect liquids that containing heat-labile components, including serum and other blood products, vaccines, drugs, enzymes and media. In addition, filtration can sterilize milk and beer without altering their flavor. It is also an important step in water purification. However, it is unable to remove soluble molecules (toxins) that can cause disease. For microorganisms smaller than the pore size, it is not considered to be effective.

5.8.1.4 Drying and Low Temperature

Drying in air is not conducive to the growth of many bacteria, because moisture is an indispensable part of the bacterial growth. However, this method can't inactivate spores. And the effect of low temperatures on microorganisms is related to the kinds of microbe and the intensity of the application. Low temperature is often used to preserve them for limited periods of time rather than kill most microorganisms by itself. Most microorganisms die slowly due to their environmental temperature below their growth range; and the lower the temperature, the more slowly they die.

Slow freezing is more harmful to bacteria than rapidly attained the subfreezing temperature, which tends to render microbes dormant but not necessarily kill them, while slow freezing results in the form and growth of ice crystals which disrupt the cellular and molecular structure of the bacteria. Bacterial cultures can be conserved by rapid freezing, sometimes with the addition of DMSO (dimethyl sulfoxide), glycerol or milk to protect proteins from denaturation and minimize the number of cells killed by freezing.

5.8.2   Chemical Methods

Heating is a reliable way to rid objects of microorganism but can damage heat-sensitive materials such as biological materials, fiber optics and many plastics. In these situations, chemicals can be used as sterilants. At present, there are approximately 10,000 different antimicrobial chemical agents, about 1,000 of which are used routinely in the health care and home environments. Antimicrobial chemicals have liquid, gaseous or even solid state. In most situations, solid or gaseous antimicrobial chemicals are dissolved in water, alcohol or a mixture. They are used for disinfectants, antiseptics, sterilants (chemicals that sterilize) or preservatives (chemicals that inhibit the deterioration of substances). While there are various actual clinical practices of chemical decontamination, some desirable qualities in germicide have been identified, such as efficient action, broad-spectrum microbicidal effect, low toxicity to human, long-term stability, not easily inactivated and so on. Though some chemicals can be considered as bactericide, only chlorhexidine and hydrogen peroxide carry out most of those qualities and approach the ideal. And several chemical compounds are widely used to sterilize bacteria listed in Table 5−3.

It should deserve our concern that the materials to be sterilized ought to be chemically compatible with the sterilant being used. In addition, the properties that make chemicals effective sterilants are usually harmful to humans, which should arouse our attention.

Table 5−3   Characteristics of commonly used disinfectants

Agent	Mechanism of Action	Target Microbes
Alcohols	Denature protein	Most bacteria, viruses, fungi
Iodine	Oxidative denaturation of bacterial proteins	Sporicidal (slowly)
Chlorine	Releases available chlorine in water, inactivating microbial enzymes	Sporicidal (slowly)
Glutaraldehyde	Denature protein	Sporicidal
Formaldehyde	Denature protein, inactivating enzymes	Sporicidal
Hydrogen peroxide	Cellular poisons	Sporicidal
Ethylene oxide gas	Block both DNA replication and enzymatic actions	Sporicidal
Phenolics	Cellular poisons / inactivate enzyme systems	Some bacteria, viruses, fungi

Chapter 6

Introduction of Medical Virology

What can be found in the ancient records (Figure 6-1) illustrates the evidence of a viral disease, smallpox. The Egyptianhieroglyph shows the characteristic of smallpox, a typical withered leg and pustular lesionson the face which Figure out the consequences of poliovirus infection. The poliovirus was possibly endemicin the Ganges river basin and succeedingly spread to other parts of the world.

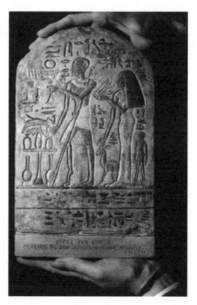

Figure 6-1　An Egyptian stone tablet from the 18th dynasty (1580—1350B. C.)

However, there is no fundamental conception of virusuntil thelate nineteenth century. The scientists made extracts (containing tobacco mosaic virus as we know now) from diseased plants andpassed the extracts through filters. The filtrates were able to infect plants, but no bacteria could be found. Eliminating the possibility of toxin, the scientists called the infective agent a virus (Latin for "poison") and such term has been used ever since.

Viruses are obligate intracellular microorganisms using cellular machinery of living host cells to create progeny virus particles. Comparing other microorganisms(Table 6-1), viruses lack any cellular organelles forthe generation of metabolic energy or protein synthesis out side host cells. Besides, viruses are known to infect all living forms, from eukaryotes (vertebrate animals, invertebrateanimals, plants, fungi) to prokaryotes (bacteria and archaea).

Table 6-1 Viruses vs. other microorganisms

	Virus	Normal Bacteria	Mycoplasma	Rickettsia	Chlamydia	Fungus
Microorganism types	Acellularmicroorganisms	Prokaryotic microorganisms	Prokaryotic microorganisms	Prokaryotic microorganisms	Prokaryotic microorganisms	Eukaryotic microorganisms
Visualized with light microscope	No	Yes	Yes	Yes	Yes	Yes
Passedthrough 0.45 μm filter	Yes	No	Yes	No	Yes	No
cell wall present	No	Yes	Yes	Yes	Yes	Yes
Ribosomes present	No	Yes	Yes	Yes	Yes	Yes
Nuclear acid material	DNA or RNA	DNA+RNA	DNA+RNA	DNA+RNA	DNA+RNA	DNA+RNA
Growth on artificial media	No	Yes	Yes	No	No	Yes
Division by binary fission	No	Yes	Yes	Yes	Yes	No
Sensitive to antibiotics	No	Yes	Yes	Yes	Yes	Yes
Sensitive to Interferon	Yes	No	No	No	No	No

Abroad variety of viruses contribute to human disease, ranging from the trivial common colds to the lethal rabies and viruses also play important roles in the development of several types of cancer. As well as causing individuals to suffer, virus diseases can also affect the well-being of societies. Smallpox had a great impact in the past and AIDS is having a great impact today. There is therefore a requirement to understand the nature of viruses, how viruses replicate and how viruses cause disease.

6.1 General Properties of Viruses

6.1.1 Viral Morphology

6.1.1.1 Viral Size

Viruses are the smallest infectious microorganisms, vary in size from 20 nm to 300 nm and can only be seen by electron microscopy. By contrast, bacterial are typically around 1,000 nm in diameter and the cells of higher organisms a few tens of micrometers (Figure 6-2).

6.1.1.2 Viral Structure

Outside the host cells, viruses survive as infectious particles, also known as virions. The virion is actually a gene delivery systemto protect the genome until it can be delivered into a cell in which it can replicate. All virions consist of two (naked viruses) or three parts (enveloped viruses). ①The viral genome (DNA or RNA) contains genetic information. ②The protein coat, called the capsid, encloses and protects the viral genome. Moreover, the capsid together with the enclosed viral genome is called the nucleocapsid. Some virus families have. ③An outer envelope, which is alipid bilayer surrounding the viral capsid.

The capsid contains many small errepeating subunits which are called capsomere sencoded by the viral genomeserving as the basis for morphological distinction. Such capsomereswill self-assemble to form a capsid. In general, there are three main viral morphological types: helical, icosahedral (20-sided) or complex (Figure 6-3).

(1) Helical

These viruses are composed of a single type of capsomere stacked around a central axis to form a helical structure, which may have a central cavity or tube. This arrangement results in rod-shaped or filamentous virions which can be short and highly rigid or long and very flexible. The genetic material is bound into the protein helix by electrostatic interaction between the negative charged nucleic acid and the positive charged protein. Overall, the length of a helical capsid is related to the length of the nucleic acid contained within it and the diameter is dependent on the size and arrangement of capsomeres. The well-studied tobacco mosaic virus is an example of a helical virus.

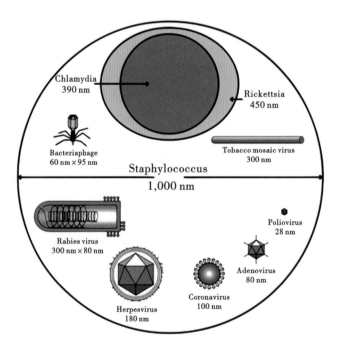

Figure 6-2　Shapes and sizes of virus particles

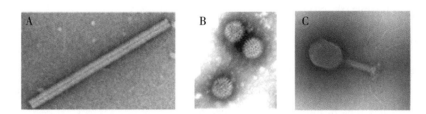

Figure 6-3　Electron micrographs of viruses of different morphological types.

A. Helical particle of tobacco mosaic virus; B. Icosahedral particles of human rotavirus; C. Complexparticle ofbacteriophage T4

（2）Icosahedral

Most animal viruses are icosahedral or near-spherical with chiral icosahedral symmetry. A regular icosahedron is the optimum way of forming a closed shell from capsomeres. The minimum number of identical capsomeres required for each triangular face is 3, which gives 60 for the icosahedron. Many viruses, such as rotavirus, have more than 60 capsomeres and appear spherical but retaining this symmetry. To achieve this, the capsomeres at the apices are surrounded by five other capsomeres and are called pentons. Capsomeres on the triangular faces are surrounded by six others and are called hexons. Hexons are in essence flat and pentons, which form the 12 vertices, are curved. The same protein may act as the subunit of both the pentamers and hexamers or they may be composed of different proteins.

（3）Complex

These viruses possess a capsid that is neither purely helical nor purely icosahedral and that may possess extra structures such as protein tails or a complex outer wall. Some bacteriophages, such as Enterobacteria phage T4, have a complex structure consisting of an icosahedral head bound to a helical tail, which may have a hexagonal base plate with protruding protein tail fibers. This tail structure acts like a molecular syringe, attaching to the bacterial host and then injecting the viral genome into the cell.

（4）Viralenvelope

Some species of virus envelop themselves in a modified form of one of the cell membranes, mainly from the outer membrane of an infected host cell, in some cases from internal membranes such as nuclear membrane or endoplasmic reticulum, during virions release（budding）from the infected cell. The exterior of the bilayer is studded with transmembrane proteins coded by viral genome, revealed as glycoprotein spikes or knobs. The lipid membrane itself and any carbohydrates present originate entirely from the host. The influenza virus and HIV use this strategy. Most enveloped viruses are dependent on the envelope for their infectivity.

6.1.2　Viralfunctional Compositions

6.1.2.1　Viral Genomes

By definition, the nucleic acid in the virion is the viral genome. In somecases, viral genomes can participate in the replication cycle directly. In others, viral genomes must first be modified and then participate in the replication cycle. For each strategy, the viral genomes contain the following essential information：genome structure, degree of dependence on host for replication, gene expression strategies and noteworthy features of the interaction with the host. It is clear that the viral genome determines the heredity and variation of viruses and the method of packaging and replication.

Any one virus haseither a DNA or an RNA genome, called a DNA virus or an RNA virus, respectively. Unlike the complementary paired double-stranded DNA of cells, each genome of virionsis eithersingle-stranded（ss）or double-stranded（ds）, giving four categories of virus genome：double-stranded DNA（dsDNA）, single-stranded DNA（ssDNA）, double-stranded RNA（dsRNA）and single-stranded RNA（ssRNA）.

For most viruses with RNA genomes, the single strands are said to be either positive-sense or negative-sense. Some genomes of RNA viruses are in the same sense as viral mRNA and thus function directly as messenger RNA（mRNA）without further modification, so called positive-sense［（+）strand］RNA. In other RNA viruses, the RNA is a complementary copy of mRNA and thus must be converted to positive-sense RNA by an RNA-dependent RNA polymerase before translation, so called negative-sense［or the（-）strand］RNA. Besides, the genomes of RNA viruses may be present as a single strandas in paramyxoviruses or as two copies as in the retroviruses or exist as a specific number of fragmentsas in the orthomyxoviruses and reoviruses.

Generally, virus genomes are much smaller than cell genomes. The amount of nucleic acid in virions is constant for a particular virus but shows considerable variation in size. The smallest virus known is tobacconecrosis satellite virus, with an ssRNA genome of 1,239 bases, while there are 375 kilobase pairs in the largest poxviruses. However, all viruses lack the genetic information necessary to generate metabolic energy or protein synthesis. The viral genomes rarely have intronsand code for more than the few protein snecessary for replication or physical structure.

6.1.2.2 Viral Proteins

As the size of thevirus genome increases, so the number of proteins tends to increase. With smallgenome, the virion of tobacco mosaic virus contains only one kind of protein. However, the virions of herpessimplex virus 1 (HSV-1) contain 50 proteins. Analysis of such proteins produced in a cell during viral infection shows that some proteins are the essential components of the viruses. Based on whether the virion contains the proteins, such proteins are divided into two groups, the structural proteins and non-structural proteins.

The structural proteins include enzymes and capsid proteins as well as basic core proteins that are necessary to package the nucleic acid. Additionally, the essential steps of virus attachment and penetration to the host cellare known to depend on the outer proteins, such as the apical fibers and knobs of naked virus adenoviruse or the glycoproteins (spike) of enveloped viruses, such as in fluenza A and B (HA, NAand M2) and the human immunodeficiency virus (HIV) (gp120 and gp41). Many viruses carry essential enzymes in the virion. An RNA-dependentRNA polymerase or transcriptase is a fundamental component of the negative-strand RNA viruses. And the hepadnaviruses have a virionpolymerase complex that has similarity to the reverse transcriptase of theretroviruses.

Suchstructural proteins haveto carry out a wide range of functions, including:

1) protection and packaging of the virus genome

2) attachment of the virion to a host cell (for many viruses)

3) fusion of the virion envelope to a cell membrane (for enveloped viruses)

4) involving in the process of replication cycle; e. g. reverse transcriptase

5) formation of ion channels in viral and cell membranes; e. g. M2 in influenza A virus

Other proteins suchas enzymes are needed for the production of viral components but are not part of the virion, called the non-structural proteins. Generally, such non-structural proteins may be expressed after the step of virus penetration and have additional roles, including:

1) enzymes, e. g. protease

2) transcription factors

3) interference with the immune response of the host

Moreover, there is no standard nomenclature system for viral proteinson account of different groups of viruses. However, the following system has been adoptedfor quite a number ofviruses. The proteins are numbered indecreasing order of size:

1) structural proteins: VP1, VP2, VP3···(VP, virus protein)

2) non-structural proteins: NSP1, NSP2, NSP3···

Many virus proteins arenamed by an abbreviation of one or two letters, which mayindicate:

1) a structural characteristic: G (glycoprotein), P (phosphoprotein), M (matrix protein)

2) a functional characteristic: F (fusion protein), RT (reverse transcriptase), P (polymerase)

6.1.2.3   Viral Membranes

Enveloped viruses have an outer surface with lipid membrane component. This structure is known as an envelope and it encloses the nucleocapsid of the enveloped viruses. For the lipid membraneis a modified form derived from one of the host cell membranes, theenvelope of viruses is prone to fuse with host cell membranes.

In most of these viruses, the membrane is studded with one or more kinds ofviral proteins. Most of these proteins are O-and/or N-glycosylated. Many of the glycoproteins in virion envelopes are multimers. For example, the envelope of influenzaA virus contains two glycoproteins: hemagglutinin (trimers) and neuraminidase (tetramers). There is also a third protein(M2) that is not glycosylated. Some surface glycoproteins of enveloped viruses perform the function of fusing the virion membrane to a cell membrane during the replication cycle. These fusion proteins have an additional hydrophobic region that plays a major rolein the fusion process.

Many enveloped viruses have a layer of proteins between the envelope and the nucleocapsid. This protein is often called amatrix protein. In some viruses, however, such as yellow fever virus, there is no such layer and the nucleocapsid interacts directly with the internal tails of the integral membrane protein molecules.

6.1.3   Replication Cycle (Life Cycle)

The aim of a virus is to replicate itself to make thousands more by entering the host cell, making new copy of the viralgenome, encoding viral proteins which assemble to form new virus particles (Figure 6-4). Ingeneral, the replication cycle of viruses differs between species but there are six basic stages in the life cycle of viruses: Attachment, Penetration, Uncoating, Biosynthesis, Assemblyand Release. These are used here for convenience in explaining the replication cycle of a nonexistent "typical" virus. Regardless of their hosts, all viruses must undergo each of these stages in some form to successfully complete their replication cycles. Not all the stages are distinctly detecTable for all viruses and some appear to occur almost simultaneously.

6.1.3.1   Attachment

Viral infection is initiated by a collision between the virion and the cell governed by chance. Therefore, a higher concentration of virus particles increases the probability of infection. However, a virion may not infect every cell it encounters. Attachment is specific binding between outer viral proteins and specific receptors on the host membrane, like a key fitting in its lock. This specificity determines the host range of a virus. It has been found that some viruses need to bind to a second type of cell surface molecule (co-receptor) in order to infect the host cell. In at least some cases, binding to a receptor causes a conformational change in the viral protein that enables it to bind to the co-receptor. For example, the HIV infects only human T cells, because viral surface proteins, gp120 and gp41, can only react with the receptor CD4 and the co-receptor CXCR4 or CCR5 on the T cellular surface, respectively.

Some cell surface molecules used by viruses as receptors are sugars, but most are glycoproteins. Some-examples are given in Table 6-2.

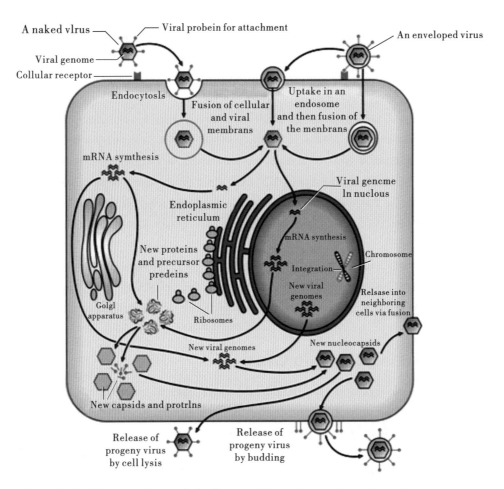

Figure 6-4　Diagram of a cell indicating possible pathways for various viruses may use during their replication cycles

Table 6-2　Examples of cell receptors, virus proteins involved in attachment

Virus	Viral protein involved in attachment	Host cell receptor
Poliovirus	VP1 + VP3	CD155
Rhinovirus	VP1 + VP3	ICAM-1
ECHO virus	VP1 + VP3	VLA-2 integrin
Influenza virus A and B	Hemagglutinin	Sialic acid
HIV-1	gp120, gp41	CD4, CCR5, CXCR4
EBV	gp320	CD21
Measles virus	Hemagglutinin	CD46

6.1.3.2　Penetration

Penetration of the host cell normally occurs a very short time after attachment of the virus to its receptor in the cell membrane. Unlike attachment, penetration is generallyan energy-dependent process by receptor-mediated endocytosis for most naked viruses or membrane fusion for most enveloped viruses.

There are a number of endocytic mechanisms, including clathrin-mediated endocytosis and caveolin-mediated endocytosis. For example, adenoviruses and vesicular stomatitis virus penetrate the host cell by clathrin-mediated endocytosis. Molecules of clathrin accumulate onthe inner side of the plasma membrane at the site where the virion attached. The clathrin forces the membrane to bend around the virion to form a pit, which ispinched off to form a clathrin-coated vesicle. The clathrin is lost fromthe vesicle leaving the virion in an endosome. Some viruses, such as simian virus 40, are endocytosed at caveolin-coated regions of the plasma membrane and the virionsend up in caveolin-coated endosomes.

Fusion of the virus envelope with the cell membrane, either directly at the cell surface or following endocytosis in acytoplasmic vesicle, requires the presence of a specific fusionprotein in the virus envelope, for example, influenza hemagglutinin or retrovirus transmembrane (TM) glycoproteins. These proteins promote the joining of the cellular and viral membranes which results in the nucleocapsid being deposited directly in the cytoplasm.

6.1.3.3   Uncoating

Uncoatingis a general term for the events that occur after penetration and happens inside the cell when the viral capsid is completely or partially removed. This may be by degradation by viral enzymes or host enzymes or by simple dissociation, thereby exposing the viral genomic nucleic acid, usually in the form of a nucleoprotein complex. It should be noted that successful entry of a virion into a cell is not always followedby virus replication. The host's intracellular defenses, such as lysosomalenzymes, may inactivate infectivity before or after uncoating. In some cases the virus genome may initiate a latent infection rather than a complеtereplication cycle.

The product of uncoating depends on the structure of the virus nucleocapsid. In some cases, it might be relatively simple (e. g. , picornaviruses have a small basicprotein of approximately 23 amino acids [VPg] covalently attached to the 5′ end of the viral RNA genome) or highly complex (e. g. , retrovirus cores are highly ordered nucleoprotein complexes that contain, in addition to the diploid RNA genome, the reverse transcriptase enzyme responsible for converting the virus RNA genomeinto the DNA provirus). The structure and chemistry of the nucleocapsid determines the subsequent steps in replication.

6.1.3.4   Biosynthesis

Biosynthesis is the stage involving primarily multiplication of the genomes and synthesis of viral messenger RNA (mRNA)to produce viral proteinsby the synthesis abilities of the host cell. In this respect, all viruses can be divided into seven groups based on the genome replication and the expression of genes. A schematic overview of the major events during replication of the different virus genomes is shown in Figure 6–5.

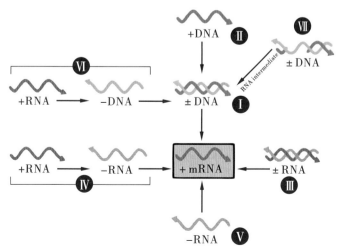

Figure 6–5   Replication of virus genomes in the seven Baltimore Classes

1) Class Ⅰ : Double-stranded DNA. This class can be subdivided into two further groups : (a) replication is exclusively nuclear , so replication of these viruses is relatively dependent on cellular factors and (b) replication occurs in cytoplasm (Poxviridae) , in which case the viruses have evolved (or acquired) all the necessary factors for transcription and replication of their genomes and are therefore largely independent of the cellular machinery. This class involves synthesis of viral mRNA from "early" genes , viral protein synthesis , then viral genome replication mediated by early or regulatory protein expression. This may be followed by one or more further rounds of mRNA synthesis : "late" gene expression is , in general , of structural or virion proteins.

2) Class Ⅱ : Single-stranded DNA. Replication occurs in the nucleus , involving the formation of a double-stranded intermediate which serves as atemplate for the synthesis of single-stranded progeny DNA and viral mRNA.

3) Class Ⅲ : Double-stranded RNA. These viruses have segmented genomes. Each segment is transcribed separately to produce individual monocistronic mRNAs.

4) Class Ⅳ : Single-stranded (+) sense RNA. Viruses with complex transcription , for which two rounds of translation are necessary to produce the genomic RNA. The genomes of viruses are replicated by synthesis of complementary strands of RNA that are then used as templates for synthesis of new copies of the genome. As with most viruses inthis class , the genome RNA forms the mRNA and is translated to form apolyprotein product , which is subsequently cleaved to form the mature proteins.

5) Class Ⅴ : Single-stranded (−) sense RNA. The genomes of these viruses can be divided into two types : ①Nonsegmented genomes (order Mononegvirales) , for which the first step inreplication is transcription of the (−) sense RNA genome by the virion RNA dependent RNA polymerase to produce monocistronic mRNAs , which also serve as the template for subsequent genome replication. ②Segmented genomes (Orthomyxoviridae) , for which replication occurs in the nucleus , with monocistronic mRNAs for each of the virus genes produced by the virus transcriptase from the full-length virus genome.

6) Class Ⅵ : Single-stranded (+) sense RNA with DNA intermediate. Retrovirus genomes are (+) sense RNA but unique in that they are diploid andthey do not serve directly as mRNA , but as a template for reverse transcriptioninto DNA. This DNA is then incorporated into the host's own DNA and copied into mRNA by the normal pathways.

7) Class Ⅶ : Double-stranded DNA with RNA intermediate. This group of viruses also relies on reverse transcription , but , unlike the retroviruses (class Ⅵ) , this process occurs inside the virus particle during maturation. On infection of a new cell , the first event to occuris repair of the gapped genome , followed by transcription. Both of thesemodes of genome replication involve reverse transcription (class Ⅵ and Ⅶ) , which has two major steps : synthesis of (−) DNA from a (+) RNA template followed by synthesis of asecond DNA strand. Both steps are catalyzed by a reverse transcriptase that is encoded by the virus.

6.1.3.5　Assembly

Assembly involves the collection of all the components necessary forthe structure-mediated self-assembly of the mature virion at a particular site in the cell. The formation of virus particles may be a relatively simple process which is driven only by interactions between the subunits of the capsid and controlled by the rules of symmetry. In other cases , assembly is a highly complex , multistep process involving not only virus structural proteins but alsovirus-encoded and cellular scaffolding proteins that act as templates to guide theassembly of virions. The encapsidation of the virus genome may occur either earlyin the assembly of the particle (e. g. , many viruses with helical symmetry are nucleated on the genome) or at a late stage , when the genome is stuffed into an almost completed protein shell.

In spite of considerable study, the control of virus assembly is not well understood. However, the site of assembly depends on the site of replication in the host cell and on the mechanism by which the virus is eventually released from the cell and varies for different viruses. In the case of picornaviruses, poxviruses and reoviruses, assembly occurs in the cytoplasm; in adenoviruses, polyomaviruses and parvoviruses, it occurs in the nucleus. Following the self-assembly, some modification of the proteins, at which the virus becomes infectious (sometimes called maturation), often occurs. Maturation usually involves structural changes that may result from specific cleavages of capsid proteins to form the mature products or conformational changes in proteins during assembly. For some viruses, assembly and maturation occur inside the cell and are inseparable, whereas for others maturation events may occur only after release of the virus particle from the host cell-such as HIV.

In general, it is thought that rising intracellular levels of virus proteins and genome molecules reach a critical concentration and that this triggers the process. Many viruses achieve high levels of newly syn the sized structural components by concentrating these into subcellular compartments, visible in light microscopes, which are known as inclusion bodies. These are a common feature of the late stages of infection of cells by many different viruses. The size and location of inclusion bodies in infected cells is often highly characteristic of particular viruses. For example, rabies virus infection results in large perinuclear 'Negri bodies', first observed by Adelchi Negri in 1903. Alternatively, local concentrations of virus structural components can be boosted by lateral interactions between membrane-associated proteins. This mechanism is particularly important in enveloped viruses released from the cell by budding.

6.1.3.6   Release

Release occurs when the new viruses escape from the cell by either sudden rupture of the cell or gradual extrusion (budding) of enveloped viruses through the cell membrane. Nearly all viruses escape the cell by one of the two mechanisms. For lytic viruses (such as most naked viruses), release is a simple process that the infected cell breaks open and releases the virus. Release of virus particles in this way may be highly damaging to the host cell.

Enveloped viruses (e. g. , HIV) typically are released from the host cell by budding and acquire the envelope but the cells survive by the replication process. The envelope is a modified piece of the host's cytoplasmic membrane or intracellular vesicle membrane. In most cases, budding involves cytoplasmic membranes (retroviruses, togaviruses orthomyxoviruses, paramyxoviruses, bunyaviruses, coronaviruses, rhabdoviruses, hepadnaviruses). But in some cases budding can involve the nuclear membrane (herpesviruses). Besides, virion envelope proteins are picked up during this process as the virus particle is extruded. As with the early stages of replication cycle, assembly and release are usually simultaneous processes for viruses released by budding.

6.1.3.7   Abnormalities During Infection

▶▶ *Abortive infection*

As already stated above, host cells must be both susceptible and permissive if an infection is to be successful. For viruses that bind to the host cell surface as the first step in infection, the cell must have appropriate receptors that the virus can bind to. Furthermore, all the requirements of the virus must either be present in the cell or be inducible. These requirements include proteins, such as transcription factors and enzymes. This mechanism has evolved to favor those viruses that only infect proper cells (permissive cell) in which they are capable of proliferation. In some cases, specific binding can be side-stepped by nonspecific orinappropriate interactions between virus particles and cells. It is possible that virus particles can be 'accidentally' taken up by cells via processes such as pinocytosis orphagocytosis. However, the improper cell (nonpermissive cell) doesn't allow the virus to circumvent its defenses and reproduce into more infectious viruses, which is so called abortive infection.

(1) Defectiveviruses

Defective virusesare virus particles that contain in sufficient nucleic acid to provide for production of all essential viral components. Such a virus may, however, replicate and produce progeny in the presence of another non-defective virus called a helper virus that can provide the missing function(s). Hepatitis B virus (HBV) is an example of a helper virus that helps Hepatitis D virus (HDV) (a replication defective, helper dependent ssRNA virus) to replicate. For HDV, it requires the surface antigen of HBV (HBsAg) for the encapsidation of its own genome. The envelope proteins on the outer surface of HDV are entirely provided by HBV.

(2) Virusinterference

Virus inter ference is the inhibition of the replication of a virus by a previous infection with another virus. The two viruses may be unrelated, related or identical. In some cases, virus interference may take place even if the first virus was inactivated. Several mechanisms of interference can be distinguished: ①Inactivation of cell receptors by one virus may prevent subsequent adsorption and penetration by another virus. ②The first virus may inhibit or modify cellular enzymes or proteins required for replication of the superinfecting virus. ③The first virus may generate destructive enzymes or induce the cell to synthesize protective substances which prevent superinfection. ④ The first virus may generate defective interfering particles (DIPs) or mutants which may inhibit the replication of the infecting virus by competing with it for a protein (or enzyme) available in limited quantities. This interfering nature is becoming more and more important for future research on virus therapies. It is thought that because of their specificity, DIPs will be targeted to sites of infection. In one example, scientists have used DIPs to create "protecting viruses", which attenuated the pathogenicity of an influenza A infection in mice to a point that it was no longer lethal.

6.1.4　Mutations Ingenes and Resulting Changes to Viruses

Sometimes, during replication cycle, mutations may occur. Deletion mutations can remove anentire gene in replication and produce truncated gene products. Insertion mutations can be made by the addition of unrelated sequences or sequences derived from a closely related virus. Substitution mutations, which can correspond to one or more nucleotides, are often made in coding or noncoding regions. Included in the latter class are nonsense mutations, in which a termination codon is introduced and missense mutations, in which a single nucleotide or a codon is changed, resulting in the production of a protein with a single amino acidsubstitution. The introduction of a termination codon is frequently exploited to cause truncation of a membraneprotein so that it is secreted or to eliminate the synthesis of a protein without changing the size of the viral genome or mRNA.

Because of rapidgenome replication, relative enzymes of viruses are often error prone with appreciablefrequency, which is a process called antigenic drift where individual bases in the DNA or RNA mutate to other bases. For example, amismatched A : C pair could be formed during replication of DNA instead of A : T or an A : T pair could bemiscopied into G : T. More rarely, a piece of nucleic acid could be lost due to some slippage of polymerase. Like HIV, the polymerase can generate one point mutation for every 10,000 basestranscribed so that many changes are generated. However, most of these point mutations are "silent", which do not change the protein that the gene encodes, but others can confer evolutionary advantages such as resistance to antiviral drugs or the immune system of host.

By natural selection, antigenic shiftmay occur when there is a major change in the genome of the virus. This can be a result of recombination or reassortment. Or point mutations accumulate and lead to the generation of small antigenic differences between strains or serotypesover long time spans. Manyaccumulated mutations lead to changes in virulence of thevirus, that is, changes in the severity of symptoms and course of viral infection in the host. Like influenza viruses, different strains with segmented genome can shuffle and combine genes and produce progeny viruses that might result in pandemics potentially (Figure 6-6). On the contrary, whena disease-causing virus is passaged for long times in cell cultures or in a non-natural animal host, attenuation of virus strains may occur and allow the generation of live-virus vaccines.

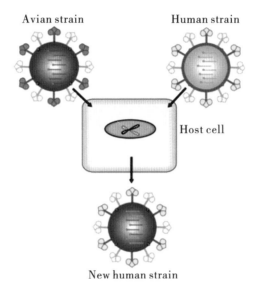

Avian strain   Human strain

Host cell

New human strain

Figure 6 - 6   How antigenic shift or reassortment, can result in novel and highly pathogenic strains of influenza viruse

6.1.5 Stability and Viability

6.1.5.1 Temperature

Mostviruses are cold-resistant. The temperature below 0 ℃, especially at the dry ice temperature (-70 ℃) and liquid nitrogen (-196 ℃), can maintain its infectivity for a long time. Most viruses are inactivated at 50-60 ℃ for 30 minutes. The inactivation of virus by heat is mainly due to the degeneration of capsid protein and the change of virus coated glycoprotein spike, which prevents virus from attachment on host cells. Heat can also destroy the enzymes needed for virus replication, so that the virus can not be shelled.

6.1.5.2 pHvalue

Most of the viruses were relatively stable in the range of pH 5-9, but rapidly inactivated under pH 5 or above pH 9. But different viruses had different tolerance to pH value. Many enteric viruses are more stable at pH 3-5 than at pH 9 and above. Adenoviruses and rotaviruses are delicate to pH 10 or greater and lead to inactivation.

6.1.5.3 Rays

Gamma ray, beta-ray and ultraviolet (UV) raycan induce molecular changes in a process called irradiation. Applications of theserays can sterilize medical equipment (as an alternative to autoclaves or chemical methods). Also, they can be used to inactivate virus particles. And the UV ray can induce the dimerization of nucleic acids, so that the virus particles can't replicate their genomes.

6.1.5.4　Fatsolvent

Enveloped virus contains lipid components, which are easily dissolved by ether, trichloromethane, deoxycholate and other fat solvents. Therefore, the enveloped virusescan berapidly destroyed by the bilein the digestive tract. As one of the fat solvents, ether can be used to identify the enveloped or naked virus forits damage to the virus envelope.

6.1.5.5　Other Chemical Components

Many disinfectant, such as Phenol and its derivatives, oxidants and halogens, are protein denaturants, so they can be used to inactive viruses.

6.1.5.6　Antibiotics

Antibiotics have no inhibitory effect on the viruses. However, they can inhibit the bacteria and fungi in the specimens to be examined, so that it is beneficial to isolate and test the viruses.

6.1.6　Virus Vlassification

Viruses are mainly classified by phenotypic characteristics, such as morphology, nucleic acid type, mode of replication, host organisms and the type of diseases they cause. The International Committee on Taxonomy of Viruses (ICTV) began to devise and implement rules fora single, universal taxonomic scheme for all the viruses infecting animals (vertebrates, invertebrates and protozoa), plants (higher plants and algae), fungi, bacteria and archaea since 1970s.

Viral classification starts at the level of order and continues as follows, with the taxon suffixes given in italics:

Order (*-virales*)

　Family (*-viridae*)

Subfamily (*-virinae*)

　Genus (*-virus*)

　　Species

The establishment of an order is based on the inference that the virus families it contains have most likely evolved from a common ancestor. The majority of virus families remain unplaced. As of 2016, 9 orders, 125 families and 4,404 species of viruses have been defined by the ICTV (Some examples in Table 6-3 and Table 6-4). Descriptions of virus satellites, viroids and the agents of spongiform encephalopathies (prions) of humans and several animal and fungal species are included.

Table 6-3　DNA viruses

Virus family	Examples (common names)	Virion naked/enveloped	Capsid symmetry	Nucleic acid type	Group of baltimore classes
Adenoviridae	Adenovirus	Naked	Icosahedral	ds	I
Parvoviridae	Papillomavirus	Naked	Icosahedral	ds circular	I
Poxviridae	Smallpox virus	Enveloped	Complex	ds	I

Continue to Table 6-3

Virus family	Examples (common names)	Virion naked/enveloped	Capsid symmetry	Nucleic acid type	Group of baltimore classes
Herpesviridae	Herpes simplex virus, Varicella-zoster virus, Cytomegalovirus, Epstein-Barr virus	Enveloped	Icosahedral	ds	I
Parvoviridae	Parvovirus B19	Naked	Icosahedral	ss	II
Hepadnaviridae	Hepatitis B virus	Enveloped	Icosahedral	circular, partially ds	VII

Table 6-4   RNA viruses

Virus family	Examples (common names)	Virion naked/enveloped	Capsid symmetry	Nucleic acid type	Group of baltimore classes
Reoviridae	Reovirus, rotavirus	Naked	Icosahedral	ds	III
Flaviviridae	Dengue virus, Hepatitis C virus, Yellow fever virus	Enveloped	Icosahedral	ss	IV
Picornaviridae	Enterovirus, Rhinovirus, Poliovirus, Coxsackievirus	Naked	Icosahedral	ss	IV
Coronaviridae	Corona virus	Enveloped	Helical	ss	IV
Rhabdoviridae	Rabies virus	Enveloped	Helical	ss(−)	V
Filoviridae	Ebola virus, Marburg virus	Enveloped	Helical	ss(−)	V
Orthomyxoviridae	Influenza Avirus, Influenza Bvirus, Influenza Cvirus	Enveloped	Helical	ss(−)	V
Paramyxoviridae	Measles virus, Mumps virus, Respiratory syncytial virus	Enveloped	Helical	ss(−)	V
Retroviridae	HIV, HTLV	Enveloped		Two copies of ss	VI

Subviral agents are smaller than viruses but have only some of their properties, including viroids, satellite viruses and prion.

Viroids are the smallest known agents of infectious disease. Conventional viruses are made up of nucleic acid encapsulated in protein (capsid), whereas viroids are uniquely characterized by the absence of a capsid. In spite of their small size, viroid ribonucleic acids (RNAs) can replicate and produce characteristic disease syndromes when introduced into cells. Viroids thus far identified are associated with plants.

Satellite viruses, which are most commonly associated with plants, but are also found in mammals, arthropods and bacteria, have the components to produce their own protein shell to enclose their genetic material, but rely on a helper virus to replicate. Most viruses have the capability to use host enzymes or their own replication machinery to independently replicate their own viral RNA. Satellite viruses in contrast, are completely dependent on a helper virus for replication. The symbiotic relationship between a satellite and a helper virus to catalyze the replication of a satellite viral genome is also dependent on the host to provide components like replicases to carry out replication.

Prions are infectious agents composed entirely of a protein material that can fold in multiple, structurally abstract ways, at least one of which is transmissible to other prion proteins, leading to disease in a manner that is epidemiologically comparable to the spread of viral infection. Prions composed of the prion protein (PrP) are believed to be the cause of transmissible spongiform encephalopathies (TSEs) among other diseases.

6.2 Viral Infection and Antiviral Immunity

In considering virus diseases, two aspects are involved, the direct effects ofvirus replication (viral infection) and the effects of body's responses to the infection (antiviral inmuunity). The extentand severity of viral infection is determined similarly. In some cases, most of the pathologic symptoms observed are not directly causedby virus replication but are to the side effects of the immune response. Inflammation, fever, headaches and skin rashes are not usually caused by viruses themselves but by the cells of the immune system due to the release of potent chemicals such as interferons and interleukins. It is possible that none of the pathologic effects of certain diseases is caused directly by the virus, except that its presence stimulates activation ofthe immune system. Above all, it is the delicate and dynamic balance between the virus infection and the host defenses.

In the past few decades, molecular analysis has contributed enormously toour understanding of virus pathogenesis. Nucleotide sequencing and site-directed mutagenesis have been used to explore molecular determinants of virulence in many different viruses. Specific sequences and structures foundonly in disease-causing strains of virus and not in closely related attenuatedor avirulent strains have been identified. Sequence analysis has also led to the identification of T-cell and B-cell epitopes on virus proteins responsiblefor their recognition by the immune system. Unfortunately, these advances do not automatically lead to an understanding of the mechanisms responsible for pathogenicity.

6.2.1 Virus Infection

In general, virions must first enter cells at a body surface. Common sites of entry include the mucosal linings of therespiratory, alimentary and urogenital tracts, the outer surface of the eyes (conjunctival membranes or cornea) and the skin (Figure 6-7).

6.2.1.1 Transmission

The chain of infection can be maintained only by spreading from one susceptible host to another (transmission). Viruses need to be able to spread from one host to another in order to survive. The only other possibility for the survival of virusis to be maintained in cells as nucleic acids, which could be replicated and passed on to off spring cells with cell division. Virus properties in fluence the way they are transmitted.

Some viruses such as enteroviruses, hepatitis A and rotavirus, secreted in humanfeces, are resistant and can survive for many weeks in the environment, which allow viruses to be often ingested again whenpeople eat with contaminated hands, eatcontaminated food or drinkcontaminated water. Some viruses such as many paramyxoviruses and HIV are quickly inactivated by drying out and need close contact to be transmitted between humans by inhalingvirus-containing droplets or by sexual activities. Besides, the arboviruses replicate inboth the arthropod host (usually inthe salivary glands) and the vertebratehost with the arthropods transmitting these viruses from the one vertebratehost to the other. Viral infections are transmitted among hosts in specific way (Table 6–5). Horizontal transmission, which relies on a high rate of infection to maintain thevirus population, refers to the direct or indirect host-to-host transmission of viruses. And Vertical transmission refers to the transfer of infection between parentand off spring directly. This may occur by infection of the fetusbefore (intrauterine infection), during (obstetric infection) or after birth (e. g. , by breast feeding). More rarely, it may involve direct transfer of the virus via the germ line itself(e. g. , retroviruses). In contrast to horizontal transmission, this strategy relies on long-term persistence of the virus in the host rather than rapid propagation and dissemination of the virus.

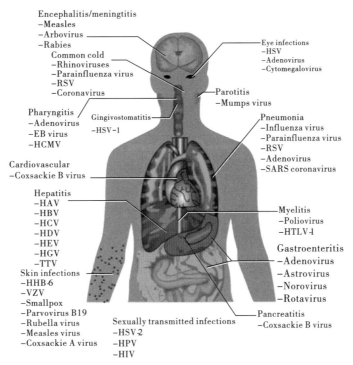

Figure 6–7   An overview of the main types of viral infection and the most notable species involved

Table 6–5   Routes of pathogenic virus transmission

Routeof transmission	Nature of transmission	Examples
Horizontal transmission		
	Close contact: kissing	Herpes simplex virus and Epstein-Barrvirus
	Respiratory droplets	Paramyxoviruses, rubella virus
	Blood and blood products	HIV, Hepatitis B virus, Hepatitis C virus
	Sexual contact	Herpes simplex viruses, HIV
Human-to-humantransmission	Abrasions	HPV
	Contaminated hands: virus excreted infeces	Hepatitis A virus, rotavirus
	Contaminated hands: virus in respiratorysecretion	Rhinovirus

Continue to Table 6-5

Routeof transmission	Nature of transmission	Examples
Human-to-environment-to-human	Virus excreted in feces: contaminated food, surfaces, water	Hepatitis A virus, enteroviruses, rotavirus, caliciviruses
	Contaminated surfaces respiratory secretions	Rhinovirus
	Aerosolized virus from respiratory secretions	In fluenza virus
Animal-human viaa vector to human: arboviruses	Mosquito-borne	West Nile virus, JEV
	Tick-borne	TBEV
Direct animal-to-human	Animal bites	Rabies virus
Vertical transmission		
mother-to-child	Intrauterine	Rubella virus, HIV
	During the birth process	Hepatitis B virus, HIV
	Breastfeeding	HIV, HTLV

After entering to the potential host, the virus must initiate an infection by penetrating a susceptible cell (primary replication). In some cases, virus spread is controlled by infection of polarized epithelial cells and the preferential release of virus from either the apical (e. g. , influenza virus, alocalized infection in the upper respiratory tract) or basolateral (e. g. , rhabdoviruses, a systemic infection) surface of the cells. In addition to direct cell-cell contact, there are two main mechanisms for spread throughout the host, via the bloodstream (viremia) or via the nervous system.

Following primary replication at the site of infection, the next stage may be spread throughout the host. The spread of the virus to various parts of the body is controlled to a large extent by its cell or tissue tropism. Tissue tropism is controlled partly bythe route of infection but largely by the interaction of the viral spikeprotein with its specific receptor on the cellular surface and has considerable effect on pathogenesis.

6.2.1.2 Pathogenesis

Virus pathogenesis, the capacity of the virus to cause disease, is a complex and variable process leading to a departure from the normal physiological parameters of the host. This could range from a temporary and minor condition, such as a slightly raised temperature or lack of energy, to chronic pathologic conditions thatresult in death eventually. Here, three major aspects of virus pathogenesis are considered, direct cell damage resulting from virus replication, damage resulting from immune activation or suppression and cell transformation caused by viruses.

(1) Cellular Injury

Virus infection often results in a number of changes that are detectable by visual or biochemical examination of infected cells. These changes result from the production of virus proteins and nucleic acids, but also from alterations of infected cells. A number of common phenotypicchanges can be recognized in virus-infected cells. These changes are often referred to as the cytopathic effects (CPE) of a virus and include:

(2) Altered Shape

Adherent cells that are normally attached to other cells(*in vivo*) or an artificial substrate (*in vitro*) may change from their normal flattened appearance to a rounded shape after virus infection. The regular structural formation (extensions of the cell surface) involvedin attachment or mobility are withdrawn into the cell.

(3) Detachment from the Substrate

For adherent cells, this is the stage of cell damage that follows above altered shape. Both of these effects are caused by partial degradation or disruption of the cytoskeleton that is normally responsible for maintaining the shape of the cell.

(4) Lysis

This is the most extreme cellularinjury, where the entire cell breaks down. With loss of membrane integrity, the cell may swell because of the absorption of extracellular fluid. Lysis is beneficial to a virus for releasing progeny virus particles from the infected cell. However, it is important to realize that cell lysisis mainly induced by naked viruses. There are alternative ways of releasing progeny viruses, such as budding (most enveloped viruses).

(5) Membrane Fusion

Membrane fusion is the result of virus-encoded proteins required for infection of cells, typically, the spike proteins of enveloped viruses. The spikes induce the fusion of the viral envelope to the cell membrane. Besides, the spikes could further fuse the membranes of adjacent cells, resulting in a merged giantcell with more than one nucleus (depending on the number of cells) , known as asyncytium. Production of syncytia is a common feature of HSV infection. Fused cells are short lived and subsequently lyse.

(6) Membrane Permeability

A number of viruses cause an increase inmembrane permeability, allowing an influx of extracellular ions such assodium. Some processes of viral mRNAs translation are resistant to highconcentrations of sodium ions, permitting the expression of viral proteins instead of the cellular proteins.

(7) Inclusion Bodies

These are areas where virus components have accumulated in the host cell. They are usually the sites of virus assembly and some cellular inclusions consist of crystalline arrays of virus particles. It is not clear how inclusion bodies damage the cell, but they are frequently associated with cell lysis by viruses, such as herpesviruses and rabies virus. Inclusion bodies are detectable by visual cytological identification via some special staining methods.

(8) Apoptosis

Many cells undergo apoptosis in response to viral infection, with a consequent reduction in the release of progeny virus. However, virus infection may inhibit (by viral gene products) or trigger (as a defense against viral infections) apoptosis, depending on the specific mechanism involved in the replication of different viruses.

(9) Transformation and Oncogenesis

The proliferation of cells is a strictly regulated process. Oncogenic viruses can induce changes thataffect cell proliferation and cause cancer, for example, retroviruses that may activate the oncogenesand viral proteins that may inactivate tumor suppressor genes. In many cases, the host cells transformed by viruses *in vivo* can form tumors.

(10) Immunopathology

The clinical symptoms of viral disease in the host (e. g. , fever, tissue damage, pains and nausea) result primarily from the host response to infection. However, at least two groups of viruses, retroviruses and herpesviruses, directly infect the cells of immune system. Damage involved in the immune system is called immunopathology and it may be at the expense of the host to eliminatethe viruses.

(11) Caused by CTLs

The best characterized example of CTL-mediated immunopathology occurs during the infection of mice-with lymphocytic choriomeningitis virus. Infection is not cytopathic and induces tissue damage only in immunocompetent animals. The mechanism by which these cells cause damage is not clear, but may be a result oftheir cytotoxicity. CTLs may also release proteins that recruit inflammatory cells to the site ofinfection, which in turn elaborate proinflammatory cytokines.

(12) Caused by B Cells

Virus-antibody complexes accumulate toa high concentration when the complexes are not eliminated efficiently by the reticuloendothelial system and continue to circulate in the blood. They become deposited in the capillaries andcause lesions that are exacerbated when the complement system is activated. Deposition of such complexes in blood vessels, kidneys and brainmay result in vasculitis, glomerulonephritis and mentalconfusion, respectively. Antibodies may also cause an enhancement of viral infection. This mechanism probably accounts for the pathogenesis of dengue hemorrhagic fever.

(13) Caused by $CD4^+$ T Cells

$CD4^+$ T lymphocytes produce far more cytokines and activate more nonspecific effector cells than CTLs. Such inflammatory reactions are usually called delayed-type hypersensitivity responses. Most of the recruited cells are neutrophils and mononuclear cells, which are protective but also can cause tissue damage. Immunopathology is the result of release of reactive free radicals such as peroxide and nitric oxide, proteolytic enzymes and cytokines such as TNF-α.

(14) Caused by Superantigens

Some viruseshave extremely powerful T-cell mitogens known as superantigens. The superantigens bind to MHC class II molecules on antigen-presenting cells and interact with the particular Vβ chain of the T-cell receptor. For approximately 2% to 20% of all T cells produce the Vβ chain, superantigens short-circuit the interaction of MHC class IImolecules. Rather than activation of only 0.001% to 0.01% of T cellsby a given antigen, all subsets of T cells producing the Vβ chain are activated and proliferate. Superantigens clearly interfere with a coordinated immune response and divert thehost's defenses.

(15) Caused by Viral Infection-induced Immunosuppression

Immunosuppression by viral gene products can range from a mild and rather specific attenuation to aremarkable inhibition of the response with a variety of mechanisms. Immunosuppression can result from the direct effects of viral replication on lymphocyte functions. Either all classes of lymphocytes can be affected, as occurs in measles or the effect can be restricted to a cell subtype, as is the case with human T cell-lymphotropic virus type III. Moreover, the activity of soluble factors of viral or host origin released from infected cells can affect immunosuppression. A third mechanism results from viral infection of macrophages and affects the function of these cells in natural and acquired immunity. Finally, immunosuppression may result from viral triggering of an imbalance in immune regulation, which culminates in the over-activity of suppressor cells.

(16) Caused by Systemic Inflammatory Response

An important principle of immune defense is that when virus replication exceeds a certain threshold, immune defenses are mobilized and amplified. Generally the immune response is well tolerated. However, if the immune response is not proportionalto the infection, the large-scale production and systemicrelease of inflammatory cytokines and stress mediators can overwhelm and kill the infected host.

(17) Caused by Autoimmune

Autoimmune disease is caused by an immune responsedirected against host tissues. Amodified version of hypothesis proposes that infection leads to exposure of cellular self-antigens normally hidden from the immune system. Cytokines or even virus-antibody complexes that modulate the activity of proteases inantigen-presenting cells, might cause the unmasking of self-antigens. Cytokines produced during infection may stimulate inappropriate surface expression of host membrane proteins that are recognized by host defenses. Another possibility is that during virus assembly, host proteinsnormally not exposed to the immune system are packagedin virions; these host proteins are delivered to cells during infection and are recognized bythe immune system. A popular hypothesis for virus-induced autoimmunitystates that viral and host proteins share antigenic determinants.

(18) Virusesescape of Immuneresponses

Viruses have evolved various mechanisms that enable them to escape and survive in the immuneresponse. Some viruses mutate rapidly changing their surface proteins to escape immune pressure. HIV evades the immune system by constantly changing the amino acid sequence of the proteins on the surface of the virion. This is known as "escape mutation" as the viral epitopes escape recognition by the host immune response. These persistent viruses evade immune control by sequestration, blockade of antigen presentation, cytokine resistance, evasion of natural killer cell activities, escape from apoptosis and antigenic shift. Other viruses, called neurotropic viruses, hide from the immune system by infecting immune privileged sites such as the brain where the immune system may be unable to reach.

6.2.1.3   Patterns of Infection

Virus infections in populations differ from infections in cultured cells of the laboratory. In the former, initiation of the infection rest upon complex variables such as composition of the host population, the environment and host defenses. Despite such complexity of viruses and hosts, certain patterns of infection occur. In general, natural infections can be rapid and self-limiting (acute infections) or long-term (persistent infections). These patterns can be stable overtime and characteristic for different virus families(Figure 6-8). It can be argued that all patterns begin with an acute infection and differences in the subsequent results of infections.

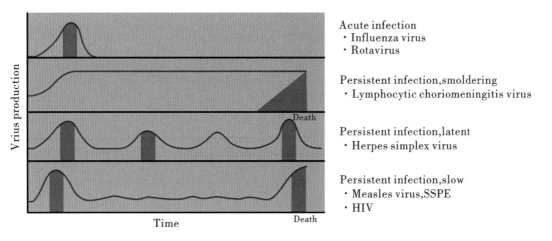

Figure 6-8   General patterns of infection. Relative virion production is plotted as a function of time afterinfection (blue line). The time when symptoms appear is indicated by the red shaded area

The top panelis the typical profile of the acute infection, in which virions are produced, symptoms appear and the virions are eliminated within 7 to 10 days after infection. The second is the typical profile of the smoldering persistent infection, in which virion production continues during the life of the host. Symptoms may or may not appear just before death, depending onthe virus. The bottom two panels are variations of the profile of the persistent infection. The third panelis the latent infection in which an initial acute infection is followed by a quiescent phase and repeated bouts of reactivation. Reactivation may or may not be accompanied by symptoms, but generally resultsin the production of virions. The fourth panel depicts the slow virus infection, in which a period of years intervenes between a typical primary acute infection and the usually fatal appearance of symptoms. The production of infectious particles during the long period between primary infection and fatal outcome maybe continuous (e. g. , HIV) or absent (e. g. , measles virus SSPE).

(1) Abortiveinfection

Abortive infection occurs when a virus infects a cell (or host) but cannot complete the full replication cycle, so this is a nonproductive infection.

(2) Acute Infection

This pattern is familiar for many common virus infections (e. g. , colds). In these infections, the virus is usually eliminated completely bythe immune system. Typically, in acute infections, virus replication occurs before the onset of symptoms (e. g. , fever), which are the result not only of virus replication but also of the activation of the immune system. Acute infections present a serious problem for the society and are thepattern most frequently associated with epidemics (e. g. , influenza, measles).

(3) Chronic Infection

The chronic infections have a protracted course (i. e. , prolonged and stubborn), characterized by a lesser degree of inflammation and reduced immune response. The virus must persist in the host for a significant period. To the clinician, there is no clear distinction among chronic, persistent and latent infections and the terms are often interchangeably used. But for virologists, there are significant differences in the events that occur during these infections. In chronic infections, the virus is usually eventually eliminated by the host (unless the infection isfatal).

(4) Persistent Infection

Compared to chronic infections, in persistent infections the virus may continue to be present and to replicate in the host for its entire life time. The mechanisms that control these events are not completely understood, but evidently there is a delicate balance between the virus and the host, in which ongoing virus replication occurs but the virus adjusts its replication and pathogenicity to avoid killing the host. Usually, persistent infections may result from the production of defective interfering particles. The presence of DIP can profoundly influence the course and the outcome of a virus infection. In some cases, they appear to moderate pathogenesis, whereas in others they potentiate the risk of disease. Moreover, as DIPs cause restricted gene expression (because they are genetically deleted), they may also lead to a persistent infection by a virus that normally causes an acute infection.

(5) Latent Infection

In a latentinfection, the virus is able to enter an inactive state with strictly limited gene expression and without ongoing virus replication. Latent virus infections typically persist for theentire life of the host. An example of such an infection in humans is HSV. Infection of sensory nerves serving the mucosa results in localized primary replication. Subsequently, the virus travels into the nervous systemvia axon transport mechanisms. Then, it hides in dorsal root ganglia, such as the trigeminal ganglion, establishing the latent infection. The nervous system is an immunologically privileged site, but the major factor in latency is the ability of the virus to restrict its gene expression, which eliminates the possibility of recognition by the immune system. After reactivated by certain stimuli, HSV could travel down the sensory nerves to cause peripheral manifestations such as cold sores or genitalulcers. Sometimes, periodic reactivation establishes the pattern of infectionwith painful reappearance of symptoms for the host's life. Even worse than this, immunosuppression later in life can cause the latent infection to flare up (the immune system has a certain role in suppressing the latent infections), resulting in a very severe infection.

(6)Slow Infection

Infection by retroviruses may result in aslow infection. Integration of the provirus into the host genomecertainly results in the persistence of the virus for the lifetime of the host. Similarto HIV, the victims infected by measles virus have an uneventful recovery, but a characteristic systemic immuno suppressive effect lasts for one week or two after the infection is resolved. Measles virus can enter the brain in infected lymphocytes that traverse the body during the viremia following primary infection. Such a secondary infection of a tissue with reduced immune surveillance has a number of consequences. One is acute postinfectiou sencephalitis, which occurs in about 1 in 3,000 infections. The other is a rare, but delayed and often lethal, braininfection called subacute sclerosing panencephalitis(SSPE).

(7)Transforming Infection

Transforming infection is a special class of persistent infection. The cell infected by certain DNA viruses or retroviruses may exhibit altered growth properties and begin to proliferate faster than uninfected cells. In some cases, this changeis accompanied by integration of viral genetic information. In others, replication is in concert with the cell. Virus particles may no longer be produced, but some or all of their genetic material generally persists. This pattern of persistent infection could be considered as transforming because of the change in cell behavior. It is also considered oncogenic because some transformed cells cause cancer in the host.

6.2.2　Antiviral Immunity

The cascade of antiviral defense starts by the reactions of a single infected cell. Despite single cell defenses, if viral replication continues unabated, a thresholdfor more active and global defenses would be crossed. Subsequently, the antiviral immunity begins. The immune response to viral infection consists of an innate (nonspecific)andan adaptive (specific)defense. The innate imuunity is the first line of immune defense, because it functions continually in a normal host without any prior exposure to the invading virus. Indeed, most viral invasions are repelled by intrinsic defenses and the innate immune systembefore viral replication outpaces host defense. However, once this threshold is passed, second-line defenses (the adaptive immunity)must be mobilized for survival of the host. The adaptive immunity consists of the an tibody response and the lymphocyte-mediated response, often called the humoral immunity and the cell-mediated immunity, respectively.

Besides, the cellular agents of the innate and adaptive immuneresponses are the myelomonocytes (monocytes, macrophages, dendritic cells and a variety of granulocytes)and the lymphocytes (natural killer, T and B cells). One aspect of the immune system is that its effector cells are dispersed throughout the body, the response can be promptly directed to the site ofinfection. And the cytokines can coordinate the antiviral immunity.

6.2.2.1　Innate Immunity

The innate immunesystem, also known as the non-specific immune system or in-born immunity system, provide the first line of defense against infectious disease. Unlike the adaptive immune system, the innate immune system does not provide long-lasting immunity to the host and provide immediate defense against infection. Engagement of innate immunesystem leads to triggering of signal pathways to promote inflammation, ensuring that invading viruses remain in check while the specific immuneresponse is either generated or upregulated.

The innate immunity comprises anatomic and physiologic barriers, cytokines released from infected cells, local sentinel cells (dendritic cells and macrophages), a complex collection ofserum proteins termed complement and cytolytic lymphocytes called natural killer cells (NK cells). Neutrophils and other granulocytic white blood cells also play important roles in response to the initialburst of cytokines from dendritic cells, macrophages andinfected cells.

(1) Anatomic and Physiologic Barriers

Anatomic and physiologic barriers include physical, chemical and biological barriers. The epithelial surfaces form a physical barrier that is impermeable to most infectious agents, acting as the first line of defense against invading viruses. Lack of blood vessels and inability of the epidermis to retain moisture and presence of sebaceous glands in the dermis provide an environment to prevent many types of viruses from infecting the host. In the gastrointestinal tract, the acidity of the contents destroys many viruses that have been swallowed. The flushing action of tears and saliva helps prevent infection of the eyes and mouth.

(2) Cellularagents

When the viruses overcome the above barriers and enter the host, other innate defenses prevent the spread of infection in the host. As a type of white blood cell, macrophages undergo the process of phagocytosisto engulf and digest viruses. Besides, they play a critical role in innate immunity and also help initiate adaptive immunity by recruiting other immune cells such as lymphocytes. In humans, dysfunctional macrophages cause severe diseases such as persistent viremia that result in frequent infections. As another critical part of innate immunity, NK cells provide rapid responses to viral-infected cells, acting at around 3 days after infection, somehow like the cytotoxic T cells in the adaptive immune response.

(3) Interferon

The important innate immune response to an invading virus is producing a special signaling glycoprotein called interferon (IFN) which protects other cellsof the same species from attack by a wide range ofviruses. It is now clear that this activity is mediated by members of a family of regulatory proteins.

In human, as in a number of other species, there are three main interferons: interferon-α (IFN-α), produced mainly by peripheral blood mononuclear cells; interferon-β (IFN-β), produced predominantly by fibroblasts; and interferon-γ (IFN-γ), a lymphokine produced by antigen-activated T lymphocytes and NK cells. IFN-α and IFN-β are known as type Ⅰ interferons and are considered part of the innate defenses whereas IFN-γ is referred to as type Ⅱ interferon. The production of interferons is under strict inducible control. IFN-α and IFN-β are produced in response to the presence of viruses and certain intracellular bacteria. However, IFN-γ has an extensive role in the control of immune responses.

To exert their biological effects these interferonsmust interact with cell surface receptors. IFN-α and IFN-β share a common receptor, whereas IFN-γ binds to its own specific receptor. After binding to thecell surface receptors, interferons act by rapidly and transiently inducing or upregulating some cellulargenes and down regulating others. The overall effect isto inhibit viral replication and activate host defense mechanisms. The antiviral activity is mediated by the interferon released from a virus-infected cell binding to aneighboring cell and inducing the synthesis of antiviral proteins (Figure 6–9).

Interferons are extremelypotent in this function, acting at femtomolar (10^{-15} M) concentrations. They can inhibit many stages of the viralreplication cycle, attachment, uncoating, biosynthesis and release. Many new proteins can be detected in cellsex posed to interferon, but major roles have been proposed for two enzymes that inhibit protein synthesis: 2′, 5′-oligoadenylate synthetase (2,5-A synthetase) anda protein kinase. The activity of both of these enzymesis dependent on double-stranded RNA (dsRNA) provided by viral intermediates in the cell. The proteinkinase is responsible for the phosphorylation of histones and the protein synthesis initiation factor eIF2. This leads to the inhibition of protein synthesis with in interferon-stimulated cells as a result of inhibition of ribosome assembly. The 2,5-A synthetase is stronglyinduced in human cells by all three types of interferon and forms $2',5'$-linked oligonucleotides of adenosine from a-denosine triphosphate (ATP). These oligonucleotides activate a latent cellular endonuclease that degrades both messenger and ribosomal RNA, with are sultant inhibition of protein synthesis. The requirement for the presence of dsRNA for the full expression of these responses safe guards uninfected cells from the damaging effects of the enzymes. Apart from these well characterized changes, many other change soccur in cells treated with interferons. Some viral proteins can inhibit the interferon response.

Interferons are able to modify immune responses by altering the expression of cell surface molecules, altering the production and secretion of cellularpro-teins and enhancing or inhibiting effector cell functions. One of the main ways in which interferons controlimmune responses is by the induction or enhance-mentof major histocompatibility complex (MHC)-en-codedmolecules. Class I MHC genes are upregulated by all types of interferon, as is the production of $\beta2$-microglobulin. IFN-γ induces and increases the

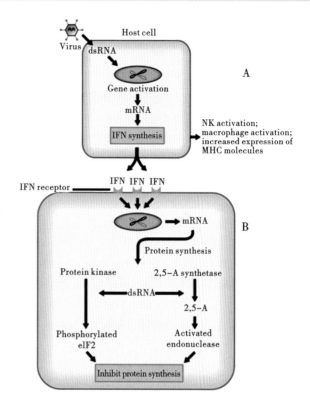

Figure 6-9   Proposed mechanisms of an induction of synthesis of IFN-α and IFN-β and production of resistance to virus infection. 2,5-A,$2',5'$-oligoade-nylate;dsRNA,double-stranded ribonucleic acid;elf, eukaryotic initiation factor;MHC, major histocompatibility complex; mRNA, messenger RNA; NK, natural killer cells

expression of MHC class II antigens. In addition, interferons can induceor enhance the expression of Fc receptors and receptors for a number of cytokines. These activities increase the efficiency of antigen recognition and lead to a more effective immune response.

Interferons have also been implicated in the controlof B cell responses. When added in vitro or in vivo they can suppress or enhance primary or secondary antibody responses, depending on the dose and time of addition. The regulatory effects seem to be on theB cells themselves, on increased antigen presentationand through an effect on regulatory T cells.

A number of immune effector cells act by killing infected target cells. The cytotoxicity of macrophages, neutrophils, T cells and NK cells is enhanced by interferons. IFN-γ produced by T lymphocytes is capable of activating macrophages. This lymphokine has all the activities of the molecule that used to be known as macrophage-activatingfactor (MAF). NK cells are able to destroy a range of syngeneic, allogeneic and xeno-geneic cells in an MHC-unrestricted fashion. All three types of interferon increase NK cell activity in vitro and in vivo, not only by recruiting pre-NK cells to become actively lytic but also by increasing the spectrum ofcells lysed. The mechanisms by which interferon smake cells cytotoxic are not clear, but it is of interest that interferons can stimulate the production of cytotoxins such as TNF.

The interferon response is rapid and helps to protect the host until acquired responses develop. Interfer-onsinduce a febrile response and this may also be important in inhibiting viral growth in some infections with viruses that have a low ceiling temperature for growth.

6.2.2.2 Adaptive Immunity

The adaptive immune system, also known as the acquired immune system or, more rarely, as the specific immune system, is a subsystem of thetotal immune system that is composed of highly specialized cells and processes that prevent and eliminate viruses. Adaptive immunity can create immunological memory after an initial response to a specific virus and leads to an enhanced response to subsequent encounters with the samevirus. This process of acquired immunity is the basis of vaccination. When a viral antigen that is not part of the antigen repertoire of the host is presented to the immune system by an antigen-presenting cell (APC), both B cell immunity (humoral immunity) and T cell immunity (cell-mediated immunity) aremobilized.

B cells produce antibodies that are secreted proteins able to combine with the antigenic determinants specifically. Immune T cells have antigen-binding sites on their surfaces and interact with antigen-bearing cells, resulting in lysis of thevirus infected cells. Together, these two parts of the immune system allow the host to detect and destroy both free viruses and virus-infected cells with viral proteins at the surface. A general outline of the interaction between the immune system and an antigenic pathogen is shown in Figure 6-10.

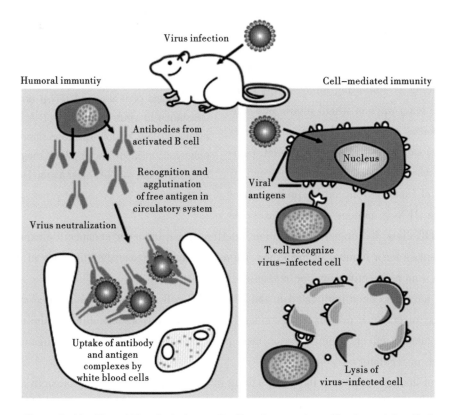

Figure 6-10   B and T cells in immunity. B cells secrete antibody proteins that bind to antigenic determinants to neutralize infectivity of virus. T lymphocytes play the central role in evokingthe immune response. Activated by interaction with a specific antigenic determinant, they proliferate and carry out the function of lysis

(1) Humoralimmunity

There are several ways by which antibody can protect the host from virus infection. Antibodies can't enter cells and therefore are ineffective against viruses in cells or those that spread from cell to celldirectly.

However, they bind to extracellular viral epitopes which can be on intact virions or on the surface of infected cells. Antibodies can block binding between the virions and the host cell membrane and thus stop attachment and penetration of virions. The immunoglobulins IgG and IgM have this important function in serum and body fluids and IgA can neutralize viruses by a similar mechanism onmucosal surfaces. Antibody can also work at stages after penetration. Uncoating, via the release of viralnucleic acid into the cytoplasm, can be inhibited if the virion is covered by antibody. Antibody can also cause aggregation of virus particles, thus limiting the spread of the infectious particles and forming a complex that is readily phagocytosed. Complement can aid in the neutralization process by opsonizing the virus or directly lysing enveloped viruses.

The efficiency of antibody dependson whether the virus passes through the blood stream outside host cells to reach its target organ. Poliovirus crosses the intestinal wall, enters the bloodstream to cause viremia and passes to thespinal cord and brain for its replication. Antibodies in the blood can neutralize thevirus before it reaches its target cells of the nervous system. However, the viruses, such as in fluenza virus and rhinovirus, localize in the respiratory mucous membranes instead of passing through the bloodstream. So, a high level of antibody in the blood is relatively ineffective. The antibody must be present in the mucous secretions during the infection. There are very low levels of IgG or IgM in secretions and IgA has been shown to be responsible for neutralizing activity against respiratory tract viruses.

Humoral immunity is probably the predominant form of immunity responsible for protection from reinfection. Passively administered antibody, before or soon after exposure, can protect against several human infections, including measles, hepatitis A and B. Immunity to many viral infections is lifelong because that antibodies could be boosted by re-exposure to the virus.

(2) Cell-Mediatedimmunity

The destruction of virus infected cells is an important mechanism in the eradication of virus from the host. Antibody can neutralize free virions, but other strategies are employed after virus penetration. The destruction of an infected cell by cell-mediated immunity is an effective way of terminating a viral infection. Varioustypes of effector cell have evolved tomediate the process of recognizing the infected cells.

As viralproteins are synthesized in the cell, some of the proteins are hydrolyzedinto small peptides. These endogenously produced antigen fragments are associated with MHC class I molecules and the complex is then transported to the cellsurface to be the recognition unit for cytotoxic T lymphocytes(CTLs). Most CTLs have a receptor that binds to fragments of the virus in thecleft of an MHC class I molecule. This T cell has the CD8 molecule on its surface. Some T cells are restricted in their recognition of antigen by MHC class II molecules and therefore have the CD4 molecule. $CD4^+$ and $CD8^+$ T cells can produce variouslymphokines when stimulated by antigens, including molecules that are active in the elimination of virus (e. g. IFN-γ and TNF) and others that generally increase the effectiveness of the immune system by attracting cells to the site of infection, stimulating the production of more cells and supporting their growth.

Besides, some of virus-encoded molecules (spikes of enveloped virus) are inserted into the host cell membrane, often very early during the replication cycle. If antibody binds to the spikeson cell surface, the infected cell can be destroyed by antibody-dependent cell-mediated cytotoxicity. The effector cells have an Fc receptor that recognizes the Fc portion of immunoglobulin boundto the spikes. All these interactions inducevirus infected cell lysis directly or indirectly.

6.3 Diagnosis, Treatment and Control of Viral Infection

The large number of possible virions causing a given disease precludes the use of one simple test as diagnostic for a specific virus infection. However, laboratory diagnosis is usually performed under the assumption of clinical disease spectrum, relying on symptoms and epidemiologic data. Base on the results of diagnosis, treatment against viral infection makes use of chemotherapeutic agents that are effective to control infection and disease. Besides, vaccination (immunoprophylaxis) induces a primed state so that later exposure to a pathogen generates a rapid immune response, leading to accelerated elimination of the virions and protection against onset of viral disease.

6.3.1 Diagnostic Procedures

Sometimes clinical observations alone are sufficientfor diagnosis, allowing for therapeutic intervention prior tovirus identification. The identification of a virus froma clinical specimen relies on general characteristics such as certain phenotypes in cell culture, induced immunity responses toviral antigens and extracted viral RNA or DNA.

6.3.1.1 Specimen Collection and Handling

The importance of proper specimen collection must be emphasized. Appropriate specimen collection is vital for viruses that cause infections to be rapidly isolated and identified.

1) Collect specimens as soon as possible after the onset of symptoms to improve its positive ratio. The chance is best during the first 3 days after onset and is greatly reduced beyond 5 days with many viruses.

2) If possible, clinicalviral specimens should be administrated antibioticsto inhibition of bacteria and fungi growth. Most specimens from normally sterile sites can be collected directly into a sterile container.

3) Samples should be transported to the laboratory and plated within 2 hours post-collection. If this is not possible, specimens should be placed into transport media and kept cool on ice or refrigerated to maintain viability for extended periods of time.

4) Both an acute serum sample from early acute stage and a convalescent serum specimen from postonset should be collected. Such paired serum specimens, which show a four-fold increase or a rising titers of IgG antibody enzyme-linked immunosorbent assay (IgG-ELISA) are indicative of a recent infection.

6.3.1.2 Cultivation of Viruses

In the vast majority of cases, it is necessary to supply the virus with appropriate cells in which it can replicate. Viruses may be propagated in whole organisms, such as mice, which may be genetically modified. Transgenic mice areused in studies of hepatitis B and hepatitis C viruses. Some viruses are propagated in eggs containing chick embryos. For the most part, however, animal viruses are grown in cultured animal cells.

The index of virus proliferation includes:

1) Cytopathic effect or cytopathogenic effect (CPE) refers to structural changes in host cells that are caused by viral invasion. The infecting virus causes lysis of the host cell or when the cell dies without lysis due to an inability to reproduce. Both of these effects occur due to CPEs. If a virus causes these morphological changes in the host cell, it is said to be cytopathogenic. Common examples of CPE include rounding of the infected cell, fusion with adjacent cells to form syncytia and the appearance of nuclear or cytoplasmic inclusion bodies.

2) Hemadsorption is the adherence of red blood cells to other cells or surfaces; a process in which a substance or an agent, such as certain viruses and bacilli, adheres to the surface of an erythrocyte. The process occurs naturally or it may be induced for laboratory identification of specimens.

6.3.1.3   Virus quantification

Virus quantification involves counting the number of viruses in a specific volume to determine the virus concentration. It is utilized in both research and development in commercial and academic laboratories.

50% tissue culture infective dose ($TCID_{50}$) is the measure of infectious virus titer. This endpoint dilution assay quantifies the amount of virus required to kill 50% of infected hosts or to produce a cytopathic effect in 50% of inoculated tissue culture cells. This assay may be more common in clinical research applications where the lethal dose of virus must be determined or if the virus does not form plaques. When used in tissue culture cells, host cells are plated and serial dilutions of the virus are added. After incubation, the percentage of cell death (i. e. infected cells) is manually observed and recorded for each virus dilution and results are used to mathematically calculate a $TCID_{50}$ result. Due to distinct differences in assay methods and principles, $TCID_{50}$ and PFU/mL or other infectivity assay results are not equivalent. This method can take up to a week due to cell infectivity time.

Plaque-based assays are the standard method used to determine virus concentration in terms of infectious dose. Viral plaque assays determine the number of plaque forming units (PFU) in a virus sample, which is one measure of virus quantity. This assay is based on a microbiological method conducted in petri dishes or multi-well plates. Specifically, a confluent monolayer of host cells is infected with the virus at varying dilutions and covered with a semi-solid medium, such as agar or carboxymethyl cellulose, to prevent the virus infection from spreading indiscriminately. A viral plaque is formed when a virus infects a cell within the fixed cell monolayer. The virus infected cell will lyse and spread the infection to adjacent cells where the infection-to-lysis cycle is repeated. The infected cell area will create a plaque (an area of infection surrounded by uninfected cells) which can be seen visually or with an optical microscope. Plaque formation can take 3–14 days, depending on the virus being analyzed. Plaques are generally counted manually and the results, in combination with the dilution factor used to prepare the plate, are used to calculate the number of plaque forming units per sample unit volume (PFU/mL). The PFU/mL result represents the number of infective viruses within the sample and is based on the assumption that each plaque formed is representative of one infective virus.

The hemagglutination assay (HA) is a common non-fluorescence protein quantification assay specific for influenza. It relies on the fact that hemagglutinin, a surface protein of influenza viruses, agglutinates red blood cells (i. e. causes red blood cells to clump together). In this assay, dilutions of an influenza sample are incubated with a 1% erythrocyte solution for one hour and the virus dilution at which agglutination first occurs is visually determined. The assay produces a result of hemagglutination units (HAU), with typical PFU to HAU ratios in the 10^6 range. This assay takes about 1–2 hours to complete and results can differ widely based on the technical expertise of the operator.

6.3.1.4   Diagnosis of Virus Infection

Virological diagnosis is based either on demonstration of the virus or its components (antigens or genome) or on demonstration of a specific antibody response. In some infections antibodies are detectable at the onset of clinicaldisease (e. g. poliomyelitis, hepatitis B (anti-HBc) or the antibody appearance may be delayed by days (rubella), weeks or months (hepatitis C, HIV infection). Whenever an early diagnosis is important for the institution of antiviral therapy or some other interference measures, the possible use of methods that demonstrate the virus should be considered.

(1) Structural Investigations of Viruses

1) Light microscopy: The sizes of most virions are beyond the limits of resolution of light microscopes, but light microscopy has useful applications in detecting and studying virus-inducedchanges in cells, for example observing cytopathic effects.

2) Electron microscopy: Many investigations of the structure of virions or of virus-infected cells involveobservations at large magnifications using transmission electron microscopes. The specimen may be a preparation of virions, a virion component, virus-infected cellsor an ultra-thin section of a virus-infected cell. In order to observe detail in the specimen it is either negatively stained or cooled to a very low temperature orboth. Cryo-electron microscopy techniques are more recent. For these techniques wetspecimens are rapidly cooled to a temperature below -160 ℃, freezing the water as a glass-like material. The images are recorded while the specimen is frozen. They require computer processing in order to extract maximum detail anddata from multiple images are processed to reconstruct three-dimensional images of virus particles. This may involve averaging many identical copies or combining images into three-dimensional density maps.

(2) Detection of Virus Components

1) Detection of virus antigens: Virus antigens can be detected using virus-specific antisera or monoclonalantibodies. In most techniques positive results are indicated by detecting the presence of a label, which may be attached either to the anti-virus antibody (directtests) or to a second antibody (indirect tests). Several virus antigen tests are available for rapid diagnosis of virusinfections. Methods most commonly used are immunofluorescence or immunoperoxidase for respiratory viruses, ELISA for HBsAg, HIV androtavirus, latex agglutination for rotavirus and reverse passive haemagglutination for HBsAg. Immunofluorescence and immunoperoxidase procedures depend on the sampling and preservation of infected cells, requiring rapidtransport of cooled material. Alternatively, preparation of the slide has to bemade locally. Blood (serum) and faeces can be sent in the usual way.

2) Detection of Virusgenomes: Viral genomes can be demonstrated by various nucleic acid hybridizationtechniques, either *in situ* or in tissue extracts (slot blot, Southern blot, *in situ* hybridization) using labelled DNA or RNA probes or by methods that include amplification of the viral nucleic acid such as polymerase chain reaction (PCR) and ligase chain reaction (LCR), Both PCR and LCR are extremely sensitive, requiring strict precautions in the laboratory to avoid contamination. The gene technology methods are of particular importance for rapid diagnosis ofinfections that are accessible to antiviral treatment (herpes simplex encephalitis, CMV infection), for diagnosis of infection with viruses that cannot be cultivated (human papillomaviruses) or viruses that grow slowly in culture(enteroviruses), as well as in clinical situations where a definite diagnosis cannot be made by other means (possible HIV infection and hepatitis B or C innewborns and infants).

3) Detection of Antiviral Antibodies: Antibody molecules are secreted glycoproteins that have the capacity to recognize and combine with specificportions of viral. Antibody examinations are mostly performed with serum. Anticoagulants added to whole blood may interfere with complement activity and enzymefunctions and should be avoided. In certain situations (SSPE, herpes simplex encephalitis) antibody titration is performed on cerebrospinal fluid.

(3) Specific IgM Tests

Acute infection is diagnosed by demonstrating a rise in titre, seroconversion orspecific IgM (or IgA). A rise in titre may be seen both in primary infections andin reinfection or after reactivation. A positive IgM test usually indicates aprimary infection, but lower concentrations of specific IgM are found inreactivations (CMV infections and zoster) and reinfections (rubella). A variety of methods (complement fixation (CF), haemagglutination inhibition (HI), enzyme-linked immunosorbent assay (ELISA), immunofluorescence (IF)) are available for demonstration of antibodies and the choiceof test will depend on the virus and whether the clinical problem is the immunestatus or diagnosing an acute infection. Blood samples for demonstration of seroconversion or titrerise (paired sera) are taken 1–3 weeks apart, depending on the time of exposureor onset of symptoms.

(4) Neutralization Tests

Some methods to measure the reaction between specific antibody molecules and an antigen involve the loss of specificfunctions by the target virus. Many antibodies will block the ability of a virus to initiate an infection in a cultured cell and thus block the formation of virus plaque. And the inhibition of plaque formation is termed an infectivity neutralization or neutralization of avirus. Here, a target virus with a known titer is incubated with test antibody dilutions. The more concentrated and specific the antibody, the more the initial antibody solution can be diluted and still block viral infectivity (and thus formation of plaques). Neutralization is illustrated schematically in Figure 6–10.

Figure 6–10 Antibody neutralization of virus infectivity. Specific types of antibody molecules, called neutralizing antibodies, can bind to surface proteins of the virus and block one or another aspect of the early events of virus-cell recognition or effective internalization of the virus.

(5) Hemagglutination Inhibition

Some methods for the measurement of antibody against viruses are based on the ability of the antibody to block certain property of the virus. For example, it has been known that many envelopedviruses will stick to red blood cells and cause haemagglutination. This property can be used as a crude measure of viral particle concentration in solution. Many antibodies against enveloped viruses will inhibit virus-mediated agglutination of red blood cells and this hemagglutination inhibition (HI) test can be used to measure antibody levels. If a virus that can cause hemagglutination is preincubated with an antibody, the virus will be physically masked by antibody and will not be able to stick to the red blood cells.

An experiment utilizing HI test is shown in Figure 6–11. All that is required to measure a patient's immune response is a standard virus stock and blood serum. Agglutination is characterized by a diffuse red or salmon-pink solution. If the red blood cells do not agglutinate, the cells' pellet forms a red "button" atthe bottom of the wells by gravity. Low dilutions of serum result in sequestering the virus so that it is not available for hemagglutination. Higher dilutions of the antiserum dilute the antibody concentration to a point where enough virions remain to causea positive hemagglutinin reaction. If there were more antibodies in the serum, a higher dilution would be required to accomplish this. Therefore, the HI titer of the serum is a measurement of how far it can be diluted with still blocking of the hemagglutinin reaction. In the example shown in Figure 6–10, a 1∶3,200 dilution of the original sample (asterisks) is the lastone in which agglutination is inhibited. Since a 1∶3,200 dilution was the

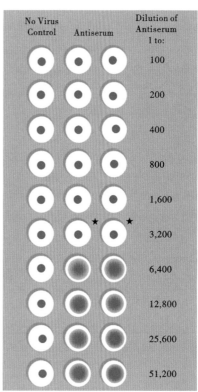

Figure 6–11　The hemagglutination inhibition assay for measuring antibody against a virus in serum. The assay is carried out by mixing constant amounts of a known hemagglutinating viruswith serial dilutions of serum; then the virus-serum mixture is added to red blood cells

endpoint, there are 3,200 hemagglutination inhibition units in the original stock.

The HI test is not accurate enough. However, it is relative fast, easy and low cost of performance, which is very important in small clinical laboratories.

6.3.2 Prevention of Viral Infection

The human immune system provides protection against foreign antigens, many of which are from infectious viruses. However, until the body has been exposed to a new virus, it has to rely on innateimmunity for prevention. The adaptive immunity can forma specific immune response and formmemory cells to respond morerapidly to reexposure to the infectious virus. Exposingan in dividual to a harmless form of the viral antigens, a similar immune response can be induced without risk of viral disease. This is what occurs during activeimmunity or vaccination. In contrast, passive immunit yintroduces the products of the immuneresponse (e. g., antibodies or stimulated immune cells) obtained from the appropriate donor(s) directly into thepatient. Such prevention of viral infection can be accomplished to eliminate the spreadof the virus or prevention its transmission.

6.3.2.1 Active Immunity

Active immunity is the induction of immunity before exposure to infectious viruses. The most effective approaches are vaccinations to provide active acquired immunity to virus infection. Vaccines contain biological substances intended to induce an immune response for providing prevention against a specific viraldisease. The purpose of most vaccines is to induce long-term immunity against the virus by establishing B cell and T cell memory that will be triggered if the virus invades the body. Several types of (potential) vaccines exist ranging from live viruses to DNA that products certain proteins of the virus.

(1) Inactivated Vaccine

Most of the successful vaccines produced in the last century utilized inactivated virus inactivated with chemicals, heat or radiation to maintain the viral antigenicity. Originally, the highly successful Salk poliovirus vaccine was a formalin-inactivated preparation of the three virus serotypes. An advantage of the inactivated vaccines is absence of the virus's capacity to revert to virulence, since there is noviral replication during immunization. Further, inactivated vaccines can be stored more easily than live attenuated vaccines. On the contrary, these are the facts that the vaccines must be injected, multiple rounds of immunization are generally required and vaccination does not result in whole immunity because a real infection does not occur.

(2) Live Attenuated Vaccine

Many of attenuated vaccine are active viruses that have been cultivated under certain conditions that disable their virulent properties. Such mutants are produced by serial passage of the virulent strainsin cell or animal. The process of attenuation introduces a number of point mutations, essentially mutating functions not required for replication but rather for pathogenesis. This technique was used to produce the Sabin strains of oral vaccine against the three serotypes of poliovirus. Live attenuated vaccines typically provoke more durable immunological responses and are the preferred type for healthy adults. But they may not be safe for use in immunocompromised individuals and may rarely mutate to a virulent form and cause disease.

(3) Subunit Vaccine

Since the desired immune response is most often directed against a critical surface protein of a virus, such protein could be used as a vaccine if it were properly presented to the immune system. A subunit vaccine can be prepared by purification of the protein subunit from the viral particle or by recombinant DNA cloning and expression of the viral protein in a suitable host cell, either bacteria or yeast. Direct administration of a protein will not induce a cell-mediated response the way a live attenuated vaccine would. Theadvantages of a subunit vaccine include the lack of any potential infectivity, either mild in the case of theattenuated strains or severe in the case of the virulent strains. In addition, subunit vaccines may servewhen the virus probably is extremely virulent or when it can not be cultured.

(4)Genetically Engineering Vaccine

If a specificviral antigen or set of viral antigenscan be identified, the genes for those antigens can be inserted into other organisms, e. g. brewer's yeast(*Saccharomyces cerevisiae*)in the case of hepatitis B surface antigen. After cultivation of brewer's yeast, the expressed antigens can be purified and applied for immunization. This vaccinehas been successfully used and appears to reduce the incidence of primary liver cancer.

(5)Recombinant Vector Vaccine

Recombinantvector viruses are currently being tested for use as vaccines. It is possible to use the process of genetic recombination to introduce the genes for viral proteins inducing protective immunity into the genome of another virus, which itself might be avirulent. Such are combinant virus could then be used to vaccinate an individual, leading to generation of immunity against the viral proteins. Since the vector-virus would be able to replicate, it would hopefully be able to generate a full repertoire of immune responses against the proteins. Possible candidate vectors include poxviruses, herpesviruses and adenoviruses, but vaccinia virus has been subjected to the majority of developmental studies to date.

(6)DNA Vaccine

Naked DNA may be injected or delivered in other ways, into the skin or muscle. This DNAis taken up by the cells and the proteins it codes for may be produced. Immunity against viral proteins can beinduced in this way. However, no DNA vaccines are currently available commercially.

6.3.2.2　Passive Immunity

In some cases, artificially passive immunity is another method to protect the health care worker exposed to infectious viruses. Naturally, passive immunity is transferred from mother to child across the placenta, providing immunity for the firstmonths of life. For the same reason, testing for IgG in infants may merely indicate maternal IgG and not anacquired immunity in the infant.

Viral infections were initially often treated with antibodies. Today antibodies, either normalhuman immunoglobulin (totalimmunoglobulin) or hyperimmuneglobulin (organism-specific), are still an important part of prophylaxisagainst certain viral infections such as hepatitis A, hepatitis B, rabies, measles, varicella and respiratory syncytial virus(RSV). In the modern era of laboratory-synthesized monoclonal antibodies, RSV can be prevented with palivizumab, a recombinant human-mouse monoclonal and monoclonal antibodies for other viruses, such asfor avirumab and rafivirumab for rabies, are in development. Passive immunityhas also shown some effect inpreventing mortality in cases of Ebola.

6.3.3　Treatment of Viral Infection

Some viral infections can be controlled effectively by public health measuresand vaccines. However, for many others, these measures have no effect or cannot be applied. Antiviral drugs are intended to fill a portionof this void. Treatment of virus infection can involve methods to encourage the body's own highly evolved antiviral mechanisms to deploy before virus infection leads to serious damage.

Inhibitors of viral replication can be subdivided into two groups: nucleoside analogues and non-nucleoside inhibitors. Nucleoside analogues compete with natural nucleotides, bind to the active center of polymerases and inhibit the function of the enzyme. In addition to this form of competitive inhibition, a nucleoside analogue can also be used as a substrate by the enzyme, i. e. it can be introduced into a growing viral nucleic acid chain. If it is incorporated, it disturbsthe habitual structure of DNA or RNA, which there after cannot be replicated and transcribed correctly or it can lead to chain termination during replication. However, despite almost 50 years of research, the armamentarium of such drugs remains small. The current arsenal comprises fewerthan 50 drugs and most of these are directed against human immunodeficiency virus (HIV) and herpesviruses.

6.3.3.1   Inhibitors of Viral Replication

Treatment can be mediated byspecific antiviral agents designed to selectively blockevery stage of virus replication in the host (Table 6-6).

Table 6-6   Steps in virus replication that are susceptible to inhibitors

Target	Antiviral drugs	Virus/infection
Virus attachment	Dextran sulphate	HIV-1
	CD4 (receptor)	HIV-1
Virus penetration and uncoating	Amantadine	Influenza A
	Rimantadine	Influenza A
	Gp41 peptides	HIV-1
Reverse transcriptase	Zidovudine	HIV-1
	Zalcitabine	HIV-1
	Didanosine	HIV-1
	Stavudine	HIV-1
	Lamivudine	HIV-1
	Delavirdine	HIV-1
	Nevirapine	HIV-1
	Efavirenz	HIV-1
DNA polymerase	Aciclovir	HSV
	Penciclovir	HSV
	Ganciclovir	Cytomegalovirus
	Trifluorothymidine	HSV
	Foscarnet	CMV
	Cidofovir	Pox viruses
Protease	Saquinavir	HIV
	Indinavir	HIV
	Nelfinavir	HIV
	Ritonavir	HIV
Virus release	Zanamivir	Influenza A and B
	Oseltamivir	Influenza A and B
Viral protein synthesis	Interferon	Many viruses
Free virus particle	Pleconaril	Rhinoviruses

(1) Attachment Inhibitor

One anti-viral strategy is to interfere with the ability of a virus to attach the host cell. This stage of viral replication can be inhibited by using agents which mimic the virus-associated protein (VAP) to bind the cellular receptors or using agents which mimic the cellular receptor to bind the VAP.

(2) Penetration Inhibitor

A number of penetration-inhibiting drugs are being developed to inhibit HIV. HIV infects a host cell through fusion with the cell membrane, which requires two different cellular molecular receptors, CD4 and a chemokine co-receptor (CCR5 or CXCR4). Approaches to blocking this virus/cell fusion have shown some promise in preventing entry of the virus into a cell.

(3) Uncoating Inhibitor

Inhibitors of uncoating have also been investigated. Amantadine and rimantadine have been introduced to combat influenza by blocking viral uncoating. Moreover, pleconaril works against rhinoviruses, which cause the common cold, by blocking a pocket on the surface of the virus that controls the uncoating process.

(4) Biosynthesis Inhibitor

This approach is to target the processes that synthesize virus components after a virus invades a cell.

(5) Reverse Transcription

A number of anti-viral drugs are synthetic compounds structurally similar tonucleosides. When viruses mistakenly incorporate such nucleoside analogs into their genomes during replication, the replication-cycle of the virus is halted because the newly synthesised DNA is inactive. The first successful antiviral, aciclovir, is a nucleoside analogue and is effective against herpesvirus infections. The first antiviral drug to be approved for treating HIV, zidovudine (AZT), is also a nucleoside analogue. An improved knowledge of the action of reverse transcriptase has led to better nucleoside analogues to treat HIV infections. One of these drugs, lamivudine, has been approved to treat hepatitis B, which uses reverse transcriptase as part of its replication process. Another target being considered for HIV antivirals include RNase H, which is a component of reverse transcriptase that splits the synthesized DNA from the original viral RNA.

(6) Transcription

Once a virus genome becomes operational in a host cell, it generates messenger RNA (mRNA) molecules that direct the synthesis of viral proteins. Production of mRNA is initiated by proteins known as transcription factors. Several antivirals are now being designed to block attachment of transcription factors to viral DNA. Ribavirin is a guanosine analog used to stop viral RNA synthesis and viral mRNA capping.

(7) Translation/Antisense

Genomics has not only helped find targets for many antivirals, it has provided the basis for an entirely new type of drug, based on "antisense" molecules. These are segments of DNA or RNA that are designed as complementary molecule to critical sections of viral genomes and the binding of these antisense segments to these target sections blocks the operation of those genomes. A phosphorothioate antisense drug named fomivirsen has been introduced, used to treat opportunistic eye infections in AIDS patients caused by cytomegalovirus and other antisense antivirals are in development. An antisense structural type that has proven especially valuable in research is morpholino antisense.

(8) Translation/Ribozymes

Another antiviral technique inspired by genomics is a set of drugs based on ribozymes, which are enzymes that will cut apart viral RNA or DNA at selected sites. In their natural course, ribozymes are used as part of the viral manufacturing sequence, but these synthetic ribozymes are designed to cut RNA and DNA at sites that will disable them.

(9) Protease Inhibitors

Some viruses include an enzyme known as a protease that cuts viral protein chains apart so they can be assembled into their final configuration. HIV includes a protease and so considerable research has been performed to find "protease inhibitors" to attack HIV at that phase of its replication cycle. Protease inhibitors became available in the 1990s and have proven effective, though they can have unusual side effects, for example causing fat to build up in unusual places. Improved protease inhibitors are now in development.

(10) Release Inhibitors

The final stage in the replication cycle of a virus is the release of completed viruses from the host cell and this step has also been targeted by antiviral drug developers. Two drugs named zanamivir (Relenza) and oseltamivir (Tamiflu) that have been introduced to treat influenza prevent the release of viral particles by blocking neuraminidase that is found on the surface of influenza viruses and also seems to be constant across a wide range of strains.

6.3.3.2　Viral Resistance to Antiviral Inhibitors

Virusvariants, with the resistance to antiviral drugs, are cumulatively selected under the selection pressure of such different compounds. The selection applies especially to viral species with an RNA genome. Being involved in genome replication of different RNA viruses, polymerases such as reverse transcriptase, RNA-dependent RNA polymerase and the cellular RNA polymerases, have no proof reading activity to check whether the newly synthesized sequences are accurately complementary with the original template. Therefore, mutations occur with a statistical probability of 10^{-4} during viral genome replication. Such resistant viruses have been found in AIDS patients treated with reverse transcriptase inhibitors. In addition, influenza A virusesalso generate virus variantsa short time after patients have been previously treated with amantadine or with neuraminidase inhibitors. The underlying mutations mainly affect the regions of the enzyme which interacts with the inhibitors.

Forthe various inhibitors of reverse transcriptase differ from each other, a change of drug is applied after the first occurrence of resistant HIV variants inpatients. Nowadays, combinations of at least three or four inhibitors with differing molecular targets are used in highly active antiretroviral therapy (HAART) at the beginningof therapy. By HAART, it should be impossible to mutate all targeted regions for the virus to develop a multi-resistant HIV. Besides, developing new antiviral inhibitors by using different experimental approaches, based on new molecular targets and bio-functions, is in progress.

Chapter 7

Introduction of Medical Mycology and Main Mycoses

7.1 General Properties of Fungi

The fungi (plural form of fungus) are a large and diverse eukaryotic microorganisms group most are widely distributed in soil and water. They contain no chlorophyll with no differentiation of root, stem and leaf. Fungi are the great recyclers which are one of the important members of earth ecosystem. If they were lacking, the biochemical cycles of matter in nature would have a different quality, one that would not sustain our biosphere as we know it.

At present, the status of fungi in the biological world has not been unified, Ainsworth's classification systemthat is kingdom fungi is classified into *Myxomycota* and *Eumycota* two phyla and *Eumycota* is classified into the following subphyla: *Mastigomycotina*, *Zygomycotina*, *Ascomycotina*, *Basidiomycotina* and *Deuteromycotina* (Imperfect fungi), has been accepted by most scholars. Most of *Zygomycetes* containing *Mucor* and *Rhizopus* are saprophytes, which are usually found in soil and animal feces. They can also be acted as parasites in plants, animals and humans. *Ascomycotina* is the largest group of fungi. Most of them are saprophytes and a few are opportunistic pathogens. It includes *Blastomyces*, *Histoplasma* and *Trichophyton*, etc. For *Basidiomycotina*, some are useful, such as edible mushrooms and medicinal ganoderma. It also includes some others which are harmful, such as some plant-disease causing pathogens-smut fungus and rust fungus and some human-disease causing pathogens-*Crytococcus* and *Malassezia furur*. For Imperfect fungi, members in it are distributed into *Ascomycotina* and *Basidoomycotina* at first. It is called as Imperfect fungi because only asexual stage has been observed at present or sexual stage is difficult to be observed in nature environment. For some members of Imperfect fungi, their asexual stage and sexual stage are actually classified into different subphyla followed by different names. Most fungi which are important in medicine are imperfect fungi, such as *Coccospora*, *Candida albicans*, *Aspergillus* and various dermatophytes. Latest fungal classification is to classify Kingdom Fungi into the following divisions: *Zygomycota*, *Basidiomycota*, *Ascomycota* and *Chytridiomycota*. Members in *Deuteromycotina* are distributed into the former three and *Myxomycota* has been canceled.

Fungi are closely relative with human life. Fungi are greatly beneficial to humankind in food brewing,

Pharmaceutical and chemical industry and agriculture. But at the same time, fungi can also do serious harm to human due to causing human, animal and plant diseases and corruption of organisms. It is estimated that there are about 1.5 million fungi in the world, but only a few hundred of them can cause human diseases and 90 percent of human fungal diseases are caused by only a few dozen fungi. With the application of broad spectrum antimicrobial drugs, immunosuppressants and antitumor drugs and the development and application of organ transplantation, tracheal intubation and radiation technology, in recent years, the fungal infections, especially the opportunistic fungal infections are in obviously rising trend. Therefore, it is very important to know about biological characteristic and pathogenesis of fungi and to develop effective prevention and treatment measures of fungal infection.

7.1.1　Morphology of Fungi

Fungi are eukaryotic microorganisms. They are usually greatly different from each other in their shape and size. At present, the properties of fungal morphology still play a very important role in identification of fungi. According to the differences of fungal morphology and structure, fungi can be classified into unicellular fungi and multicellular fungi. Unicellular fungi are usually round or oval, such as yeast. But Most of fungi are multicellular and make up of hyphae and spores. Hyphae and spores intertwine and file up together into a mass called as filamentous fungus or mold. A few fungi can appear as yeast type or filamentous fungus in different environmental condition. It is called as dimorphic fungus. The transformation of dimorphic fungus' morphology is closely related to the pathogenicity of fungi.

7.1.1.1　Unicellular Fungi

The simplest fungi are unicellular. A cell means all, carrying out all processes of the whole life of fungi. Unicellular fungiusually reproduce themselves by budding and fission. Most are round or oval shape. It includes two types: yeast type and yeast-like type.

7.1.1.2　Multicellular Fungi

The morphology of multicellular fungi is complex and it consists of two basic structures: hypha and spore.

(1) Hypha

In a suitable environment, a fungal spore elongates gradually, forming a filamentous structure. This filamentous structure is called as hypha. Hypha growsout a lot of branches, forming a woven, intertwining mass of them that make up the body or colony of a mold. The woven, intertwining mass of hypha is called as mycelium. The mycelium of different fungi are usually different from each other (Figure 7-1). It can be used to identify different fungi.

According to the difference of hyphal structure, hypha can be classified into septatehypha and aseptate hypha (Figure 7-2). Septate hypha usually locates in higher fungi and aseptate hypha usually locates in lower fungi. In septate hypha, there are some septa which can divide hypha into several cells. Every cell contains one to several nuclei. There are some pores in septum by which cytoplasm can flow from one cell to another. The septum is a part of the cell wall that is directly related to mitosis. Aseptate hypha refers to those with no septum. The hypha of most pathogenic filamentous fungi is septate hypha.

According to the particularfunction of hypha, hypha can be classified into the following three (Figure 7-3): ①Vegetative mycelium-Vegetative mycelia are those penetrating the supporting medium and being responsible for absorption of nutrients. ②Aerial mycelium-Aerial mycelia are those projecting above the surface of mycelium. ③Reproductive mycelium-Reproductive mycelium is the part of aerial mycelium which give rise to structures. These hyphae are responsible for the production of fungal reproductive bodies or spores.

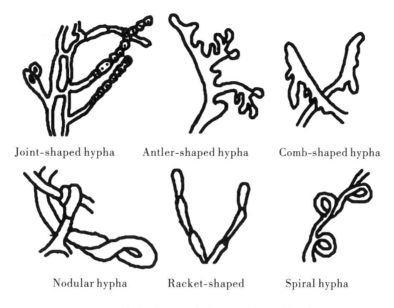

Joint-shaped hypha   Antler-shaped hypha   Comb-shaped hypha

Nodular hypha   Racket-shaped   Spiral hypha

Figure 7-1   Different shapesof fungal hypha

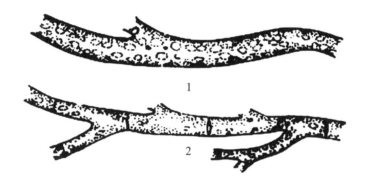

Figure 7-2   Septate hypha and aseptate hypha

1. aseptate hypha;2. septate hypha

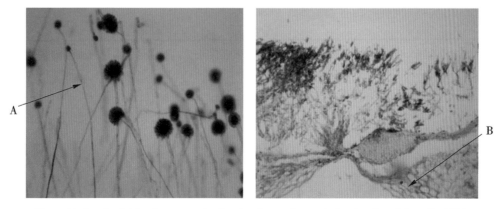

Figure 7-3   Aerial hypha,reproductive hypha and vegetative hypha of fungi(×100)

A. aerial hypha and reproductive hypha;B. vegetative hypha

（2）Spore

Spore is a reproductive form of fungi produced by reproductive mycelium. Fungal spores' function is not only in multiplication but also in survival, providing genetic variation and dissemination. Because of their compactness and relative light weight, spores of fungi are dispersed widely through the environment by air, water and living things. Upon encountering a favorable environment, a spore will germinate and produce a new fungal colony in a very short time. The spores of different fungi may be obviously different from each other in their shape, size, movement properties and surface signs. It is closely related with its functions. It is also important basis of fungal identification and classification. The spore of fungi can be generated asexually or sexually.

Asexual spore is derived directly from hyphal cells but not from cell fusion of sexual cell. There are three kinds of them:①Thallospore（Figure 7-4）. It is produced directly in reproductive mycelium, including blastospore, arthrospore and chlamydospore. Blastospore is a round or oval spore produced by budding. The bud usually becomes separate cell from its parental cell. But some remain attached in a row, forming pseudohypha. Because of its manner of formation, it is not a true hypha like that of molds. Arthrospore is produced by hyphal cells when mycelia cell wall thickened, producing septum and breaking into rectangular segments. They usually arrange in a chain and appear in old culture of fungi. Chlamydospore is a kind of dormant cells of fungi, forming from the top or the middle section of hypha by concentration of cytoplasm, thickening of cell wall and becoming round when fungi are in an environment with poor nutrients. Arthrospore can germinate in a favorable condition. ②Conidium. Conidium forming from the terminal or the branches of reproductive mycelium by cell division or concentration is the common one of asexual spores. It includes macroconidium（Figure 7-5）and microconidium（Figure 7-6）. Macrconidium is made up of more than one cell, appearing as spindle or pear-shaped, etc. The properties of their shape, size, structure and color can be acted as the basis of their identification and classification. Microconidium is smaller and unicellular. Because most multicellular fungi can produce microconidium, microconidium has little significance in the identification of fungi. ③Sporangiospore（Figure 7-7）. The terminal of reproductive mycelium enlarges into a cystic structure called as sporangium. Cytoplasm in sporangium separates from each other, transforming into a sporangiospore with a nucleus involved in it. Spores in sporangium can be released after maturation and form new mycelium.

Sexual spore is produced by the fusion and meiosis of two cells in the same fungus or in different fungi. There are 4 kinds of sexual spores:①Oospore ②Zygospore ③Ascospore ④Basidiospore.

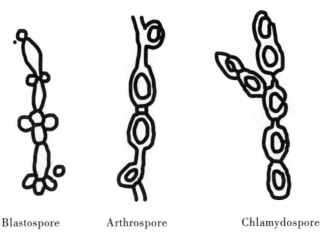

Blastospore   Arthrospore   Chlamydospore

Figure 7-4 **Thallospore**

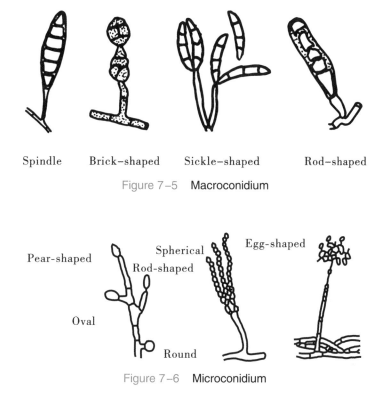

Spindle   Brick-shaped   Sickle-shaped   Rod-shaped

Figure 7-5   **Macroconidium**

Pear-shaped   Spherical   Egg-shaped
Rod-shaped
Oval   Round

Figure 7-6   **Microconidium**

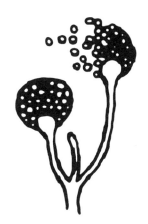

Figure 7-7   **Sporangiospore**

7.1.2   Structure of Fungi

Fungiis eukaryotic cellswith typical nuclear structure(nuclear membrane, nuclear pore, nucleus small body and linear chromosome). Besides microtubules composed of microtubules proteins, there is cytoskeleton made up of microfilaments which is mainly composed of actins in cytoplasm. There are also a variety of organelles such as mitochondria, endoplasmic reticulum, ribosome, etc. But Golgi apparatus is uncommon. The fungal cell membrane contains a large amount of sterols, which is different from the main components of human cell membrane-cholesterol. Sterol of fungus is mainly ergosterol, which is the target of antifungal drugs.

7.1.2.1   Cell Wall of Fungi

The cell wall of fungus is very solid, being related to glucan. The cell wall of fungus can play very important roles in life cycle of fungus. It includes: maintaining the appearance of cells, protecting cells free from the influence of osmotic pressure, regulating the absorption of nutrients, regulating secretion of metabolites and being antigenic components of fungi.

The fungal cell wall can be divided into four layers from the outside to the inside, the outermost layer is the amorphous glucan layer, the second layer is the glycoprotein layer, the third layer is the protein layer and the innermost layer is chitin microfiber layer. Different from bacterial cell walls, fungal cell walls are largely composed of chitin, a polymer of N-acetyl glucosamine, rather than peptidoglycan, which is a characteristic component of bacterial cell walls. All fungal cell walls have two kinds of components-fibrous and amorphous. The fibrous components mainly include chitin and glucan. The amorphous component is mainly composed of polysaccharides, most soluble, including aglucan and mannose glycoprotein. The amorphous component is often mixed in the microfilament fiber net, which can make the cell wall permeable.

7.1.2.2   Septum of Fungi

In most fungi, the hyphais divided into segments by cross walls or septa. The nature of the septa varies from solid partitions with no communication between the compartments to partial walls with small pores that allow the flow of organelles and nutrients between adjacent compartments. Aseptate hypha consists of one long, continuous cell not divided into individual compartments by septa. With this construction, the cytoplasm and organelles in it can move freely from one region to another and each hyphal element can have several nuclei. The appearance of fungal septa is an adaptable form of fungi to changing environment conditions. The septa of different fungi are usually different from each other. The structures of septa are also important basis of fungal classification.

7.1.2.3   Nucleus of Fungi

The function of fungal nucleus is to carry genetic information, control cell proliferation and metabolism. Compared to other eukaryotic cells, the nuclei of fungi are round, but relatively small. A cell or mycelium segment can have one or two nuclei, some even up to 20 to 30. There is usually one to several nuclear pores in the nuclear membrane, which is the channel of material exchange between nucleus and cytoplasm. The number and size of fungal chromosomes were determined usually by using the pulse field gel electrophoresis (PFGE) technique. The fungal genome is between the genome of the prokaryotes and the higher creatures-plants and animals. The gene sequences of many fungi, including ribosomal genes, mitochondrial genes and the genes encoding proteins, have been sequenced. In particular, ribosomal genes are of great significance in the classification and evolution of fungi.

7.1.3   Culture of Fungi

7.1.3.1   The Reproduction of Fungi

There are a variety of ways of fungal reproduction, such as budding, binary fission and breaking of hypha, etc. They all can be classified as asexual reproduction and sexual reproduction.

Sexual reproduction of fungi is characterized by the fusion of two nuclei followed by meiosis. It includes the following stages: ①The stage of cytoplasm fusion; ②The stage of nucleus fusion; ③Meiosis of fused nucleus. Most medicine fungi have no sexual reproduction.

A sexual reproduction is the main reproductive method of fungi. It is the reproduction of new individuals without the fusion of two heterosexual cells. It includes the following four: ①Budding. Reproductive mycelium or spores germinate forming blastospores and every blastospore transformed into a new individual. Most yeasts reproduce by budding. ②Binary fission. The production of offspring cell are in the form of binary fission. Only a few of dimorphic fungi reproduce in this way when they are in organism such as *Schizosaccharomyces pombe*. ③Septa. A septum is formed in a certain segment of conidiophore and the protoplast is then condensed into a new spore. The spore can reproduce independently. ④The breaking of hypha. In the process of fungal reproduction, reproductive mycelium can break into many small fragments and each fragment can germinate into a new hypha in a favorable environment.

7.1.3.2   Culture of Fungi

Most of fungi are not picky in nutritional requirement. They can occur in nature and grow readily on simple sources of nitrogen and carbohydrate. Traditionally, Sabouraud's agar containing glucose and modified peptone which inhibit the growth of bacteria but not most fungi because of its low pH has been used to cultivate most fungi, especially pathogenic fungi. Most fungi grow slowly and take longer to develop colony, so some antibiotics are often added to the medium to inhibit bacterial growth. Most fungi grow well under 22–28 ℃. But for some systemic infection fungi, their optimum growth temperature is 37 ℃ and their optimum pH scale is 4.0–6.0. In Sabouraud's agar, fungi can form the following three types colony (Figure 7–8) : ①yeast type colony. After cultivation, most unicellular fungi appear as yeast type colony. They are usually similar to S type colony of bacteria. But they are usually bigger and cream-colored. ②yeast-like colony. The appearance of yeast-like type colony is similar to yeast type. But under microscope, there are some pseudohyphae growing into the medium which is different from yeast type colony. ③filamentous type colony. The appearance of multicellular fungal colony is filamentous. They are usually bigger and are made up of mycelium and spores. The appearance of filamentous type colony is powdery, villous or flocky. The center and the edge, the front and the back of the colony can be different in color and its color can change with its culture time, which can be an important basis for the identification of fungi.

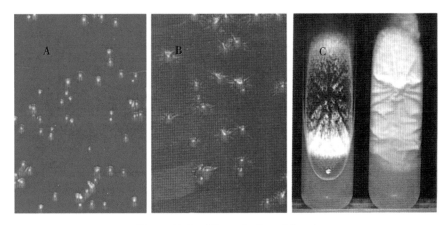

Figure 7-8   **The colonies of fungi**

A. yeast type colony   B. yeast-like colony   C. filamentous type colony

7.1.4   Variation and Resistance of Fungi

A variety of variations are easily to take place in the process of fungal growth and reproduction. After a long time artificial cultivation, the variations of fungal morphologies, colony characteristics, the number of spores and virulence were appeared. Clinically, there is an upward trend in fungal drug resistance.

The resistance of fungi is not strong and most of them can be killed under 60–70 ℃ for 1 hour. Most fungi grow in neutral or weakly acidic environments and they are resistant to drying-out, sunlight, ultraviolet rays and a variety of chemical disinfectants. However, they are usually sensitive to 2.5% tincture, 2% crystal violet, 1% –3% carbolic acid and 10% formaldehyde. The fungus is not sensitive to most antibacterial drugs and clotrimazole, ketoconazole, nystatin and 5-flucytosine have inhibitory effects on a variety of fungi.

7.2 Diagnosis and Treatment of Fungal Infection

7.2.1 Laboratory Diagnosis of Fungal Infection

Laboratory diagnosis of fungal infection includes the detection of etiology and the detection of infected ones' immune response to fungi. Laboratory procedures used in the diagnosis of fungal infection in human are same as the diagnosis of bacterial infection which includes the following: ①Morphologic identification. ②Cultivation and identification. ③serological diagnosis. ④Detection of nucleic acid.

7.2.1.1 The Collection of Specimen

Specimens may be different in different diseases and different stages of a disease. In the superficial infection, the hair, dandruff, fingernail (nail), etc., in the area of the lesion, can be taken as specimens. And the secretions, the blood, lymph, cerebrospinal fluid, etc., in the area of the lesion, can be taken as specimens in systemic infection. There are the following notices in specimen collection: ①Exact collection location. It is usually taken from the exact location of the infection to ensure that the fungi in the vegetative state can be obtained. ②Enough and appropriate specimen. It can not only satisfy the needs of identification but also avoid of damage to human tissue or waste. ③Free from pollution. Whether aseptic locations or opening location, to free from specimen pollution, some aseptic operations are necessary.

7.2.1.2 Morphologic Identification

Microscopic detection of stained or unstained specimens is a relatively simple and inexpensive but much less sensitive method than culture. Before observation under microscope, specimens unstained must be treated with a solution of 10% potassium hydroxide, which can dissolve or clear the tissue (epithelial cells, leukocytes, debris) surrounding the fungal mycelia to allow a better view of the hyphal forms. If spores or mycelium can be observed, the initial diagnosis of mycosis can be sure of. In addition to a few species of fungi, most species can not be identified. In order to improve the detection rate for liquid specimens, the microscopic examination of sediment should be taken after centrifugation. Staining examination of fungi was usually used in the detection of systemic infection fungi, especially their tissue specimens. The common ones include the hematoxylin and eosin method, the silver impregnation method, gram stain, periodic acid-Schiff staining method, etc. After primary isolation of fungi, lactophenol cotton blue staining method or gram stain are usually used to distinguish fungal growth and to identify organisms by their morphology.

7.2.1.3 Cultivation and Identification

The fungal culture is often used in the following conditions: fungal infection can still not be sure of after microscopic examination or determining the species of fungi. After isolation and cultivation, pure culture of fungi is conducive to the researches on their morphologic classification, the properties of their physiological and biochemical characteristics, pathogenicity and drug sensitivity to antifungal drugs, etc. The most commonly used medium for cultivation fungi is Sabouraud's agar. The optimum temperature of cultivation is usually 25 ℃ (filamentous type fungi) or 37 ℃ (yeast type and yeast-like type fungi). The objective fungi can be identified according to the morphologic characteristics of their spores and hyphae after cultivation.

Besides morphologic identification methods above, there are some special identification methods such as CHROM agar identification culture of fungi based on their biochemical properties and special yeast rapid identification system(API-20C AUX) and so on. Compared to some traditional identification methods such as microscopic detection and cultivation, they are more rapidly and accurately.

7.2.1.4   Serological Diagnosis

The laboratory diagnosis of mycoses mainly depends on the finding of fungal mycelia, spores and other structures in clinical specimens or pathological tissue. But for some patients with negative results of fungal microscopic detection and cultivation in their clinical specimens and pathological tissue, who can be determined into fungal infection based on their clinical manifestation, serological identification is important to their laboratory diagnosis. The commonly used serological identification methods include enzyme immunoassays(EIA), including enzyme-linked immunosorbent assay (ELISA) and latex agglutination test, immunofluorescence assay(IFA) and complements fixation test(CF), etc. At present, serological identification are usually used in the antigen or antibody detection of fungal systemic infection because of the complexity of fungal antigens, cross reaction, etc.

7.2.1.5   Detection of Nucleic Acid

Because of limitations of phenotype classification, the application of molecular biology techniques to elucidate the relationship between members in different fungi species or members in the same specie has been widely used in the classification and identification of medical fungi. It includes G+C mol% determination of nucleic acid, a variety of polymerase chain reaction(PCR) techniques, restrictive fragment length polymorphism analysis(RFLP) of nucleic acid, random amplified polymorphic DNA(RAPD), DNA chip technology, etc.

7.2.2   Antifungal Chemotherapy

There are many substances with antifungal activity in nature. But most of them can't be available for treatment of fungal infection in clinic. Because fungi are eukaryotes just like human. Many of cellular and molecular processes of fungi are similar tothat human, resulting in poor selective toxicity of antifungal agents to fungal cells and human cells. And this is one of the main difficulties in the development of antifungal agents. Besides this, poor diffusion into tissues, narrow antifungal spectrum and most just with bacteriostatic effects, they all are the limitations of antifungal agents in current clinical application. The antifungal agents currently used in clinic include polyenes, azoles, allylamines, echinocandins, thiocarbamates and morpholines, etc. They can play their antifungal effects mainly by influencing fungal cell membrane such as amphotericin B, nystatin and azoles, the damage to fungal cell wall such as caspofungin, nikkomycin and pradimicin, influencing the synthesis of fungal nucleic acids such as griseofulvin, flucytosine. The main anti-fungal agents and their features are listed in Table 7−1.

Table 7−1   Features of Antifungal Agents

Agent	Mechanism of action	Mechanism of resistance	Route	Clinical use
Polyenes				
Nystatin	Membrane disruption	Sterol modification	Topical	Most fungi
Amphoteri-cin B	Membrane disruption	Sterol modification	Intravenous	Most fungi

Continue to Table 7-1

Agent	Mechanism of action	Mechanism of resistance	Route	Clinical use
Azoles				
Ketoconazole	Block of Lanosterol 14α-demethylase of rgosterol synthsis	Active efflux, demethylase alteration or over production	Oral	*Candida*, *Crytococcus*, dimorphic fungi
Fluconazole	Block of Lanosterol 14α-demethylase of rgosterol synthsis	Active efflux, demethylase alteration or over production	Oral, intravenous	*Candida*, *Crytococcus*, dimorphic fungi
Itraconazole	Block of Lanosterol 14α-demethylase of rgosterol synthsis	Active efflux, demethylase alteration or over production	Oral, intravenous	*Candida*, *Crytococcus*, dimorphic fungi, invasive molds (*Aspergillus*)
Clotrimazole	Block of Lanosterol 14α-demethylase of rgosterol synthsis	alteration of binding target or increase of target enzyme	Topical	*Candida*, some other yeasts
Miconazole	Block of Lanosterol 14α-demethylase of rgosterol synthsis	Active efflux, alteration of binding target or increase of target enzyme	Topical	*Candida*, some ergosterol other yeasts
Voriconazole	Block of Lanosterol 14α-demethylase of rgosterol synthsis	Unknown	Oral, intravenous	*Candida*, some other yeasts and molds
Allylamines				
Terbinafine	Block of squalence epoxidase	Active efflux		Dermatophytes, combined with azoles for *Candida*, *Aspergillus*
Naftifine	Block of squalence epoxidase	Unknown	Topical	Dermatophytes
Flucytosine	Block of thymine synthase and RNA modifying	Permease or *Crytococcus*, enzymes absent or decreased	Oral	*Candida* and synthsis resistance emerges in monotherapy
Echinocandins				
Caspofungin	Block of β-(1,3)-D-glucan synthase	Unknown	Intravenous	*Aspergillus*, *Candida*
Griseofulvin	Microtubule disruption	The absence of cytosine deaminase or guanosine phosphate ribosyltransferase	Oral	Dermatophytes
Potassium Iodide	Probable activation of phagocytes	Unknown	Oral	
Tolnaftate	Unknown	Unknown	Oral	Dermatophytes

Chapter 8

Bacteriology

8.1 Cocci

8.1.1 *Staphylococcus*

Staphylococcus cells are Gram-positive microorganism, spherical in shape, 0.5 – 1.5 μm in diameter, occurring in pairs, in tetrads or in short chains (3 – 4 cells) and characteristically dividing in more than one plane to form irregular grape-like clusters. The genus *Staphylococcus* currently comprises more than 50 species. These small, hardy bacteria are normal inhabitants of skin, skin glands and mucous membranes of warm-blooded animals including humans. Some organisms may be isolated from a variety of animal products and environment sources. Some species are opportunistic pathogens of humans and/or animals. Staphylococci can be divided into two big groups by catalase test: catalase-positives/variable staphylococci (CoPS) and catalase-negative staphylococci (CoNS) (Table 8–1).

Table 8–1　Clinical and epidemiological schema of staphylococcal species

Group	Human associated	Animal associated
catalase-negative staphylococci (CoNS)	*S. epidermidis*-like "group":	*S. carnosus* subsp. *carnosus*
	S. epidermidis,	*S. felis*
	S. haemolyticus,	*S. caprae*
	S. capitis,	*S. lentus*
	S. hominis,	others
	S. pettenkoferi,	
	S. simulans,	
	S. warneri,	
	others	
	S. saprophyticus subsp. *saprophyticus*	
	S. lugdunensis	

Continue to Table 8-1

Group	Human associated	Animal associated
catalase-positives/variable staphylococci (CoPS)	S. aureus subsp. aureus	S. pseudintermedius
		S. intermedius
		S. hyicus
		S. aureus subsp. Anaerobius
		others

8.1.1.1　*Staphylococcus Aureus*

(1) Biological Character

1) Morphology and Cultural characteristics: *Staphylococcus aureus* is nonmotile, non-spore-forming, Gram-positive cocci. Cells are 0.5-1.5 μm in diameter, occurring singly and forming pairs and clusters. Colonies are raised, smooth, glistening and translucent, with entire margins. Pigmentation varies from gray to yellow to orange. May produce capsules. Facultatively anaerobic. The optimum temperature is 30-37 ℃. Strains grow well in medium containing 10% NaCl, poor at 15% NaCl.

2) Biochemical characteristics: Positive reactions: acetoin production, alkaline phosphatase, arginine dihydrolase, caseinase, catalase, clumping factor, coagulase, fibrinolysin, gelatinase β-glucosidase heat-stable nuclease (thermonuclease), hemolysin, lipase, esterases, nitrate reduction and urease. Acid produced aerobically from fructose, galactose, glucose, glycerol, lactose, maltose, mannitol, mannose, ribose, sucrose, trehalose and turanose, but no gas produced.

3) Antigen: Staphylococcal protein A. Staphylococcal protein A (Spa), a cell wall component, is ubiquitous in *S. aureus* and is often used in strain typing. As Spa interact with the Fc fragment region of immunoglobulins from most mammalian species, this protein has also been used for quantitative and qualitative immunological techniques.

Capsular polysaccharide antigen. Polysaccharide antigen located in cell wall and has group specificity. The majority of clinical isolates of *S. aureus* express a surface polysaccharide, mainly dominated by serotype 5 or 8. The capsule enhances staphylococcal virulence by impeding phagocytosis, resulting in bacterial persistence in the bloodstream of infected hosts. *S. aureus* isolated from infections expresses high levels of polysaccharide but rapidly loses it upon laboratory subculture.

4) Genomes: The genome size of the *S. aureus* strains is 2.82-2.9 Mbp. Comparisons of whole genomes revealed *S. aureus* genome are highly diverse and populations are clonal, with 10 dominant lineages colonizing and infecting humans. The lineages differ in hundreds of genes that are present/absent or have variant regions within genes, including surface proteins, gene regulators and immune evasion pathways. The mobile genetic elements (MGE) occupy 15%-20% of the *S. aureus* genome, including bacteriophage, pathogenicity islands, plasmids, transposons and staphylococcal cassette chromosomes (SCC). Horizontal gene transfer of MGEs between isolates of the same lineage is key to the evolution of new clones that adapt to new niches and cause novel clinical and economic problems.

5) Molecular typing techniques: Spa typing. Single locus DNA sequencing of the repeat region of staphylococcal protein A can be used for reliable and accurate typing of *S. aureus*. The sequences of polymorphic X region of *spa* gene are used in this mothed. On the basis of series of r-codes identified, a *spa* type can be defined. The homology score can be calculated based on the relationship between *spa* types.

Multilocus sequence typing (MLST). MLST is a highly discriminatory mothed of characterizing bacterial isolates based on the sequence of seven house-keeping genes (*arc*, *aro*, *glp*, *gmk*, *pta*, *tpi*, *yqi*). The different sequences are assigned as distinct alleles for each gene and each isolate is defined by the alleles at each of the seven housekeeping loci (sequence type, ST). The online database of MLST (http://saureus. beta. mlst. net) make it possible for comparations between *S. aureus* sequences described in different parts of the world.

Pulsed-Field Gel Electrophoresis (PFGE). PFGE is one of the most commonly used mothed for bacterial molecular typing. The following steps are involved: embedding organisms in agarose, lysing the organisms in situ, digesting the chromosomal DNA with restriction endonucleases (*Sma* I for *S. aureus*) and separating the fragments by gel electrophoresis in an alternating electrical filed. Although PFGE is an adequate technique to study outbreak, it is not sufficient for long-term or global epidemiological study (Table 8-2).

(2) Pathogenicity

1) Factors of the pathogenicity: *S. aureus* expresses many cell surface-associated and extracellular proteins that are potential virulence factors.

Table 8-2　Virulence factors of *S. aureus*

Category	Virulence factors	Function
Components of the cell wall	Capsular polysaccharide	Impede phagocytosis
	Protein A	Binds Fc domain of immunoglobulin and TNFR-1 Binds complement protein C3 and promotes C3-C3b conversion
	Teichoic acids	Contribute to colonization Protection against cell damage
toxins	α toxin	Cytolytic pore-forming toxin
	β toxin	Sphingomyelinase with cytolytic activity
	Leukotoxins	Kill leukocytes Bi-component pore-forming leukotoxins
	Enterotoxins	Gastroenteric toxicity Immunomodulation via superantigen activity
	Toxic shock syndrome toxin-1	Endothelial toxicity (direct and cytokine-mediated) Superantigen activity
Enzymes and other proteins	Coagulase	Binds and activates prothrombin Promotes conversion of fibrinogen to fibrin
	Staphylokinase	Plasminogen activator (plasminogen-serine protease plasmin conversion)
	Catalase	Inactivate hydrogen peroxide Pivotal for nasal colonization

Capsular polysaccharide. The capsular polysaccharides expressed by *S. aureus* are clearly important in the pathogenesis of staphylococcal infections. They enhance staphylococcal virulence by impeding phagocytosis, resulting in bacterial persistence in the bloodstream of infected hosts and promoting abscess formation.

Teichoic acids. The cell wall teichoic acidsare one of the most important factors contributing to *S. aureus* colonization of abiotic surface and nasal colonization. It's also proposed to protect *S. aureus* against cell damage by enabling resistance to cationic antimicrobial peptides (CAMPs), antimicrobial fatty acids, lysozyme and other factors, controlling protein machineries in the pathogens' cell envelope, serving as phage receptor.

α-toxin is released by 95% of S. aureus strains as a water-soluble monomer with pore-forming and pro-inflammatory properties. α-toxin destroys a variety of host cells, including epithelial cells, erythrocytes, fibroblasts, monocytes, macrophages and lymphocytes, but not neutrophils.

β-toxin is a sphingomyelinase which damages membranes rich in this lipid. The classical test for β-toxin is lysis of sheep erythrocytes. The majority of human isolates of S. aureus do not express β-toxin.

The classical Panton and Valentine (PV) leukocidin (PVL) has potent leukotoxicity and is non-hemolytic. Only a small fraction of S. aureus isolates expresses the PVL. The pore-forming leukocidin can lyse cells of the myeloid lineage, including macrophages and neutrophils, which is considered important for S. aureus immune evasion. There is a close epidemiological linkage between PVL and chronic or recurrent skin and soft tissue infections (SSTIs) as well as necrotizing pneumonia.

The staphylococcal enterotoxins (SEs) and SEs-like toxins (SEls) are considered to be major virulence factors of S. aureus in particular in the context of food safety. These toxins have become to be a superfamily with 23 types including the staphylococcal enterotoxins A-E, G-J and R-T (SEA-SEE, SEG-SEJ, SER-SET) and the staphylococcal enterotoxin-like toxins K-Q and U-X (SElK-SElQ, SElU-SElX). Both of SEs and SEls have superantigenic activity.

Toxic shock syndrome toxin. The other type of staphylococcal toxin with superantigen activity is toxic shock syndrome toxin (TSST-1). TSST-1 is responsible for 75% of toxic shock syndrome (TSS), including all menstrual cases. TSS is an acute, life-threatening condition associated with infections by S. aureus or Streptococcus pyogenes in susceptible individuals. Clinically, thesyndrome is characterized by fever, rash, hypotension, desquamation of the skin upon recovery and involvement of three or more of the following organ systems: gastrointestinal, renal, hepatic, central nervous system, mucous membranes, muscular and hematologic.

Coagulase is an extracellular protein which binds to prothrombin in the host to form a complex called staphylothrombin. S. aureus is distinguished clinically from less pathogenic strains of staphylococci by the coagulase test. Inoculation of calcium chelated plasma or blood with S. aureus results in rapid clotting. Staphylocoagulase generated fibrin networks may display unique structural, biochemical and physiological attributes that enable staphylococci to form a pseudo-capsule and escape opsonophagocytic clearance in host tissues. Moreover, Staphylococcal coagulation generates thromboembolic events that promote bacterial dissemination into all organ systems.

Staphylokinase (Sak) is secreted by many isolates of S. aureus, acting as a plasminogen activator. In addition, Staphylokinase is also showed to be able to inactivate several defensins by binding. In vivo, staphylococcal strains producing Sak were protected against the bactericidal effect of α-defensins.

2) Disease: In humans, S. aureus has a niche preference for the anterior nares, especially in the adult. Nasal carrier rates range from less than 10% to more than 40% in normal adult human populations residing outside of the hospital. However, S. aureus is also an important pathogen of humans and animals. In principle, there are two kinds of S. aureus-caused diseases: pyogenic and/or systemic infections, which can affect virtually all organ and organ systems, respectively and toxin-mediated diseases.

Pyogenic and/or systemic infections caused by S. aureus including: folliculitis, furuncles, carbuncles, limited/severe cellulitis, necrotizing fasciitis, wound infection, mastitis, meningitis, arthritis, bursitis, osteomyelitis, hematogenous osteomyelitis and others.

Toxin-mediated diseases caused by S. aureus including: staphylococcal toxic shock syndrome caused by

TSST-1 and SEs, SE-caused food poisoning (SFP) and staphylococcal skin syndrome caused by exfoliative toxins (ETs).

(3) Laboratory Diagnosis

Microscopy. Staphylococci are Gram-positive cocci about 0.5–1.0 μm in diameter, growing in clusters or pairs. The appearance of clusters helps to distinguish staphylococci from streptococci, which usually grow in chains.

Isolation and identification. The clinical specimen can be plated on blood agar or mannitol salt agar containing 7.5% sodium chloride. The Gram stain of the suspected colony could be performed. Catalase and coagulase detection should also be conducted. Another very useful test for S. aureus is the production of thermostable deoxyribonuclease. Positive reactions of hemolysis, catalase, coagulase, thermostable deoxyribonuclease could be found for S. aureus.

Susceptibility testing. The clinical strains of S. aureus are often resistance to many different antibiotics, therefore susceptibility testing should be performed to find the clinically useful drugs.

SEs testing. For food poisoning cases, the vomit, faeces and residual food should be cultivated for bacterial culture and identification. Enzyme-linked immunosorbent assay (ELISA) can be used for the SEs-containing detection.

(4) Prevalence, Treatment and Prevention

S. aureus is carried mostly in the nose, but also in the throat, gut and skin folds of humans. Carriage increases the risk of developing a staphylococcal infection and healthcare-associated infections are usually caused by the strains carried in the patient nose.

Identification of the organism is recommended to assess antimicrobial susceptibility. In general, β-lactam family antibiotics are the first choice for the treatment of Methicillin-susceptible Staphylococcusaureus (MSSA) infections. Vancomycin has been the antibiotic of choice for the treatment of methicillin-resistant strainsfor decades.

Prevention of S. aureus infections relies on implementation of recommended contact precautions and adequate principles of infection control. Hand hygiene is one of the most cost-efficient interventions to prevent S. aureus infections within and outside the health care setting. Bundles of care orientated to improving adherence to quality of care indicators have shown to be effective in preventing S. aureus infections. The use of mupirocin 2% ointment in surgical patients with nasal S. aureus carriage has significant benefit in reducing the infection rate with S. aureus.

8.1.1.2　Coagulase Negative Staphylococci

Coagulase-negative staphylococci (CoNS) constitutes a major component of the normal microflora of the human and now represent one of the major nosocomial pathogens, with S. epidermidis and S. haemolyticus being the most significant species.

(1) Biological Character

Gram-stain-positive. Coagulase-negative. Typically, most CoNS species display nonpigmented, smooth, entire, glistening and opaque colonies. Strong slime producers may display a mucoid colony appearance. CoNS consists of more than 30 species, including S. epidermidis, S. haemolyticus, S. saprophyticus, S. capitis. The most common ones are S. epidermidis and S. saprophyticus.

(2) Pathogenicity

1) Factors of the pathogenicity: In general, CoNS isolates lack the virulence determinants responsible for aggression. In comparison with S. aureus, clearly less is known about the virulence mechanisms in CoNS. The colonization of the polymer surface of a medical device by formation of a multilayered biofilm has been

considered the critical factor in the pathogenesis of foreign body-associated infections caused by CoNS. A-mong the CoNS, *S. epidermidis* is by far the species recovered most often from biofilm-associated infections.

2) Disease: The dominant *Staphylococcus* species on skin is *S. epidermidis*, which is considered to be a universal colonizer and part of a panmicrobiota. Across different body sites, a substantial proportion of the skin community comprises coagulase-negative staphylococci (CoNS), including *S. hominis*, *S. haemolyticus*, *S. saprophyticus*, *S. capitis*, *S. warneri*, *S. simulans* and *S. cohnii*. While most CoNS interactions with skin are likely to be commensal, they can caus eopportunistic infections.

Infections associated with medical devices: *S. epidermidis* is the leading causative organism colonized and infected the inserted or implanted foreign body. Originating from bacteremia or other systemic spread of causative organisms and depending on the nature and localization of the foreign body, the following clinical manifestations may result: sepsis, endocarditis, meningitis, joint sepsis, vertebral abscesses and other local manifestations. Local inflammation signs include erythema, warmth, swelling, tenderness and purulent drainage, which characterize exit-site infections.

Native valve endocarditis: CoNS have emerged as being responsible forinfective endocarditis (IE), not only prosthetic valve infective endocarditis (PVIE) but also native valve infective endocarditis (NVIE). CoNS causing both endocarditis have been identified as *S. epidermidis* (71.4%), followed by *S. lugdunensis* (8.8%), *S. hominis*, *S. capitis*, *S. haemolyticus* and others.

Bacteremia/septicemia in neutropenic patients: Especially with chemotherapy-induced neutropenia, *S. epidermidis* is the main cause of septicemia in febrile patients.

Urinary tract infection (UTI): *S. saprophyticus* subsp. *saprophyticus* is the second most frequent causative microorganism of uncomplicated lower UTI in young, sexually active women.

(3) Diagnosis and Treatment

Coagulase test, pigment detection are the traditional methods for distinguish *S. aureus* from CoNS. Identification of *S. epidermidis* can be confirmed by commercial biotyping kits. For methicillin-susceptible isolates, treatment with β-lactamase resistant penicillin and cephalosporins (first or second generation) is advisable. Unfortunately, the vast majority of clinically recovered isolates are methicillin resistant. Thus, most infections by *S. epidermidis* require treatment with glycopeptides, with vancomycin given preference.

8.1.2 *Streptococcus*

Streptococci are Gram-positive, nonmotile, non-spore-forming, catalase-negative cocci. *Streptococcus* strains are normally spherical or ovoid in shape, occurring in chains or pairs. Older cultures may lose their Gram-positive character. *Streptococcus* genus currently consists of over 50 recognized species which, for the most part, exit as commensals or parasites on mucosal surfaces in the oral cavity, upper respiratory tract and gastrointestinal tract of human and animals. Some species can cause localized and systemic infections under appropriate conditions. Thereinto, group A streptococci together with *Streptococcus pneumoniae* are the major pathogens.

Generally, streptococci are classified based on the following ways: colony morphology, hemolysis, serologic specificity and biochemical reactions.

Hemolysis. Streptococci are divided into three groups by the type of hemolysis on blood agar:

1) α-hemolytic: *Streptococcus* (commonly called viridans streptococci) is characterized by a zone of greenish discoloration occurs around the colony, usually 1–3 mm in width and the margin is indistinct. Most *S. pneumoniae* are α-hemolytic but can cause β-hemolysis during anaerobic incubation.

2) β-hemolytic: *Streptococcus* (also called *Streptococcus* hemolytic) is characterized by a sharply defined

zone of clearing around the colonies with the zone size varying from strain to strain. This type of streptococci shows a high virulence, leading to a variety of disease.

3) γ-hemolytic: *Streptococcus* has no effect on blood agar.

Serologic specificity. The serological classification is based on the group-specific polysaccharides antigens associated with the cell wall. According to the cell-wall associated group antigen, the strains are designated by a letter of the alphabet (A-H and K-V). Among these, Group A streptococci is most commonly pathogen associated with human disease. The serogroups A (*Streptococcus pyogenes*), B (*Streptococcus agalactiae*) and *S. dysgalactiae* subsp. *equisimilis* (group C and G) are generally defined as β-hemolytic streptococci(Table 8-3).

Table 8-3　Streptococci of medical importance

Species	Serogroup	Hemolytic type	Host	Human disease
S. pyogenes	A	β-hemolytic	common	Acute pharyngitis and more severe conditions
S. agalactiae	B	β-hemolytic	Cattle, human	Miscarriages, premature birth and neonateinfection in the form of sepsis, pneumonia or meningitis
S. bovis	D	γ-hemolytic	Animal, human	Endocarditis, bacteremia, sepsis, meningitis
S. viridans	–	α/γ-hemolytic	human	Caries, endocarditis
S. pneumoniae	–	α-hemolytic	human	Pneumonia

8.1.2.1　Group A *Streptococcus* (GAS)

Streptococcus pyogenes constitutes group A *Streptococcus* (GAS), colonizing on the throat or skin epithelial surfaces and causing a wide variety of clinical manifestations.

(1) Biological Character

1) Morphology and Cultural characteristics: Cells are spherical in shape, 0.5-1.0 μm in diameter and growth in chains of short or moderate length. Ovoid forms may occur usually in older cultures and growth in pairs with long chains frequently observed in broth culture. The typical appearance of *S. pyogenes* colonies after 24 hours of incubation at 35-37 ℃ is dome-shaped with a smooth or moist surface and clear margins. After overnight culture on blood agar, three major visual colony types may form: mucoid, matte or glossy and β-hemolysis. The optimum temperature for growth is 37 ℃. Growth is enhanced by supplementation with blood and serum.

2) Biochemical characteristics: Glucose is the primary carbon source for obtaining energy. Acid is produced, but no gas. Unlike staphylococci, *S. pyogenes* lacks catalase.

3) Antigen: Polysaccharide antigen. The antigenic components essential in classification and diagnosis are located mainly in the cell wall. The group A specificity of *S. pyogenes* is represented by a polysaccharide, owns a multibranch structure and composed of N-acetylglucosamine and rhamnose, which is considered as the grouping basis of *Streptococcus*.

M-protein antigen. The M protein, essentially a long α-helical coiled coil anchored in the bacterial membrane and extending from the surface of the cell, coats the surface of GAS and acts as a primary antigen. M protein is essential for GAS virulence. More than 80 different serological M protein types within GAS are recognized.

T-protein antigens. The T protein antigen is a relatively stable, trypsin-resistant surface protein of unknown function but is well defined in>95% of GAS, which provides a valuable additional strain characteristic for epidemiological studies.

(2) Pathogenicity

1) Factors of the pathogenicity: GAS possesses various cell-surface components such as hyaluronic acid (HA), M and T proteins and proteins binding to host components such as fibronectin (FN), laminin, immunoglobulins (Igs), lipoteichoic acid (LTA) and peptidoglycan, which may contribute to pathogenesis. Additionally, GAS produces extracellular enzymes including streptokinase (Ska), proteinases, hyaluronidase, nucleases and neuraminidase and toxins such as streptolysins, pyrogenic exotoxins (Spe) and streptococcal superantigens, some of which induce fever and shock.

Hyaluronic acid (HA). GAS is surrounded with polysaccharide capsules composed of hyaluronic acid (HA), which consists of glucuronic acid and N-acetylglucosamine repeating units. The hyaluronic acid capsule is weakly immunogenic due to antigenic similarity with the host and provides protection against phagocytosis by cells of the immune system.

M protein. M protein plays an important role in pathogenesis. It owns anti-phagocytic properties against neutrophils and promotes the adhesion/invasion of GAS into host cells.

Fibronectin. Fibronectin is a primary target of the streptococcal adhesion. It plays an important role in connecting bacterial adhesins to integrin receptors on the surface of eukaryotic cells.

Lipoteichoic acid (LTA). LTA is an amphipathic molecule associated with M proteins. It is thought to account for around 60% of the adhesion of GAS to epithelial cells. LTA is reported to mediate the first-step of adhesion and have little cellular specificity.

Streptokinase. Streptokinase is plasminogen activator protein, secreted by group A, C and G streptococci. The generation of plasmin from plasminogen may facilitate streptococci to spread from its primary or initial site of infection into surrounding sites.

Hyaluronidase. The hyaluronidase-type enzymes have the ability to aid in the spread of the organism or its proteins and toxins.

Streptolysins. *S. pyogenes* secretes two well-known hemolysins, streptolysin S (SLS) and streptolysin O (SLO). They are involved in the breakdown of host tissues and cells and are able to lyse red blood cells, inhibit normal cell function and destroy cells and tissues. The oxygen-stable SLS is secreted by 99% of all GAS isolates at stationary phase. The oxygen-sensitive SLO is secreted by nearly all GAS isolates during exponential and early stationary growth phases.

Pyrogenic exotoxins. Pyrogenic exotoxins A, B and C are associated with invasive disease. Exotoxins A, B and C are probably important in the clinical manifestations of streptococcal toxic-shock syndrome (STSS). They are also responsible for the signs seen in cases of scarlet fever, including rash, strawberry tongue and desquamation of the skin. Exotoxin B may contribute to survival of GAS in the host through increased resistance to phagocytosis and dissemination to organs.

2) Disease: GAS is an important human pathogen which colonizes the throat or skin, causing a broad spectrum of disease, from severe invasive infections and the poststreptococcal complications of acute rheumatic fever (ARF) and acute post-streptococcal glomerulonephritis (APSGN) to mild superficial infections of the throat or skin. According to the estimation of the World Health Organization (WHO), approximately 18.1 million people currently suffer from a serious GAS disease, another 1.78 million new cases occur each year and these diseases are responsible for over 500,000 deaths each year(Table 8-4).

Table 8-4   The spectrum of GAS infection

Illness resulting	Manifestations
Direct infection	Skin and soft tissue infection (pyoderma, impetigo, cellulitis, erysipelas)
	Bone and joint infection
	Pharyngitis/tonsillitis
	Bacteremia
	Other invasive infection
Immune-mediated disease	Acute post-streptococcal glomerulonephritis
	Acute rheumatic fever(rheumatic heart disease)
Toxin-mediated disease	Scarlet fever
	Streptococcal toxic shock syndrome (STSS)
	Necrotizing fasciitis

(3) Laboratory Diagnosis

Isolation and Culture. Laboratory diagnosis of GAS infections still largely relies on culturing bacteria from clinical specimens (such as throat, pharyngeal and pus swabs). To detect streptococci (and especially *S. pyogenes*) in clinical samples, the material is most often cultured on blood agar plates at 37 ℃.

Morphology. After 24 hours incubation at 37 ℃, typical appearance may form: dome-shaped with a smooth or moist surface and clear margins, white-greyish color, >0. 5 mm in diameter, β-hemolysis. Microscopically, *S. pyogenes* appears as Gram-positive cocci, arranged in chains.

PYR test. The PYR test is a rapid colorimetric method based on the activity of the enzyme pyrrolidonyl aminopeptidase, which hydrolyzes L-pyrrolidonyl-β-naphthylamide (PYR) to β-naphthylamide. It is often used to distinguish *S. pyogenes* from other β-hemolytic streptococci with a similar morphology (such as *S. dysgalactiae* subsp. *equismilis*).

Serologic tests. Since antibody development takes about one to two weeks after the onset of acute infection to be detectable in serum samples, serologic tests is rarely useful in acute infections diagnosis. One of the most widely used antibodies for the diagnosis of poststreptococcal diseases are anti-streptolysin O. Antibody levels against streptolysin O (ASO) start rising after one week of infection and reach maximum levels at about three to six weeks of infection. The upper limits of normal (IU/mL) of ASO are 276 in the pediatric age group 5-14 years and 238 in the age group 15-24. More than 85% of patients presenting with ARF have a titer of ASO above the threshold 80% value.

(4) Prevalence, Treatment and Prevention

The estimates of WTO suggest that GAS causes a substantial burden of disease and death on a global scale. This is not surprising, given that all of these diseases are related to poverty and hence are most common in less developed countries and that GAS causes such a broad spectrum of acute and chronic disease. Penicillin remains the drug of choice for *S. pyogenes*. Prevention can be conceptualized at levels described as primordial (improved social health determinants), primary (vaccination or treatment of GAS pharyngitis), secondary (antimicrobial prophylaxis after ARF e. g., monthly benzathine penicillin) and tertiary (medical and surgical management of rheumatic heart disease).

8. 1. 2. 2   *Streptococcus Pneumoniae*

Streptococcus pneumoniae, also known as *pneumococcus*, is a significant human pathogen causing meningitis, sepsis and pneumonia. Risk groups include young children, elder people and patients with immunodeficiencies.

(1) Biological Character

1) Morphology and Cultural characteristics: Cells are Gram-positive, oval or spherical in shape, 0. 5-1. 25 μm in diameter, typically in pairs, occasionally singly or in short chains. The distal end of each pair of cells tends to be pointed or lance-shaped. Gram-positive reaction may be lost in older cultures.

α-hemolysis on blood agar when cultures are incubated aerobically, while β-hemolysis when anaerobic incubation is applied. Mucoid colonies result from copious capsular polysaccharide synthesis. Smooth colonies are glistening, dome-shaped and reflect decreased capsular polysaccharide. "Phantom" colonies reflect early and rapid partial autolysis of a mucoid colony, which is suppressed by incubation under increased CO_2 tension.

2) Biochemical characteristics: Acid is produced from glucose, galactose, fructose, sucrose, lactose, maltose, raffinose, glycogen, trehalose and inulin, but no gas produced. Bile-solubility test can be used to differentiate pneumococci from other streptococci.

3) Antigen: Pneumococcal capsules. Pneumococcal capsules are generally composed of repeating oligosaccharide units consisting of 2-10 monosaccharides. There are ninety-eight reported pneumococcal serotypes classified on biochemical and genetic differences in the structure of the capsular polysaccharide (CPS). The specific distribution of pneumococcal serotypes and serogroups has been associated with age, site of infection, pre-existing medical condition, social status and geographic region.

C-polysaccharide antigen. The C-polysaccharide antigen is attached to the peptidoglycan backbone and is uniformly distributed over the cell surface. C-Polysaccharide is responsible for pneumococcal reaction with C-reactive protein, an acute-phase human serum protein and also for the bacterium's susceptibility to pneumococcal autolysin.

M protein antigen. M protein antigen of *S. pneumoniae*, a serotype specific antigen, is not related to the virulence.

(2) Pathogenicity

1) Factors of the pathogenicity: Several factors of *S. pneumoniae*, most found at the cell surface, contribute to escape the host immune system and involve in the inflammation resulting from infection. These factors include capsules, cell-wall polysaccharide, IgA1 protease, pneumolysin, autolysin, neuraminidase and hyaluronidase.

Capsules. The virulence of *pneumococcus* is largely due to the polysaccharide capsule. Around 20 to 30 serotypes of the more than 90 show significant invasiveness. Although capsule can increase invasiveness in many different ways (influencing biofilm formation, sensitivity to neutrophil extracellular traps and interaction with the epithelium), its primary role in virulence is to shield the cell wall from reacting with host antibodies and complement.

Pneumolysin. Pneumolysin is directly toxic for a wide variety of host cells and tissues, elicits strong inflammatory responses at the site of infection and activates complement via antibody binding of the Fc region. In pneumococcal meningitis, the majority of the damage to the blood-brain barrier has been attributed to pneumolysin.

Cell-wall polysaccharide. The cell wall layer, consisting of polysaccharides and teichoic acid, serves as an anchor for cell-wall-associated surface proteins. The polysaccharides induce inflammatory responses in the host by activation of the alternative complement pathway and stimulation of interleukin-1 production by monocytes.

Neuraminidase. Neuraminidase improves colonization by cleaving N-acetylneuraminic acid from mucin, decreasing the viscosity of the mucus.

2）Disease：Human are the main reservoir for the *pneumococcus*. The asymptomatic carriage in the naso-pharynx is widely prevalent in healthy people. In some cases, colonization is followed by disease when *pneumococcus* gains access to normally sterile body sites. According to the estimations of WHO, about 1.2 million children aged below 5 years die each year as a result of pneumonia, for which the main casual factor is *S. pneumoniae*. It is also the causal agent of meningitis, otitis media and some less frequent conditions such as abscesses, conjunctivitis, pericarditis and arthritis（Table 8-5）.

Table 8-5　Generalities on pneumococcal disease

Disease	Symptom
Otitis, Sinusitis	Fever, pain and discharge from ears, tenderness over sinuses and/or persistent discharge from the nose
Pneumonia	Fever with or without shaking or chills, cough, rapid breathing, chest wall indrawing
Meningitis	Fever, headaches, sensitivity to light, neck stiffness, sometimes confusion or altered consciousness
Bacteraemia, sepsis	Fever, chills, altered consciousness, septic shock

（3）Laboratory Diagnosis

A preliminary diagnosis of *S. pneumoniae* can be made on the basis of morphology and Gram stain: on a blood agar plate, colonies of *S. pneumoniae* appear as small, grey, moist（sometimes mucoidal）colonies and characteristically produce a zone of α-hemolysis（green）. Under a microscope, the cells are Gram-positive, lancet-shaped, capsule-forming cocci or diplococci. The following test can be used to distinguish *pneumococcus* from viridans streptococci:

Quellung（capsular swelling）reaction. In this reaction, antibodies bind to the bacterial capsule of *S. pneumoniae*. Under a microscope, the capsule becomes opaque and appears to enlarge.

Bile solubility. *S. pneumoniae* is bile soluble whereas all other α-hemolytic streptococci are bile resistant. Sodium deoxycholate（2% in water）will lyse the pneumococcal cell wall.

Optochin inhibition. *S. pneumoniae* strains are sensitive to the chemical optochin（ethylhydrocupreine hydrochloride）. Optochin sensitivity allows for the presumptive identification of α-hemolytic streptococci as *S. pneumoniae*, although some pneumococcal strains are optochin-resistant. Other α-hemolytic streptococcal species are optochin-resistant.

（4）Prevalence, Treatment and Prevention

Pneumococcus spreads mainly through coughing or sneezing with air droplets and causes disease among children under two years of age and older adults or those with underlying risk factors. It is important to vaccinate children against pneumococcal disease. Moreover, besides vaccination, breastfeeding and proper hygiene help children to develop a healthy immune system. Treatment is usually with penicillin. As treatment is not always efficient and vaccines do not work against all types of pneumococcal disease, control of pneumococcal disease can only be achieved by a combination of strategies to prevent, protect and treat.

8.1.2.3　Other medical Important Streptococci

（1）Group B *Streptococcus*

Streptococcus agalactiae（Group B *Streptococcus*, GBS）is a Gram-positive encapsulated bacterium, found in the digestive and vaginal tracts of 20% -30% healthy individuals. It is the leading cause of neonatal invasive infection, including pneumonia, meningitis and sepsis. GBS is acquired by the baby via vertical transmission from the birth canal around the time of birth.

The GBS-associated syndromes were divided into two major types in neonates, the early-onset disease (EOD) and the late-onset disease (LOD). EOD usually occurs in the first week of life (age 0–6 days) where prolonged rupture of the membranes and chorioamnionitis features pneumonia, septicemia or meningitis. LOD occurs after (age 7 days-3 months), features septicemia, meningitis and other foci of infection and reportedly associates with capsular serotype Ⅲ clones.

(2) Group D *Streptococcus*

Group D *Streptococcus* is Gram-positive microorganisms. On blood agar, the majority of strains produce α-hemolytic reaction of varying intensity or γ-hemolytic reaction. Group D *Streptococcus*, dominated by *S. bovis* and *S. equinus*, is a group of human and animal derived streptococci that are commensals (rumen and gastrointestinal tract), opportunistic pathogens or food fermentation associates. As reported, Group D *Streptococcus* are part of bowel flora in 2% –12% of healthy adults but may be more prevalent in patients with gastrointestinal carcinoma. Group D *Streptococcus* are important etiologic agents of urinary tract infections and infections associated with biliary tract procedures, as well as cases of disseminated infection, bacteremia and endocarditis.

(3) Viridans *Streptococcus*

Viridans *Streptococcus* are gram-positive microorganisms that can form α-hemolytic reaction on blood agar. Modern classifications divide these species into five groups termed Mitis, Mutans, Salivarius, Sanguinis and Anginosus. They reside as normal flora in oral cavity, respiratory, gastrointestinal, urogenital tract and on skin. Viridans *Streptococcus* associated with a number of important clinical syndromes, including bacteremia, endocarditis, meningitis and septicemia following dental procedures.

8.1.3 *Enterococcus*

The genus *Enterococcus* was initially grouped within the genus *Streptococcus* and then officially named *Enterococcus* in 1984. The genus consists of non-sporulating gram-positive bacteria which usually inhabit the intestinal tracts of humans, animals and insects, as well as the environments (plants, soil and water). Enterococci are also leading opportunistic hospital pathogens, causing infections. The vast majority of clinical isolates are *Enterococcus faecalis* that account for 80% –90% of clinical strains, followed by *Enterococcus faecium* that account for 5% –10%.

8.1.3.1 Biological Character

Cells are ovoid, occur singly, in pairs or in short chains and are frequently elongated in the direction of the chain. Enterococci are Gram-positive, catalase-negative, non-spore-forming, facultative anaerobic bacteria. Hemolytic activity is variable and largely species-dependent. Optimal growth of most species at 35–37 ℃. The following characteristics are common to most of the species: Lancefield group D antigen, resistance to 40% bile, resistance to 0.4% sodium azide or 6.5% NaCl, growth at 10 ℃ and 45 ℃.

8.1.3.2 Pathogenicity

(1) Factors of the Pathogenicity

Aggregation substance (AS). AS is an LPXTG-containing surface protein that encoded by antibiotic-resistance plasmids. AS is an important component of pheromone-responsive plasmid transfer systems of *E. faecalis*. Induction of AS expression promotes effective mating pair formation, a first step in plasmid transfer. During infection, AS increases vegetation size and severity of *E. faecalis* experimental endocarditis and promotes internalization of bacteria by cultured enterocytes. AS also assist the bacteria to adhere and persist on tissues and medical devices by forming biofilm.

Extracellular surface protein (Esp). Esp is a cell-wall-associated protein that is thought to promote adhesion, colonization and evasion of the immune system. Esp also contributes to enterococcal biofilm formation, which could lead to resistance to environmental stresses and adhesion to eukaryotic cells such as those of the urinary tract.

Cytolysin. Cytolysin is a pore-forming exotoxin that expressed by highly virulent strains of *E. faecalis*. it lyses both bacterial and eukaryotic cells in response to quorum signals.

A group of hydrolytic enzymes including hyaluronidases, gelatinase and serine protease are also involved in the virulence of *Enterococcus* species.

(2) Antibiotic Resistance

Multidrug-resistant (MDR) enterococci are important nosocomial pathogens and a growing clinical challenge. Resistance among the enterococci can be either intrinsic or acquired. Enterococci are intrinsically resistant to many β-lactams, fluoroquinolones, lincosamides, trimethoprim-sulfamethoxazole and low concentrations of aminoglycosides.

β-lactam resistance. Intrinsic tolerance to the action of β-lactams is associated with the presence of a species-specific class B PBP, which possesses low binding affinity for ampicillin and the cephalosporins. Ampicillin resistance is also mediated by a β-lactamase that inactivates the antibiotic through the cleavage of the β-lactam ring.

Aminoglycoside resistance. Enterococci generally exhibit a moderate level of intrinsic aminoglycoside resistance that has been attributed to poor uptake of antibiotics. Only two aminoglycosides (gentamicin and streptomycin) are reliably used in clinical practice (for synergism with β-lactams) due to the fact that these compounds are not readily affected by intrinsic enzymes produced by enterococci. However, high-level resistance to aminoglycosides, which is usually acquired on a mobile element that encodes an aminoglycoside-modifying enzyme, abolishes the synergistic effect of these compounds.

Glycopeptide resistance. The biochemical basis for vancomycin resistance derives from modification of the antibiotic target. Nine distinct vancomycin resistance clusters have been described in enterococci (*vanA*, *vanB*, *vanC*, *vanD*, *vanE*, *vanG*, *vanL*, *vanM* and *vanN*).

(3) Disease

During the past few decades, enterococci have emerged as important healthcare-associated pathogens and cause a series of disease.

Urinary Tract Infections. Urinary Tract Infections is the most common type of enterococcal infection. Lower urinary tract infections (such as cystitis, prostatitis and epididymitis) are frequently seen in older men. Enterococcal urinary tract infections are more likely to be acquired in hospital or long-term care settings.

Intra-Abdominal, Pelvic and Soft Tissue Infections. Enterococci are often recovered from cultures of intra-abdominal, pelvic and soft tissue infections.

Bacteremia. Enterococci are currently the second leading cause of healthcare-associated bacteremia.

Endocarditis. Endocarditis is one of the most serious enterococcal infections.

Uncommon Infections. Other infections less commonly or rarely seen due to enterococci include meningitis, hematogenous osteomyelitis, septic arthritis, central nervous system infections, otitis, sinusitis, pneumonia, endophthalmitis and burn wounds.

8.1.3.3 Laboratory Diagnosis

The following approach can be used for species identification: catalase-negative, Gram-positive cocci, showing good growth on *Enterococcus*-selective media containing 0.4% sodium azide and able to grow in

6. 5% NaCl broth. Isolates with these characters can be identified presumptively as belonging to the genus *Enterococcus*.

8.1.3.4 Prevalence, Treatment and Prevention

Enterococci is normal flora in the gastrointestinal (GI) tract of humans. They are also routinely recovered from beach sands, freshwater and marine water sediments, soil and aquatic and terrestrial vegetation. Transmission of enterococcal strains has been documented within medical units, between hospitals and even from state to state. Enterococci become a nosocomial pathogen associated with both endogenous colonization and patient-to-patient spread. Hospitalized patients may have a greater incidence of enterococcal infection.

For susceptible isolates, ampicillin and penicillin remain the drugs of choice for enterococcal infections in nonallergic patients. Monomicrobial enterococcal infections, such as urinary tract infections or non-endocarditis bacteremia, can be treated with penicillin or ampicillin alone. For endocarditis caused by *E. faecalis*, combination of a cell wall-active agent and an aminoglycoside remains the standard of care. Of the available aminoglycosides, gentamicin is generally preferred over streptomycin, as the synergistic agent used with either an aminopenicillin or a glycopeptide.

Vancomycin-resistant enterococci (VRE) represent a major problem in healthcare settings worldwide. Each healthcare facility needs a comprehensive infection control program that can decrease the transmission of VRE among patients. Hospital Infection Control Practices Advisory Committee (HICPAC) suggested the following measures to reduce cross-transmission among hospitalized patients: restriction of vancomycin use; education of hospital staff and the promotion of handwashing with antiseptic soap or a waterless antiseptic agent; routine screening for vancomycin resistance among isolates from clinical samples; contact isolation for patients with VRE colonization or infection; and rectal surveillance cultures. Recommended treatment for VRE includes streptogramins (quinupristin/dalfopristin for E. faecium only) and oxazolidinones (linezolid, tedizolid).

8.1.4 *Neisseria*

Neisseria is Gram-negative, aerobic or facultatively anaerobic cocci, occurring singly but often in pairs. Capsules and fimbriae (pili) may be present. Endospores are not present. As a significant component of the human microbiome, most of the species other than *Neisseria meningitidis* and *Neisseria gonorrhoeae* have negligble infection rates. *N. meningitidis* is a frequent asymptomatic colonizer of the human upper respiratory tract, causing serious blood and brain infections of susceptible people. *N. gonorrhoeae* is always considered to be pathogenic and cause disease.

8.1.4.1 *Neisseria Meningitidis*

N. meningitidis, also known as *meningitidis*, is a well-known agent of epidemic meningitis.

(1) Biological Character

1) Morphology and Cultural characteristics: *N. meningitidis* is Gram-negative, non-pigmented cocci. Cells are 0.6–1.9 μm in diameter, arranged in pairs. Capsules and fimbriae (pili) are present. Growth can be enhanced with an atmosphere containing 3% –10% CO_2 and high relative humidity. Optimal temperatures are 36–37 ℃. After 18–24 h incubation, the size of the colonies is ≥1.0 mm in diameter. Colonies are small, round, smooth, glistening, sometimes mucoid and translucent on Mueller-Hinton agar and are often iridescent. Due to autolysis with age, colonies become more butyrous and rubbery to the touch of an inoculating needle.

2) Biochemical characteristics: Oxidase positive. Catalase positive. *N. meningitidis* produce acid from glucose by oxidation, not fermentation.

3）Antigen：Polysaccharide capsules. Based on antigenic differences in capsular polysaccharides, 13 meningococcal serogroups have been identified, including A, B, C, H, I, K, L, X, Y, Z, W135 and 29E. The majority of disease is caused by organisms with capsule types A, B, C, Y or W-135.

Porin. Meningococcal outer membranes contain trimeric proteins that form hydrophilic pores (porins) termed Por. The Neisserial porin proteins are important as serotyping antigens, putative vaccine components and proposed to play a role in the intracellular colonization of humans. Meningococcal strains express two porin molecules, PorA (or class Ⅰ protein) and PorB (or class Ⅱ protein).

Lipo-oligosaccharide (LOS). At least 12 *N. meningitidis* LOS immunotypes (L1-L12) have been identified on a serological basis.

（2）Pathogenicity

1）Factors of the pathogenicity：Capsule. The capsule of *N. meningitidis* functions as a virulence factor based on its antiphagocytic properties.

Lipo-oligosaccharide (LOS). *N. meningitidis* releases large amounts of the potent LOS through blebs or lysis. LOS may shield bacterial surfaces from the host innate and adaptive immune effector mechanisms.

Fimbriae (pili). Pili are hair-like projections and are considered primary adhesion factors utilized by Gram-negative and Gram-positive bacterial species. Meningococcal pili belong to the type 4 pilus family and mediate the attachment of *N. meningitidis* to nasopharyngeal cells.

IgA1-protease. IgA1-protease, which is present only in pathogenic *Neisseria* species, degrades and inactivates immunoglobulin of the IgA1 subtype, which exist in mucosal secretions and serum.

2）Disease：Normally, meningococci are transient visitors of the human nasopharynx and most adults are resistant to infection through acquired immunity. However, on occasion they can cause serious blood and brain infections such as septicaemia and meningitis in susceptible individuals.

Once in the bloodstream *N. meningitidis* can either be responsible for a deadly septic shock leading to purpura fulminans and/or cross the blood-brain barrier (BBB) to invade the meninges.

Compared with the carriage rate, meningococcal disease is rare and disease rates vary in different geographic regions of the world. In endemic situations, it is prevalent in two age groups：children under 1 year of age and young adults between 15-19 years of age.

（3）Laboratory Diagnosis

In cases of suspected meningococcal disease, specimens of blood, cerebrospinal fluid and nasopharyngeal secretions can be collectedfor Gram stain and microscopic diagnosis.

The blood and nasopharyngeal secretions can be inoculated into broth media supplemented with serum for enrichment. The presence of oxidase-positive and Gram-negative diplococci provides a presumptive identification of *N. meningitidis*. Production of acid from glucose and maltose but not sucrose, lactose or fructose may be used for confirmation. The serologic group may be determined by a slide agglutination test, using first polyvalent and then monovalent antisera.

（4）Prevalence, Treatment and Prevention

N. meningitidis strains are considered as normal in the oro-and nasopharynx of adults and children. The rate increases gradually after birth and reaches a peak in teenagers. Treatment of choice for meningococcal disease is parenteral administration of β-lactam antibiotics, such as cephalosporins and penicillin. Capsule-based vaccines against several serogroups are available for meningococcal disease prevention.

8.1.4.2　*Neisseria Gonorrhoeae*

Neisseria gonorrhoeae, also known as *gonococcus*, is the agent of gonorrhea that specifically infect humans.

(1) Biological Character

1) Morphology and Cultural characteristics: *N. gonorrhoeae* is Gram-negative, nonpigmented cocci. Fimbriae (pili) are present. Capsules are not present. Cells are 0.6-1.9 μm in diameter, arranged in pairs. *N. gonorrhoeae* is fastidious and requires glutamine for primary isolation of approximately 20% of strains and co-carboxylase for 1% of strains. Iron is an essential growth factor for *N. gonorrhoeae*. After 48 h incubation, the colonies are 0.6-1.0 mm in diameter, opaque, grayish white, raised, finely granular, glistening, convex and become mucoid with further incubation.

2) Biochemical characteristics: Oxidase positive. Catalase positive. *N. gonorrhoeae* use glucose as the only carbohydrate energy source and produce acid by oxidation.

3) Antigen

Outer membrane protein. Outer membrane protein of Gonococci is constituted of protein I (Porins, PI), protein II and protein III. Porins is the dominant component of the gonococcal outer membrane protein. Gonococci express one of two classes of porins, termed PIA and PIB or PorA and PorB, which are encoded by alleles of the same gene. Antigenic heterogeneity in the PIA and PIB molecules provides the basis for gonococcal serotyping. PI has been considered as a potential vaccine candidate against gonococcal disease.

Lipo-oligosaccharide (LOS). As the corresponding molecule of lipo-oligosaccharide (LPS), LOS of the pathogenic *Neisseria* spp. lacks the repeating O-antigen polysaccharides.

Pili. Pili have been found on the surface of *N. gonorrhoeae*, which is essential for infectivity and disease.

(2) Pathogenicity

1) Factors of the pathogenicity: Outer membrane protein. PI (Porins) is specifically associated with increased bacterial invasiveness for human cells. PII (Opa) contributes to autoagglutination and adherence.

Fimbriae (pili). Fimbriae have been found on the surface of *N. gonorrhoeae* and mediate the attachment of *N. gonorrhoeae* to a wide range of different cell types. It is essential for infectivity and disease.

IgA1-protease. IgA1-protease degrades and inactivates immunoglobulin of the IgA1 subtype found in mucosal secretions and serum.

LOS. The resemblance of the lactoneoseries glycolipids in gonococcal LOS to human glycolipids appear to represent a form of host mimicry that may play a role in immune evasion.

2) Disease: Gonorrhoea, caused by *N. gonorrhoeae*, is the second most common bacterial sexually transmitted infections (STI) and results in substantial morbidity and economic cost worldwide. *N. gonorrhoeae* primarily infects the urogenital tract, giving rise to intense local inflammation and a range of clinical manifestations. The manifestations of uncomplicated gonococcal infection are urethritis in men and mucopurulent cervicitis in women. Gonococcal infections are often asymptomatic in women. This may lead to unrecognized and untreated infection and result in serious complications, including pelvic inflammatory disease, ectopic pregnancy and infertility. Untreated urethral infection in men can lead to epididymitis, urethral stricture and infertility. Infants of mothers with gonococcal infection can contract neonatal conjunctivitis, which may lead to blindness if left untreated.

(3) Laboratory Diagnosis

Gram stain can be employed to diagnosis the clinical specimens of urethral, cervical and rectal specimens. A presumptive diagnosis of gonorrhea may be made if Gram-negative diplococci are observed within leukocytes.

N. gonorrhoeae can also be diagnosed by culture. Specimens should be inoculated onto appropriate media and incubated immediately after collection at 35 to 36.5 ℃ in a CO_2 enriched atmosphere. The combination of oxidase-positive colonies and Gram-negative diplococci provides a presumptive identification of *N. gonorrhoeae*. Fluorescent-antibody staining, coagglutination, specific biochemical tests and nucleic acid amplification tests (NAATs) may be used for confirmation.

(4) Prevalence, Treatment and Prevention

The estimated 27 million prevalent cases of gonorrhea in 2012 translates to a global prevalence of gonorrhea of 0.8% among females and 0.6% among males aged 15-49 years, with the highest prevalence in the WHO Western Pacific and African Regions. Penicillin and Bleomycin can be used for the gonococcal infection. Unfortunately, the treatments turn to be complicated as the antimicrobial susceptibility patterns of *N. gonorrhoeae* are changing rapidly. WHO has provided six treatment guidelines for the following conditions caused by *N. gonorrhoeae*: genital and anorectal infections oropharyngeal infections, retreatment of gonococcal infections after treatment failure and gonococcal ophthalmia neonatorum. Prostitution prohibition and STI education of the public can be an effective strategy for the prevention of gonococcal infection.

8.1.4.3   Other Medical *Neisseria*

Although less virulent than *N. meningitidis* and *N. gonorrhoeae*, commensal *Neisseria* can be opportunistic pathogens in humans (Table 8-6).

Table 8-6   Infections attributed to commensal *Neisseria* species

Species	Colony Morphology	Infections
N. cinerea	small (1.0-1.5 mm in diameter), grayish white with entire edges, slightly granular	Peritonitis, Neonatal conjunctivitis, Bacteraemia, Proctitis
N. lactamica	small, smooth, translucent, slightly butyrous, often have a yellowish tinge	Arthritis and septicaemia, Cavitary lung disease, Bacteraemic pneumonia
N. mucosa	large, mucoid and often adherent	Meningitis, Endocarditis, Visceral botryomycosis
N. subflava	smooth, transparent or opaque, often adherent	Meningitis and septicaemia, Bacteraemia, Endocarditis
N. flavescens	Smooth, opaque with golden yellow pigment.	Endocarditis, Septicaemia
N. sicca	large (up to 3 mm), grayish white, opaque, dry, wrinkled, adherent	Endocarditis, Meningitis, Conjunctivitis

8.2   Enteric Bacilli

1) The enteric bacilli are a collection of medically important gram-negative rods, among of which *E. coli*, *Salmonella*, *Shigella* and *Klebsiella* are the most famous.

2) The diagnostic serotyping scheme is based on the distribution of O, H and K antigens.

3) *E. coli* can be pathogenic both within and outside of the gastrointestinal (GI) tract.

4) *E. coli* can produce every kind of toxin found among enteric bacilli, including α-hemolysin, shiga toxin, labile toxin and stable toxin.

5) The enterovirulent *E. coli* are divided into 4 groups: Enteropathogenic (EPEC), Enterotoxigenic (ETEC), Enteroinvasive (EIEC) and Enterohemorrhagic (EHEC).

6)The known *Salmonella* serovars currently can be classified to three clinical forms of salmonellosis: gastroenteritis, septicemia and enteric fevers.

7)The vast majority of *salmonella* are chiefly pathogenic in animals that constitute the reservior for human infection: poultry, pigs, rodents, cattle, pets and many others.

8)*Shigella* causes disease in primates (eg. humans and gorillas), but not in other mammals.

9)Klebsiella, belonging to pathogens outside the enteric tract, are usually opportunistic pathogens that cause nosocomial infection, especially pneumonia and urinary tract infections.

The enteric bacilli are the largest and most heterogeneous collection of medically important gram-negative rods, inhabiting in the intestinal tract of human and animals and are commonly isolated from clinical specimens. The organisms are facultative anaerobes or aerobes, ferment a wide range of carbohydrates, posses complex antigenic structure [cell membrane (O) antigens, flagellar (H) antigens and capsular (K) antigens] and produce a variety of toxins (endotoxins and/or exotoxins) and other virulence factors.

There are at least 14 genera that have been described to cause human infection. Some are opportunistic pathogens and a few are true pathogens. *E. coli* is the most important intestinal organism and a few of its strains are pathogenic. *Salmonella* is a significant cause of food poisoning. *Shigella* is the causative agent of dysentery. Other important genera include *Proteus*, *Klebsiella*, *Enterobacter*, *Citrobacter*, *Serratia* and *Yersinia*.

8.2.1　General Features of Enteric Bacilli

8.2.1.1　Morphology

The enteric bacilli are among the largest bacteria, measuring 2-4 μm long and 0. 4-0. 6 μm in diameter, with parallel sides and rounded ends. Forms range from large coccobacilli to elongated, filamentous rods. The organisms do not form spores or demonstrate acid fastness.

8.2.1.2　Culture and Growth Characteristics

Most of the enteric bacilli, including *E. coli*, form circular, convex, smooth colonies with distinct edges. The colonies of the organisms are similar but somewhat mucoid. The *salmonella* and *Shigella* produce colonies similar to *E. coli* but ferment lactose. Some strains of *E. coli* produce hemolysis on blood agar.

Enteric bacilli grow readily on simple media, often with single carbon energy source. Growth of Enteric bacilli is rapid under both aerobic and anaerobic conditions, producing 2-5 mm colonies on agar media and diffuse turbidity in broth after 12 to 18 hours incubation. All enteric bacilli ferment glucose, reduce nitrates to nitrites and are oxidase negative.

Carbohydrate fermentation patterns and the activity of amino acid decarboxylases and other enzymes are used in biochemical differentiation. Some tests, e. g. the production of indole from tryptophan, are commonly used in rapid identification systems, while others, e. g. the Voges-Proskauer reaction (productionof acetylmethylcarbinol from dextrose), but used less often. Culture on "differential" media that contain special dyes and carbohydrates distinguishes lactose-fermenting (colored)from non-lactose-fermenting colonies (non-pigmented)and may allow rapid presumptive identification of enteric bacilli.

Many complex media have been designed to help identification of enteric bacilli. One such medium is triple sugar iron (TSI)agar, which is often used to help differentiate *Salmonella* and *Shigella* form other enteric gram-negative rods in stool cultures.

8.2.1.3　Antigenic Structures

The antigenic composition of the enteric bacilli is complex, with more than 170 cell membrane (O)antigens, more than 56 flagellar (H) antigens and numerous capsular (K) antigens described (Figure 8-1).

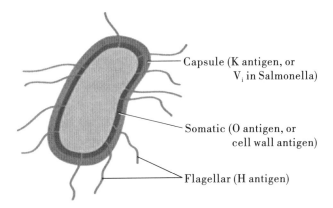

Figure 8-1   Antigenic structure of gram-negative enteric bacteria

(1) O Antigens

O antigens are the most external part of the cell wall lipopolysaccharide and consist of repeating units of polysaccharide. O antigens are resistant to heat and alcohol and usually are detected by bacterial agglutination. Antibodies to O antigens are predominantly IgM.

While each genus of Enterobacteriaceae is associated with specific O groups, a single organism may carry several O antigens. Thus, most *Shigella* species share one or more O antigens with *E. coli* and *E. coli* may cross-react with some *Klebsiella* and *Salmonella* species.

(2) K Antigens

Not all enteric bacilli are associated with K antigens. Some are polysaccharides, including the K antigens of *E. coli* and others are proteins. K antigens may interfere with agglutination by O antisera and they may be associated with virulence. For example, *E. coli* strains producing K1 antigen are prominent in neonatal meningitis and K antigens of *E. coli* cause attachment of the bacteria to epithelial cells prior to gastrointestinal or urinary tract invasion.

(3) H Antigens

H antigens are located on flagella and could be denatured or removed by heat or alcohol. They are preserved by treating motile bacterial variants with formalin. Such H antigens agglutinate with anti-H antibodies, mainly IgG. The determinants in H antigens are a function of amino acid sequence in flagellar protein (flagellin). The organism tends to change from one phase to the other, which is called phase variation. H antigens on the bacterial surface may interfere with agglutination by anti-O antibody.

8.2.1.4   Classification

Enteric bacilli have the following characteristics: they are gram-negative rods, either motile with peritrichous flagella or nonmotile; they grow on peptone or meat extract media without addition of sodium chloride or other supplements; grow well on MacConkey's agar; grow aerobically and anaerobically (are facultative anaerobes); ferment rather than oxidize glucose, often with gas production; are catalase-positive, oxidase-negative and reduce nitrate to nitrite; and have a 39% –59% G+C DNA content. Examples of biochemical tests used to differentiate the species of Enterobacteriaceae are presented.

The major groups of enteric bacilli are described and discussed briefly in the following paragraph. Specific characteristics of *salmonella*, *Shigella* and the other medically important enteric gram-negative rods and the diseases they cause are discussed separately later in this chapter.

Genus and species designations are based on phenotypic characteristics, such as patterns of carbohydrate fermentation and amino acid breakdown. The O, K and H antigens are used to further divide some species into multiple serotypes. These types are expressed with letter and number of the specific antigen, such as *Escherichia coli* O157 ： H7, the cause of numerous food-borne outbreaks.

8.2.2　Escherichia Coli

Escherichia coli are part of the normal flora of the colon in humans and other animals but can be pathogenic both within and outside of the gastrointestinal (GI) tract. Cells are typically rod-shaped and are about 2. 0 μm in length and 0. 25–1. 0 μm in width. The differences in the degree of virulence of various *E. coli* strains are correlated with the acquisition of plasmids, integrated prophages and pathogenicity islands. *E. coli* has fimbria or pili that are important for adherence to host mucosal surface and different strains of the organism may be motile or nonmotile. Most strains can ferment lactose in contrast to the major intestinal pathogens (eg. *Salmonella* and *Shigella*), which cannot ferment lactose. *E. coli* produces both acid and gas during fermentation of carbohydrates.

8.2.2.1　Biological Character

(1) Morphology

E. coli is a Gram-negative and non-sporulating bacteria. Cells of *E. coli* are typically rod-shaped and are about 2. 0 μm long and 0. 25–1. 0 μm in diameter, with a cell volume of 0. 6–0. 7 μm^3. *E. coli* stains Gram-negative because its cell wall is composed of a thin peptidoglycan layer and an outer membrane. During the staining process, *E. coli* picks up the color of the counterstain safranin and stains pink. The outer membrane surrounding the cell wall provides a barrier to certain antibiotics such that *E. coli* are not damaged by penicillin.

Strains that possess flagella are motile. The flagella have a peritrichous arrangement. It also attaches and effaces to the microvillus of the intestines via an adhesion molecule known as intimin.

(2) Cultural Characteristics

Optimum growth of *E. coli* occurs at 37 ℃, but some laboratory strains can multiply at temperatures up to 49 ℃. *E. coli* grows in a variety of defined laboratory media, such as lysogeny broth or any medium that contains glucose, ammonium phosphate, monobasic, sodium chloride, magnesium sulfate, potassium phosphate, dibasic and water. Growth can be driven by aerobic or anaerobic respiration, using a large variety of redox pairs, including the oxidation of pyruvic acid, formic acid, hydrogen and amino acids and the reduction of substrates such as oxygen, nitrate, fumarate, dimethyl sulfoxide and trimethylamine N-oxide. *E. coli* is classified as a facultative anaerobe. It uses oxygen when it is present and available. However, *E. coli* can continue to grow in the absence of oxygen using fermentation or anaerobic respiration. The ability to continue growing in the absence of oxygen is an advantage to bacteria because their survival is increased in environments where water predominates.

(3) Biochemical Character

E. coli form circular, convex, smooth colonies with distinct edges. *E. coli* colonies are usually similar and some strains produce hemolysis on blood agar.

E. coli typically produces positive tests for indole, lysine decarboxylase and mannitol fermentation and produces gas from glucose. An isolate from urine can be quickly identified as *E. coli* its hemolysis no blood agar, typical colonial morphology with an iridescent "sheen" on differential media such as EMB agar and a positive for β-glucuronidase using the substrate 4-methylumbelliferyl-β-glucuromide (MUG). Isolates from anatomic sites other than urine, with characteristic property (including negative oxidase tests) often can be confirmed as *E. coli* with positive MUG test.

More specialized pili are found in subpopulations of *E. coli*. P pili (also called Pap or Gal-Gal) bind to digalactoside (Gal-Gal) moieties present on certain mammalian cells, including uroepithelial cells and erythrocytes of P blood group. Other pili bind to intestinal cells and have their own set of specificities. Those binding to human enterocytes are called colonization factor antigens (CFAs) or bundle-forming pili (BFP), depending on the pathogenic type of E. coli involved and possibly the cell type in the gastrointestinal tract (Figure 8-2).

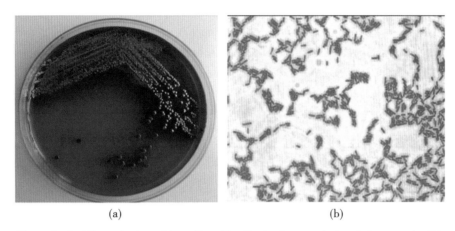

(a)   (b)

Figure 8-2   The colonies of *E. coli on* MacConkey's agar (a) and Gram stain (b)

The genetics of pilin expression is complex. The genes are organized into multicistronic clusters that encode structural pilin subunits and regulatory function. Pili of different types may coexist on the same bacterium and their expression may vary under different environment conditions. Type Ⅰ pili expression can be turned "on" or "off" by inversion of a chromosomal DNA sequence containing the promoter responsible for initiating the transcription of the pili gene. Others genes control the orientation of this switch.

Typical biochemical properties of *E. coli* are: ①Lactose fermentation (red colonies and red colored agar around colonies on Endo); ②D-mannitol fermentation (red colored agar and colonies around mannitol tablet); ③Negative cellobiose fermentation (colorless colonies and agar on Endo around cellobiose tablet); ④ Acid from glucose with gas; ⑤Hydrogen sulfide negative; ⑥ Indole production (positive); ⑦Voges-Proskauer test (negative); ⑧Simmons citrate (negative); ⑨Malonate utilization (negative).

(4)Antigen

The differentiation of *E. coli* strain is usually based on difference of the three antigens: O antigen, H antigen and K antigen. The O antigens (cell wall antigens) are found on the polysaccharide portion of the lipopolysaccharide (LPS). These antigens are heat stable and may be shared among different Enterobacteriaceae genera. O antigens are commonly used to serologically type many of the enteric gram-negative rods. The H antigens are associated with flagella and, therefore, only flagellated Enterobacteriaceae such as *E. coli* have H antigen. The K antigens are located within the polysaccharide capsules. Among *E. coli* species, there are many serologically distinct O, H and K antigens. For example, a serotype of *E. coli* possessing O157 and H7 (designated O157 ∶ H7) causes a severe form of hemorrhagic colitis.

8.2.2.2   Pathogenicity

E. coli can produce every kind of toxin found among enteric bacilli, including a pore-forming cytotoxin, inhibitors of protein synthesis and a number of toxins that altering messenger pathways in host cell.

(1)α-hemolysin

Alpha-hemolysin is a pore-forming cytotoxin that inserts into the plasma membrane of wide range of host cells in manner similar to streptolysin O and *Staphylococcus aureus* α-toxin. The toxin causes leakage of cytoplasmic contents and eventually cell death.

(2) Shiga Toxin

Shiga toxin is named for the microbiologist who discovered *shigella* dysenteriae and this toxin was once believed to be limited to that species. It is now recognized to exist in at least two molecular forms released by multiple *E. coli* and *Shigella* strains on lysis of the bacteria. Shiga toxins are of the AB type. The B unit directs binding to a specific glycolipid receptor present on eukaryotic cell it internalized in an endocytotic vacuole. Inside the cell, the subunit crosses the vacuolar membrane in the trans-Golgi network, exits to the cytoplasm and enzymatically modifies 28S-ribosomal RNA of 60S-ribsomal subunit by removing an adenine base. This prevents the enlongation-factor-1-dependent binding of aminoacyl tRNA to the ribosome blocking protein synthesis, leading to cell death.

(3) Labile Toxin (LT)

Labile toxin is also an AB toxin. Its name relates to the physical property of heat lability, which was important in its discovery and contrasts with the heat-stable toxin described below. The B subunit binds to the cell membrane and the A subunit catalyzes the ADP-ribosylation of a regulatory G protein located in the membrane of intestinal epithelia cell. This inactivation of part of the G protein causes permanent activation of the membrane-associated adenylate cyclase system and a cascade of events, the net effect of which depends on the biological function of stimulated cell. If the cell is an enterocyte, the result is the stimulation of chloride secretion out of the cell and the blockage of NaCl absorption. The net effect is the accumulation of water and electrolytes into the bowel lumen.

(4) STable Toxin (ST)

ST toxin is a small (17-to 18-amino acid) peptide that binds to glycoprotein receptor, resulting in the activation of a membrane-bound guanylate cyclase. The subsequent increase in cyclic GMP concentration causes an LT-like net secretion of fluid and electrolytes into the bowel lumen.

8.2.2.3　Disease

The three principal kinds of disease are urinary tract infections, neonatal meningitis and diarrheal diseases.

(1) Urinary Tract Infections

E. coli is responsible for 90% of infections in anatomically normal unobstructed urinary tracts. The uropathogenic strains are present in the stool and subsequently colonize the vaginal and periurethral region. The bacteria may then ascend into the bladder. Females are more prone to UTIs than males because of their shorter urethra.

(2) Neonatal Meningitis

E. coli is the most common cause of neonatal meningitis, affecting 1 in 2,000 to 4,000 infants. Approximately 80% of the isolates synthesize the K1 capsular polysaccharide. *E. coli* meningitis is best treated with a beta-lactam antibiotic.

(3) Intestinal Diseases

The majority of *E. coli* strains in the GI tract are harmless unless they are displaced to other parts of the body such as the urinary tract or meninges. The pathogenic or enterovirulent *E. coli* are divided into 4 groups according to their action in the body:

1) Enteropathogenic (EPEC): Enteropathogenic (EPEC) is responsible for severe infantile diarrhea. They cause outbreaks of diarrhea in infant nurseries and rarely adult diarrhea. The most common O serotypes involved are O55, O111, O119, O127 and O128. EPEC cause either watery or bloody diarrhea, the for-

mer is due to the attachment to and physical alteration of the integrity of the intestine. Bloody diarrhea is associated with attachment and an acute tissue-destructive process, caused by a toxin similar to that of verotoxin. Occasionally, the diarrhea is prolonged, leading to dehydration, electrolyte imbalance and death. EPEC is highly infectious for infants and the dose is very low. Common foods implicated in EPEC outbreaks are raw beef and chicken, although any food exposed to faecal contamination is strongly suspect. EPEC outbreaks most often affect infants, especially those who are bottle fed, suggesting that contaminated water is used to rehydrate milk powder feeds in underdeveloped countries.

The distinction of EPEC from other groups of pathogenic *E. coli* isolated from patient's stool involves serological and cell culture assays. Serotyping, although useful, is not strict for EPEC. The isolation and identification of *E. coli* in foods follow standard enrichment and biochemical procedures. Serotyping of isolates to distinguish EPEC is laborious and requires high quality, specific antisera. The total analysis may require 7–14 days.

2) Enterotoxigenic (ETEC): Enterotoxigenic (ETEC) produces a heat labile (LT) or heat stable (ST) toxin. Both may be produced by the same organism. They are responsible for cases of paediatric diarrhea, severe cholera-like illness and traveler's diarrhea. The symptoms consist of watery diarrhea, abdominal cramps, low-grade fever, nausea and malaise. A relatively large dose (10^2 to 10^{10} bacteria) is required to cause an infection. Infants and travelers to developing countries are most at risk of infection. ETEC is not considered as a serious foodborne disease hazard in countries and/or regions with high sanitary standard. Contamination of water with human sewage may lead to the contamination of foods. Infected food handlers may also contaminate more foods. These organisms are infrequently isolated from dairy products.

Heat labile toxin is an 8.6 kDa protein and is structurally and functionally very similar to cholera toxin. Heat stable toxin, of which there are several types, are small polypeptides ranging in size from 18 to 50 amino acids. They are structurally related and some ST genes reside on a transposon. At least half the cases of traveler's diarrhea are caused by ETEC that elaborate only 1 toxin.

During the acute phase of infection, large numbers of organisms are excreted in faeces. These strains are differentiated from nontoxigenic *E. coli* present in the bowel by a variety of in vitro, immunochemical, tissue culture or NA probe tests designed to detect either the toxins or genes that encode for these toxins. The diagnosis can be completed in 3 days. With the availability of a gene probe method, foods can be analyzed directly for the presence of enterotoxigenic *E. coli* and the analysis can be completed in 3 days. Alternative methods which involve enrichment and plating of samples for isolation of *E. coli* and confirmation as toxigenic strains require at least 7 days.

3) Enteroinvasive (EIEC): Enteroinvasive (EIEC)-pathogenicity is due to invasion of the gut mucosa. They give rise to a dysentery-like illness. The EIEC strains responsible for this illness are closely related to *Shigella*: they resemble *Shigella* in their pathogenic mechanisms and the kind of clinical illness they produce. Moreover, like *Shigella*, they are non-motile and lactose-negative. Their pathogenicity is conferred by a large 140 Mb plasmid. This plasmid is similar but not identical to the plasmids seen in *Shigella* species. The infective dose of EIEC is thought to be as few as 10 organisms (same as *Shigella*). It is currently unknown what foods may harbor EIEC, but any food contaminated with human faeces directly or indirectly through contaminated water could cause disease. Outbreaks have been associated with hamburger meat and unpasteurized milk.

The signs and symptoms of the EIEC infection are similar to that caused by *Shigella* dysenteriae. The dysentery occurs 12 to 72 hours following the ingestion of contaminated food. The disease is characterized by abdominal cramps, diarrhea, vomiting, fever, chills and malaise. The disease may be complicated by hemolytic uremic syndrome (HUS).

The culturing of the organism from the stools of infected individuals and the demonstration of invasiveness of isolates in tissue culture in a suitable animal model is necessary to diagnose dysentery caused by this organism. More recently, genetic probes for the invasiveness genes of both EIEC and *Shigella* spp. have been developed. Foods are examined as stool cultures. Detection of this organism in foods is extremely difficult because undetectable levels may cause illness.

4) Enterohemorrhagic (EHEC): Enterohemorrhagic (EHEC) is responsible for bloody diarrhea and colitis. It differs from bacillary dysentery in that fever is not prominent and the bloody discharges are copious rather than scanty. This diarrhea syndrome is distinct from the bacillary dysentery caused by *Shigella* and EIEC. *E. coli* O157 : H7 is the causative organism and it cause disease through the production of large quantities of one or more related toxins. Two toxins appear to be important. Toxin 1 is identical to the toxin produced by *Shigella* and is known as Shiga toxin. Toxin 2 appears to be related to severe disease.

Hemorrhagic colitis is the name of the disease caused by *E. coli* O157 : H7. The illness is characterized by severe abdominal cramps and diarrhea which is initially watery but becomes grossly bloody. Occasionally vomiting occurs. The illness is usually self-limited and lasts for an average of 8 days. Some individuals exhibit watery diarrhea only. Some victims, particularly the very young, develop hemolytic uremic syndrome (HUS) characterized by renal failure and hemolytic anemia. Up to 15% of hemorrhagic colitis victims may develop HUS. In the elderly, HUS plus two other symptoms, fever and neurological symptoms constitute thrombotic thrombocytopenic purpura (TTP). This illness can have a mortality rate in the elderly as high as 50%. The infective dose is unknown but may be similar to that of *Shigella* (i. e. as few as 10 organisms). All people are believed to be susceptible to hemorrhagic colitis but larger outbreaks have occurred in institutional settings.

Hemorrhagic colitis is diagnosed by the isolation of *E. coli* O157 : H7 from diarrheal stools. Alternatively, the stools can be tested directly for the verotoxins. *E. coli* O157 : H7 will form colonies on agar media that are selective for *E. coli*. However, the high temperature growth procedure normally performed to eliminate background organisms before plating cannot be used because of the inability of these organisms to grow at temperatures of 45 ℃ that support the growth of most *E. coli*. The use of molecular methods to detect verotoxins 1 and 2 is most sensitive method available.

5) Enteroaggregative (EAEC): EAEC is now recognized as an emerging enteric pathogen. In particular, EAEC are reported as the second most common cause of traveler's diarrhea, second only to Enterotoxigenic *E. coli* and a common cause of persistent diarrhea amongst pediatric populations. The pathogenesis of EAEC involves the aggregation of and adherence of the bacteria to the intestinal mucosa, where they elaborate enterotoxins and cytotoxins that damage host cells and induce inflammation that results in diarrhea. Adherence to the small intestine is mediated by aggregative adherence fimbriae. The adherent rods resemble stacked bricks and result in shortening of microvillus. EAEC strains produce a heat-stable toxin that is plasmid encoded. EAEC trains could acquire the phage-encoded gene to produce Shiga-like toxin 2. The resulting strains were capable of tight adherence to the small intestine in addition to toxin production (Table 8-7).

Table 8-7   Characteristics of intestinal infections caused by *Escherichia coli*

E. coli strains	Abbreviation	Syndrome	Therapy
Enteropathogenic *E. coli*	EPEC	Watery diarrhea of a long duration, mostly in infants	Antibiotics may be need
Enterotoxigenic *E. coli*	ETEC	Watery diarrhea	Antibiotics may be need
Enteroinvasive *E. coli*	EIEC	Bloody diarrhea	Antibiotics may be avoided
Enterohemorrhagic *E. coli*	EHEC	Bloody diarrhea; hemorrhagic colitis and hemolytic uremic syndrome	Rehydrate and correct electrolyte abnormalities
Enteroaggregative *E. coli*	EAEC	Persistent watery diarrhea in children	Rehydrate and correct electrolyte abnormalities

Undercooked or raw hamburger (ground beef) has been implicated in nearly all documented outbreaks and in other sporadic cases. Raw milk has also been implicated in other outbreaks. These are currently the only two demonstrated food causes of disease, but other meats may contain *E. coli* O157 : H7.

8.2.2.4   Laboratory Diagnosis

In testing water supplies, it is important to distinguish *E. coli*, which is an index of faecal contamination, from Enterobacter which is widely found in plants. Four metabolic tests (indole, methyl red, Voges-Proskauer and citrate utilization) collectively referred to as the IMVIC tests were originally used to distinguish Enterobacter from *E. coli*. Only the latter produces indole in media containing tryptophan. The methyl red test distinguishes heavy and light production of acid, because this indicator shifts from yellow to red below pH 4.5 and in glucose-peptone broth cultures incubated for 48 hours, only the mixed acid fermentation produces enough acid to turn the indicator red. The Voges-Proskauer reaction is a color test for acetoin, a product of butylene glycol type of fermentation. Citrate can serve as the sole carbon source for Enterobacter but not for *E. coli*.

8.2.2.5   Prevalence, Treatment and Prevention

(1) Prevalence

Transmission of pathogenic *E. coli* often occurs via fecal-oral transmission. Common routes of transmission include: unhygienic food preparation, farm contamination due to manure fertilization, irrigation of crops with contaminated greywater or raw sewage, feral pigs on cropland or direct consumption of sewage-contaminated water. Dairy and beef cattle are primary reservoirs of *E. coli* O157 : H7 and they can carry it asymptomatically and shed it in their feces. Food products associated with *E. coli* outbreaks include cucumber, raw ground beef, raw seed sprouts or spinach, raw milk, unpasteurized juice, unpasteurized cheese and foods contaminated by infected food workers via fecal-oral route.

According to the U. S. Food and Drug Administration, the fecal-oral cycle of transmission can be disrupted by cooking food properly, preventing cross-contamination, instituting barriers such as gloves for food workers, instituting health care policies so food industry employees seek treatment when they are ill, pasteurization of juice or dairy products and proper hand washing requirements.

Shiga toxin-producing *E. coli* (STEC), specifically serotype O157 : H7, have also been transmitted by flies, as well as direct contact with farm animals, petting zoo animals and airborne particles found in animal-rearing environments.

（2）Treatment

The mainstay of treatment is the assessment of dehydration and replacement of fluid and electrolytes. Administration of antibiotics has been shown to shorten the course of illness and duration of excretion of enterotoxigenic *E. coli* (ETEC)in adults in endemic areas and in traveler's diarrhea,though the rate of resistance to commonly used antibiotics is increasing and they are generally not recommended. The antibiotic used depends upon susceptibility patterns in the particular geographical region. Currently,the antibiotics of choice are fluoroquinolones or azithromycin,with an emerging role for rifaximin. Oral rifaximin,a semisynthetic rifamycin derivative,is an effective and well-tolerated antibacterial for the management of adults with non-invasive traveler's diarrhea. Rifaximin was significantly more effective than placebo and no less effective than ciprofloxacin in reducing the duration of diarrhea. While rifaximin is effective in patients with *E. coli*-predominant traveler's diarrhea,it appears ineffective in patients infected with inflammatory or invasive enteropathogens.

Maintenance of fluid and electrolyte balance is of primary importance in treatment of diarrhea caused by *E. coli*. For patients with more severe symptoms (for example,high fever,bloody diarrhea,worsening illness or illness of more than 1 week's duration),antibiotics should be administered. Extraintestinal diseases require antibiotic treatment,e. g. ciprofloxacin,trimethoprim/sulfamethoxazole,cefotaxime and aminoglycosides. Antibiotic sensitivity testing of isolates is necessary to determine the appropriate choice of drugs.

（3）Prevention

Intestinal disease can best be prevented by care in selection,preparation and consumption of food and water. ETEC is the type of *E. coli* that most vaccine development efforts are focused on. Antibodies against the LT and major CFs of ETEC provide protection against LT-producing,ETEC-expressing homologous CFs. Oral inactivated vaccines consisting of toxin antigen and whole cells,i. e. the licensed recombinant cholera toxin B subunit (rCTB)-WC cholera vaccine Dukoral®,have been developed. There are currently no licensed vaccines for ETEC,though several are in various stages of development. In different trials,the rCTB-WC cholera vaccine provided high (85% –100%) short-term protection. An oral ETEC vaccine candidate consisting of rCTB and formalin inactivated *E. coli* bacteria expressing major CFs has been shown in clinical trials to be safe,immunogenic and effective against severe diarrhea in American travelers but not against ETEC diarrhea in young children in Egypt. A modified ETEC vaccine consisting of recombinant *E. coli* strains over-expressing the major CFs and a more LT-like hybrid toxoid called LCTBA,are undergoing clinical testing.

Other proven prevention methods for *E. coli* transmission include handwashing and improved sanitation and drinking water,as transmission occurs through fecal contamination of food and water supplies. Additionally,thoroughly cooking meat and avoiding consumption of raw,unpasteurized beverages,such as juices and milk are other proven methods for preventing *E. coli*. Lastly,avoid cross-contamination of utensils and work spaces when preparing food.

8.2.3 *Salmonella*

Salmonella is one of the most common causes of food poisoning over the world,often by the oral route. They are transmitted from animals and animal products to humans,where they cause enteritis,systemic infection and enteric fever. Usually,symptoms last 4–7 days and most people get better without treatment. But, *Salmonella* can cause more serious illness in older adults,infants and persons with chronic diseases.

Salmonella species are gram-negative,flagellated facultatively anaerobic bacilli characterized by O,H and Vi antigens. There are over 1,800 known serovars which current classification considered to be separate species three clinical forms of salmonellosis: gastroenteritis, septicemia and enteric fevers. This chapter focuses on the two extremes of the clinical spectrum—gastroenteritis and enteric fever. Salmonellosis includes several syndromes, such as gastroenteritis, enteric fevers, septicemia, focal infections and an asymptomatic carrier state. Most non-typhoidal *salmonella* e enter the body when contaminated food is ingested. Person-to-person spread of *salmonella* e also occurs. To be fully pathogenic, *salmonella* e must possess a variety of attributes called virulence factors, including the ability to invade cells, a complete lipopolysaccharide coat, the ability to replicate intracellularly and possibly the elaboration of toxins. After ingestion, the organisms colonize the ileum and colon, invade the intestinal epithelium and proliferate within the epithelium and lymphoid follicles. The mechanism by which *salmonella* e invade the epithelium is partially understood and involves an initial binding to specific receptors on the epithelial cell surface followed by invasion. Invasion occurs by the organism inducing the enterocyte membrane to undergo "ruffling" and thereby to stimulate pinocytosis of the organisms

8. 2. 3. 1   Biological Character

（1）Morphology

Salmonella species are non-spore-forming, predominantly motile enterobacteria with cell diameters between about 0. 7 μm and 1. 5 μm, lengths from 2 to 5 μm and peritrichous flagella (all around the cell body). Most isolates are motile with peritrichous flagella. *Salmonella* grow readily on simple media, but they almost never ferment lactose or sucrose. They form acid sometimes gas from glucose and mannose. They usually produce H_2S from sulfur-containing amino acids. They survive freezing in water for long periods. *Salmonella* are resistant to certain chemicals (e. g. brilliant green, sodium tetrathionate, sodium deoxycholate) that inhibit other enteric bacteria; such compounds are therefore useful for inclusion in media to isolate *salmonella* form feces (Figure 8-3).

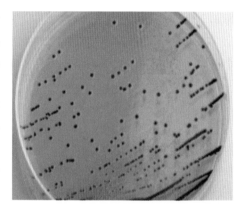

Figure 8-3   the black colonies of *Salmonella* on *Salmonella-Shigella* agar (SS agar)

Salmonella possess multiple types of pili, one of which is morphologically and functionally similar to the E. coli type Ⅰ pili, which bin D-mannose receptors on various eukaryotic cell types. Most strains are motile through the action of their flagella.

（2）Cultural Characteristics

They are chemotrophs, obtaining their energy from oxidation and reduction reactions using organic sources. They are also facultative anaerobes, capable of generating ATP with oxygen when it is available; or when oxygen is not available, using other electron acceptors or fermentation. *Salmonella enterica* subspecies are found worldwide in all warm-blooded animals and in the environment. *Salmonella bongori* is restricted to cold-blooded animals, particularly reptiles.

（3）Classification

There are more than 2,500 serotypes of *salmonella*, including more than 1,400 in DNA hybridization group Ⅰ that can infect human. Four serotypes of *salmonella* that cause enteric fever can be identified in clinical laboratory by biochemical and serological tests. These serotypes should be routinely identified because of their clinical significance. They are as follows: *salmonella* paratyphi A (serogroup A), *salmonella* paratyphi B (serogroup B), *salmonella* choleraesuis (serogroup C_1) and *salmonella* typhi (serogroup D). The more than other *salmonella* that are isolated in clinical laboratories are serogrouped by their O antigens as A, B, C_1, C_2 and E; some are then sent to reference laboratories for definitive serologic identification. This allows public health officers to monitor and assess the epidemiology of *salmonella* infections on a statewide and national basis.

8.2.3.2 Pathogenicity

Salmonella typhi, *salmonella* choleraesuis and *salmonella* paratyphi A and *salmonella* paratyphi B are primarily infective for humans and infection with these organisms implies acquisition from a human source. The vast majority of *salmonella*, however, are chiefly pathogenic in animals that constitute the reservoir for human infection: poultry, pigs, rodents, cattle, pets (from turtles to parrots) and many others.

The organisms almost always enter via the oral route, usually with contaminated food or drink. The mean infective dose to produce clinical or subclinical infection in humans is $10^5 - 10^8$ *salmonella* (perhaps as few as 10^3 *salmonella* typhi organisms). Among the host factors that contribute to resistance to *salmonella* infection are gastric acidity, normal intestinal microbial flora and local intestinal immunity. *Salmonella* produce three main types of disease in human (i. e. enteric fevers, septicemias, gastroenterocolitis), but mixed forms are frequent.

8.2.3.3 Disease

Salmonella invade epithelial cells of the small intestine. Disease may remain localized or become systemic, sometimes with disseminate foci. The organisms are facultative, intracellular parasites that survive in phagocytic cells. *Salmonella* infection can cause both intestinal and extraintestinal diseases.

(1) Gastroenteritis

The localized disease (also called salmonellosis) is caused primarily by serovars Enteritidis and Typhimurium. Salmonellosis is characterized by nausea, vomiting and diarrhea (usually non-bloody), which develop gently within 48 hours of ingesting contaminated food or water. Fever and abdominal cramping are common. In comprised patients, disease is generally self-limiting (about 48-72 hours), although convalescent carriage of organism may persist for a month or more. More than 95% of cases of *salmonella* infection are foodborne and salmonellosis accounts for approximately 30 percent of deaths resulting from foodborne illness over the world.

(2) Enteric of Typhoid Fever

This is a severe, life-threatening systemic illness, characterized by fever and, frequently, abdominal symptoms. It is primarily caused by serovar Typhi. Nonspecific symptoms may include chill, sweats, headache, anorexia, weakness, sore throat, cough, myalgia and either diarrhea or constipation. About 30 percent of patients have a faint and evanescent (transient) maculopapular rash on the trunk (rose spots). The incubation period ranges from 5 to 21 days. Untreated, mortality is approximately 15 percent. Among survivors, the symptoms generally resolve in 3 to 4 weeks. Timely and appropriate antibiotic therapy reduces mortality to less than 1 percent and speeds resolution of fever. Complications can include intestinal hemorrhage and/or perforation and, rarely, focal infections and endocarditis. A small percentage of patients become chronic carriers.

(3) Other Sites of *Salmonella* Infection

Sustained bacteremia is often associated with vascular *salmonella* infections that occur when bacteria seed atherosclerotic plaques. *Salmonella* can also cause abdominal infections (often of the hepatobiliary tract and spleen), osteomyelitis, septic arthritis and, rarely, infections of other tissues or organs. Chronic carriages of non-typhoidal serovars may develop, although this is rare.

8.2.3.4 Laboratory Diagnosis

In patients with diarrhea, *salmonella* can typically be isolated from stools on MacConkey's agar or selective media. For patients with enteric fever, appropriate specimens include blood, bone marrow, urine, stool and tissue from typical rose spots.

(1) Bacteriological Method

1) Differential medium cultures: EMB, MacConkey's or deoxycholate medium permitthe rapid detection of non-lactose fermenters(e. g. *salmonella*, *shigella*, proteus, serratia and pseudomonas). Gram-positive organisms are somewhat inhibited. Bismuth sulfite medium permits rapid detection of *salmonella* which form black colonies because of H_2S production. Many *salmonella* stainsproduce H_2S.

2) Selective medium cultures: The specimen is plated on *salmonella-shigella* (SS) agar, Hektoen enteric agar, XLD or deoxycholate-citrate agar, which favor growth of *salmonella* and *shigella* over other Enterobacteriaceae.

3) Enrich cultures: The specimen (usually stool) also is put into selenite For tetrathionate broths, which both inhibit replication of normal intestinal bacteria and permit multiplication of *salmonella*. After incubation for 1-2 days, this is plated on differential and selective media.

4) Final identification: Suspect colonies from solid media are identified by biochemical reaction patterns and slide agglutination tests with specific sera.

(2) Serologic Methods

Serologic techniques are used to identify unknown cultures with known sera and many also be used to determine antibody titers in patients with unknown illness, although the letter is not very useful in diagnosis of *salmonella* infections.

1) Agglutination test: In this test, known sera and unknown culture are mixed on slide. Clumping, when it occurs, can be observed within a few minutes. This test is particularly useful for primarily identification of cultures. There are commercial kits available to agglutinate and serogroup *salmonella* by their O antigens: A, B, C_1, C_2, D and E.

2) Tube dilution agglutination test: Serum agglutinins rise sharply during the second and third weeks of *salmonella* infection. At least two serum specimens, obtained at intervals of 7-10 days, are needed to produce a rise in antibody titer. Serial dilutions of unknown serum are tested against antigens from representative *salmonella*. The results are interpreted as follows: ①High or rising titer of O ($\geq 1 : 160$) suggests active infection is present. ②High titer of H ($\geq 1 : 160$) suggests past immunization or past infection. ③High titer of antibody to Vi antigen occurs in some carriers. Results of serologic tests for *salmonella* infection must be interpreted cautiously. The possible presence of cross-reactive antibodies limits the use of serology in the diagnosis of *salmonella* infections.

8.2.3.5   Prevalence, Treatment and Prevention

Salmonella are widely distributed in nature. Serovar typhi is an exclusively human pathogen, whereas other strains are associated with animals and foods (e. g. eggs and poultry). Fecal-oral transmission occurs and *salmonella* serovar typhi may involve chronic carriers. Pet turtles have also been complicated as sources of infection. Young children and older adults are particularly susceptible to *salmonella* infection. Individuals in crowded institutions may also be involved in *salmonella* epidemics.

For gastroenteritis in uncompromised hosts, antibiotic therapy is often not needed and may prolong the convalescent carrier state. For enteric fever, appropriate antibiotics include β-lactams and fluoroquinolones. Prevention of *salmonella* infection is accomplished by proper sewage disposal; correct handling of food and good personal hygiene. Two different vaccines are available to prevent typhoid fever: one vaccine is delivered orally and consists of the Vi capsular polysaccharide and is delivered parenterally. Vaccination is recommended for people who travel from developed countries to endemic areas including Asia, Africa and Latin

America.

8.2.4 *Shigella*

Shigella species causes shigellosis (bacillary dysentery), a human intestinal disease that occurs most commonly among young children. *Shigella* is nonmotile, unencapsulated and Lac⁻. Most strains do not produce gas in a mixed-acid fermentation of glucose.

The causative agent of human shigellosis, *Shigella* causes disease in primates, but not in other mammals. It is only naturally found in humans and gorillas. During infection, it typically causes dysentery.

Shigella is one of the leading bacterial causes of human diarrhea worldwide, causing an estimated 80 – 165 million cases per year. The number of deaths it causes each year is estimated at between 74,000 and 600,000. It is in the top four pathogens that cause moderate-to-severe diarrhea in African and South Asian children.

8.2.4.1 Biological Character

Shigella strains are slender gram-negative rods; coccobacillary forms occur in young cultures. *Shigella* species are facultative anaerobes but grow best aerobically. Convex, circular, transparent colonies with intact edges reach a diameter of 2 mm in 24 hours. All *shigella* ferments glucose. With the exception of *Shigella sonnei*, they do not ferment lactose. The inability to ferment lactose distinguishes *shigella* on different media. *Shigella* produces acid from carbohydrates but rarely produce gas. They also can be divided into those that ferment mannitol and those that do not.

8.2.4.2 Pathogenicity

(1) Endotoxin

Endotoxins are large molecules consisting of a lipid and a polysaccharide composed of O-antigen, outer core and inner core joined by a covalent bond. Upon autolysis, all shigella releases the toxic lipopolysaccharide. This endotoxin probably contributes to the irritation of bowel wall. Endotoxins are rarely fatal, although they often cause fever (Figure 8–4).

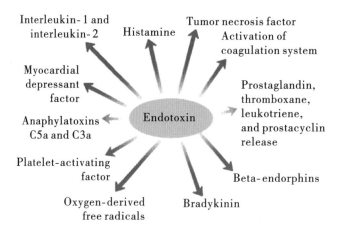

Figure 8–4　Results of endotoxin release

(2) Exotoxin

Shigella dysenteriae type 1 (*shigella* bacillus) produces a heat-labile exotoxin that affects both the gut and the central nervous system. The exotoxin is a protein that is antigenic (stimulating production of antitoxin) and lethal for experimental animals. Acting as an endotoxin, it produces diarrhea as does the *E. coli* verotoxin, perhaps by the same mechanism. In humans, the exotoxin also inhibits sugar and amino acid absorption in the small intestine. Acting as a "neurotoxin", this material may contribute the extremely severity and fatal nature of *S. dysenteriae* infections and to the central nervous system reactions observed in them (i. e. meningismus, coma). Patients with *Shigella flexneri* or *Shigella sonnei* infections develop antitoxin in vitro. The toxic activity is distinct from the invasive property of *shigella* in dysentery. The two may act in sequence, the toxin producing an early nonbloody, voluminous diarrhea and invasion of the large intestine resulting in later dysentery with blood and pus in stools.

Shigella, unlike Vibrio cholerae and most *salmonella* species, is acid-resistant and survives passage through the stomach to reach the intestine. Once there, the fundamental pathogenic event is invasion of the human colonic mucosa. This triggers an intense acute inflammatory response with mucosal ulceration and abscess formation. Invasion and spread is a multistep process, which is the same in *shigella* and EIEC.

Shigella initially crosses the mucosal membrane by entering the follicle-associated M cells of the intestine, which lack highly organized brush borders of absorptive enterocytes. This *Shigella* adheres selectively to M cells and can transcytose through them into the underlying collection of phagocytic cells. Bacteria inside M cells and phagocytic macrophages are able to cause their demise by activating normal programmed cell death (apoptosis). Bacteria released from the M cell contact the basolateral side of enterocytes and initiate a multistep invasion progress mediated by a set of invasion plasmid antigens (IpaA, IpaB and IpaC). On contact with the enterocyte, these antigens are injected by a contact secretion system and each has its individual action. These include cell attachment, cytoskeleton reorganization, actin polymerization and induction of apoptosis. Rather than create A/E lesions as with EPEC and EHEC, this cytoskeleton modification process involves accumulation of filamentous actin underneath the host cell cytoplasmic membrane, including engulfment and internalization of the bacterium into the host cell by endocytosis.

Some *Shigella* produce shiga toxin, which is not essential for disease, but does contribute the severity of the illness. The original and most potent producer of Shiga toxin, *S. dysenteriae* type 1, is the only *shigella* with a significant mortality rate among the previously healthy individuals. This is probably due to systemic effect of the toxin, which can be the same as described above for the EHEC, including HUS. Enterotoxins have also been described that may be the basis of the watery diarrhea sometimes observed in the early phases.

All virulent *Shigella* and EIEC carry a very large plasmid that has several genes essential for the attachment and entry process, including the Ipa genes. The characteristics of *shigella* entry and interaction with cellular elements are very similar to those observed with *Listeria monocytogenes*, which is Gram-positive, motile and prefers livsstock to humans. Finding that such dissimilar bacteria through similar tactics to infect their preferred host suggests that this represents a common thread in the selective pressure for microbe to become a "successful" enteric pathogen.

Shigella infections are almost always limited to the gastrointestinal tract; bloodstream invasion is quite rare. *Shigella* is highly communicable; the infective dose is on the order of 10^3 organisms (whereas it usually is 10^5-10^8 for *Salmonella* and Vibrio). The essential pathologic process is invasion of the mucosal epithelial cells by induced phagocytosis, escape from the phagocytic vacuole, multilocation and spread within the epithelial cell cytoplasm and passage to adjacent cells. Microabscesses in the wall of large intestine and terminal ileum lead to necrosis of the mucous membrane, superficial ulceration, bleeding and formation of a "pseudomembrane" on the ulcerated area. This consists of fibrin, leukocytes, cell debris, a necrotic mucous membrane and bacteria. As the process subsides, granulation tissue fills the ulcers and scar tissue forms.

After a short incubation period (1-2 days), there is a sudden onset of abdominal pain, fever and watery diarrhea. The diarrhea has been attributed to an exotoxin acting in the small intestine. A day or so later, as the infection involves the ileum and colon, the number of stools increases; they are less liquid but often contain mucus and blood. Each bowel movement is accompanied by straining andtenesmus (rectal spasms), with resulting lower abdominal pain. In more than half of adult cases, fever and diarrhea subside spontaneously in 2−5 days. However, in children and the elderly, loss of water and electrolytes may lead to dehydration, acidosis and even death. The illness due to *S. dysenteriae* may be particularly severe.

On recovery, most persons shed dysentery bacilli for only a short period, but a few remain chronic intestinal carriers and may have recurrent bouts of the disease. Upon recovery from the infection, most persons develop circulating antibodies to *shigella*, but these do not protect against reinfection.

8.2.4.3   Laboratory Diagnosis

(1) Specimens

Specimens include Fresh stool, much flecks and rectal swabs. Large numbers of fecal leukocytes and some red blood cells often are seen microscopically. Serum specimens, if desired, must be taken 10 days apart to demonstrate a rising in titer of agglutinating antibodies.

(2) Culture

The materials are streaked on differential media (e. g. MacConkey's or EMB agar) and on selective media (Hektoen enteric agar or *salmonella-shigella* agar), which suppress other Enterobacteriaceae and Gram-positive organisms. Colorless (lactose-negative) colonies are inoculated into triple sugar iron agar. Organisms that fail to produce H_2S, that produce acid but not gas in the butt and an alkaline slant in triple sugar medium and that are nonmotile should be subjected to slide agglutination by specific *shigella* antisera.

(3) Serology

Normal persons often have agglutinins against several *shigella* species. However, serial determinations of antibody titers may show s rise in specific antibody. Serology is not used to diagnose *shigella* infections.

(4) Immunity

Shigella infection produces relatively short-lived immunity to reinfection with homologous serogroups. There is no consensus on the mechanisms involved. Infection is followed by a type-specific antibody response. Injection of killed *shigella* stimulates production of antibodies in serum but fails to protect human against infection. IgA antibodies in the gut may be important in limiting reinfection; these may be stimulated by live attenuated strains given orally as experiment vaccines. Serum antibodies to somatic *shigella* antigen are IgM.

8.2.4.4   Prevalence, Treatment and Prevention

(1) Prevalence

Shigellosis is strictly human disease with no animal reservoirs. In the United States, the number of reported cases has remained in the range of 8−12 cases per 100,000 persons for over 30 years. Worldwide, it is consistently one of the most common causes of infectious diarrhea in both developed and developing countries and it is estimated to cause 600,000 deaths per year. The organism can be readily transmitted by the fecal-oral route through person-to-person contact or by contamination of food or water. This mode of spread is efficient; the infecting dose of is less than 200 organisms in volunteer studies. The secondary attack rates among family members are as high as 40%.

(2) Prevention

Shigella strains are transmitted by food, fingers, feces and flies from person to person. Most cases of *shigella* infection occur in children less than 10 years of age. *S. dysenteriae* can spread widely. Mass chemoprophylaxis from limited periods of time has been tried, but resistant strains of *shigella* tend to emerge rapidly. Since humans are the main recognized host of pathogenic *shigella*, control efforts must be directed at eliminating these organisms from this reservoir by: ① sanitary control of water, food and milk; sewage disposal; and fly control; ② isolation of patients and disinfection of excreta; ③ detection of subclinical cases and carriers, particularly food handlers; ④ antibiotic treatment of identified individuals.

(3) Treatment

Ciprofloxacin, ampicillin, doxycycline and trimethoprim-sulfamethoxazole are most commonly inhibitory for *shigella* isolates and suppress acute clinical attacks of dysentery and shorten the duration of symptoms. They may fail to eradicate the organisms from the intestinal tract. Multiple drug resistance can be transmitted by plasmids and resistant infections are widespread. Many cases are self-limited. Opioids should be avoided in *shigella* dysentery.

8.2.5　*Klebsiella*

The genus *Klebsiella* consists of non-motile, aerobic and facultatively anaerobic, Gram negative rods, comprising *K. pneumoniae* subsp. pneumoniae, *K. pneumoniae* subsp. ozaenae, *K. pneumonia* e subsp. *rhinoscleromatis*, *K. oxytoca*, *K. ornithinolytica*, *K. planticola* and *K. terrigena*. *Klebsiella*, are usually opportunistic pathogens that cause nosocomial infection, especially pneumonia and urinary tract infections. The most distinctive bacteriologic features of the *klebsiella* genus are the absence of motility and the presence of polysaccharide capsule. This gives colonies a glistening, mucoid character and forms the basis of serotyping system. Over 70 capsular types have been defined, including some that cross-react with those of other encapsulated pathogens, such as *Streptococcus pneumoniae* and *Haemophilus influenzae*. Limited studies suggest that the capsule interferes with complement activation in a way similar to other encapsulated pathogens. Several types of pili are also present on the surface and probably aid in adherence to respiratory and urinary epithelium.

8.2.5.1　Biological Character

Klebsiella are frequently found in the large intestine but are also present in soil and water. Those organisms have very similar properties are usually distinguished on the basis of several biochemical reaction and motility. *Klebsiella pneumoniae* is the species most often involved in human infections. *K. pneumoniae* has a very large capsule, which gives its colonies a striking mucoid appearance. This organism is also able to cause classic lobar pneumonia, which is also a characteristic of other encapsulated bacteria. Most Klebsiella pneumonias are indistinguishable from those produced by other members of the enterobacteriaceae. Of all the enterobacteriaceae, *Klebsiella* species are now among the most resistant to antimicrobials.

8.2.5.2　Pathogenicity

Compared to other Enterobacteriaceae, *K. pneumoniae* is more likely to be a primary, non opportunistic pathogen; this property is related to its antiphagocytic capsule. As with many other gram-negative rods, the pathogenesis of septic shock caused by *K. pneumoniae* is related to the endotoxins in their cell walls.

Urinary tract infection and pneumonia are the usual clinical entities associated with *K. pneumoniae*. Pneumonia caused by *Klebsiella* produces thick, bloody sputum and may progress to necrosis and abscess formation. There are other two species of *Klebsiella* that cause unusual human infections rarely seen over the world. *Klebsiella ozaenae* is associated with atrophic rhinitis and *Klebsiella rhinoscleromatis* causes a destructive granuloma of the nose and pharynx.

8.2.5.3　Laboratory Diagnosis

The members of the genus *Klebsiella* are gram-negative, nonmotile, facultative anaerobic rods ranging from 0.3−1.0 μm in width and 0.6−6.0 μm in length. Most strains grown readily on standard media, although occasionally cysteine requiring urinary isolates of *K. pneumoniae* are encountered. These strains will appear as pinpoint colonies on routine media and require supplementation of media with cysteine for more adequate growth. The vast majority of *Klebsiella* species are encapsulated. The *Klebsiella* which has been linked to the invasive syndrome presenting as liver abscess have a mucoid appearance.

The organisms produce lactose-fermenting (colored) colonies on differential agar such as MacConkey's or EMB and also can be differentiated by the use of biochemical tests. In practice, *K. pneumoniae* and *K. oxytoca* are distinguished by indole production by *K. oxytoca* but not *K. pneumoniae*. However, it should be noted that *K. ornitholytica* is also an indole producer. The five clinically important species can be distinguished by tests for indole production ornithine decarboxylase production, Voges-Proskauer reaction, malonate utilization and O-nitrophenyl-β-D-galactopyranoside (ONPG) production (Figure 8-5, Figure 8-6).

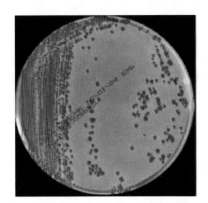 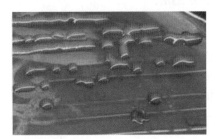

Figure 8-5　The colonies of klebsiella on McConkey's agar

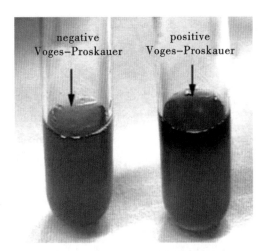

Figure 8-6　Results of Voges-Proskauer (VP) test

8.2.5.4　Prevalence, Treatment and Prevention

Although this organism is a primary pathogen, patients with *K. pneumoniae* infections frequently have predisposing conditions such as advanced age, chronic respiratory disease, diabetes or alcoholism. The organism is carried in the respiratory tract of about 10% of healthy people, who are prone to pneumonia if host defenses are lowered. *Klebsiella* infections are clearly related to hospitalization, especially to invasive procedures such as intravenous catheterization, respiratory intubation and urinary tract manipulations.

Outbreaks of *Klebsiella* infections, particularly in neonatal intensive care units, have been known for more than 30 years. *Klebsiella* species has a propensity for survival on human hands for several minutes, which is enough to enable transfer of organisms from one patient to another. As is shown in some molecular epidemiologic studies, genotypic evidence existed of horizontal transfer of *Klebsiella* from patient to patient. Outbreaks emanating from a common environmental source have been described but are extremely uncommon. Some outbreaks are monoclonal, but in some hospitals a more complicated situation exists in which multiple strains are circulating at any one time. *Klebsiella* infections may also occur in nursing homes. As is the case with acute-care hospitals, patient to patient spread of the organisms is a frequent occurrence in nursing homes. Nursing homes may also serve as a reservoir of infection for the acute-care hospitals to which they send patients. Interventions similar to those used in acute-care hospitals would appear warranted in some nursing homes.

Restriction of third generation cephalosporins or eventhe entire class of cephalosporins has been implemented as a control strategy, which may improve the antibiotic susceptibility of *Klebsiella* andreduce infection-related hospital mortality in critically ill patients. Besides, replacement of extended-spectrum cephalosporins with piperacillin/tazobactam has also been advocated in the treatment of *Klebsiella* infection. Several measures can be adopted to prevent the *Klebsiella* infection, such as changing the site of intravenous catheters, removing urinary catheters when they are no longer needed and taking proper care of respiratory therapy devices. Nowadays, there is no vaccine for *Klebsiella* infection.

8.3   Vibrios

Vibrios are among the most common bacteria in surface watersthroughout the world. They are curved, aerobic and gram-negative rods. They are actively motile with a polar flagellum, none-spore forming and oxidase positive. There are 56 species of the genus *Vibrio*, at least 12 species of which are related to human infections. *Vibrio cholerae* (Vibrionaceae family) is belonging to the gamma subdivision of the phylum Proteobacteria. *V. cholerae* serogroups O1 and O139 cause cholera in humans, while other vibrios may cause enteritis or sepsis. Besides *V. cholerae*, the *Vibrio* genus includes other important human pathogens, i. e. *V. parahemolyticus*, *V. vulnificus* and *V. hollisae*. The medically important vibrios are listed in Table 8−8.

Table 8−8   The medically important vibrios

Organism	Human Disease
V. cholerae serogroups O1 and O139	Epidemic and pandemic cholera
V. cholerae serogroups non-O1/non-O139	Cholera-like diarrhea; mild diarrhea; rarely, extraintestinal infection
V. parahaemolyticus	Gastroentertis, perhaps extraintestinal infection
V. mimicus, *V. vulnificus*, *V. hollisae*, *V. fluvialis*, *V. damsela*, *V. anginolyticus*, *V. metschnikovii*	Ear, wound, soft tissue, other extraintestinal infections, all uncommon

8.3.1   *Vibrio Cholerae*

Cholera is an acute gastrointestinal disease which is caused by *V. cholerae*. The epidemiology of cholera is closely related to the recognition of *V. cholerae* transmission in water and the development of sanitary water systems. Since recorded history, "Asiatic cholera", as it was sometimes called, has been endemic in South Asia, especially the Ganges delta region. People have been worried about it because it regularly occurred in epidemics with high mortality rates. In Kolkata, a cholera temple named Ola Beebe ("our lady of the flux") was built for protection against the disease. In 1817, the first cholera pandemic occurred outside the Indian subcontinent, spreading along trade routes to the west as far as southern Russia. A second pandemic started in 1826 and then reached major cities of Europe by the early 1830s. In 1831, the pandemic reached the United Kingdom of Great Britain and Northern Ireland (UK). The response was important in that it led to the establishment of local Boards of Health and a "Cholera Gazette", which served as a clearinghouse for tracking the epidemic.

At that time, it was thought that cholera was spread by the "miasma" (a fog) coming from the river. In 1854, an English physician John Snow (1813 to 1858) in London conducted a classic epidemiological study, suggesting the association of the disease with contaminated drinking water before any bacteria were known to exist. He described the process of the outbreak, managed to understand its paths of transmission and proposed effective measures to stop its spread, which was leading to modern infectious disease epidemiology. Continuing up to 1925, three more pandemics occurred in Africa, Australia, Europe and all the Americas. The pathogen of *V. cholerae* was not discovered until 1884 in Kolkata during the fifth pandemic. The origins and end of the earlier pandemics are unclear. However, cholera did not continue to exist in any new geographical regions that it had invaded but prevailed as an endemic disease in the Ganges delta.

The cholera was seen as a major public-health disaster requiring governmental intervention as a result of the high numbers of cases and deaths during these pandemics. In 1866, the epidemic of cholera in New York led to the creation of the first Board of Health in the United States (USA) and cholera became the first disease to be reported. Six additional major pandemics (worldwide epidemics) of cholera occurred during the 19th and 20th centuries most probably caused by *V. cholerae* O1 of the classical biotype.

The current (seventh) pandemic now has involved almost worldwide. This pandemic began in Indonesia, rather than the Ganges delta. The pathogen was a biotype of *V. cholerae* serogroup O1 called El Tor. It was first isolated in 1905 from Indonesian pilgrims traveling to Mecca at a quarantine station in the village of El Tor, Egypt. It was found again in 1937 in Sulawesi, Indonesia. Then in 1960, for unknown reasons, this strain began to spread around the world. It invaded India in 1964, Africa in 1970, southern Europe in 1970 and South America in 1991. The disease has now become endemic in many of these places, especially in South Asia and Africa. Millions of people have had cholera in this pandemic. Since 1973, a focus of El Tor *V. cholerae* similar but not identical to the pandemic strain has persisted in the Gulf of Mexico of the USA, causing sporadic cases of cholera associated with seafood in the summer.

In 1992, a newly described non-O1 serogroup of *V. cholerae*, named O139 (the 139th serotype in the typing scheme for *V. cholerae*) Bengal, caused an unusual outbreak of cholera in India and Bangladesh. Before the discovery of *V. cholerae* O139, only serogroup O1 was known to cause epidemic cholera, so the O139 serotype was essentially a "new" cause of cholera. Currently, serogroups of O139 Bengal and O1 co-exist and continue to cause massive cholera outbreaks in India and Bangladesh. The O139 serogroup may be the cause of the next (eighth) cholera pandemic. In spring 2002, serotype O139 caused an estimated 30,000 cases in Dhaka, Bangladesh, exceeding the number of short-term cases associated with El Tor.

Unlike many other infectious diseases, such as plague, smallpox and poliomyelitis, cholera becomes a huge public health problem worldwide, despite the existence of effective prevention and treatment methods. Cholera is spreading rapidly in places where hygienic conditions are unsatisfactory and where already fragile sanitation and health infrastructure have collapsed as a result of natural disasters or humanitarian crises.

8.3.1.1 Biological Characteristics

(1)Morphology and Identification

Upon first isolation, *V. cholerae* is a halophilic, comma-shaped, curved rod 2–4 μm long. It is actively motile through a polar flagellum. Vibrios may become straight rods that resemble the gram-negative enteric bacteria after prolonged cultivation. Only strains of *V. cholerae* that produce toxigenic are associated with cholera and only a small number of *V. cholerae* isolates which are toxigenic in the environment cause cholera. Environmental *V. cholerae* is often closely related with zooplankton and shellfish, which are capable of utilizing chitin as a source of carbon and nitrogen. The presence of chitin induces the natural ability of *V. cholerae* via a quorum sensing-dependent pathway.

(2)Culture

V. cholerae produces convex, smooth, round colonies that are opaque and granular in transmitted light. *V. cholerae* and most other vibrios grow well at 37 ℃ on many kinds of media, including defined media containing mineral salts and asparagines as carbon and nitrogen sources. *V. cholerae* grows well on thiosulfate-citrate-bile-sucrose (TCBS) agar, on which it produces yellow colonies that are easily visible against the dark-green background. Vibrios are oxidase-positive, which differentiates them from enteric gram-negative bacteria. Characteristically, vibrios grow at a very high pH (8.5–9.5) and are rapidly killed by acid. As a result, cultures containing fermentable carbohydrates quickly become sterile.

In areas where cholera is prevalent, it is appropriate to culture stool directly on selective media such as TCBS and to enrich cultures in alkaline peptone water. However, in areas where cholera is rare, it is not necessary or cost-effective to rout stool cultures on special media such as TCBS generally.

V. cholerae regularly ferments sucrose and mannose generally, but it does not ferment arabinose. A positive oxidase test is a key step in the preliminary identification of *V. cholerae* and other vibrios. *Vibrio* species are sensitive to the compound O/129 (2,4-diamino-6,7-diisopropyl pteridine phosphate), which distinguishes them from Aeromonas species, which are resistant to O/129. Most *Vibrio* species are halotolerant and NaCl often stimulates their growth. Moreover, some vibrios are halophilic, requiring the presence of NaCl to grow. Another difference between vibrios and Aeromonas species is that vibrios grow on culture media containing 6% NaCl, whereas Aeromonas does not.

(3)Antigentic Structure & Biologic Classification

Many vibrios share a single heat-labile flagellar H antigen. H antigen antibodies may not be involved in the protection of susceptible hosts.

The serological classification of *V. cholerae* is based on the composition of different O antigens. The O antigen specificity is derived from the O-specific polysaccharide on the outermost layer of the lipopolysaccharide (LPS). While more than 200 serogroups of *V. cholerae* have been identified, only serogroups O1 and O139 have been associated with epidemic cholera. *V. cholerae* strains which do not belong to serum group O1 or O139 are usually collectively referred to as non-O1/O139 *V. cholerae*. Non-toxigenic, non-O1/O139 *V. cholerae* may not cause cholera-like illness, but may cause sporadic cases of gastroenteritis and septicemia. Antibodies to the O antigens tend to protect laboratory animals against infections with *V. cholerae*.

The *V. cholerae* O1 serogroup is further divided into two biotypes. El Tor and classical biotypes are distinguished by biochemical differences and susceptibility to specific bacteriophages. In conventional microbiologic tests, classical strains of *V. cholerae* O1 are sensitive to polymyxin B. They also have a negative Voges-Proskauer test and do not agglutinate chicken red blood cells. The E1 Tor strains of *V. cholerae* O1 produce a hemolysin, give positive results on the Voges-Proskauer test and are resistant to polymyxin B. Molecular techniques can also be used for the type of *V. cholerae*. Typing is used for epidemiologic studies and tests usually are done only in reference laboratories.

During the current cholera pandemic, the El Tor biotype completely replaced the circulating classical biotype, which is now thought to be extinct in nature. Recent cholera epidemics caused by a *V. cholerae* O1 El Tor strain harboring a CTXΦ previously associated with the classical biotype strain appears to confer a more virulent phenotype than a pure biotype El Tor *V. cholerae*.

The *V. cholerae* serogroup O1 antigen has determinants that make further typing possible. The two dominant serotypes are *V. cholerae* O1 Inaba and *V. cholerae* O1 Ogawa. The Inaba and Ogawa serotypes were different due to the addition of the single 2-O-methyl group in the non-reducing terminal saccharide of the Ogawa O-specific polysaccharide. The transition from Ogawa to Inaba resulted from mutations in the WbeT methyltransferase and may play an important role in evading host immunity.

V. cholerae O139 is very similar to *V. cholerae* O1 E1 Tor biotype. *V. cholerae* O139 does not produce the O1 lipopolysaccharide. And also *V. cholerae* O139 does not have all the genes necessary to make this antigen. Like other non-O1 *V. cholerae* strains, *V. cholerae* O139 makes a polysaccharide capsule, while *V. cholerae* O1 does not.

V. cholerae O139 emerged in 1992 and it has been a major cause of epidemic cholera for 15 years. However, *V. cholerae* O139 as a major cause of cholera has since disappeared. Therefore, *V. cholerae* O1 is still the predominant cause of global cholera.

V. cholerae possess long filamentous pili, forming bundles on the surface of bacterial and belonging to a family of pili. Its chemical structure is similar to those of the gonococcus and a number of other bacterial pathogens. All strains capable of causing cholera produce a colonizing factor known as the toxin-coregulated pilus (TCP) because its expression is modulated along with cholera toxin (CT).

Genome

Like other members of the *Vibrio* genus, the *V. cholerae* genome consists of two circular chromosomes. This was first confirmed by pulsed-field gel electrophoresis (PFGE) in 1998 and demonstrated in the first full whole genome sequencing of the *V. cholerae* O1 El Tor strain N16961. The published N16961 sequence contains one large chromosome (chromosome I) of 2.91 Mb with a 46.9% G+C content and one small chromosome (chromosome II) of 1.07 Mb with a 47.7% G+C content. Although the origin of the bipartite chromosome is unclear, the universality of this feature across all vibrios suggests the possibility that the small chromosome was originally produced as a large plasmid and eventually acquired genes with essential functions.

While chromosome I contains a greater number of genes and has a clearly defined role in pathogenesis and other essential cell functions, chromosome II contains a much smaller number of such genes with a very large integron that comprises genes with multiple functions. Integrons are genetic elements that act as gene capture systems by integrating exogenous mobile DNA, usually in the form of individual gene cassettes. The *V. cholerae* chromosome integron, unlike many of the mobile integrons in pathogenic bacteria that harbor important antibiotic resistance genes, is quite large and does not itself move. This type of integron, first discovered in *V. cholerae*, is commonly known as a superintegron. For example, the superintegron of sequenced N16961 reference genome contains at least 215 open reading frames (ORFs) and approximately 12% of the genetic material is located on chromosome II or 3% of the entire *V. cholerae* genome. Over the last century, replication, loss and gain of cassettes within the superintegron may have led to the diversity of *V. cholerae*. The integron consists of a highly repeated sequence of 123-126-bp termed VCR (*V. cholerae* repeats), representing the integration sites within the superintegron.

In addition to the superintegron on chromosome II, the genome of *V. cholerae* may harbor other horizontally acquired gene clusters which play important roles in the pathogenesis and evolution of the organism. Selected genomic regions of importance in *V. cholerae* include:

CTXΦ: The lysogenic bacteriophage CTX, which includes the genes that encode CT and phage integration, replication and morphogenesis as well as accessory toxin.

VPI: The TCP and CTXΦ receptors are located in an area called the TCP island or vibrio pathogenicity island (VPI). Colonization of the human intestine requires TCP, whose expression is up-regulated in coordination with CT. VPI contains putative, integron-like elements. Its genomic architecture suggests it originated from horizontal gene transfer. VPI contains genes that encode TCP and the ToxR regulator which regulate the CT and TCP coordinated expression. Thus VPI and CTXΦ are both essential for virulence and the evolution of virulence in non-toxigenic strains of *V. cholerae* includes continuous acquisition of VPI followed by CTXΦ.

SXT/R391 ICE: The SXT/R391 integrative and conjugative element (ICE) was first identified in *V. cholerae* O139. Subsequently, this horizontally acquired region was found in pandemic *V. cholerae* O1 El Tor which predated the origin of *V. cholerae* O139. SXT is a mobile transposon-like element that confers important antibiotic resistance phenotypes.

VSP1 and VSP2: Strains of *V. cholerae* O1 El Tor associated with the seventh pandemic harbor horizontally acquired gene clusters are known as Vibrio seventh pandemic island 1 and 2 (VSP1 and VSP2). VSPs were initially thought to exist only in O1 and O139 strains of *V. cholerae*, however, whole-genome sequencing studies have shown significant variations in VSPs, including partial deletion of VSP2 and duplication or deletion of VSP1 in pathogenic strains.

rfb encoding region: *V. cholerae* O139 originated from the substitution of a genomic island, the rfb region, which includes the genes required for synthesis of the O139 lipopolysaccharide antigen, but is otherwise virtually identical to previously circulating strains of *V. cholerae* O1 El Tor. A possible mechanism for this conversion was discovered when single step exchange of large fragments of DNA was observed experimentally in 2007 through co-culturing seawater and O1 and O139 strains within a biofilm on a chitin surface.

Plasmids: Several plasmids have been identified in *V. cholerae* strains. However, these have not been implicated in virulence, with the exception of some plasmids belonging to the C incompatibility class that have carried antibiotic resistance phenotypes.

8.3.1.2　Pathogenesis & Immunity

(1) Pathogenesis

Under natural conditions, *V. cholerae* is only pathogenic for humans. A person with normal gastric acidity may have to ingest as many as 10^{10} or more *V. cholera*. Persons can only be infected when the vehicle is water because the organisms are susceptible to acid. When the vehicle is food, as few as 10^2-10^4 organisms are necessary due to the buffering capacity of food. Any medication or condition that decrease stomach acidity makes a person more susceptible to infection with *V. cholerae*.

Cholera is not an invasive infection. The organisms do not enter the bloodstream, but remain within the intestinal tract. Virulent *V. cholerae* organisms attach to the microvilli of the brush border of epithelial cells. They multiply and liberate cholera toxin and perhaps mucinases and endotoxin.

The heat-labile enterotoxin produced by *V. cholerae* and related vibrios has a molecular weight of about 84,000, consisting of subunits A (MW 28,000) and B. The structure and mechanism of action of CT have been studied extensively. CT is an A-B type ADP-ribosylating toxin. Its molecule is an aggregate of multiple polypeptide chains organized into two toxic subunits (A1, A2) and five binding (B) units. The B units bind to a GM1-ganglioside receptor found on the surface of many types of cells. Once bound, the A1 subunit is released from the toxin molecule through the reduction of the disulfide bond that binds it to the A2 subunit and then it enters the cell by translocation. In the cell, it exerts its effect on the membrane-associated adenylate cyclase system at the basolateral membrane surface. The toxic target A1 subunit is a guanine nucleotide (G) protein, Gsα and it regulates activation of the adenylate cyclase system. CT catalyzes the ADP ribosylation of the G protein, making it impossible to dissociate from the active adenylate cyclase complex. This leads to a persistent activation of intracellular adenylate cyclase, which in turn stimulates the conversion of adenosine triphosphate to cyclic adenosine 3′,5′-monophosphate (cAMP). The net effect is the excessive accumulation of cAMP at the cell membrane, resulting in hypersecretion of chloride, potassium, bicarbonate and associated water molecules out of the cell. Strains of *V. cholerae* other than the two epidemic serotypes may or may not produce CT. Diarrhea occurs—as much as 20−30 L/d-with leading to dehydration, shock, acidosis and death. The genes for *V. cholerae* enterotoxin are on the bacterial chromosome. Cholera enterotoxin is antigenically associated with LT of *Escherichia coli* and can stimulate the production of neutralizing antibodies. However, the exact role of antitoxic and antibacterial antibodies in protection against cholera is unclear.

The fluid loss caused by the adenylate cyclase stimulation of cells depends on the balance between the amount of bacterial growth, toxin production, fluid secretion and fluid absorption in the entire gastrointestinal tract. The outflow of fluid and electrolytes is greatest in the small intestine, where the secretory capacity is high and absorptive capacity is low. The diarrheal fluid can reach many liters per day, with approximately the same sodium content as plasma, but two to five times the concentrations of potassium and bicarbonate. The result is isotonic fluid loss (dehydration), potassium loss (hypokalemia) and bicarbonate loss (metabolic acidosis). Since *V. cholerae* does not invade or otherwise injure the enterocyte, the intestinal mucosa remains unchanged except for some hyperemia. Mutants lacking CT may still cause mild diarrhea due to the recently discovered accessory toxins which cause fluid secretion or increase intestinal permeability.

(2) Clinical Findings

Although the typical clinical presentation is severe diarrhea, the fact is that most individuals infected with *V. cholerae* have no symptoms or only mild diarrhea, indistinguishable from other mild diarrhoeal diseases. About 60% of infections with classic *V. cholerae* and about 75% of infections with the E1 Tor biotype are asymptomatic. The incubation period is between 18 h and 5 days and symptoms are generally abrupt, including watery diarrhea and vomiting. The most striking feature of cholera is the painless purging of voluminous stools similar to rice-water. The stools are sometimes described as having a fishy odor. The vomitus is generally a clear, watery, alkaline fluid. In adults with severe cholera, the rate of diarrhea may quickly reach 500−1000 mL/h, leading to severe dehydration, circulatory collapse and anuria. Symptoms of severe dehydration include absent or low-volume peripheral pulse, undetectable blood pressure, poor skin swelling, sunken eyes and wrinkled hands and feet (as soaking in water for long periods). At first, patients are restless and extremely thirsty, but as shock develops, they become numb and may lose consciousness. Many patients also show respiratory signs of metabolic acidosis with Kussmaul's respiration, a kind of very deep, gasping, desperate breathing. Most patients do not urinate until the dehydration has been corrected. With such a rapid rate of loss of fluid, the patient is at risk of death within a few hours of onset and most deaths occur during the first day. However, if rehydration fluids are provided in insufficient quantities, the patient may survive temporarily and die a few days later. The mortality rate without treatment is between 25% and 50%. In the event of an epidemic, there is no problem with the diagnosis of a full-blown outbreak of cholera presents. However, sporadic or mild cases are not easily distinguished from other diarrheal diseases. The E1

Tor biotype is more likely to cause milder disease than the classical biotype.

There are several complications occurring with cholera, but these are generally caused by improper treatment. They include acute renal failure due to protracted hypotension if adequate fluids are not provided. Most cholera patients have low blood glucose concentrations and a few have severe hypoglycemia. If the intravenous fluids are administered improperly, electrolyte imbalance can occur, especially hypokalaemia. Miscarriage or premature delivery can be a complication of shock and poor placental perfusion in pregnant women. These obstetric emergencies are becoming less frequent with good hydration, but cholera treatment centers must be prepared for them. Severe muscle cramps of arms and legs are common. They may be due to the electrolyte imbalance, although the exact explanation is unclear. They recede within a few hours of treatment.

(3)Immunity

Nonspecific defenses such as gastric acidity, gut motility and intestinal mucus play an important role in preventing colonization with *V. cholerae*. For example, the attack rate of clinical cholera is higher in persons who lack gastric acidity (gastrectomy or achlorhydria from malnutrition).

Natural infection can provide long-lasting immunity. The immune state has been associated with IgG directed against the cell wall LPS and with the production of secretory IgA by lymphocytes in the subepithelial areas of the gastrointestinal tract. The exact protective mechanisms have yet to be established. An attack of cholera is followed by immunity to reinfection, but the duration and degree of immunity are also unknown. In experimental animals, specific IgA antibodies appear in the intestinal cavity. Similar antibodies are produced in the serum after infection, but only for a few months. Vibriocidal antibodies in serum (titer $\geqslant 1 : 20$) have been associated with protection against colonization and disease. The presence of antitoxin antibodies has not been associated with protection.

8.3.1.3   Laboratory Diagnosis

The initial suspicion of cholera depends on recognition of the typical clinical features in an appropriate epidemiologic setting. A bacteriologic diagnosis of *V. cholerae* isolated from the stool can be accomplished.

(1)Specimens

The culture specimens consist of mucus flecks from stools.

(2)Smears

There was no obvious difference in the microscopic appearance of smears made from stool samples. Dark-field or phase contrast microscopy may show the fast-moving vibrios.

(3)Culture

Peptone agar, blood agar with a pH near 9.0 or TCBS agar are suitable for growth rapidly and typical colonies can be picked within 18 hours. For enrichment, a few drops of stool can be incubated for 6−8 hours in taurocholate peptone broth (pH 8.0−9.0). It led to the result that organisms from this culture can be stained or subcultured. Once isolated, the organism can be readily identified by biochemical reactions.

(4)Specific Tests

V. cholerae organisms are further identified by slide agglutination tests using anti-O group 1 or group 139 antisera and by biochemical reaction patterns.

8.3.1.4   Epidemiology, Prevention & Treatment

(1)Epidemiology

Cholera is often described as the classic water-borne disease because it is usually associated with water. This description oversimplifies the transmission of *V. cholerae*, which can also be transmitted through contaminated food. Contaminated water is frequently mixed with food and both can serve as vehicles. For more developed countries, contaminated food (especially undercooked seafood) is the usual medium for transmission, while contaminated water is more common in less developed countries.

Cholera has pronounced seasonality. In Bangladesh, the disease is endemic with two peaks each year that correspond to the warm seasons before and after the monsoon rains. In Peru, epidemics are strictly confined to the warm season. It seems to be that vibrios are more suitable for rapid growth in warm environmental temperatures. Other than shellfish and plankton, there are no animal reservoirs. In endemic areas, annual incidence rates of disease vary widely, possibly as a result of environmental and climate changes. The better understanding of the relation to climate will help public-health officials better plan for epidemics.

The ratio of cases to *V. cholerae* infections ranges from one in three to one in 100. The severity of the infection depends on a number of factors, particularly including local intestinal immunity (from previous natural exposure or vaccination), the size of the inoculum ingested, the adequacy of the gastric-acid barrier and the patient's blood types. For unknown reasons, people with O blood type have a much higher risk of severe cholera from El Tor vibrios than those with other blood types. This susceptibility to cholera may account for the lower than normal proportion of people with this blood type in the Ganges delta area.

In areas where cholera is endemic, the incidence is highest in children aged 2-4 years. In contrast, in newly invaded areas, the rates of attack are similar for all ages. However, because of exposure to contaminated food and water, the disease generally first appears in adult men. Patterns of Water-use in different regions affect the spread of the disease. In some cities in Peru, cholera vibrios were transmitted through the municipal water system, resulting in very high rates of infection in the urban population. In rural areas, where rivers or open wells are used for drinking water, cases tend to cluster among people living near contaminated water and drinking water sources. Secondary cases sometimes occur during funeral feasts because of traditional but unsanitary burial practices in some parts of the world.

When cholera outbreaks can become massive epidemics, they must be reported to national health authorities. If possible, suspected cases of cholera should be confirmed by bacteriology. Even without laboratory confirmation, cases should be reported if they meet the WHO definition: a cholera outbreak should be suspected if a patient older than 5 years develops severe dehydration or dies from acute watery diarrhea or if there is a sudden increase in the daily number of patients with acute watery diarrhea, especially patients who pass "rice water" stools typical of cholera.

(2) Prevention and Control

Cholera is endemic in India and Southeast Asia. From these centers, it is carried along shipping lanes, trade routes and pilgrim migration routes. The disease is spread by contact with individuals having mild or early illness as well as by water, food and flies. Contaminated food and water are both the main vehicles of transmission of *V. cholerae* and many measures can be taken to keep transmission rates to a minimum. These measures include ensuring a safe water supply, particularly for municipal water systems, improving sanitation, making food safe for consumption by thoroughly cooking of high-risk foods (especially seafood) and health education through mass media. During outbreaks, some important messages for the media include the importance of purifying water and seafood, washing hands after defecation and before food preparation, recognition of the signs of cholera and locations where treatment is available to avoid delays in case of illness. The long-term prevention of cholera will require improvements in water and sanitation facilities, but these improvements are not happening rapidly in most regions where cholera is prevalent. In many cases, only 1%-5% of susceptible people who are exposed to it will develop disease. The carrier state seldom exceeds 3-4 weeks and true chronic carriers are rare. *Vibrios* survive in water for up to 3 weeks. Control depends on education and improved sanitation, particularly of food and water.

Patients should be isolated, their excreta disinfection is required and contacts are followed up. Chemo-prophylaxis with antimicrobial drugs may have a place. Soon after the discovery of *V. cholerae* in the 1880s, an inactivated injectable vaccine containing either lipopolysaccharides (LPS) extracted from vibrios or dense vibrio suspensions was developed shortly and widely used worldwide. Vaccination was even a requirement for international travelers, who mistakenly believe that it might prevent international spread of cholera. This vaccine may be probably suitable for those who could afford it during the early part of the 20th century when treatment was ineffective and sanitation standards were low. As a public health intervention, however, it was not cost-effective because protection was short-lived (just 6 months). It was associated with local inflammatory reactions to pain and it does not prevent the spread of disease. Vaccination was not practicable and was too expensive for people who might benefit from it. Those who could afford it no longer needed it and they did not like the side-effects. As a result, the whole-cell injectable vaccine is no longer recommended for any purpose, although it is still licensed. Current interest includes live attenuated vaccine strains that may have the potential to stimulate the local sIgA immune response.

New oral cholera vaccines are expected to provide substantial protection without side-effects. The inactivated oral vaccine (Dukoral) is composed of killed *V. cholerae* organisms and the cholera B subunit and therefore it can stimulate both antibacterial and antitoxic immunity. Two doses are given 1–6 weeks apart. The other vaccine (Orochol) is a non-toxic mutant of *V. cholerae*, strain CVD103HgR, given as a single-dose, lyophilized oral vaccine. Both are licensed in several countries, but not yet in the USA.

Dukoral has been effective in field trials in less developed countries and it is currently recommended for use in refugee environments at risk of cholera. Its cost-effectiveness in endemic areas is still unclear. Orochol has a highly protective effect in volunteer studies, though its use in endemic areas is not yet known. Other live and inactivated oral vaccines are also being developed and may become useful in the future. One of the main problems in developing these new oral vaccines will be to make them cheap enough and to develop a formulation that can be readily distributed to huge populations at risk. Each of the new oral vaccines may require booster doses and the formulations will need to be sufficiently simple that the vaccine might even be self-administered in the event of risk.

The new oral vaccines will not prevent all cases of cholera because local intestinal immunity can be overcome with high-dose vaccinations, but they should reduce the risk by as much as 80% if used regularly. In addition, a vaccine programme could work synergistically with sanitation programmes. The numbers of vaccinations needed to cause disease would be raised and the numbers of pathogenic organisms entering the environment would be decreased. Therefore, vaccines and sanitation programmes should not be seen as alternative preventive strategies, but as complementary and perhaps even synergistic ones.

(3) Treatment

Without treatment, the case-fatality rate for severe cholera is about 50%. However, treatment is very effective and simple, which is based on the concept of replacing fluids as quickly as they are being lost. The most important part of therapy is the replacement of water and electrolyte to correct the severe dehydration and salt consumption. Initially, the fluids must be supplied sufficiently rapidly to make up for the lost volume to restore circulating blood volume. Additional maintenance fluids must then be given to continue to replace continuing losses as they occur. Almost all deaths can be avoided if fluids are given in time. However, effective treatment is not always available in remote areas where cholera occurs and thus, cholera deaths are still common.

In order to facilitate clinical evaluation and management of patients, dehydration is divided into three categories according to the clinical symptoms and patients signs: no dehydration, moderate dehydration and severe dehydration. Signs of dehydration are not clinically significant unless the patient has already lost about 5% of his or her body weight. The degree of dehydration guides directly the treatment of the patient. A patient with severe dehydration requires emergency intravenous polyelectrolyte solution for rehydration, followed by oral rehydration solution (ORS) for maintenance hydration. For milder cases, ORS is used for both rehydration and maintenance. The principles of rehydration therapy are: rapid replacement of fluid deficits; correction of the metabolic acidosis; correction of potassium deficiency; and replacement of continuing fluid losses. These aims are all achieved through appropriate rehydration fluids. Due to the acidosis, the serum potassium concentration may be normal or even high and the potassium deficiency may not be obvious. As the acidosis is corrected, the serum potassium concentration will fall to dangerously low values unless additional potassium is provided.

Patients who are severely dehydrated are assumed to have lost 10% of their body weight and this is the volume that needs to be replaced. Patients who have no pulse or blood pressure should receive the fluid as rapidly as possible and more than one intravenous line may be needed to inject the fluid rapidly enough to restore the pulse. The total quantity should be given within 2–4 h. The most common error in the treatment of cholera is the slow rate of intravenous infusion, which leaves the patient in a state of shock for a long period. If peripheral veins cannot be found, infusion via the femoral vein may be necessary.

For patients with mild degrees of dehydration, ORS can effectively replenish water. The volume should also be calculated to replace the fluid deficit to ensure that adequate volumes are provided. For individuals with moderate dehydration, at least 5.0%–7.5% of the body weight in ORS should be given just to make up for the deficiency and additional ORS should be given to compensate for the sustained losses.

The intravenous fluid should be kept constant with salts. Ringer's lactate is the best commercially available intravenous fluid, although other polyelectrolyte solutions containing additional potassium provide even better balance with the composition of the stool losses. Since Ringer's lactate contains only 4 mmol/L potassium, patients should be given ORS containing 20 mmol/L potassium as soon as the patient can drink. If polyelectrolyte solution is not available, normal saline can be used in emergency situations, but ORS should be provided as soon as possible to compensate for the acidosis and potassium deficiency. Dextrose and water do not provide the salts needed and are not appropriate.

ORS is the preferred therapy for patients without significant or moderate dehydration. It is also used to maintain hydration to compensate for continuing losses of intravenous fluids after severe dehydration has been corrected. Packaged oral rehydration solutes, containing carbohydrate and the correct salts, are now widely available throughout the world. For cholera, it is even better to use ORS rather than glucose because it reduces the rate of purging and this form is also available in packets to be mixed with water. Recently, the preferred formulation of ORS has changed and the sodium concentration has been reduced to 75 mmol/L. This hypo-osmolar solution is acceptable for cholera, although ORS solutions with sodium concentrations lower than this do not contain sufficient sodium and could lead to severe hyponatremia. In the absence of ORS packets, the following simple ingredients can be added to 1 L water to prepare ORS: 2.6 g sodium chloride, 2.9 g trisodium citrate, 1.5 g potassium chloride and 13.5 g glucose (or 50 g boiled and cooled rice powder). The purest water that is available should be used for making ORS and the remaining solution should be discarded after 24 h.

Clinically significant cholera patients should receive a 1–3 day course of antibiotics to shorten the illness and lessen the purging of diarrhea. Antibiotics can not only cure the illness, they also decrease the need for rehydration fluids and shorten the length of hospital stay. These effects are especially important because cholera outbreaks typically occur in areas lacking intravenous fluid and other supplies. In most cases, doxycycline is the preferred antibiotic. Oral tetracycline tends to reduce stool output in cholera and shortens the excretion period of vibrios. In some endemic areas, tetracycline resistance has emerged in *V. cholerae*, which can transmit plasmids carrying. For outbreaks caused by tetracycline-resistant strains, other clinically effective antibiotics include erythromycin, co-trimoxazole, ciprofloxacin and azithromycin. Trimethoprim-sulfamethoxazole and erythromycin are alternative medicines for children and pregnant women. Patients with mild diarrhea need not receive antibiotics even during cholera outbreaks. Without antibiotic treatment (as long as rehydration is given), patients will recover within 4−5 days. Antibiotic use can shorten the recovery time to about 2−3 days. Asymptomatic contacts should not use antibiotics. Prophylactic use of antibiotics greatly increases the risk of developing resistance and is not cost-effective.

8.3.2 Vibrio Parahaemolyticus

Vibrio Parahaemolyticus is a halophilic bacterium that causes acute gastroenteritis after eating contaminated seafood, such as raw fish or shell fish. Symptoms such as nausea and vomiting, abdominal cramps, fever and watery bloody diarrhea can occur after an incubation period of 12−24 hours. Fecal leukocytes are often observed. Enteritis tends to subside spontaneously within 1−4 days, with no treatment other than restoration of water and electrolyte balance. Enterotoxin has not yet been isolated from this organism. The disease occurs worldwide and the incidence is highest in areas where people eat raw seafood. *V. Parahaemolyticus* does not grow well on some different media used to grow *salmonellae* and *shigellae*, but it does grow well on blood agar. It also grows well on TCBS, where it produces green colonies. *V. Parahaemolyticus* is usually identified by its oxidase-positive growth on blood agar.

8.3.3 Vibrio Vulnificus

Vibrio vulnificus can cause serious wound infections, bacteremia and even gastroenteritis. It is a free-living estuarine bacterium that lives on the Atlantic, Gulf and Pacific Coasts of the United States. Korea has reported the cases of infections and the organism may be distributed throughout the world. *V. vulnificus* is particularly apt to be found in oysters, especially during warm months. Bacteremia with no focus of infection occurs in persons who have consumed infected oysters and who have alcoholism or liver disease. In places where the bacterium is present, normal or immunocompromised persons who are in contact with water may infect the wounds. Infection often proceeds rapidly and develops into severe disease. About 50% of the patients with bacteremia die. Wounds infections may be mild, but often proceed rapidly (over a few hours), developing bullous skin lesions, cellulitis and myositis with necrosis. Because of the rapid progression of the infection, appropriate antibiotics are usually required for treatment before culture confirmation of the etiology can be obtained. Diagnosis is performed by culturing the organism on standard laboratory media. TCBS is the preferred medium for stool cultures, in which most strains produce blue-green (sucrose-negative) colonies. Tetracycline seems to be the preferred drug for *V. vulnificus* infection; ciprofloxacin may also be effective based on in vitro activity.

8.3.4 Other Vibrios

Several other vibrios can also cause human diseases: *Vibrio mimicus* can cause diarrhea after eating uncooked seafood, particularly raw oysters. *Vibrio hollisae* and *Vibrio fluvialis* can also cause diarrhea. *Vibrio alginolyticus* can cause infections in eye, ear or wound after exposure to seawater. *Vibrio damsela* can also cause wound infections. Other *vibrios* are a very rare cause of disease in humans.

8.4 Anaerobes

Anaerobes, also calledanaerobic bacteria, are bacteria that do not surviveor grow in the presence of oxygen. Anaerobes can be classified into two categories: *Clostridium* and non-spore-forming anaerobes.

The genus *Clostridium* includes all anaerobic gram-positive bacilli capable of forming endospores. Although most members of the genus are strict anaerobes, some species are aerotolerant (e. g. , *Clostridium histolyticum* and *Closiridium tertium*) and can grow on agar media exposed to air. Some clostridia consistently stain gram-negative(e. g. , *Clostridinm clastridiiforme*, *Clostridium ramosum*) and sporesare only rarely demonstrated insome species (e. g. , *C. ramosum*, *Clostridium perfringens*). The clostridia are ubiquitous, being present in soil, water and sewage and as part of the normal microbial population in the gastrointestinal tracts of animals and humans. The bacteria produce spores when the environment becomes stressed. Most clostridia are harmless saprophytes, but some are well-recognized human pathogens with a clearly documented history of causing diseases, in their vegetative form, these bacteria secrete powerful exotoxinssuch as tetanus(*Clostridium tetani*), food poisoning(*C. perfringens*), botulism(*Clostridium barati*, *Clostridium butyricm*), diarrhea and colitis (*Clostridium difficile*) and mynecrosis or gas gangrene (*C. perfringen* s, *Clostridium septicum*, *Clostridium novyi*, *Clostridiumsordellii*, *C. histolyticum*). Despite the notoriety of these diseases, we now know that clostridia are more commonly associated with skin and soft tissue infections, food poisoning and antibiotic-associated diarrhea and colitis. The remarkable capacity of clostridia to cause diseases is attributed to the following features: ①rapid growth in a nutritionally enriched, oxygen-deprived environment, ②ability to survive adverse environmental conditions through spore formation and ③production of numerous histolytic toxins, enterotoxins and neurotoxins. The four clinically important species of *Clostridium* will be discussed here: *C. tetani*, *C. perfringens*, *C. botulinum* and *C. difficile*.

Non-spore-forming anaerobes are members of the indigenous flora in humans and animals, including gram-positive and gram-negative cocci and rods. Anaerobes are present in large numbers in the intestine, but also at other areas of the body, such as the skin, the mucosal surfaces, the mouth, the upper respiratory tract and the genitourinary tract. These organisms are primarily opportunistic pathogens, typically responsible for endogenous infections and are usually recovered in mixtures of aerobic and anaerobic bacteria. Additionally, many of these anaerobes have fastidious nutritional requirements and grow slowly on laboratory media. Thus, the isolation and identification of individual strains are difficult and frequently time-consuming. Fortunately, the appropriate management and treatment of most infections with these organisms can be based on the knowledge that a mixture of aerobic and anaerobicorganisms is present in the clinical specimen and does notrequire isolation and identification of the individual organisms. An exception to these general rules is infections caused by *Bacteroides fragilis*, a rapidly growing gram-negative rod and a prototypical endogenous anaerobic pathogenthat can produce life-threatening disease. Anaerobic bacteria can cause an infection when a normal barrier(such as gums, skin or intestinal wall) is damaged due to surgery, injury or disease.

8.4.1 *Clostridium*

8.4.1.1 Clostridium Tetani

(1) *General Features of* Clostridium Tetani

C. tetan i is bacterium that grows in a wound and secretes a toxin that invades systemically and causes tetanus in humans. The disease occurs primarilyin elderly patients with waning immunity. Tetanus is still responsible for causing many deaths in people living in less developed areas where vaccination is unavailable or medical practices are lax. Risk is greatest for people with inadequate vaccine induced immunity. It is estimated that more than one million cases occur worldwide, with mortality rate ranging from 20% to 50%. At least half the deaths occur in neonates. Disease does not induce immunity. This organism is ubiquitous and it is found in fertile soil and colonizes the gastrointestinal tracts of many animals including humans. Spores may be highly resistant to adverse conditions, can survive 75−80 ℃ for 10 minutes and remain alive in dry soil or dust for many years, but are destroyed at 100 ℃ for an hour.

(2)*Biological Characteristics*

C. tetani is a slender [about $(0.5-1.7)$ μm×$(2.1-18)$ μm], motile, spore-forming anaerobic rod. The organism produces round, terminal spores that giving it a characteristic of a drumstick appearance. Although it is gram-positive, gram-negative forms are usually found in stained smears. Most strains are motile with peritrichous flagella colonies often swarm on blood agar plate with β-hemolysis. *C. tetani* is difficult to grow because the organism is extremely sensitive to oxygen toxicity; when growth is detected on agar media, it typically appears as a film over the surface of the agar rather than discrete colonies. The bacteria are proteolytic but unable to ferment carbohydrates and difficult to isolate from clinical specimens.

(3)*Pathogenic Features*

Although being punctured by a rusty nail is a common source of an infection, infections can also occur from a burn, a wound, a compound fracture, an ulcer, drug injection or operative wounds (acquired during operations). If an anaerobic environment is present, such as necrotic tissue where blood supply is poor the spores will germinate and form vegetative cells. The vegetative cells of C. tetani die rapidly when exposed to oxygen, but spore formation allows the organism to survive in the most adverse conditions. The organism itself is not invasive and thus remains in the local wound, but exotoxins secreted by the organism invade systemically and causes muscle spasms.

C. tetani produces two toxins: tetanolysin, an oxygen-labile hemolysin that is inactivated by cholesterol and has an uncertain role in pathogenesis and tetanospasmin, a plasmid-encoded, heat-labile spasmogenic toxin responsible for the classical symptoms of tetanus.

Tetanolysin is serologically related to hemolysins produced by C perfringens and Listeria monocytogenes and the streptolysin O; however, the clinical significance of tetanolysin is unknown because it is inhibited by oxygen and serum cholesterol.

Tetanospasmin is a neurotoxin deadly poisonous which responsible for the clinical manifestations of tetanus. It is produced during the stationary phase of growth and released when the cell is lysed. The toxin is heat labile being destroyed at 65 ℃ in 30 minutes and is O_2 labile. The estimated minimum human lethal dose is 2.5 ng/kg of body weight or 175 ng for a 70 kg human.

Tetanospasminis synthesized as a 150,000-Da peptide. It is made up of two parts: a 100,000-Da heavy or H-chain and a 50,000-Da light or L-chain. Two chains are connected by a disulfide bond and noncovalent forces. The H-chain mediates attachment to specific sialic acid receptors (e.g., polysialogangliosides) in peripheral nerve terminals such as adjacent glycoproteins on the surface of motor neurons; subsequently the intact toxin molecules are internalized in endosomal vesicles and moves to the central nervous system by retrograde axonal transport and trans-synaptic spread. Once inside the central nervous system, the L-chain, a zinc endopeptidase, act by selective cleavage of a protein component of synaptic vesicles, synaptobrevin II (an essential component of synaptic vessels needed for fusion and release of neurotransmitters) and this prevents presynaptic release of inhibitory neurotransmitterglycine and γ-aminobutyric acid (GABA), causing sustained excitatory discharge of disinhibited α-motor neurons and muscle spasms of tetanus. The toxin exerts its effects on the spinal cord, peripheral nerves, brain stem, neuromuscuiar junctions and directly on muscles. The toxin binding is irreversible, sorecovery depends on whether new axonal terminals form.

(4) Clinical Diseases

The human disease associated with *C. tetani* is tetanus. Disease is characterized by muscle spasms and involvement of the autonomic nervous system. The duration of the incubation period seems to directly depend on the distance of the infection site from the central nervous system. The incubation period for tetanus varies from a few days to weeks, with an average of eight days. In neonates the average latent period is about a week.

Tetanus can be initiated in two different ways, resulting in either generalized or local tetanus. Generalized tetanus is the most common form. In generalized tetanus (also called descending tetanus), all of the toxin cannot be absorbed by local nerve endings; therefore, it passes into the blood and lymph with subsequent absorption by motor nerves. The most susceptible centers are the head and neck: the first symptom in most patients is usually involvement of the masseter muscles (trismus or lockjaw), withmuscle spasms descending from the neck to the trunk and limbs. The characteristic sardonic smile that results from the sustained contraction of the facialmuscles is known as *risus sardonicus*. Other early signs are drooling, irritability, sweating and persistent back spasms (*opisthotonos*). As the disease progresses, the spasms increase in severity, becoming very exhausting and painful. During spasms, the upper airway can become obstructed, resulting in respiratory failure. Spasms often are initiated by environmental stimuli that may be as insignificant as the sound of a footstep or the flash of a light. The autonomic nervous system is involved in patients with more severe disease; the signs and symptoms include dehydration, cardiac arrhythmias, profound sweating and fluctuations in blood pressure. In the localized form of tetanus(alsocalled ascending tetanus)toxins travel along the neural route(peripheral nerves)in which the disease remains confined to the musculature at thesite of primary infection, causing a disease confined to the extremities and seen most often in inadequately immunized persons. Infection may precede generalized disease. Localized tetanus may last for months but usually resolves spontaneously. Another unusual form of a variant tetanus is called cephalic tetanus which results from head particularly ear wounds and affects the face, most commonly the muscles innervated by lower cranial nerves. In contrast to the prognosis for patients with localized tetanus, the prognosis for patients with cephalic tetanus is very poor. This disease causes the cranial nerve, especially the seventh cranial nerve, isolated or combined involvement. The outcome is typically poor, but mild cases (often associated with otitis media)have more favorable outcomes. Neonatal tetanus (tetanus neonatorum)is seen in newborns when the mother lacks immunity and the umbilical stump becomes contaminated with spore that progresses to become generalized. The mortality in infants exceeds 90% and developmental defects are present in survivors.

(5) Laboratory Diagnosis

The diagnosis of tetanus, as with that of most other clostridial diseases, is based on the clinical signs and symptoms only. Laboratory diagnosis such as the microscopic detection or isolation of *C. tetani* is useful but frequently unsuccessful. The bacteria often cannot be recovered from the wound of patients with tetanus and conversely, can be isolated from the skin of an individual who does not have tetanus. Culture results are positive in only about 30% of an individual who has tetanus, because disease can be caused by relatively few organisms and the slow-growing bacteria are killed rapidly when exposed to air. Neither antibody to the toxin nor tetanus toxin is detecTable in the patient.

(5) Prevention and Treatment

The highest mortality associated with tetanus is in newborns and in patients in whom the incubation period is shorter than one week. Tetanus is completely preven Table by active immunization. In China for primary immunization of children, tetanus toxoid is recommended as part of the diphtheria, tetanus and acellular pertussis(DTP)series; Three injections are given in the first year of life at 3,4,5 months and a booster is given about year later and again at 7 years of age. After this, in cases of potentially dangerous wounds, a booster of toxoid should be injected immediately. In some countries, booster doses are recommended every 10 years to ensure preventing tetanus.

Debridement of the primary wound which may appear innocuous is important to eradicate spores and change anaerobic conditions for germination. Treatment of tetanus requires vaccination with tetanus toxoid, use of metronidazole and passive immunization with human tetanus immunoglobulin. With wounds that involve the possibility of tetanus contamination, a patient without a history of primary immunization needs a dose of tetanus antitoxin (TAT,3,000–5,000 IU)as soon as possible; Tetanus toxoid should also be given simultaneously. Special treatment of tetanus includes antitoxin and antibiotics therapies. Antitoxin can bind to and inactivate the toxin before it attacks muscles and nerves, should be given as early as possible. A single intramuscular dose of 200,000 to 200,000 units is generally recommended for children and adults, with part of the dose infiltrated around the wound if it can be identified. *C. tetani* itself can be killed easily with penicillin. Supportive measures, such as respiratory assistance and intravenous fluids, are often critical topatient survival. The antitoxin antibodies work by binding free tetanospasmin molecules and wound care and metronidazole therapy eliminate the vegetative bacteria that produce toxin. Metronidazole and penicillin have equivalent activity against *C. tetani*; however, penicillin, such as tetanospasmin, should not be used, because it inhibits GABA activity. Toxin bound to nerve endings is protected from antibodies. Thus, the toxic effects must be controlled symptomatically until the normal regulation of synaptic transmission is restored.

8.4.1.2 *Clostridium perfringens*

(1)*General features of* Clostridium Perfringens

C. perfringens is widely distributed in the environment and frequently occurs in the intestines of humans and animals. The organism is involved in a variety of human diseases. *C. perfringens* type A is the major cause of both gas gangrene and food poisoning. Strains of types B through E do not survive in soil but rather colonize the intestinal tracts of animals and occasionally humans.

1) Biological characteristics: *C. perfringens* is a relatively large, rectangular, gram-positive bacillus [about $(0.6-2.4)\mu m\times(1.3-19.0)\mu m$] with stubby round ends. It is capsulated and nonmotile, spores are oval, subterminal in position, narrower than the cell, rarely observed either in vivo or after in vitro cultivation. This organism is one of the few nonmotile clostridia, but rapidly spreading growth on laboratory media(resembling the growth of motile organisms)is characteristic. The organism grows rapidly in tissues and in culture, is hemolytic and is metabolically active, features that make possible its rapid identification in the laboratory. *C. perfringens* has been classified into five toxigenic types(A through E)on the basis of its ability to produce the major lethal toxins(α toxins, β toxins, ε toxins and τ toxins). Within the genus *C. perfringens* type A is the primary pathogen and occurs in soil and also the intestinal tracts of humans and animals. The types B, C, Dand E seem to be obligate intestinal parasites of animals. *C. perfringens* was the third most common cause of confirmed outbreaks and cases of food-borne illness. The illness is caused by an enterotoxin produced during sporulation and the vehicles of infectionare typically meat and poultry products, usually those found in food service settings

C. perfringens is an aerotolerant anaerobe with an optimum temperature for growth of 45 ℃ (growth temperature 20–50 ℃). It presents rapid spreading growth mimics growth of motile organisms and produces a distinctive double-zone of hemolysis on blood agar: a narrow zone of β-type hemolysis due to ε-toxin near the colony surrounded by a wider zone of incomplete hemolysis due to α-toxin. *C. perfringens* can be identified by the Nagler reaction, which detects the presence of α-toxin (phospholipase-C) on egg yolk medium; colonies are surrounded by an area of opacity, the effect is specifically inhibited if *C. perfringens* antiserum containing α antitoxin is added to the medium. In an aerobically grown Litmus Milk cultures, enzymes of *C. perfringens* will attack the proteins and carbohydrates of the milk producing a "stormy fermentation" with clotting and a large amount of gas formation.

C. perfringens was one of the most common causes of confirmed outbreaks and cases of food-borne illness. The illness is caused by an enterotoxin produced during sporulation and the vehicles of infection are typically poultry products and meat, usually those found in food service settings.

2) Pathogenic features: *C. perfringens* produces more than 10 exotoxins, some of them are extracellular enzymes. α-Toxin, produced by all five types and is the predominant product of *C. perfringens* type A. It exhibits lecithinase activity in addition to its lethal and necrotic activities. It lyses cell membrane lecithins, disrupting cell membranes and causing lysis of erythrocytes, platelets, leukocytes, fibroblasts and muscle cells, resulting in hemolysis, tissue necrosis, myocardial and liver function affected and an increase in vascular permeability, the common and often fatal feature of gas gangrene. β-Toxin is responsible for intestinal stasis, loss of mucosa with formation of necrotic lesions and progression to necrotizing enteritis. ε-Toxin, a protoxin, is activated by trypsin and increases the vascular permeability of the gastrointestinal wall. τ-Toxin, produced by type E *C. perfringens*, has necrotic activity and increases vascular permeability.

C perfringens produces enterotoxin, primarily by type A strains, a minority of type C and type D strains. It is heat labile and may be instantaneously destroyed at 100 ℃. Its activity is enhanced three fold by treatment with trypsin. The enterotoxin is produced during the phase transition from vegetative cells to spores and is released in the alkaline environment of the small intestine when the cells undergo the terminal stages of spore formation (sporulation). The released enterotoxin binds to receptors on the brush border membrane of the small intestine epithelium in the ileum (primarily) and jejunum but not duodenum insertion of the toxin into the cell membrane leads to altered membrane permeability and loss of fluids and ions. The enterotoxin also acts as a superantigen, stimulating T-lymphocyte activity.

3) Clinical diseases: Infection with *C. perfringens* can cause a variety of diseases.

Gas gangrene: *C. perfringens* type A is the most common cause of gas gangrene and is present in 60% –80% of cases, although other species (e. g, *C. septicum*, *C. histolyticum*, *C novyi*) can also produce this disease. This is a life-threatening disease that illustrates the full virulence potential of histotoxic clostridia. Gas gangrene generally occurs at the site of trauma, war wound or a recent surgical wound, as a result of infection by Clostridia that, under anaerobic conditions, produce toxins that cause the tissue necrosis and associated symptoms.

The onset of gas gangrene is sudden and dramatic with an average incubation period is 8 –48 h. Gas Gangrene is an acute disease with a poor prognosis and often fatal outcome. Initially trauma to the host tissue damages muscle and impairs the blood supply. This lack of oxygenation causes oxidation-reduction potential to decrease and allows the growth of anaerobic clostridia bacteria. As the clostridia bacterium multiply, various exotoxins are released into the surrounding tissue causing more local tissue necrosis and systemic toxemia. Infected muscles are discolored and edematous and produce a foul smelling exudates; gas bubbles form from the products of anaerobic fermentation. As capillary permeability increases, the accumulation of fluid increases and venous return eventually ends. As more tissue becomes involved, the clostridia multiply within the increasing area of dead tissue, releasing more toxins into the local tissue and the systemic circulation. Gram stain of tissue or exudates collected from the wound of a patient with *C. perfringens* myonecrosis will reveal abundant rectangular gram-positive rods in the absence of inflammatory cells resulting from lysis by clostridial toxins. Because ischemia plays a significant role in the pathogenesis of gas gangrene, the muscle groups most frequently involved are those in the extremities served by one or two major blood vessels. Without treatment, gas gangrene is invariably fatal.

Clostridial food poisoning: this is a relatively common but underappreciated bacterical disease that results from ingestion of meat products contaminated with large numbers of enterotoxin-producing type A *C. perfringens*. The common form of perfringens food poisoning is characterized by intense abdominal cramps and watery diarrhea but no fever, nausea or vomiting, which begin 8 – 22 hours after consumption of foods contaminated by *C. perfringens* bacteria. The illness is usually over within 24 hours.

Necrotizing enteritis: also called enteritis necroticans, is a rare, acute necrotizing process in the jejunum characterized by abdominal vomiting, pain, shock, bloody diarrhea and peritonitis. The mortality in patients with this infection approaches 50%. β-Toxin-producing *C. perfringens* type C is responsible for this disease. Risk factors for the disease are exposure to large numbers of organisms and malnutrition (with loss of the proteolytic activity that inactivates the enterotoxin).

4) Laboratory diagnosis: Gas gangrene is rapidly progressive and often lethal. Immediate diagnosis is required. The laboratory performs only a confirmatory role in the diagnosis of clostridial soft-tissue diseases, because therapy must beinitiated immediately in affected patients. The microscopic detection of gram-positive rods in clinical specimens, usually in the absence of leukocytes, can be a very useful finding because these organisms have a characteristic morphology. It is also relatively simple to culture these anaerobes. Under appropriate conditions, *C. perfringens* divides every 8 to 10 minutes, so growth on agar media or in blood culture broths can be detected after incubation for only a few hours. The role of *C. perfringens* in food poisoning is documented by recovery of more than 10 organisms per gram of food or more than 10^6 bacteria per gram of feces collected within one day of the onset of disease. Immunoassays have also been developed for detection of the enterotoxin in fecal specimens; however, clostridial food poisoning is a clinical diagnosis and culture or immunoassays are not commonly used.

5) Prevention and Treatment

Prevention of *C. perfringens* infections is difficult because of the ubiquitous distribution of the organisms. Disease requires introduction of the organism into devitalized tissues and maintenance of an anaerobic environment favorable for bacterial growth. Thus, proper wound care and the judicious use of prophylactic antibiotics can do much to prevent most infections.

C. perfringens soft-tissue infections, such as suppurative myositis and myonecrosis, treatment must be aggressively and immediately with surgical debridement and high-dose penicillin therapy. If extremities are extensively involved, amputation should be performed. Intravenous antibiotics are used before, during and after abdominal surgery to prevent postoperative infection. There are no vaccines to prevent clostridia infection. Hyperbaric oxygen treatment has been used to manage these infections; however, the results are inconclusive. Despite all therapeutic efforts, the prognosis in patients with these diseases is poor, with mortality reported from 40% to almost 100%. Less serious, localized soft-tissue infections can be successfully treated with debridement and penicillin.

8.4.1.3 *Clostridium botulinum*

(1) General features of *Clostridium Botulinum*

C. botulinum is commonly isolated in soil and water samples throughout the world. It is the causative agent of botulism. The followingfour forms of botulism have been identified: ①classic or foodborne botulism; ②infant botulism; ③wound botulism; ④inhalation botulism.

1) Biological characteristics: *C. botulinum* is a gram-positive anaerobic bacillus (about 5 μm×1 μm) with peritrichous flagella. Its spores are oval and subterminal. Seven toxigenic types of the organism exist, each producing an immunologically distinct form of botulinum toxin. The toxins are designated A,B,C1,D, E,F and G; human disease is associated with types A,B,E and F. Only one toxin is produced by most individual isolates. In China type A is the most significant cause of botulism. Types C and D most commonly cause animal botulism. Type G, which is found solely in the soil, has no outbreaks associatedwith it. *C. botulinum* can also be divided into four groups(i-iv)taxonomically, which is mainly based on type of toxin produced and proteolytic activity. The *C. botulinum* toxin is heat labile and can be destroyed in one minute if boiled.

2) Pathogenic features: The botulinum toxin is one of the most potent toxins in existence. Its intraperitoneal LD_{50} in mice is bout 0.006,25 ng. The botulinum toxin is very similar in structure and function to the tetanus toxin, differing only in the target neural cell. *C. botulinum* toxin is a 150,000−165,000 Da progenitor protein (A-B toxin) consisting of the neurotoxin subunit (light or A chain) and one or more nontoxic subunits (heavy or B chain). Each nontoxic subunit protects the neurotoxin from being inactivated by stomach acids. The heavy chain of the toxin mediates binding to presynaptic receptors and then the toxin (A fragment) enters the cell by receptor mediated endocytosis. Once inside a neuron, inhibit acetylcholine release. The affected cells fail to release a neurotransmitter, thus producing flaccid paralysis of the motor system. *C. botulinum* also produces a binary toxin consisting of two components that combine to disrupt vascular permeability.

3) Clinical Diseases: Foodborne botulism: sausages, meat products, canned vegetables products have been the most frequent vehicles for human botulism. Patients with foodborne botulism typically become weak and dizzy 1 to 3 days after consuming the contaminated food. Botulinum toxin causes flaccid paralysis by blocking motor nerve terminals at the myoneural junction. The flaccid paralysis progresses symmetrically downward, usually starting with the eyes and face, to the throat, chest and extremities. The initial signs include blurred vision with fixed dilated pupils, dry mouth (indicative of the anticholinergic effects of the toxin), constipation and abdominal pain. Fever is absent. When the diaphragm and chest muscles become fully involved, respiration is inhibited and death from asphyxia results and death is most commonly attributed to respiratory paralysis. Despite aggressive management of the patient's condition, the disease may continue to progress, because the neurotoxin is irreversibly bound and inhibits the release of excitatory neurotransmitters for a pro-longed period. Complete recovery in patients frequently requires many months to years or until the affected nerve endings regrow. Mortality in patients with foodborne botulism, which once approached 70% has been reduced to 10% through the use of better supportive care, particularly in the management of respiratory complications.

Infant botulism: infant botulism is due to infection caused by *C. botulinum*. Although adults certainly are exposed to the organism in their diet, *C. botulinum* cannot survive and proliferate in their intestines. In the absence of competitive bowel microbes, however, the organism can become established in the gastrointestinal tracts of fants. The disease occursin infants 5−20 weeks of age that have been exposed to foods such as honey, presumably the source of infection (spores). It is characterized by constipation, weak cry and weak sucking ability and generalized weakness. *C. botulinum* can apparently establish itself in the bowel of infants at a critical age before the establishment of competing intestinal bacteria (normal flora). Production of toxin by bacteria in the gastointestinal tract induces symptoms. This "infection-intoxication" is restricted to infants.

Wound botulism: wound botulism is a rare disease, can be initiated by contamination of a wound by *C*.

botulinum. Although the symptoms of disease are identical to those of foodborne disease, the incubation period is generally longer(4 days or more) and the gastrointestinal tract symptoms are less prominent.

4)Laboratory diagnosis: The clinical diagnosis of foodborne botulism is confirmed if toxin activity is demonstrated in the implicated food or in the patients' serum, feces or gastric fluid. Infant botulism is confirmed if toxin is detected in the infants' feces or serum or the organism cultured from feces. Wound botulism is confirmed if toxin is detected in the patients' serum or wound or if the organism is cultured from the wound. Toxin activity is most likely to be found early in the disease.

5)Prevention and treatment: Botulinum toxin is heat-labile, boiling food for a few minutes will eliminate toxin contamination. Therefore the best way to control botulism food poisoning is to use adequate food preservation methods and to heat all canned food before eating.

Once a case of wound botulism or food poisoning has been diagnosed, therapy has four objectives: to eliminate the source of the toxin, to eliminate any unabsorbed toxin, to neutralize any unbound toxin with specific antitoxin and to provide general supportive care.

Patients with botulism require the following treatment measures: ① Adequate ventilatory support. ②Elimination of the organism from the gastrointestinal tract through the judicious use of gastric lavage and metronidazole or penicillin therapy. ③The use of trivalent botulinum antitoxin versustoxins A, B and E to bind toxin circulating in the blood stream.

Ventilatory support is extremely important in reducingmortality. Infant botulism has been associated with the consumption of honey contaminated with *C. botulinu* spores, so children younger than one year shouldnot eat honey.

8.4.1.4　*Clostridium difficile*

▶▶ General features of *Clostridium difficile*

C. difficile is a motile bacterium that can be part of the natural intestinal flora. When the normal flora of the intestine is altered by antibiotic therapy, this organism-which is present in the gastrointestinal tract of many babies-can grow and colonize.

(1)Biological Characteristics

C. difficile is a large $[(0.5-1.9)\,\mu m \times (3.0-17)\,\mu m]$ anaerobic rod that freely forms spores in vivo and in culture. The organism grows rapidly in culture, although the vegetative cells die rapidly when exposed to oxygen. *C. difficile* produces a variety of volatile fatty acids that produce a characteristic "barnyard" smell in culture.

(2)Pathogenic Features

C. difficile produces two toxins: an enterotoxin(toxin A)and a cytotoxin (toxin B). The enterotoxin is chemotactic for neutrophils, stimulating the infiltration of polymorphonuclear neutrophils into the ileum with release of cytokines. Toxin A also produces a cytopathic effect, resulting in disruption of the tight cell-to-cell junction, increased permeability of the intestinal wall and subsequent diarrhea. The cytotoxin causes actin to depolymerize, with resultant destruction of the cellular cytoskeleton both in vivo and in vitro. Although both toxins appear to interact synergistic all in the pathogenesis of disease, enterotoxin a negative isolates can still produce disease. In addition, production of one or both toxins alone does not appear to be sufficient for disease (e. g. carriage of *C. difficile* and high levels of toxins are common in young children, although disease is rare). Bacterial "surface layer proteins" are important for the binding of *C. difficile* to the intestinal epithelium, leading to localized production of toxins and subsequent tissue damage.

(3) Clinical Diseases

C. difficile is part of the normal intestinal flora in a small number of healthy people and hospitalized patients. For most of these patients, they have a recent history of exposure to a health care facility, where they were presumably exposed to *C. dificile* and antibiotic use. The disease develops in people taking antibiotics, because the drugs alter the normal enteric flora, either permitting over growth of these relatively resistant organisms or making the patient more susceptible to exogenous acquisition of *C. difficile*. The disease occurs if the organisms proliferate in the colon and produce their toxins.

(4) Laboratory Diagnosis

Isolation of the *C. difficile* in stool culture documents colonization but not disease, so the diagnosis of diseaseis confirmed by demonstration of the enterotoxin or cytotoxin in a stool specimen from a patient with compatible clinical symptoms or detection of the *C. difficile* toxin genes directly in clinical specimens by nucleic acid amplification techniques. Commercial assays with high sensitivity and specificity are now available that provide results within a few hours of sample collection.

(5) Prevention and Treatment

Discontinuation of the implicated antibiotic (e. g. , ampicillin, fluoroquinolones, clindamycin) is generally sufficient to alleviate mild disease. However, specific therapy with metron-dazole or vancomycin is necessary for the management of severe diarrhea or colitis. Because only the nutritional form of *C. difficile* is killed by antibiotics; the spores are resistant and as many as 20% to 30% of patients may relapse after treatment. A second course of treatment with the same antibiotic is frequently successful, although multiple relapses are well documented in some patients. One novel approach to treat recurrent disease is to infuse fecal contents from a healthy donor (repopulate) into the intestines of the ill patient. Remarkable success with these "fecal transplants" has been demonstrated, illustrating the fact that *C. difficile* does not become established when a healthy enteric population of bacteria is present. It is difficult to prevent the disease, because the organism commonly exists in hospitals, particularly in areas adjacent to infected patients (e. g. , bathrooms, beds). The spores of *C. difficile* are difficult to eliminate unless thorough housekeeping measures are used. Thus the organism can contaminate an environment for many months and can be a major source of nosocomial outbreaks of *C. difficile* disease.

8.4.2　Non-spore-forming Anaerobes

8.4.2.1　Introduction and Classification

Non-spore-forming anaerobes are members of the indigenous flora in humans and animals, including gram-positive and gram-negative rods and cocci. Anaerobes are present in large numbers in the intestine (95% –99% of total bacterial mass), but also at other areas of the body (80% –90%), such as the mouth, the skin, the upper respiratory tract and the genitourinary tract. The organisms are primarily opportunistic pathogens, typically responsible for endogenous infections and are usually recovered in mixtures of aerobic and anaerobic bacteria. Anaerobic bacteria can cause an infection when a normal barrier (such as gums, skin or intestinal wall) is damaged due to surgery, disease or injury. Many of these anaerobes have fastidious nutritional requirements and grow slowly on laboratory media. Fortunately, the appropriate management and treatment of most infections with these organisms can be based on the knowledge that a mixture of aerobic and anaerobic organisms is present in the clinical specimen and does notrequire isolation and identification of the individual organisms. An exception to these general rules is infections caused by *Bacteroides fragilis*, a rapidly growing gram-negative rod that can produce life-threatening disease.

（1）Anaerobic Gram-positive Rods

The non-spore-forming gram-positive rods are a diverse collection of facultatively anaerobic or strictly anaerobic bacteria that colonize the skin and mucosal surfaces. *Actinomyces*, *Propionibacterium*, *Lactobacillus* and *Mobiluncus* are well-recognized opportunistic pathogens, whereas other genera such as *Bifidobacterium* and *Eubacterium* can be isolated in clinical specimens but rarely cause human disease.

（2）*Actinomyces*

Actinomyces organisms are facultatively anaerobic or strictlyanaerobic gram-positive rods. They are not acid-fast（in contrast to the morphologically similar *Nocardia* species）, they grow slowly in culture and they tend to produce chronic slowly developing infections. They typically develop delicate filamentous forms or hyphae, similar to fungi, inclinical specimens or when isolated in culture. However, these organisms are true bacteria in that they lack mitochondria and a nuclear membrane, reproduce by fissionand are inhibited by penicillin but not antifungal antibiotics. *Actinomyces* colonize the upper respiratory tract, female genital tract and gas-trointestinal tract. These bacteria are not normally present on the skin surface. The organisms have a low virulence potential and cause disease only when the normal mucosal barriers are disrupted by trauma, infection or surgery.

Almost 50 species have been described and many have been implicated in human disease. Disease caused by actinomyces is termed actinomycosis. Actinomycosis is characterized by the development of chronic granulo-matous lesions that become suppurative and form abscesses connected by sinus tracts. Macroscopic colonies of organisms resembling grains of sand can frequentle seen in the abscesses and sinus tracts. These colonies, called sulfur granules because they appear yellow or orange, are masses of filamentous organisms bound together by calcium phosphate. The areas of suppuration are surrounded by fibrosing granulation tissue, which gives the surface overlying the involved tissues a hard or woody consistency. Most actinomycetes infections are cervicofacial, developing in patients who have poor oral hygiene or have undergone an invasive dental procedure or oral trauma. In these patients, the Actinomyces present inthe mouth invade into the diseased tissue and initiate the infectious process. The disease may occur as an acute pyogenic infection or as a slowly evolving, relatively painless process. Abscesses may form in the lung tissue early in the disease and then spread into adjoining tissues as thedisease progresses. Pelvic actinomycosis can occur as are latively benign form of vaginitis or, more commonly, therecan be extensive tissue destruction, including development of tuboovarian abscesses or ureteral obstruction. The most common manifestation of central nervous system actinomycosis is a solitary brain abscess, but meningitis, subdural empyema and epidural abscess are also seen Actinomycosis in patients with chronic granulomatous disease, presenting as a nonspecific febrile illness, has recently been described. Abdominal actinomycosis can spread throughout the abdomen, potentially involving virtually every organ system. Symptoms of thoracic actinomycosis are nonspecific.

Laboratory confirmation of actinomycosis is frequently difficult. Care must be used during collection of clinical specimens that they not become contaminated with actinomyces that are part of the normal bacterial population on mucosal surfaces.

Actinomyces are fastidious and grow slowly under anaerobic conditions; it can take 2 weeks or more for the organisms to be isolated.

Treatment for actinomycosis involves the combination of surgical debridement of the involved tissues and the prolonged administration of antibiotics. Actinomyces are uniformly susceptible to penicillin（considered the antibiotic of choice）as well as carbapenems, macrolides and clindamycin. Most species are resistant to metronidazole and the tetracyclines have variable activity. The clinical response is generally good even in patients who have suffered extensive tissue destruction. Maintenance of good oral hygiene and the use of appropriate antibiotic prophylaxis when the mouth or gastrointestinal tract is penetrated can lower the risk of these infections.

(3) *Propionibacterium*

Propionibacteria are small gram-positive rods that are frequently arranged in short chains or clumps. Major metabolic by product is propionic acid from fermentation of carbohydrates. They are commonly found on the skin (in contrast with the actinomyces), conjunctiva, in the oropharynx, externa ear and female genital tract. The organisms are anaerobic or aerotolerant, catalase-positive, nonmotile and capable of fermenting carbohydrates, producing propionic acid as their major product. Propionibacteria can be grown on common laboratory medium but is a slow grower and often overgrown by contaminating flora. The two most commonly isolated species are Propionibacterum acnes and Propionibacterium propionicus.

P. acnes is responsible for two types of infections: the first type is acne vulgaris(as the name implies) in teenagers and young adults and the other type is opportunistic infections in patients with prosthetic devices (e. g. , artificial heart valves or joints) or intravascular lines (e. g. , catheters, cerebrospinal fluid shunts). Propionibacteria are also commonly isolated in blood cultures, but this finding usually represents contamination with bacteria on the skin at the phlebotomy site.

The central role of *P. aces* in acne is to stimulate an inflammatory response. Production of a low-molecular-weight peptide by the bacteria residing in sebaceous follicles attracts leukocytes. The bacteria are then phagocytosed, followed by the release of hydrolytic enzyme that, together with bacterial lipases, proteases, neuraminidase and hyaluronidase, precipitate the inflamma-tory response leading to rupture of the follicle. When injected into experimental animals, *P. propionicus* causes lacrimal canaliculitis (inflammation of the tear duct).

Propionibacteria can grow on most common media although it may take 2 to 5 days for growth to appear. Care must be taken to avoid contamination of the specimen with the organisms normally found on the skin. The significance ofthe recovery of an isolate must also be interpreted in light of the clinical presentation(e. g. ,a catheter or other foreign body an serve as a focus for these opportunistic pathogens).

Acne is unrelated to the effectiveness of skin cleansing because the lesion develops within the sebaceous follicles. For this reason, acne is managed primarily through topical application of benzoyl peroxide and antibiotics. Antibiotics such as erythromycin and clindamycin have proved effective for treatment) and abscesses.

(4) *Lactobacillus*

Lactobacillus species are facultatively anaerobic or strictly anaerobic rods. They are found as part of the normal flora ofthe mouth, intestines, stomach and genitourinary tract. The organisms are most commonly isolated in urine specimens and blood cultures. Because lactobacilli are the most common organism in the urethra, their recovery in urine cultures usually is a result of contamination of the specimen, even when large numbers of the organisms are present. The reason lactobacilli rarely cause infections of the urinary tract is their inability to grow in urine. Invasion into blood occurs in one of the following three settings: ①endocarditis, ②transient bacteremia from a genitourinary source(e. g. ,after child birth or a gynecologic procedure) and ③opportunistic septicemia in an immunocompromised patient. Strains of lactobacilli used as probiotics have occasionally been associated with human infections, most commonly in immunocom promised patients.

Treatment of endocarditis and opportunistic infections is diffcult because lactobacilli are resistant to vancomycin (anantibiotic commonly active against gram-positive bacteria and are inhibited but not killed by other antibiotics. A combination of penicillin with an aminoglycoside is requiredfor bactericidal activity.

（5）*Mobiluncus*

Members of the genus Mobiluncus are obligate anaerobic, gram-variable or gram-negative, curved bacilli with tapered ends. Despite their appearance in Gram-stained specimens, they are classified as gram-positive bacilli because they ①have a gram-positive cell wall. ②lack endotoxin and ③are susceptible to vancomycin, clindamycin, erythromycin and ampicillin but resistant to colistin. The organisms are fastidious, growing slowly even on enriched media supplemented with rabbit or horse serum. Two species, *Mobilmcus curtisii* and *Mobiluncus mulieris*, have been identified in humans. The organisms colonize the genital tract in low numbers but are abunant in women with bacterial vaginosis (vaginitis). Their microscopic appearance is a useful marker for this disease, but the precise role of these organisms in the pathogenesis of bacterial vaginosis is unclear.

（6）*Bifidobacterium*

Bifidobacterium are pleomorphic, branching, nonmotile obligate anaerobes. The organisms are natural flora of the gut of mammals. *B. infantis*, *B. brevi* and *B. longum* are the largest group of bacteria in infants, shifting to the third or fourth largest group in adults. The number of Bifidobacteria decline with age. Bifidobacteria may control intestinal pH by liberating lactic acid and acetic acid which also decreases the pH and inhibits the growth of pathogenic bacteria. *B. dentium* is related to dental caries with unknown mechanism.

（7）*Eubacterium*

Eubacterium are non-branching anaerobic rods of clinical importance and are normal flora of intestine. There are 45 species of the genus. *Eggerthella lenta* and is the species most frequently associated with human infections.

（8）Anaerobic Gram-negative Rods

At present there are over two dozen genera of anaerobic gram-negative rods. The most important anaerobic gram-negative rods are in the genera *Bacteroides*, *Fusobacterium*, *Parabacteroides*, *Porphyromonas* and *Prevotella*. These anaerobes are the predominant bacteria on most mucosal surfaces. The genus *Bacteroides* is composed of more than 90 and subspecies. A characteristic common to most species in the genus *Bacteroides* is that their grow this stimulated by bile *Bacteroides* species are pleomorphic in size and shape and resemble a mixed population of organisms in a casually examined Gram stain. *Bacteroides fragilis* is the most commonly isolated species, constituting one-quarter of the total anaerobic from clinical specimens and one half of total *Bacteroides* isolates. The organism is rod shaped of variable size. It is pleomorphic and shows terminal or central swellings, vacuoles or filaments. *B. fragilis* lipopolysaccharide contains little or no lipid A, 2-ketodeoxyoctanate or heptose, exhibits little endotoxin activity. Except for *Bacteroides* species, other members of gram-negative anaerobic rods slowly on artificial medium. Members of the genus *Fusobacterium* may be spindle shaped.

▶▶ *Anaerobic Gram-positivecocci*

There are six genera of G⁺ anaerobic cocci which may be isolated from humans. The majority of man isolates are Peptostreptococcus species. Among anaerobes, they are second only to Bacteroides species in frequency of isolation from clinical specimens, which are often found in vagina. Gram-positive anaerobic cocci have been reported to account for 20% to 35% of all anaerobes isolated in clinical laboratories. Again most infections are polymicrobic. G⁺ anaerobic cocci only account for 1% cases of anaerobic bacteremia, resulting from female genital tract infections caused by Peptostrepto cocci.

The anaerobic gram-positive cocci normally colonize the oral cavity, gastrointestinal tract, genitourinary tract and skin. They produce infections when they spread from these sites to normally sterile sites. For example, bacteria in the intestines can cause intra abdominal infections; bacteria on the skin can cause cellulitis and soft-tissue infections; bacteria colonizing the upper airways can cause sinusitis and pleuropulmonary infections; bacteria in the genitourinary tract can cause endometritis, pelvic abscesses and salpingitis; and bacteria that invade the blood can produce infections in bones and solid organs.

Laboratory confirmation of infections with anaerobicbacteria is complicated by the following three factors: ①care must be taken to prevent contamination of the clinical specimen with the anaerobes that normally colonize the skin and mucosal surfaces; ②the collected specimen must betransported in an oxygen-free container to prevent loss of the organisms; ③specimens should be cultured on nutritionally enriched media for a prolonged period. In addition, some species of staphylococci and streptococci grow initially in an anaerobic atmosphere only and may be mistaken for anaerobic cocci. However, these organisms eventually grow well in air supplemented with 10% carbon dioxide (CO_2) so they cannot be classified as anaerobes.

Anaerobic cocci are usually susceptible to penicillins and carbapenems; have intermediate susceptibility to broad-spectrum cephalosporins, clindamycin, erythromycin and the tetracyclines; and are resistant to the aminoglycosides (as are all anaerobes). Specific therapy is generally indicated in monomicrobic infections; however, because most infections with these organisms are polymicrobic, broad-spectrum therapy against aerobic and anaerobic bacteria is usually selected.

(9) Anaerobic Gram-negative Cocci

The anaerobic gram-negative cocci are rarely isolated inclinical specimens except when present as contaminants. Members of the genus *Veillonella* are the predominant anaerobes in the oropharynx, but they represent less than 1% of all anaerobes isolated in clinical specimens. There are seven species of *Veillonella*, of which *Veillonella parvula* is the most commonly isolated species from human specimens and in most cases there are polymicrobic in fections. The other anaerobic cocci are rarely isolated.

8.4.2.2 Pathogensis

Non-spore-forming anaerobes are part of the normal flora of the skin, the mouth and the intestinal and genitourinary tracts of healthy individuals may cause endogenous infections when immunological and anatomical defenses of host are damaged, permitting tissue penetration by members of the indigenous flora. Proliferation of anaerobic bacteria in tissue depends on the absence of oxygen. Oxygen is excluded from the tissue when the local blood supply is impaired by trauma, obstruction or surgical manipulation.

General features of non-spore-forming anaerobic infections:

1) Non-spore-forming anaerobes are not involved in any single specific disease process, infections, may range from mild abscess and tissue necrosis to life-threatening infections such as brain abscess, septicemia;

2) Infections are caused by endogenous opportunistic pathogens, may occur in all parts of the humanbody;

3) Bacteria can be found by direct microscopic examination of exudates, but not be isolated on ordinary medium;

4) Pus or exudates are viscous, foul-smelling and pigmented, sometimes gas is produced;

5) Infections have no response to some antibiotics such as aminoglycosides.

Virulence factors:

1) Toxins including proteases, lipases, hyaluronidase, chondroitin sulfatase and neuraminidase, may play a role in infection by causing tissue destruction.

2) Some members of non-sporing anaerobes can become resistant to oxygen by producing protective enzymes. For example, many species of Bacteroides can produce superoxide dismutase.

3) Often more than one species will infect the same site. Simultaneous infection with a facultative anaerobe (which uses up the already diminished oxygen supply) also encourages growth of obligate anaerobes.

4) Surface attachment structures such as fimbriae may enable adherence to epithelial cells, are important in the initiation of colonization and infection.

8.4.2.3　Types of Infections

(1) Infections in Central Nervous System

Chronic otitis media, sinusitis or mastoiditis frequently is the primary source of the organisms and may result from a direct extension of then infection into the brain.

(2) Septicemia

With widespread use of effective antibiotics, at present anaerobes can only be isolated from 50% patients with septicemia. Anaerobic septicemia may result from in fectionsin gastrointestinal tract (50%) or female genital tract (20%). The mortality is 15% –35%.

(3) Intraabdominal Infections

They are usually associated with intraabdominal pathology such as perforated gastric or duodenal ulcers, appendicitis, diverticulitis, inflammatory bowel disease or malignancy and produce peritonitis or rank abscess formation. Primary anaerobic peritonitis has only rarely been reported, usually in patients with underlying ascites. Most infections are polymicrobial and the dominant anaerobes are those of the B. fragilis group. Before the advent of anti anaerobic prophylaxis for intestinal surgery, postoperative anaerobic wound infection, abscess formation and even septicaemia were commonly seen on surgical wards.

(4) Dental Sepsis

The anaerobic oral commensal flora is found together with various aerobic and microaerophilic oral commensal bacteria in periodontal infection, dental abscesses and other oral infections and in postoperative infections associated with maxillofacial surgery.

(5) Infections of the Female Genital Tract

Anaerobic bacteria are, with *Gardnerella vaginalis*, the cause of the malodorous vaginal discharge in the common condition now known as bacterial vaginosis. They also cause tuboovarian sepsis, Bartholin's abscess, endometritis, septicabortion and infection associated with intrauterine contraceptive devices. Anaerobic infections of the female genital tract and neonatal infections are usually caused by Prevotella spp. Porphyromonas pp, Fusobacterium spp. and Peptostreptococcus spp, very rarely by *B. fragilis*.

(6) Pulmonary Infections

Anaerobic lung infections may originate in the bronchi or the blood. Aspirations from the upper respiratory tract, which contain large numbers of anaerobic bacteria, are responsible for initiating infection in the bronchi.

8.4.2.4　Laboratory Diagnosis

Specimens such as coughed sputum, feces and vaginal swabs, could be contaminated with normal microbial flora, are unacceptable. Aspirates from abscesses or the specific sites of infections must be obtained in these cases to avoid contamination with indigenous flora components. Unless the specimen can be sent to the laboratory immediately, it is placed in an anaerobic transport tube containing oxygen-free carbon dioxide or nitrogen. Anaerobic culture is required for a definitive diagnosis. Direct microscopic examination may be helpful because of the frequently unique morphology of non-spore-forming anaerobes. Analysis of metabolic end products, especially organic acids, such as gas chromatography provides additional information useful in classifying these organisms.

8.4.2.5 Prevention and Treatment

There are two primary guidelines in preventing anaerobic infections: avoiding conditions that reduce the redox potential of the tissues and preventing the introduction of anaerobes of the normal flora to closed cavities, wounds or other sites prone to infection. Surgical intervention, particularly drainage of pus and excision of necrotic tissue, is of great importance in anaerobic infections.

Drugs active against 95% anaerobes are metronidazole, chloramphenicol, imipenem and combinations of β-lactamase drugs plus a β-lactamase inhibitor, since increasing numbers of anaerobes are showing resistance to penicillin.

8.5 Mycobacteria

Mycobacteria are a family of small, rod-shaped, aerobic bacilli that do not form spores. They are not readily stained, but after being stained, they resist decolorization by acid or alcohol and are therefore called "acid-fast" bacilli. The mycobacteria can be classified into 3 main groups: ①*Mycobacterium tuberculosis* complex (MTC or MTBC), a genetically related group of *Mycobacterium* species that can cause tuberculosis (TB) in humans or animals. It includes *Mycobacterium tuberculosis* (*M. tuberculosis*), *Mycobacterium bovis* (*M. bovis*), *Mycobacterium africanum* (*M. africanum*), *Mycobacterium microti* and *Mycbacterium canetti*. ②*Mycobacterium leprae* and *Mycobacterium lepromatosis* which cause leprosy. ③Nontuberculous mycobacteria (NTM), all the other mycobacteria, including *Mycobacterium avium* complex (MAC), *Mycobacterium kansasii* and *Mycobacterium abscessus*, *et al.* Most of them are opportunistic pathogens.

8.5.1 *Mycobacterium Tuberculosis*

8.5.1.1 Morphology and Biology

(1) Morphology

Tubercle bacilli are thin, straight rods measuring about 0.4 μm×3 μm. Cells are often seen wrapped together, due to the presence of fatty acids in the cell wall that stick together. Mycobacteria cannot be stained by Gram stain method. They can be stained by basic dyes, which cannot be decolorized by acid-alcohol. The character of acid fastness depends on the mycolic acid in cell wall and the integrity of cell envelope. In the clinic, Ziehl-Neelsen acid-fast stainis used to identify mycobacteria.

(2) Structure and Antigens

Mycobacteria possess a complex, lipid-rich cell wall, being composed of mycolic acids, complex waxes and unique glycolipids. The mycolic acids are joined to the muramic acid moiety of the peptidoglycan and to arabinogalactan. Meanwhile, the lipids are largely bound to proteins and polysaccharides. Mycolic acids can cause granuloma formation; phospholipids induce caseous necrosis. Other important cell wall components include virulence related glycolipids trehalose dimycolate (cord factor), sulfolipids and lipoarabinomannan (LAM). Mycobacteria contain a variety of polysaccharides, which can elicit the formation of antibodies.

Mycobacterial cell wall proteins and culture filter proteins elicit tuberculin reaction. The Purified Protein Derivative (PPD) skin test is used to identify the exposure to mycobacteria. The proteins can elicit the formation of a variety of antibodies.

(3) Genome

The size of mycobacterial genome is 4 million base pairs, with a high (61% to 71%) guanine plus cytosine (G+C) content in their deoxyribonucleic acid (DNA). *M. tuberculosis* strain H37Rv contains 3,959 genes, including 250 genes involved in fatty acid metabolism. In addition, about 10% of the coding capacity are taken up by the *PE /PPE* gene families encoding acidic proteins with N-terminal conserved PE (Pro-Glu) and PPE (Pro-Pro-Glu) domains.

(4) Culture

Mycobacteria are obligate aerobes. They can derive energy from the oxidation of many simple carbon compounds. Therefore, increased CO_2 tension enhances their growth. *M. tuberculosis* grow slowly with doubling time of 18–20 hours. Biochemical activities are not characteristic. Commonly used media include liquid media (e. g. , Middlebrook 7H9) and solid media. Bacteria proliferate more rapidly in Middlebrook 7H9 broth than in solid media and grow in clumps if tweens are not added. Solid media are useful for observing morphology, detecting of antimicrobial susceptibility and quantity of organism. They include semisynthetic agar media (e. g. , Middlebrook 7H11 or 7H10) and inspissated egg media (e. g. , Lowenstein-Jensen). Malachite green is included to inhibit other bacteria. It takes several weeks for visible colonies to grow on solid plates.

(5) Reaction to Physical and Chemical Agents

Because of the lipid-rich cell wall, Mycobacteria are resistant to acids, alkalis, dehydration detergents, dyes, common antibacterial antibiotics (e. g. , penicillin) and the host immune responses. In addition, they are resistant to drying and survive for 6–8 months in dried sputum. *M. tuberculosis* are killed within 15 min on exposure to hot water at 62–63 ℃. Alcohol and ultraviolet light can effectively kill Mycobacteria.

(6) Variation

Variation can occur in colony appearance, virulence, drug resistance and many other characteristics. Bacille Calmette-Guérin (BCG) vaccine is prepared from a strain of the attenuated *M. bovis* . Antibiotic resistance in *M. tuberculosis* typically occurs due to mutations in some genes. *M. tuberculosis* is considered to be multidrug-resistant (MDR TB) if it does not respond to at least isoniazid and rifampicin, the 2 most powerful anti-TB drugs.

8.5.1.2 Pathogenesis and Immunity

(1) Pathogenesis

M. tuberculosis usually infects human being through respiratory airways. The infectious particles are phagocytized by alveolar macrophages. One type of macrophages (M1 macrophage) will be activated and secrete cytokines such as interleukin (IL)-12 and tumor necrosis factor (TNF)-α. These cytokines increase localized inflammation, recruit T cells and natural killer (NK) cells into the infected area, subsequently induce T-cell differentiation into TH1 cells (T-helper cells) and secret interferon (IFN)-α, which activate the infected macrophages and kill the intracellular bacteria. In addition, TNF-α stimulates production of nitrogen reactive intermediates, leading to enhanced intracellular killing. However, in another type of macrophages (M2 macrophage), infected *M. tuberculosis* prevents fusion of the phagosome with lysosomes. Phagocytized bacteria are also able to evade macrophage killing, evade the immune system and replicate. At last, most of infected *M. tuberculosis* will be eradicated by host immunity. But small part of them will survive and persist in the body. The persistent bacteria will be reactivated once the host immunity compromised. Immunocompromised individuals are at increased risk for active TB upon mycobacterial infections.

(2) Immunity and Hypersensitivity

Following the first infection with *M. tuberculosis*, a certain resistance is acquired due to the development of cellular immunity. Meanwhile, Robert Koch observed that the response of a tuberculous animal to reinfection with tubercle bacilli marked by necrotic lesions that develop rapidly and heal quickly, which is called Koch's phenomenon. It is caused by hypersensitivity to products of the tubercle bacillus, the mechanism of which is delayed-type hypersensitivity (DTH). Hypersensitivity and resistance seems to be distinct aspects of the cell-mediated immune responses.

(3) Pathology

The development of disease and their healing or progression depends on the virulence of the organism and the state of host defenses. There are two principle lesions following *M. tuberculosis* infection. First, exudative type. This consists of an acute inflammatory reaction with edema fluid, which is seen particularly in lung tissue. The polymorphonuclear leukocytes and monocytes are activated. Second, productive (proliferative)type. Macrophages, T and B lymphocytes and fibroblasts aggregate to form granulomas, with lymphocytes surrounding the infected macrophages. Macrophages fuse together to form a giant multinucleated cell. Bacteria inside the granuloma can become dormant, resulting in latent infection. When mycobacteria establish themselves in tissue, they reside intracellularly in monocyte, reticuloendothelial cells and giant cells.

Caseous necrosis happens in the center of tubercles. If the necrosis material gets liquefied and the formed cavities are joined to the air passages bronchi, bacteria in it are resuscitated and proliferate rapidly. The material containing living bacteria can be coughed up, by which the infection is spread to other persons. Infection is usually not transmissible in the primary stage and is never contagious in the latent stage.

8.5.1.3 Epidemiology and Disease

(1) Epidemiology

The World Health Organization (WHO)estimates that one-third of the world's population are infected with *M. tuberculosis*. *M. tuberculosis* bacilli initially cause a primary infection. Most of them are latent infection and only 5-10 percent of infected people would become active disease during their lifetime. In 2016, there were an estimated 10.4 million people fell ill with TB, among them 90% were adults. The top five countries are India, Indonesia, China, the Philippines and Pakistan, which account for half of cases. Other high epidemic countries are sub-SaharanAfrica, South Africa, Eastern Europe and the countries of the former Soviet Union.

(2) Primary TB

Mycobacterium tuberculosis is typically spread by close person-to-person contact through the inhalation of infectious aerosols. Following first contacting with tubercle bacilli, an acute exudative lesion develops and rapidly spreads to the lymphatics and regional lymph nodes, which consequently undergoes massive caseation. The primary site of infection in the lungs, known as the "Ghon focus", is generally subpleural, often in the mid to lower zones. If the Ghon focus involves infection of adjacent lymphatics and hilar lymph nodes, it is known as the Ghon's complex or primary complex. Tuberculosis of the lungs may also occur *via* infection from the blood stream. The prominent symptoms of pulmonary TB are chronic, productive cough, low-grade fever, night sweats, easy fatigability and weight loss.

Beside saffecting the lungs (pulmonary TB), *M. tuberculosis* can also affect other sites (extrapulmonary TB) through direct contact transmission or gastrointestinal tract. The hematogenous transmission can spread infection to other parts of the body, inducing lymphadenitis, meningitis, etc. In young children and those with HIV, who have no immunity against *M. tuberculosis*, TB bacteria can spread throughout the body and set up many foci of infection, which is called miliary tuberculosis. This disseminated TB has a high fatality rate.

(3) Secondary TB

Most (about 95%) primary infections get latent (dormant) infection. Conditions that impair cellular immunity significantly facilitate reactivation. These conditions include coinfection with HIV, diabetes, tumor, dialysis-dependent chronic kidney disease, significant weight loss, immune suppression by drugs. In some patients, active disease develops when they are re-infected. Reinfection more likely happened in areas where TB is prevalent, while reactivation predominates in low-prevalence areas. Secondary (post-primary) TB is characterized by chronic tissue lesions, formation of tubercles, caseation and fibrosis.

8.5.1.4 Diagnosis

(1) Microscopy

Sputum, exudate or other material is examined by microscopy for acid-fast bacilli. Traditionally, the clinical specimen is stained with basic *carbolfuchsin* (Ziehl-Neelsen methods) and decolorized with an acid-alcohol solution, then counterstained. Fluorescence microscopy with auramine-rhodamine stain is more sensitive than acid-fast stain because the specimen can be scanned rapidly under low magnification. Microscopy is the most simple and rapid way to confirm mycobacterial disease. The sensitivity of this test is high for specimens which contain amount of mycobacteria ($>10^4$/mL). Therefore, a positive acid-fast stain reaction corresponds to high infectivity.

(2) Culture, Identification and Susceptibility

As for pulmonary TB, particularly disease with cavitation, early morning respiratory specimens could be collected for 3 consecutive days; then sputum should be liquefied and treated with a decontaminating reagent (e. g. ,2% sodium hydroxide) to eliminate contaminated organisms. As for disseminated disease, a large volume of fluid or tissue must be collected for cultures. Decontaminated specimens from nonsterile sites and centrifuged specimens from sterile sites can be inoculated onto selective media, such as egg-based Löwenstein-Jensen and agar-based Middlebrook media. Incubation is at 35–37 ℃. It generally takes 4–8 weeks for *M. tuberculosis* to be detected. It takes additional 4–8 weeks for the drug-susceptibility assay. Conventional methods for identification of mycobacteria include observation of rate of growth, colony morphology, pigmentation and biochemical profile. Nucleic acid-based tests are becoming replacement methods in many laboratories. The culture method requires more developed laboratory capacity which limit its use in the clinic.

(3) Nucleic Acid-Based Tests

Microscopy cannot identify the particular mycobacterial species involved and cannot provide more information on drug resistance. It is recommended to detect nucleic acid sequences such as species-specific target genes (e. g. , 16S *rRNA* gene, *SecA* gene) and drug resistance related mutations by molecular probes or nucleic acid amplification to give a rapid diagnosis of TB. Nucleic acid-based test allows rapid testing where microscopy is inaccurate and culture is not available. It has been confirmed that direct detection by molecular probes is sensitive for acid-fast smear-positive specimens. Xpert® MTB/RIF assay, which can identify *M. tuberculosis* and detect most of rifampin drug-resistance, can provide results within 2 hours.

(4) Immunodiagnosis

The traditional test to assess the patient's response to exposure to *M. tuberculosis* is the tuberculin skin test. In this test, a specific amount of antigen (5 tuberculin units of PPD) is inoculated intradermally. Skin test reactivity, one kind of DTH reaction defined by the diameter of the area of induration, is measured in 48–72 hours. Patients infected with *M. tuberculosis* may show a positive response (induration>5 mm) to the tuberculin skin test. For persons at low risk for tuberculosis, strong positive reaction (induration>15 mm) might indicate the possibility of active tuberculosis, especially for infants. However, individuals vaccinated with BCG will also have a positive reaction. The patients in early stage of mycobacteria infection and with anergic will be negative.

In vitro IFN-γ release assays have been introduced as an alternative to the tuberculin skin test. The tests use immunoassays to measure IFN-γ produced by sensitized T cells following stimulation by *M. tuber-*

culosis antigens. There are two immunoassays available now: QuantiFERON-TB Gold and T-SPOT TB. If an individual was previously infected with *M. tuberculosis*, exposure of sensitized T cells to *M. tuberculosis*-specific antigens results in IFN-γ production. The stimulating antigens currently used are early secreted antigenic target-6 (ESAT-6) and culture filtrate protein-10 (CFP-10). These *in vitro* IFN-γ release assays can discriminate between infections with *M. tuberculosis* and BCG vaccination. But they could not discriminate between active TB and latent TB satisfyingly. However, they are still very useful methods to distinguish between TB and non-TB.

8.5.1.5　Treatment, Prevention and Control

(1) Vaccination

The attenuated *M. bovis* BCG vaccine was developed from 1908—1921. It proved to be effective to prevent severe forms of TB in children. However, BCG's protective efficacy is variable in adults. Novel TB vaccine candidates being developed to include recombinant BCG (rBCG), attenuated *M. tuberculosis*, killed *M. tuberculosis* or *Mycobacterium vaccae*, adjuvanted protein subunit vaccines, viral vector-delivered subunit vaccines candidates are now in clinical trials.

(2) Treatment

Effective drug treatments streptomycin (SM) and paraaminosalicylic acid (PAS) were developed in the 1940s. Since then first-line anti-mycobacterial drugs, such as isoniazid (INH), rifampin (RMP), pyrazinamide (PZA) and ethambutol (EMB) were developed before the 1980s. Among them, INH kills rapidly growing organisms, while RMP and PZA kill the slowly growing organism. Because there are spontaneous mutations resistant to these drugs. When the drugs are used singly, the resistant bacilli emerge rapidly, resulting in the rapid development of resistance and treatment failure. Therefore, in individuals with clinical disease, the principles of drug treatment are: treating early, using drugs in combination, enough dose and completing a treatment course to prevent relapse. The short-term (6–9 months) treatment regimens begin with 2 months of INH, EMB, PZA and RMP, followed by 4 to 6 months of INH and RMP. In patients with cavitary disease or in whom the sputum culture results are still positive after 2 months of treatment, an additional 3 months of therapy should be given. As drug resistance becomes a worldwide problem, modifications to this treatment scheme should be dictated by the drug susceptibility and the situation of the patient. Treatment for MDR-TB needs longer time and requires more expensive and more toxic drugs. Novel drugs are in development and in clinical trials.

(3) Control

Prompt diagnosis tuberculosis and effective treatment of patients with active tuberculosis will reduce the transmission of TB. Eradication of tuberculosis in cattle and disinfection of milk greatly reduce *M. bovis* infection. Novel diagnostics, drugs, treatment regimens and vaccines are to play a key role in the control of tuberculosis. Meanwhile, eliminating poverty and control of HIV infection contribute to the control of TB.

8.5.2　*Mycobacterium Leprae*

M. leprae was described by Hansen in 1873, but it still has not been cultivated in cell-free cultures. *Mycobacterium leprae* cause Leprosy (also called Hansen disease). The global prevalence of leprosy has fallen dramatically.

Leprosy is spread by person-to-person contact, either through the inhalation of infectious aerosols or through skin contact with respiratory secretions and wound exudates. The bacteria multiply very slowly *in vivo* and the symptoms would be developed as long as 20 years after infection. The clinical presentation of leprosy ranges from the tuberculoid form to the lepromatous form. Patients with tuberculoid leprosy have strong cellular immune responses along with bacillary clearance. Patients with lepromatous leprosy have a specific defect in the cellular response to *M. leprae* antigens along with an abundance of bacteria in dermal macrophages and the Schwann cells of the peripheral nerves. Lepromatous leprosy is the most infectious form. Typical acid-fast bacilli are regularly found in scrapings from skin or mucous membranes in patients with lepromatous leprosy.

8.5.3   Nontuberculosis Mycobacteria

Nontuberculous mycobacteria were classified originally by Runyon by their rate of growth and pigmentation (Table 8-9). The pigmented mycobacteria produce intensely yellow carotenoids, which may be stimulated by exposure to light (photochromogenic organisms) or are produced in the absence of light (scotochromogenic organisms).

Most of nontuberculous mycobacteriaare conditional pathogenic bacteria. *Mycobacterium avium* complex (MAC) including *M. avium* and *M. intracellulare*, are the most common pathogenic acid-fast species, particularly in immunocompromised patients. Many other slow-growing mycobacteria can cause human disease: some produce disease identical to pulmonary tuberculosis (*M. kansasii*), some species commonly cause infections localized to lymphatic tissue (*Mycobacterium scrofulaceum*), and others primarily produce cutaneous infections (*Mycobacterium ulcerans*, *M. marinum*, *M. haemophilum*). Disseminated disease can be observed in patients with AIDS. It is noted that most NTM are resistant to common antimycobacterial agents.

Table 8-9   Runyon's Classification of Mycobacteria

	Runyon's Classification	Reservoir	Pigmentation	Rate of growth	Species
	TB complex	Humans		3-8 weeks	*M. tuberculosis*
		Humans, monkeys,			*M. africanum*
		Humans, cattle			*M. bovis*
Slow Growers	Group I	Fish, water	photochromogens	6-12 weeks	*M. marinum*
		Water, cattle			*M. kansasii*
		Monkey, water			*M. simiae*
	Group II	Water	scotochromogens	2-4 weeks	*M. gordonae*
		Soil, water, moist food			*M. scrofulaceum*
		Unknown			*M. szulgai*
		Water, birds			*M. xenopi*
		Soil, water			*M. flavescens*
		Soil, water, birds, fowl, swine, cattle, environment			*M. avium complex* *M. avium* *M. intracellulare*
	Group III	Unknown	nonchromogens	2-4 weeks	*M. haemophilum* *M. gastri*
		Gastric washings			*M. malmoense*
		Unknow			*M. nonchromogenicum*
		Environment			*M. terrae complex*
		Soil, water			

Continue to Table 8–9

Runyon's Classification		Reservoir	Pigmentation	Rate of growth	Species
Rapid Growers	Group IV	Soil, water, animals	nonchromogens	≤7 days	M. fortuitum group
		Soil, water, animals, marine life			M. chelonae group
		Soil, water, animals			M. abscessus
		Soil, water			M. smegmatis
		Soil			M. vaccae

8.6　Zoonotic Bacteria

Bacterial zoonoses comprise a group of diseases in humans or animals acquired by direct contact with or by oral consumption of contaminated animal materials or via arthropod vectors. The major zoonotic bacteria include *Brucella*, *Yersinia*, *Bacillus*, *Coxiella*, *Bartonella*, *Francisella*, *Pasteurella* and some others.

8.6.1　Brucella

Brucella is a Gram-negative, facultative intracellular bacterium and classified as Class 3 pathogens by the Advisory Committee on Dangerous Pathogens (ACDP). Out of 10 classified *Brucella* species, *Brucella melitensis*, *Brucellaabortus*, *Brucellasuis* and *Brucellacanis* are pathogenic to humans, causing zoonotic brucellosis. Among these, *B. melitensis* is the most virulent, followed by *B. suis*.

8.6.1.1　Biological Character

(1) Morphology and Cultural Characteristics

Brucella is small non-motile, non-spore-forming, Gram-negative intracellular coccobacilli or short rod that grows rather slowly on ordinary media. Flagella and true capsules are not produced. The cells arrange singly and, less frequently, in pairs, short chains or small groups.

Although they are aerobic, some strains require supplementary CO_2. Optimal temperature for growth is 37 ℃. Growth occurs between 20 ℃ and 40 ℃ and is improved by serum or blood. Colonies on serum-dextrose agar or other clear media are transparent, raised with an entire edge and a smooth, shiny surface. They appear a pale honey color by transmitted light.

(2) Biochemical Characteristics

Catalase positive. Acid production does not occur from carbohydrates in conventional media, except for *Brucellaneotomae*. The methyl red test is negative. Identification of *Brucella* in species can be done by Urease activity, CO_2 requirement, H_2S production, agglutination with monospecific serum and cultivating the strains in the presence of dyes(Table 8–10).

Table 8-10   Characterization of typical *brucella* species

Species	Natural host	Urease activity	Biovar	CO$_2$ requirement	H$_2$S production	Growth in presence of (Dye concentration: W/V = 1 : 50,000)		Agglutination by monospecific serum	
						Thionine	Basic fuchsin	A (abortus)	M (melitensis)
B. melitensis	Sheep, goats	+[a]	1	−	−	+	+	−	+
			2	−	−	+	+	+	−
			3	−	−	+	+	+	+
B. suis	pig	+	1	−	+	+	[−]	+	−
			2	−	−	+	−	+	−
			3	−	−	+	+	+	−
			4	−	−	+	[−]	+	+
B. abortus	cattle	+	1	[+]	+	−	+	+	−
			2	[+]	+	−	−	+	−
			3	[+]	+	+	+	+	−
			4	[+]	+	−	+	−	+
			5	−	−	+	+	−	+
			6	−	[−]	+	+	+	−
			7	−	[+]	+	+	+	+
			9	−	+	+	+	−	+

[a] Symbols: +, positive for all strains; [+], positive for most strains; [−], negative for most strains; −, negative for all strains.

(3) Antigen

In the case of smooth strains, the LPS carried two different O chains (A and M) linked to the core polysaccharide. They are nominally indicating abortus (A) and melitensis (M) antigens. It should be noted that strains of *B. abortus* and *B. melitensis* can be A-, M- or A and M-antigen positive. There are also some other antigens shown in Table 8-11.

Table 8-11   Antigenic component of *Brucella*

Antigenic component	Antigens
Surface antigens	LPS
	Other polysaccharide antigens
	Outer membrane proteins
	L7/L12 ribosomal protein
Intracellular antigens	A1, A2, A3, A4, B1, B2, C antigens
	Iron regulated proteins
In vivo antigens	Stress-related proteins

8.6.1.2 Pathogenicity

（1）Factors of the Pathogenicity

Brucella lacks some well-known bacterial virulence factors such as capsules, exotoxins, secreted proteases and fimbriae. Its virulence relies on the ability to survive and replicate in the vacuolar phagocytic compartments of macrophages. There are some *Brucella* virulent factors have been identified, such as lipopolysaccharide(LPS), *virB* operon (type Ⅳ secretion system) and the two-component system (BvrR/BvrS). They may not directly mediate clinical manifestations of brucellosis, but critical in the intracellular process of *Brucella* inside macrophages(Table 8–12).

Table 8–12 Virulence factors of *Brucella*

Virulence factor	Function
Surface antigens including LPS	Inhibition of bactericidal activity of serum and phagocytes Suppression of oxidative burst in polymorphonuclear phagocytes
Two component BvrR/BvrS system	polycation resistance, virulence, cell invasion and intracellular replication
virB operon (type Ⅳ secretion system)	Transfer the virulence factors across the bacterial membrane to the extracellular space, the hostcytosol or into other cells
Phosphatidylcholine	Act as a mimicry molecule toavoid recognition by the host
Copper-zinc superoxide dismutase	Intracellular survival
Cyclicβ-1, 2 glucans	Interference with cellular trafficking, allow intracellular *Brucella* to survive and reach its replication niche
Catalase	Protection from oxidative stress
Base excision repair	Removing oxidative lesions from bacterial DNA
Urease	Survival in acidic environment Protection of bacteria during their passage from stomach
Alkyl hyperoxide reductase	Protection against oxygen radical damage
Cytochrome oxidase	Intracellular multiplication
Nitric oxide reductase	Growth under low-oxygen conditions
Brucella virulence factor A	Establishment of the intracellular niche

（2）Disease

Brucellosis is an important infectious zoonotic disease worldwide. It's also known as remitting fever, undulant fever, Mediterranean fever, Maltese fever, Gibraltar fever, Crimean fever, goat fever and Bang disease. In the pregnant animal, *Brucella* Infection often results in placental and fetal infection and this frequently causes abortion. The organisms may gain entry into the human body through conjunctivae, inhaled aerosols, ingestion or abraded skin. In humans, the disease is more severe and displaying a collection of clinical symptoms, including fever, night sweats, anorexia, polyarthritis, meningitis and pneumonia. Incubation period of brucellosis could be 2 to 24 weeks and symptoms may persist for years in the absence of treatment. The most common clinical signs of *Brucella* infection are a chronic, low-grade relapsing fever, followed by articular, muscular and back pain resulting from pathogen-induced inflammation in the joints and vertebrae (peripheral arthritis, sacroiliitis, spondylitis). *Brucella* infection can also cause splenomegaly and hepatomegaly and less frequently can lead to endocarditis and neuropsychiatric manifestations.

8.6.1.3   Laboratory Diagnosis

Blood, uterine secretion, amniotic fluid and liver, spleen or marrow of abortive animals can be collected for pathogenic bacteria isolation and culture. All specimens should be handled while wearing gloves and gowns and worked in the biosafety cabinet.

Cultures should be performed in a biosafety cabinet and incubated in 5% to 10% CO_2. Cultures may need to be incubated for up to 1 month. Presumptive identification of cultures from morphology, metabolic characteristic and slide agglutination with specific antiserum. A Gram-negative coccobacillus with oxidase and urease tests positive should be identified preliminarily as *Brucella*. Identification can be confirmed with specific antiserum.

Coombs antiglobulin reaction (AGT). AGT is the test of very big diagnostic value and especially good for complicated and chronic cases.

Coagglutination test (COAT). COAT is the subsequent reaction used in the diagnostics of brucellosis. It allows the diagnosis of the cases of chronic brucellosis by detecting incomplete antibodies.

Burnet's skin allergy test. Burnet's skin allergy test is especially useful in cases suspected of brucellosis infection, when other serologic reactions are unclear. This reaction is carried out by injecting intradermally, on the inner side of the forearm, of 0. 05–0. 1 ml of diagnostic Brucellin. The result is read after 24 and 48 hours.

8.6.1.4   Prevalence, Treatment and Prevention

Brucellosis is endemic in a large number of developing countries, mainly those in the Mediterranean rim, the Middle East, central Asia, sub-Saharan Africa and Latin America. Infection in humans arises from direct or indirect contact with infected animals/humans or by consumption of contaminated animal products.

Humans are treated with combinations of antibiotics for 4–6 weeks. Doxycycline/tetracycline combined with rifampin form the basis, with cotrimoxazole replacing doxycycline in children.

Eradication of brucellosis from domestic animals reduces dramatically the threat to humans. Vaccines can be used intensively to reduce the level of enzootic disease, particularly in immature animals.

8.6.2   Yersinia

Yersinia is Straight Gram-negative rod or coccobacilli, (0. 5–0. 8) μm×(1–3) μm in size and includes pathogenic and nonpathogenic strains. *Yersinia* species associated with human disease include *Yersiniapseudotuberculosis*, *Yersiniaenterocolitica* and *Yersiniapestis*. both *Y. pseudotuberculosis* and *Y. enterocolitica* can result in severe gastroenteritis, with local abscess formation and death as a result of peritonitis. *Y. pestis* is the causative agent of plague.

8.6.2.1   *Yersinia Pestis*

Y. pestis is the causative agent of plague. Three pandemics of this disease killed more than 200 million people over the past 1,500 years.

(1) Biological character

1) Morphology and Cultural characteristics: *Y. pestis* is a Gram-negative, non-motile, non-spore-forming coccobacillus, (0. 5–0. 8) μm×(1–3) μm long in size and exhibits bipolar staining with Giemsa, Wright's or Wayson staining. Growth occurs on ordinary bacteriological media. Optimum growth temperature is 28–29 ℃. After incubation for 24–30 h at 30 ℃ or 37 ℃, *Y. pestis* forms minute colonies (0. 1 mm) that can be discerned only with difficulty by the naked eye. After 48 h their diameter increases to 1. 0–1. 5 mm. The

colonies are slightly opaque, butyrous, smooth, round and have somewhat irregular edges. In broth, clumps of *Y. pestis* form a deposit at the bottom of the tube while the supernatant remains relatively clear and then, after 48 hours, form a pellicle.

2) Antigen: Fraction I antigen. Fraction 1 (F1) can create a capsule on the microbe surface. The biosynthesis ability of the capsule F1 antigen is associated with plague microbe resistance to engulfment by the intact host cells (neutrophils and macrophages), survival in macrophages and *Y. pestis* antibiotic sensitivity.

Murine toxin (T-antigen, Ymt) is a species-specific antigen of plague microbe. Murine toxin is not considered to be a *Y. pestis* pathogenicity factor, but plays an important role in *Y. pestis* colonization of flea mesenteron.

V/W antigen are encoded by the gene on the plasmid pLcr. V-antigen is a multifunctional protein and participates in a formation of a needle-shaped complex on the bacterial surface. It is able to inhibit neutrophils chemotaxis in vitro and in vivo. W-antigen is a virulence-associated antigen and thought to be a complex of V-antigen.

pH 6 (PsaA) antigen. Antigen pH 6 has an antiphagocytic effect, inhibits antibody production and reaction of mitogen dependent blast transformation and mediates *Y. pestis* resistance in monocytes.

(2) Pathogenicity

1) Factors of the pathogenicity: Virulence of *Y. pestis* is associated with several factors, such as the fraction I (FI) gel-like antiphagocytic capsule or surface antigen, *V/W* antigens and pH 6 antigen.

2) Disease: *Y. pestis* generally resides with in the lymphatic system, blood or tissues of rodents. The microbe is transmitted to humans through direct contact or the bite of an infected flea, causing the bubonic form of the disease or by air, causing a primarily lung-based form.

Usually, there are three primary forms of plague: bubonic, septicemic and pneumonic.

Bubonic plague is the classic form of the disease. During the early stages of the infection, *Y. pestis* replicates within macrophages at peripheral host sites and then spread into the draining lymph nodes. Therein, they replicate and lead to the formation of buboes (hemorrhagic, swollen lymph nodes), which is the characteristic clinical feature of bubonic plague. Subsequently, *Y. pestis* can disseminate into the blood stream leading to a fulminant systemic infection and fatal septicemia.

Septicemic plague: Primary septicemic plague is generally defined as occurring in a patient with positive blood cultures but no palpable lymphadenopathy. The symptoms of febrile, chills, headache, malaise and gastrointestinal disturbances may occur.

Pneumonic Plague: This is a rare but deadly form of the disease with 1 – 3 days incubation period. Pneumonic plague is spread via respiratory droplets through close contact with an infected individual. It progresses rapidly from a febrile flu-like illness to an overwhelming pneumonia with coughing and the production of bloody sputum.

(3) Laboratory Diagnosis

Samples for analysis can include blood, bubo aspirates, sputum, cerebrospinal fluid in patients with plague meningitis and scrapings from skin lesions.

Fresh smear Staining (Gram, Giemsa, Wright or Wayson stain) can provide supportive evidence of a plague infection.

After inoculate on the appropriate plate and incubation, the suspected colonies can be picked for microscopic examination, serological tests and biochemical tests.

Fluorescent-antibody test can be used as presumptive evidence of a *Y. pestis* infection.

PCR (Polymerase Chain Reaction) can be used to detect the microbe nucleotide.

(4) treatment and Prevention

Most human cases can successfully be treated with antibiotics, such as tetracycline and streptomycin, which has been embraced by the World Health Organization Expert Committee on Plague as the'gold standard' treatment.

Plague in humans can be controlled by suppression of rodent reservoir hosts and their fleas and by early detection and treatment of cases of disease.

8.6.2.2   *Yersinia Enterocolitica*

Y. enterocolitica is a heterogeneous group of bacteria. The species have been divided into 2 subspecies (*Y. enterocolitica* subsp. *enterocolitica* and subsp. *palearctica*). Based on their O (lipopolysaccharide or LPS) surface antigen, more than 57 O serogroups have been identified. Among these, strains belong to serogroups O:3, O:5, 27, O:8 and O:9 are the most frequent human pathogen.

Y. enterocolitica is widespread in environment, including terrestrial niche, aquatic niche and animal populations, such as numerous mammals, avian species, cold-blooded species. Most environmental isolates are avirulent. Infection is typically initiated by the ingestion of contaminated food or water.

Generally, the pathogenicity of *Y. enterocolitica* depends on the presence of several virulence factors, such as adhesion/invasion factors, flagella, lipopolysaccharide (LPS) and enterotoxin Yst. These factors facilitate bacteria to enter a susceptible organism, colonize it, evade the immune system and grow under unfavorable conditions. *Y. enterocolitica* can cause a broad range of gastrointestinal diseases, from enteritis to mesenteric lymphadenitis. In children, acute enteritis is the most common presentation. Concurrent mesenteric lymphadenitis and terminal ileitis simulating appendicitis may also be present. In young adults, acute terminal ileitis and mesenteric lymphadenitis appear to be more common.

Antibiotics ampicillin, chloramphenicol and polymyxin can be used for treatment. The best prevention methods for *Y. enterocolitica* infections are adequate water purification and milk pasteurization.

8.6.2.3   *Yersinia Pseudotuberculosis*

Y. pseudotuberculosis is arare *Yersinia* species, which is responsible for mesenteric lymphadenitis, diarrhea and septicemia in humans and animals. *Y. pseudotuberculosis* survives intracellularly. The primary virulence factor is a plasmid-encoded protein that causes increased invasiveness. *Y. pseudotuberculosis* is associated with food-borne infection in humans. Orally contaminated by *Y. pseudotuberculosis* develop either a mesenteric adenitis, which simulates acute appendicitis and evolves in self-cure or, in the compromised host, a severe septicemia.

8.6.3   *Bacillus*

Bacillus species are aerobic/facultative aerobic, sporulating, Gram-positive, rod-shaped bacteria that are ubiquitous in nature.

Their range of isolation sources is very wide, includingsoil, fresh and marine waters, foods and clinical specimens. The majority of *Bacillus* species apparently have little or no pathogenic potential to humans or other animals, except *Bacillusanthracis*, *Bacilluscereus*, *Bacillusthuringiensis*, *Bacilluslicheniformis*. *B. anthracis* is the agent of anthrax and has been considered a potential agent for biological warfare or bioterrorism. *B. cereus* is another important pathogen of humans and other animals, causing food-borne illness and opportunistic infections. *B. thuringiensis* shows pathogenic to invertebrates. *B. licheniformis* has been implicated infood poisoning and other human and animal infections.

8.6.3.1   *Bacillus Anthracis*

B. anthracis is the causative agent of the disease anthrax, a serious and often fatal disease of animals and humans. Classically, anthrax can be contracted through several routes of exposure: by inhalation, cutaneously and gastrointestinally. *B. anthracis* spores are metabolically inactive and resistant to environmental stresses, such as extreme heat, cold and radiation. Outside of the laboratory, the spore is the only infectious form of *B. anthracis*.

(1) Biological Character

1) Morphology and Cultural characteristics: *B. anthracis* is a Gram-positive, endospore-forming, non-motile bacterium. The cells are rod in shape and $(1-1.5)$ μm×$(3-10)$ μm in size. Spores are generally 1 to 2 μm in length and are composed of a core.

Incubated on horse (or sheep) blood agar at 37 ℃, *B. anthracis* is non-haemolytic and forms typical white colonies with bee's eye appearance (oval, slightly granular but not dry, about 2 mm in diameter) and characteristically tacky on teasing with a loop. Colonies of the capsulate *B. anthracis* appear mucoid and the capsule can be visualized by staining smears with polychrome methylene blue (M'Fadyean stain) or India Ink.

2) Antigen: The antigens of *B. anthracis* consist of two major parts: one is the cell structure antigen, including the poly-γ-D-glutamic acid capsule antigen, spore antigen and Polysaccharide antigen; the other is toxins antigen, mainly attributing to the protective antigen (PA) protein, which may combine with lethal factor (LF) or edema factor (EF) to form lethal toxin and edema toxin separately.

(2) Pathogenicity

1) Factors of the pathogenicity: The pathogenicity of *B. anthracis* mainly depends on two virulence factors: the anthrax toxins and a poly-y-D-glutamic acid polypeptide capsule.

The anthrax toxins are encoded by the virulence plasmid pXO1 and consist by three polypeptides, namely protective antigen (PA), lethal factor (LF) and edema factor (EF). PA acts as a cell-surface binding component that binds with LF and EF to form lethal toxin and edema toxin separately. The toxins alter cell signaling pathways in the host to interfere with innate immune responses in early stages of infection and to induce vascular collapse at late stages.

The antiphagocytic polyglutamic capsule is encoded by the virulence plasmid pXO2. It protects bacilli from the immune system and then promotes systemic dissemination.

2) Disease: The cycle of infection is as follows: the spores are ingested by a grazing animal and may gain access to the lymphatics and so to the spleen. Following several days of the organism multiplying and producing toxin in the spleen, the animal suffers a sudden and fatal septicemia and collapses. Hemorrhagic exudates escape from the mouth, nose and anus and contaminate the soil, where the vegetative cells sporulate in the air. The spores remain viable in soil for many years and their persistence does not depend on animal reservoirs, so that *B. anthracis* is exceedingly difficult to eradicate from an endemic area.

The disease begins with the introduction of *B. anthracis* spores into the host organism, usually through minor abrasions of the skin or insect bites (cutaneous anthrax), through minor abrasions of the gastrointestinal tract (gastrointestinal anthrax) or through inhalation (inhalation anthrax).

Cutaneous anthrax: A cutaneous anthrax infection enters the body via an abrasion, cut or other sore on your skin, a small pimple or papule will develop within two to three days. Over the next 24 hours a ring of vesicles develops, followed by ulceration of the central papule. Usually, by the fifth or sixth day a thick black eschar, firmly adherent to the underlying tissue, has developed. Cutaneous anthrax is the most common form of anthrax infection. It is considered to be the least dangerous, since almost all patients survive after proper treatment. However, without treatment, up to 20% of people with cutaneous anthrax may die.

Gastrointestinal anthrax: This form of disease results from the ingestion of under cooked meat from animals with *B. anthracis*. The incubation period is two to five days. The characteristic eschar occurs most often on the wall of the terminal ileum or caecum. It has two clinical forms: abdominal and oro-oesophageal anthrax. In abdominal anthrax initial symptoms are nausea, vomiting and anorexia and fever. In oro-oesophageal anthrax, the clinical manifestations include sore throat, dysphagia, fever, cervical lymphadenopathy and oedema.

Inhalation anthrax: Inhalation anthrax develops when anthrax spores are breathed in. The illness begins insidiously with "flu-like" symptoms of sore throat, mild fever, fatigue and muscle aches, which may last a few hours or days after the initial exposure. This mild initial prodromal phase, which usually lasts about 48 hours, suddenly ends with the development of an acute illness characterized by acute dyspnoea, stridor, fever and cyanosis. Terminally, the pulse becomes extremely rapid and faint, dyspnoea and cyanosis worsen, the patient becomes extremely disorientated and this is quickly followed by coma and death.

(3) Laboratory Diagnosis

When collecting specimens related to suspected anthrax, individual protective equipment (disposable gloves, disposable apron or overalls, masks and boots) should be worn. If aerosols are likely to be generated, the work should be performed in a safety cabinet.

Conventional methods: They are based on morphological features, which are observed after growth and staining of microorganisms. *B. anthracis* is a Gram-positive, non-motile, non β-hemolytic on sheep or horse-blood agar plates, sensitive to penicillin and susceptible to lysis by gamma phage. Clinical specimen (vesicular fluid, fluid from under the eschar, blood, lymph node or spleen aspirates or cerebrospinal fluid) can be collected to make fresh smears. After stained with polychrome methylene blue (M'Fadyean's stain), the characteristic square-ended, blue-black bacilli surrounded by a pink capsule can be seen.

The biochemical identification methods can be used for the further confirmation, such as Intact cell mass spectrometry, affinity-based assays use ligands (antibodies, peptides or aptamers) and nucleic acid-based detection assays.

(4) Prevalence, Treatment and Prevention

The ultimate reservoir of *B. anthracis* is contaminated soil, in which spores remain viable for long periods. Humans become infected almost exclusively through contact with infected animals or animal products.

Treatment is with non-β-lactam antibiotics for Gram-positive bacteria, such as doxycycline, ciprofloxacin, levofloxacin and vancomycin. After anthrax toxins release in the body, one possible treatment is antitoxin together with other treatment options.

Control measures are aimed at breaking the cycle of infection: ①cut off infection source, dispose of anthrax carcasses correctly; ②correctly disinfect, decontaminate and dispose of contaminated materials; ③vaccinate exposed susceptible animals and humans in at-risk occupations.

8.6.3.2 *Bacillus Cereus*

B. cereus is facultatively anaerobic, Gram-positive, usually motile rod bacterium, occurring singly, in pairs or long chains. Cells are (1.0−1.2) μm×(3.0−5.0) μm in size. Spores may lie obliquely in the sporangia. When grown under aerobic conditions on 5% sheep blood agar at 37 ℃, *B. cereus* colonies are β-hemolysis, dull gray and opaque with a rough matted surface.

The natural environmental reservoir for *B. cereus* consists of soil, waters, dust, dairy products and starch products.

B. cereus is one of the major foodborne pathogenic that produces a range of virulence factors and associates mainly with food poisoning. Two distinct food poisoning types are associated with *B. cereus* : emetic and diarrhoeal. The emetic syndrome is an intoxication caused by the *B. cereus* emetic toxin (cereulide), produced in foods before ingestion. The diarrhoeal syndrome is thought to be caused by vegetative cells, ingested as viable cells or spores, producing protein enterotoxins in the small intestine. In addition to food poisoning, *B. cereus* causes a number of systemic and local infections, such as fulminant bacteremia, central nervous system (CNS) involvement (meningitis and brain abscesses), endophthalmitis, pneumonia, severe eye infections and gas gangrene-like cutaneous infections. *B. cereus* is sensitive to erythromycin, chloramphenicol and gentamicin, resistance to penicillin and sulfonamides.

8.6.4　Coxiella

Coxiella has been initially classified into the family *Rickettsiaceae* and now is placed in *Legionellales*. The genus includes *Coxiella burnetii*—the agent of Q fever—and endosymbionts of ticks and aquatic invertebrates.

8.6.4.1　Biological Character

C. burnetii is a small intracellular bacterium, rod in shape, $(0.2-0.4)$ μm×$(0.4-1)$ μm in size and without any flagella or capsule. *C. burnetii* is not stainable with the Gram technique, it can be stained by Gimenez stain. *C. burnetii* grows well in cultured cell lines and in the yolk sac of chicken embryos.

C. burnetii exhibits an antigenic variation, from a smooth-rough form called Phase Ⅰ to a rough form known as Phase Ⅱ. Phase Ⅰ is the wild virulent form, isolating from natural sources. It is characterized by full-length LPS and survives inside monocytes and macrophages. Phase Ⅱ is encountered after serial passages in cell cultures and an irreversible modification is observed in the molecular weight of *C. burnetii* d LPS.

8.6.4.2　Pathogenicity

To survive within its host, *C. burnetii* interferes with the host's antimicrobial response (immunity and phagolysosome biogenesis). For this purpose, *C. burnetii* has an arsenal of virulence factors, including LPS.

C. burnetii can infect a broad range of invertebrate and vertebrate hosts, including humans. Ticks act as vectors for the transmission of *C. burnetii* to an uninfected animal. The pathogen can be found in urine, feces, milk and birth products of these animals and transmitted to humans by these substances as well as by aerosols. In animals, the infection is asymptomatic but induces abortions in livestock.

Symptomatic infection of Q fever has two forms: acute disease and chronic disease. The acute disease has an incubation period about 20 days (14-39 days) and is a febrile illness often with headache and myalgia that can be self-limiting. The chronic disease that lasts for more than 6 months typically presents as endocarditis and can be life threatening.

8.6.4.3　Laboratory Diagnosis

C. burnetii cannot be cultured with the standard routine laboratory culture techniques. Consequently, serology is the most common method for testing for *C. burnetii* infection. Currently, detection of *C. burnetii* DNA by qPCR in various clinical samples (including blood, cardiac valves or other surgical tissue biopsy specimens) is also available.

8.6.4.4　Treatment

The normal therapy for the acute disease is a two-week course of doxycycline, whereas chronic disease requires 18-24 months of doxycycline in combination with hydroxychloroquine. Cotrimoxazole is a currently recommended alternative treatment, but quinolones, rifampin and newer macrolides may also provide some benefit.

8.6.5 Bartonella

Bartonella is small, vector transmitted, Gram-negative, intracellular bacteria that has been isolated from mammals and humans. The majority of human infections are caused by *Bartonella henselae* and *Bartonella quintana*. The former is the agent of cat-scratch disease (CSD), the latter is responsible for trench fever.

8.6.5.1 *Bartonella Henselae*

The reservoirs of *B. henselae* are domestic animals like cats, guinea pigs, rabbits and occasionally dogs. Among these, cats are the main reservoir.

B. henselae is the agent of CSD and more severe human diseases observed in severely immunosuppressed persons such as bacillary angiomatosis and peliosis hepatis. People become infected by being bitten or scratched by an infected animal. *Bartonella* infection in humans produces prolonged bacteremia in blood. The disease begins with an erythematous papule (single or in the group) at the site of inoculation, progressing through erythematous, vesicular, papular and crusted stages. In typical CSD, regional lymphadenopathy occurs 1 to 3 weeks after inoculation and lasts for up to several months. Most cases of CSD are self-limited and do not require antibiotic treatment.

8.6.5.2 *Bartonella Quintana*

B. quintana is the agent of trench fever, which is characterized by the synchronous release of bacteria at intervals of approximately 5 days. This five-day cycle is triggered by reinfection of the primary niche by bacteria that are released at the end of each cycle. The clinical manifestations of *B. quintana* bacteremia range from asymptomatic infection to severe life-threatening disease. A sudden onset of fever associated with headache, shin pain and dizziness that lasts 1–3 days is observed after an incubation period of 2–3 weeks. Although fatal cases have not been reported, the disease may persist for 4–6 weeks and result in pro-longed disability. Relapses may occur years later and, in some cases, bacteremia may exist with no clinical signs. Macrolide and doxycycline can be used for the treatment.

8.6.6 Francisella

Francisella is Short, non-motile, Gram-negative bacteria and is the only recognized genus in " *Francisellaceae* ". *Francisella tularensis* is a facultative intracellular bacterium and causes the zoonotic, vector-borne disease tularemia in humans and animals, predominantly rodents and lagomorphs. *Francisella philo miragia* is associated with septicemic and pneumonic disease in humans with immunocompromised conditions.

Strains of *Francisella* are short, rod or coccoid in shape, (0.2–0.7) μm×0.2 μm or 0.7 μm×1.7 μm in size, occurring singly. *Francisella* species are strictly aerobic. Colonies are distinct, convex, pale white and reach maximum size in 3–4 days. *F. tularensis* is oxidase negative and *F. philomiragia* oxidase positive.

F. tularensis is widely distributed in nature. Humans can acquire infection with *F. tularensis* through several routes, including arthropod bites, direct contact with infected animals/animal carcasses, ingestion of contaminated materials (contaminated water or food) or inhalation.

Many of the virulence determinants of *F. tularensis* are expressed as components of the *Francisella* pathogenicity island. Tularemia is often epidemic, both in humans and in animals. The clinical manifestations are varied and depend on the type of reservoir involved and the way of infection. Fever and acute symptoms are hallmarks of tularemia in healthy individuals. The forms of tularemia include glandular and ulceroglandular tularemia (arthropod bites), ulceroglandular tularemia (skinning infected), oculoglandular tularemia (direct inoculation of the eye) oropharyngeal tularemia (ingestion of contaminated materials) and pneumonic tularemia (inhalation).

Serology ELISA (enzyme-linked immunosorbent assay) is the standard serological test used to diagnose tularemia. Standard antimicrobial therapy is effective for the treatment of tularemia, with aminoglycosides, tetracyclines and chloramphenicol approved for treatment of *F. tularensis*.

8.6.7 *Pasteurella*

Pasteurella is Gram-negative, Coccobacilli or rods-shape bacteria that highly prevalent among animal populations. Many Pasteurella species are opportunistic pathogens that can cause endemic disease. Among these, *P. multocida* is the most prevalent isolate observed in human infections. In tissues, *P. multocida* usually forms coccoid cells or short rods on solid media containing blood and often shows bipolar staining with Giemsa or Wright' s stain.

Humans acquire *Pasteurella* infection primarily through contact with animals, most usually through animal bites, scratches, licks on skin abrasions or contact with mucous secretions derived from pets. Common symptoms of pasteurellosis in humans from animal bite wounds are swelling (edema), cellulitis (diffuse, localized inflammation with redness and pain) and bloody or suppurative/purulent exudate (drainage) at the wound site.

The primary diagnosis of *P. multocida* can be done by clone morphology and cell morphology with Giemsa stain. Further confirmation can be done by biochemical and serological identification. Broad-spectrum antibiotics that target *Pasteurella* are the preferred prophylaxis for animal bites. The recommended treatment regimen for pasteurellosis includes amoxicillin with combinate of the β-lactamase inhibitor clavulanic acid (Augmentin), doxycycline plus metronidazole for patients with penicillin allergies or clindamycin plus a fluoroquinolone (ciprofloxacin or trimethoprim-sulfamethoxazole combination for children or ceftriaxone for pregnant women).

8.7 Actinomyces, Nocardia and Corynebacterium

8.7.1 Actinomyces

8.7.1.1 Physiology and Structure

Actinomyces, with hypha diameter between 0. 5–0. 8 μm, is filamentous bacterium which is gram-positive, non-acidfast, non-spore forming and with no capsules or flagellum. It reproduces through fission and usually forms branching non-septa hyphae. Actinomycete is anaerobic or micro aerobic, which is difficult to culture. When it comes to primary isolation, adding 5% CO_2 can promote their growth. The optimum culture temperature is 37 ℃ and the growth is slow. After being cultured on glucose broth medium for 3–6 days, small spheroidal off-white particles precipitated at the bottom can be seen. After 4–6 days of culture on blood agar plate, tiny round colonies are formed, with rough surface. They show off-white or light yellow in color and do not cause hemolysis. Cobweb-shaped hyphae of various lengths can be seen under microscope.

Actinomyces are opportunistic pathogens, often cause chronic suppurative inflammation. Small yellow particles are macroscopic at the site of infection and in the pus from fistula. These particles are called sulfur granules, inside of which have bacterial colonies formed by actinomycetes. If imprint these particles or make pathological tissue slice, under microscope, radially arranged long hyphae can be seen. Hypha expands to a rod-shaped end, looking like chrysanthemum.

8.7.1.2 Pathogenesis and Immunity

Actinomycetes mainly live in tracts of body that connect the outside world, like mouth, upper respiratory tract, et al. Actinomycetes are normal body flora, but they cause endogenous infection if a person's immune system weakens oral hygiene is poor or mouth mucosa is damaged. The symptom is suppurative inflammation of tissues. Chronic Granulomatous Disease (CGD) is most often to follow if there is no secondary infection, accompanied by multiple fistulas. Sulfur granules can be found in leaking pus. Such disease is called actinomycosis. Based on the route of infection and organs being infected, clinically it is divided into orocervicofacial, thoracic, abdominal, pelvic and central nerves system actinomycosis. Orocervicofacial actinomycosis is most commonly seen, constituting 60% of all cases.

A variety of specific antibodies can be detected in the serum from patient with actinomycosis, but these antibodies provide no immune protection. Cellular immunity is mainly how the body reacts to actinomycetes.

8.7.1.3 Laboratory Diagnosis

Like various other anaerobes, Actinomyces species are fastidious and thus not easy to culture and isolate. Clinical laboratories do culture and isolate them, but a negative result does not rule out infection, because it may be due simply to reluctance to grow in vitro. Microbiological examination of actinomycosis is to take pus, sputum and tissue slice as samples and extract sulfur granules from them. After imprint, we use microscope to see if there is radial hyphae like chrysanthemum. As for isolation and culture, anaerobic culture shall be performed at temperature of 37 ℃. In 1-2 weeks' time, white rough colonies with irregular edges are formed. The surface is dry, creased or granular. After observing the colonies, take some for smear. With Gram stain or also acid fast stain, actinomyces and nocardia can be differentiated under microscope.

8.7.1.4 Treatment, Prevention and Control

The main measure to prevent actinomycosis is to practice good oral hygiene and to treat oral disease in time. Patients should undergo timely surgical debridement of their abscess and fistula and should take antibiotics in the meantime. Penicillin is the priority drug and erythromycin and lincomycin can also be used.

8.7.2 Nocardia

Nocardia widely exists in soil and does not belong to normal body flora. *Nocardia asteroids* (*N. asteroids*) and *Nocardia brasiliensis* (*N. brasiliensis*) are responsible for most human infections, resulting in nocardiosis. Nocardia often invades lung and causes suppurative inflammation and necrosis and may even spread throughout the body by blood when condition worsens.

8.7.2.1 Physiology and Structure

Nocardia is gram-positive and looks like actinomyces in form with a difference that the hypha end is not expanded. Partially are weakly acid-fast. 1% hydrochloric acid alcohol with extended bleaching time can make it acid negative. In this way, can we differentiate it from *Mycobacterium tuberculosis* (*M. tuberculosis*).

Nocardia is obligate aerobic with low nutrient demand. It grows well and develops aerial hyphae on both ordinary and sabouraud medium. It is able to grow at temperature of 22 ℃ and 37 ℃. Generally, it takes one week's time to form the colony, whose surface is dry or waxy. The color of the surface is white orange or red. When it is cultured in fluid medium, membrane is formed on the surface of the liquid without obvious turbidity.

8.7.2.2 Pathogenesis and Immunity

N. asteroids invades human body through respiratory tract or wound, causing pyogenic infection. Especially for immunocompromised persons, such as patients with AIDS, lung tumor or long-term users of immunosuppressor, *N. asteroids* can cause pneumonia and pulmonary abscess after striking the lungs. The symptom is similar to pulmonary tuberculosis and pneumomycosis. If it infects human body through skin wounds, it invades underneath skin and causes chronic pyogenic granuloma. Fistula is formed and oozes pus containing small particles, inside of which lie nocardia colonies. *N. asteroids* spreads easily through blood, causing meningitis and brain abscess.

N. brasiliensis can invade subcutaneous tissue and cause chronic pyogenic granuloma. The symptom is swell, abscess and multiple fistulas formed. Involvement of feet is common. Therefore it is called mycetoma.

8.7.2.3　Laboratory Diagnosis

Microbiological examination of nocardia is to take pus or sputum as samples and find yellow or black granular nocardia colonies in these samples. We smear or imprint the sample and carry out a microscopic examination after gram stain and acid fast stain. Gram-positive and partially acid-fast branching hyphae can be seen. As for isolation and culture, aerobic culture shall be performed at temperature of 37 ℃ or 45 ℃. Colonies can be seen in one week. The colonies are small and produce different pigments. Nocardia may result in L-variation if invades lung tissues. So operators shall take care when conducting microscopic examination.

8.7.2.4　Treatment, Prevention and Control

Currently, there is no specific method to prevent nocardiosis. Surgery can be an option for abscess and fistula. Antibiotics and sulfonamides can be used for different kinds of infection and treatment course shall be no less than 6 weeks.

8.7.3　Corynebacterium

Corynebacterium is a genus of gram-positive bacilli and has many species. Most of them are opportunistic pathogens. Human pathogens mainly include *Corynebacterium diphtheria* (*C. diphtheriae*), which produces strong exotoxin resulting in diphtheria.

8.7.3.1　Physiology and Structure

The bacteria are long, thin and slightly curved. They are club-shaped at one end or two-ends, which inspires the genus name—corynebacterium. The bacteria are not regularly arranged and usually look like letter "L", "V", "Y" or fences in shape. They are gram-positive. After a short time of methylene blue staining, the bacteria are not dyed evenly and hyperchromatic granules occur. By Neisser or Albert method, granules are stained blue black. These granules are called metachromatic granules, whose color is different from that of the bacteria. They are mainly made up of RNA and polyphosphates and can help with identification. When bacteria are aging, metachromatic granules are consumed and become less obvious. Besides, cell wall becomes thinner and decolorization happens easily. Thus, gram staining is not stable anymore.

Corynebacterium is aerobic or facultative anaerobic. Though it can grow on ordinary medium, its morphology is atypical. It grows fast on Loeffler medium and forms round grayish colonies with typical morphology and obvious metachromatic granules. For isolation and culture, $K_2TeO_2 \cdot 3H_2O$ blood agar plate is often used as medium for identifying it from others. Because *C. diphtheriae* can absorb $K_2TeO_2 \cdot 3H_2O$ and reduce it to Te, which is black metal. $K_2TeO_2 \cdot 3H_2O$ also can inhibit the growth of other bacteria, without affecting *C. diphtheriae* itself. *C. diphtheriae* forms three different types on $K_2TeO_2 \cdot 3H_2O$ blood agar plate, which are gravis, mitis and intermedius respectively. All of the three types of strains can cause diseases, but there is no obvious correlation between the type and the severity of diseases.

8.7.3.2　Pathogenesis and Immunity

The major pathogen of *C. diphtheriae* is the exotoxin it produces, namely diphtherin. Diphtherin is encoded by *tox* —the toxin genes of corynebacteriophage β. Therefore, only lysogen carrying corynebacteriophage β can produce diphtherin. When this phage invades *C. diphtheriae*, *tox* can be integrated into the chromosome of host bacteria during lysogenic phase. Host bacteria hence develop the ability to produce toxin, becoming toxigenic *C. diphtheriae*. The molecule of diphtherin is composed of fragment A and fragment B. Fragment A is stable, heat-resistant, protease-resistant and halts the synthesis of susceptible cell protein. Besides, it is also the functional area of the main toxicity. Fragment B is unstable and sensitive to acid. It has two functional areas. One is at the C-terminus, which is the receptor binding domain. The other situates at the N-terminus, which is a translocation zone embedded in cell membrane and promotes fragment A access cytoplasm. Diphtherin binds the host cell receptor through fragment B. Mediated by the translocation zone of fragment B, it releases fragment A into the host cytoplasm. After fragment A enters into the host, it promotes adenosine diphosphate ribose (ADPR) of NAD to bind elongation factor EF-2, which is necessary for peptides synthesis and results in inactivating EF-2, blocking protein synthesis and causing cell functional disorder. Diphtherin is highly toxic and is lethal toxic towards both human beings and animals.

C. diphtheriae causes diphtheria, which is transmitted through respiratory tract. The major source of infection is patient and bacteria-carrier. People are generally easy to contract diphtheria, especially children. When an individual contracts diphtheria, bacteria grow in nasal and pharyngeal mucosa and produce diphtherin. Diphtherin can spread throughout body and cause local inflammation and systemic poisoning. Bacteria and toxin can cause inflammatory exudation and necrosis in local mucosal epithelial cells. Fibrous protein from vascular exudate combines inflammatory cells, necrotic mucosal cells and bacteria together. Thus a gray-white layer is formed, which is called pseudomembrane. Pseudomembrane tightly adheres to tissues and is difficult to remove. If it expands to tracheal and bronchial mucous membrane, where cilia project, pseudomembrane will easily detach and cause airway obstruction, resulting in dyspnea and asphyxia. *C. diphtheriae* itself does not go into blood, but the exotoxin it produces is absorbed by blood and binds susceptible cells. Clinical manifestation is myocarditis, uranoplegia, hoarseness and adrenal insufficiency.

Diphtheria immunization mainly relies on the humoral immunity provided by antitoxin neutralizing exotoxin. Vaccines before and after disease can both help body obtain immunity.

8.7.3.3 Laboratory Diagnosis

Microbiological examination mainly includes two parts: bacteriological examination and toxigenicity test. Pseudomembrane and its peripheral tissue shall be taken from diseased region for smear. After methylene blue or Albert's staining, microscopy should be performed to observe the typical morphology, arrangement and metachromatic granules of *C. diphtheria*. Then combining clinical practice, primary diagnosis can be given. For isolation and culture, the sample shall be inoculated on Loeffler medium at 37 ℃ and smear microscopy be conducted after 6-12 h. Detection rate is higher than that of direct smear, which is good for rapid diagnosis. If the culture is prolonged to 12-18 h, greyish white colonies can be seen and biochemical reaction and toxigenicity test can be performed. Toxigenicity test is an important one for identifying toxigenic corynebacterium diphtheria. There are two ways to perform this test: in-vivo and in-vitro methods. In vitro-method is simple and sensitive. It usually includes Elek test and SPA coagglutination test. In-vivo method detects toxicity through animal testing. The specific prevention of diphtheria divides into artificial active immunity and artificial passive immunity.

8.7.3.4 Treatment, Prevention and Control

The most important aspect of the treatment for diphtheria is the early administration of diphtheria antitoxin to specifically neutralize the exotoxin before it is bound by the host cell. The main preventive measure is to inject diphtheria toxoid. A mixed vaccine composed of diphtheria toxoid, pertussis vaccine and tetanus toxoid is used for artificial active immunity both home and abroad and the result is good. Sensitive antibiotics such as penicillin and erythromycin should be used for diphtheria patients.

8.8　Mycoplasma

Mycoplasma refers to the filamentous nature of the organisms of some species and to the plasticity of the outer membrane resulting in pleomorphism. They are a class of fascinating wall-less and the smallest prokaryotic organisms capable of growth on bacteriologic media. *Mycoplasma mycoides* ssp. *mycoides* is the first mycoplasma to be isolated and recognized in 1898. As other pathogenic isolates accumulated from veterinary and human, they became known as pleuropneumonia-likeorganisms (PPLO), a term nowadays superseded by 'mycoplasma'. Mycoplasmas are widely found in nature as saprophytes and parasites of human, animals, plants, arthropods, soil and sewage. Ureaplasmas originally designated 'T' (for tiny) strain mycoplasma because of their small colony size, are also widely distributed among animals.

Mycoplasmas and ureaplasmas belong to the class *Mollicutes* (soft skin) in reference to their marked pleomorphism and filament formation. They also accounts for their resistance to wall-acting antibiotics (penicillin or other β-lactam antibiotics) for the absence of a cell wall containing peptidoglycan. *Mollicutes* contains 7 families, 11 genera and over 200 species. The family *Mycoplasmataceae* is subdivided intotwo genera:

1) The genus *Mycoplasma* contains more than 130 named species, 14 of which are of human origin.

2) The genus *Ureaplasma* contains seven named urea-hydrolysing species, two of which are of human origin, but clinically the most relevant as a cause of urogenital tract infection.

Sixteen species of mycoplasmas as well as ureaplasmas have been isolated in humans. They colonize mucosal surfaces of the respiratory and urogenital tracts. Most form part of the normal flora but *M. pneumoniae* is a primary pathogen and *M. hominis*, *M. genitalium*, *M. fermentans* and *U. urealyticum* have been associated with human infection. Most species reside extracellularly, but some like *M. genitalium* and *M. penetrans* may localize and survive within the cells.

8.8.1　Biological Properties

8.8.1.1　Morphology

The size of the mycoplasma is generally around 0.3−0.5 μm and normally smaller than 1.0 μm. Their morphology varies with the species, stage of the growth cycle and the environmental conditions. Light microscopy reveals pleomorphic formation, which may range from spherical through coccoid, coccobacillary, ring and dumb-bell forms, to branching filaments(Figure 8−7).

Unlik eother bacteria, mycoplasmas are bounded only by a plasma membrane without a rigid cell wall containing peptidoglycan. Therefore, mycoplasma and L type bacteria are similar: ①they both lack a cell wall and the cell is pleomorphic; ②they can both pass through an antimicrobial filter. The main differences between the two are: ①Mycoplasma are independent microbes and L-type bacteria are variants of normal bacterial cells that have a cell wall (most L-typecells will revert to their original form when the inductionfactor is eliminated); ②Mycoplasma growth requires cholesterol (10% −20% serum in the medium)while the growth of L-type bacteria does not; ③L-type bacteria fade easily after Diane staining, while Mycoplasma do not fade easily.

The mycoplasmal membrane is 7.5−10 nm wide, in which two electron-dense layers are separated by an electron-lucent layer (Figure 8-8). The electron-lucent part of the membrane contains lipids with the long chains of the phospholipids and the electron-dense layers consist of proteins and carbohydrates. Cholesterol or carotenoid/carotenol, is interspersed between the phospholipid molecules and plays an important part in maintaining membrane integrity confronting external osmotic pressures.

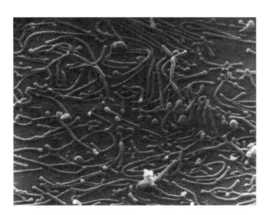

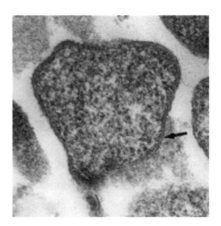

Figure 8 – 7   Electron micrograph of *M. pneumoniae*, to show pleomorphic formation

Figure 8–8   Electron micrograph of *M. pulmonis*; thinsection illustrating trilaminar membrane (arrow)

Several mycoplasmas, including *M. pneumoniae*, *M. genitalium* and *M. penetrans* have special structures at one or both ends (sometimes described as a 'nap') by which they can attach to mucosal surfaces of respiratory or genital tract (Figure 8–9). Sections of the terminal structures of the two former mycoplasmas may exhibit a dense flask-shaped appearance when viewed by electron microscopy.

8.8.1.2   Reproduction

The small and fragile cell structures of mycoplasmas hamper the analyses of division schemes. Several modes of reproduction have been proposed, including binary fission, fragmentation of an elongated cell and budding. Cytoplasmic division may not always be synchronous with genome replication, resulting in the formation of multinucleate filaments and other shapes. Subsequent division of the cytoplasm by constriction of the membrane at sites between the genomes leads to chains of beads that later fragment to give single cells. Budding occurs when the cytoplasm is not divided equally between the progeny cells.

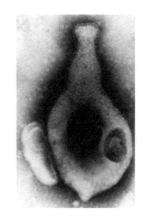

8.8.1.3   Cultivation

Mycoplasmas have limited biosynthetic abilities, so that they need a rich growth medium containing 10% –20% animal serum. The serum provides mycoplasma with the cholesterol and long-chain fatty acids required for membrane synthesis, components that the organisms cannot synthesize.

Figure 8 – 9   Electron micrograph of *M. genitalium*, to show terminal flask-shaped structure covered by extracellular 'nap'

A medium that has been widely used for isolation contains bovine heart infusion (PPLO broth or agar) with fresh yeast extract and horse serum. Besides, amodified medium designated SP-4 has been helpful in the isolation of fastidious mycoplasmas, such as *M. pneumoniae*, *M. fermentans* and *M. genitalium*, which is notoriously difficult to isolate. Although various specific formulations have been described for the isolation of ureaplasmas, most mycoplasmal media containing urea may be suitable.

The optimal pH for most mycoplasma culture is pH 7.8-8.0 for the mycoplasmal cells may die when the pH drops below pH 7.0 except *U. urealyticum* (optimal pH 5.5-6.5). Mycoplasmas are aerobic or facultative anaerobic microorganisms, but they usually grow better in an aerobic environment. The best culture environment for initial isolation is atmospheric conditions supplemented with 5% CO_2 or anaerobic conditions with 5% CO_2 and 95% N_2. The optimal temperature for growth of most mycoplasmas and ureaplasmas is 36-38 ℃. These organisms will produce color change inbroth and colonies will develop on agar within 1-3 days if sui Table growth mediaand incubation conditions are provided.

8.8.1.4　Colonial Morphology

Typical colonies of the mycoplasmas often have a 'fried egg' appearance, with an opaque central zone extending into the medium and a translucentor semitransparent peripheral zone of thin and flat on the surface (Figure 8-10). However, *M. pneumoniae* has a mulberry appearance without the peripheral zone on primary isolation. Most colonies of mycoplasmas require low-power microscopic magnification. However, the size and appearance of all mycoplasmal colonies depend on the constituents and degree of hydration of the medium, the agar concentration, atmospheric condition and age of the culture.

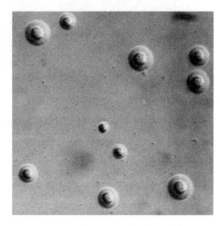

Figure 8-10　Colonies of *M. hominis* (of human origin) (up to 110 μm indiameter) with typical 'fried egg' appearance

8.8.1.5　Biochemical Reactions

Most mycoplasmas use glucose (or other carbohydrates) or arginine as a major source of energy (Table 8-13). The unique and distinctive biochemical feature of ureaplasmas is the conversion of urea to ammonia by urease.

Mycoplasma and *Ureaplasma* depend on sterol. Therefore, they fail to grow in serum-free media and are inhibited by digitonin, distinguishing them from the species that do not require sterol. In addition, most *Mycoplasma* and *Ureaplasma* species produce hydrogen peroxide, which causes some lysisof guinea-pig or other erythrocytes when these are suspended in agar over developing colonies. *M. pneumoniae* produces clear zones of β-haemolysis. About one-third of all *Mycoplasma* species display the phenomenon of haemadsorption.

8.8.1.6　Antigenic Structures

The different antigenic compositions on cell membranes of mycoplasmas and ureaplasmas consist of glycolipids and lipoproteins. Identification is often accomplished by the use of specific antisera containing antibodies that reflect their antigeni cglycolipids by ELISA and antigenic lipoproteins by complement-fixation test. Besides, the metabolic inhibition test(MIT) and growth inhibition test (GIT) are widely used for identification. The tests are based up on by specificantisera and the results demonstrated by inhibition of growth, acidproduction, arginine hydrolysis and urea metabolism.

Table 8–13   Mycoplasmas/ureaplasmas of human origin：properties of biochemical reactions

Species	Glucose	Arginine	Urea	pH	Haemadsorption
M. pneumoniae	+	–	–	7.5	+
M. hominis	–	+	–	7.3	–
M. genitalium	+	–	–	7.5	+
M. spermatophilum	–	+	–	7.5	–
M. fermentans	+	+	–	7.5	–
M. penetrans	+	+	–	7.5	+
U. urealyticum	–	–	+	6.0	+[a]

a：serovar 3 only.

For *M. pneumoniae*, the glucose-and galactose-containing membrane glycolipids of the organisms are haptens, which are antigenic only when bound to membrane protein. Glycolipids of the mycoplasma have a structure for tuitously similar to that in the human brain. The cross-reactivity of the brain glycolipids with antibodies to *M. pneumoniae* could feasibly account for the neurological manifestations of *M. pneumoniae* infection. Furthermore, the ability of the organisms to alter the I antigen on erythrocytes sufficiently to stimulate anti-I antibodies (cold agglutinins) leads to an autoimmune response and damage to erythrocytes. *M. pneumoniae* has two major surface proteins, including the P1 protein involved in attachment. Antibody to them is detected in convalescent sera and respiratory secretions.

Variable membrane lipoproteins of several mycoplasmas form an antigenic variation system that provides a means of escaping from the host immune response. And the variations are restricted to a small number of protein antigens and do not appear to alter the total cell protein profiles of the organisms.

8.8.1.7   Genome

There are currently 8 complete genome sequences and several that are in progress. *M. genitalium* is thought to have the smallest genome of any self-replicating organism, measuring only 580 kb long with just 470 open reading frames, an indication of the small amount of genetic information needed for a free-living existence and the reason why mycoplasmas have a paucity of biochemical activity and are nutritionally fastidious. The genomes of other identified species are 777–1,358 kb long.

8.8.1.8   Stability and Viability

Mycoplasmas are susceptible to disinfectants, such as phenolic disinfectants, 1% sodium hypochlorite, 70% ethanol, formaldehyde, glutaraldehyde, iodophore and peracedic acid are effective against Mycoplasmas. Mycoplasmas could be inactivated by UV, microwave, γ radiation, moist heat (121 ℃ for at least 20 min) and dry heat (165–170 ℃ for 2 h).

The presence of cholesterol renders the mycoplasmas susceptible to the agents such as saponin, digitonin and some polyene antibiotics (e. g. amphotericin B). As expected, mycoplasmas are completely resistant to β-lactam and other antibiotics that in fluence bacterial cell wall synthesis and also to lysozyme. Mycoplasmas are prokaryotes and the cytoplasm does not contain endoplasmic reticulum, but is packed with ribosomes. Ribosomal protein synthesis is inhibited by antibiotics such as tetracyclines, aminoglycosides and macrolides (Table 8–14).

Table 8-14 Susceptibility of some mycoplasmas and ureaplasmas to various antibiotics

Antibiotic	M. pneumoniae	M. hominis	M. genitalium	Ureaplasma spp
Tetracycline	+	+	+++	++
Doxycycline	++	+	+++	++
Erythromycin	+++	−	+++	++
Clarithromycin	+++	−	+++	+++
Azithromycin	+++	−	+++	−
Clindamycin	+++	+++	+	+
Cipro floxacin	±	+	−	+
Spar floxacin	+++	+++	++	+++
Moxi floxacin	++	++	+++	+

+++, extremely sensitive; ++, very sensitive; +, moderately sensitive; ±, weakly sensitive; −, insensitive.

8.8.2 Pathogenesis and Im munity

The mechanisms whereby *Mycoplasma* and *Ureaplasma* species cause disease are multifactorial and include the following:

1) Adherence of mycoplasma organisms to host cells, the adhesins of *M. pneumoniae* and *M. genitalium* being proteins P1 and MgPa, respectively.

2) The ability of some mycoplasmas to invade hostcells.

3) The production of toxins by *M. pneumoniae* and some other mycoplasmas.

4) The stimulation of pro-in flammatory cytokines.

5) Antigenic variation which enables the mycoplasma to evade the protective immune systems of the host.

6) Immunological responses of the host, for example, autoimmune ones causing disease and an exaggerated response to a repeat infection leading to worse disease.

7) The ability of mycoplasmas to develop antibioticr esistance culminating sometimes in chronic disease.

Mycoplasmas are primarily mucosally associated organisms residing in the respiratory or urogenital tracts of their hosts in close association with epithelial cells. In some species invasion of host cells occurs and the organisms reside intracellularly. Elements of the host innate immune system are activatedby mycoplasmas and the attendant inflammation accounts for many of the initial signs and symptoms accompanying the early stages of the evolving infection.

An intact humoral immune system is very important to prevent infection and dissemination by mycoplasmas. But immunity is often short-lived and humans are susceptible to repeated infections despite the development of complement-fixing and growth-inhibiting antibody responses. Cytokine production and lymphocyte activation can reduce infection and reduce inflammation or exacerbate disease through the development of immunologic hypersensitivity, resulting in damage to the epithelium and deeper tissues. Lymphoid infiltrations undoubtedly contribute to the development of inflammatory responses.

8.8.3 Major Human Mycoplasmas

The *Mycoplasma* and *Ureaplasma* species that have been isolated either from the respiratory tract (mostly the oropharynx) or from the urogenital tract, are shown Table 8–15. *M. pneumoniae*, *M. genitalium*, *M. hominis*, *M. fermentans* and *U. urealyticum* unequivocally cause disease or are strongly associated with disease.

Table 8–15   Mycoplasmas/ureaplasmas of human origin: anatomical site of detection and pathogenic roles

Species	Frequency of detection		Pathogenic role
	Respiratory tract	Urogenital tract	
M. pneumoniae	Rare[a]	Very rare	Primary atypical pneumonia, tracheobronchitis and upper respiratory tract disease. Extrapulmonary symptoms such as autoimmune responses, central nervous system complications and dermatological disorders
M. hominis [b,c]	Rare	Common	Pelvicin flammatory disease, calculi
M. genitalium[b]	Very rare	Rare[a]	Cervicitis, pelvic inflammatory diseases, endometritis, salpingitis, tubal factor infertility
M. fermentans [b]	Common	Quite common	Fibromyalgia and chronic fatigue syndrome
U. urealyticum	Rare	Common	Non-gonococcal urethritis (NGU)

[a] Rare, except in disease.

[b] Reported in rectum of homosexual men.

[c] Reported in the anal canal of women attending a genitourinary medicine clinic.

8.8.3.1   *Mycoplasma Pneumoniae*

In 1898, Nocard and Roux were the first to isolate a *Mycoplasma* species in culture from bovine. However, it was not until 1944 when *M. pneumoniae*, known then as Eaton agent, was isolated and described from a patient with primary atypical pneumonia. Initially *M. pneumoniae* was considered as a virus rather than a bacterium. Studies that followed until 1963 determined that Eaton agent was a bacterium that caused human lower respiratory tract infections.

8.8.3.2   Morphology

M. pneumoniae cells have an elongated shape that is approximately 0.1–0.2 μm in width and 1–2 μm in length. The signet-ring-shaped cell of *M. pneumoniae* is gram-negativefor having no cell wall. The extremely small cell size means they are incapable of being examined by light microscopy. Protein and lipids form the outer cell membrane and the cells are obviously pleomorphic, with spherical, rod-like, bar-like and filamentous morphologies visible under the microscope. The typical cell is shaped like a signet ring. *M. pneumoniae* cell islight purple with Giemsa stain. Colonies of *M. pneumoniae* are usually less than 100 μm in diameter and can only be observed under a light microscope at low magnificationor a dissecting microscope. Characteristic colonies are shown in Figure 8–11A and B.

M. pneumoniae could possess cholesterol in their cell membrane (obtained from the host) and possess more genes that encode for membrane lipoprotein variations than other mycoplasmas, which are thought to be associated with its parasitic lifestyle. *M. pneumoniae* cells also possess an attachment organelle "nap", which is used in the gliding motility of the organism by an unknown mechanism.

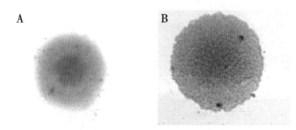

Figure 8-11 (A) *M. pneumoniae* omelet-like colonies.
(B) Mulberry-shaped colonies of *M. pneumonia*

8.8.3.3 Epidemiology

M. pneumoniae infection occurs worldwide. Although endemic in most areas, there isa preponderance of infection in late summer and early autumn in temperate climates. Spread is fostered by close contact, for example in a family. Transmission is believed to be by respiratory aerosols or droplets. 15% of family members of *M. pneumoniae*-positive indexpatients had organisms isolated from their nose or throat within 4 weeks of the index case. The frequency of transmission within families was the same regardless of the appropriateness of the antibiotic used for treatment of the indexpatient.

Overall, *M. pneumoniae* may cause only about one-sixth of all cases of pneumonia, but in certain confined populations, such as military recruits, it has been responsible for almost half of the cases of pneumonia. Children are infected more often than adults and the consequence of infection is alsoin fluenced by age. Thus, in school-aged children andteenagers, about a quarter of infections culminate inpneumonia, whereas in young adults fewer than 10% do so. Thereafter, pneumonia is even less frequent, although the severity tends to increase with the age ofthe patient. Besides, it is important to realize that *M. pneumoniae* infectioncan present as a very wide variety of clinical manifestations.

8.8.3.4 Pathogenesis

M. pneumoniae is a mucosal parasite primarily involving the upper and lower respiratory tract, but it has been isolatedand/or demonstrated by PCR in other sites including the urogenital tract, cerebrospinal fluid, synovial fluid, pericardial fluid and cutaneous lesions.

Attachment of *M. pneumoniae* to the respiratory epithelium by its specialized attachment organelle is a prerequisite for later events that culminate in production of disease. The P1 adhesin is a 170-kDa protein concentrated in the attachment tip that is now known to be the major structure responsible for interaction of *M. pneumoniae* with host cells. Close approximation of the organism to the host cells facilitated by the adhesin proteins appears to be important to facilitate localized tissue disruption and cytotoxicity. Hydrogen peroxide and superoxide radicals synthesized by mycoplasmas act in concert with endogenous toxic oxygen molecules generated by host cells to induce oxidative stressin the respiratory epithelium. Hydrogen peroxide has been known to be important as a virulence factor in *M. pneumoniae* since Somerson showed it to be the molecule that confers hemolytic activity.

Fusion of the mycoplasmal cell membrane with that of the host could result in release of various hydrolytic enzymes produced by the mycoplasma as well as insertion of mycoplasmal membrane components into the host cell membrane, a process that could potentially alter receptor recognition sites, affect cytokine induction and expression and provide a mechanism forpost-infectious autoimmune reactions.

8.8.3.5 Clinical Manifestations

Host response to *M. pneumoniae* ranges from asymptomatic infection to pharyngitis, bronchitis, bronchiolitis, croup, tracheobronchitis, pneumonitis and pneumonia. The onset of mycoplasmal pneumonia is usually insidious, in contrast to the abrupt onset of classic pneumococcal pneumonia. The symptoms include chills (55%), headache (66%), sore throat (54%), malaise (89%) and cough (99%). The disease may mimic infections caused by *C. pneumoniae*, various viral respiratory diseases such as adenovirus and influenza and even the common cold.

(1) Pneumonia

The radiographic findings in *M. pneumoniae* pneumonia can be extremely variable and mimic a wide variety of lung diseases, but sometimes the radiologic appearance coupled with clinical manifestations can give clues to a mycoplasmal etiology. The inflammatory response elicited by *M. pneumoniae* causes interstitial mononuclear inflammation in the lungs that may be manifest radiographically as bronchopneumonia.

(2) Asthma

Multiple reports suggest that *M. pneumoniae* infections are associated with asthma, although this finding is not universal. *M. pneumoniae* is known to induce a number of inflammatory mediators implicated in the pathogenesis of asthma. A variety of mediators (including IgE) is induced at high levels by mycoplasma infectionand may play a role in exacerbations of asthma.

(3) Extrapulmonary Syndromes

Reports of extrapulmonary *M. pneumoniae* complications have appeared in the literature for over 60 years. Although the complications can be grouped roughly by organ system for ease of discussion, it is important to realize that often multiple organ systems are involved and hematogenous spread to many organ systems in the same patient is well known.

1) Neurologic: CNS infections by *M. pneumoniae* can be severe and life-threatening, more commonly than generally perceived. In children, most CNS infections manifest as encephalitis (diffuse, local or expansive). However, a wide range of disease syndromes in adultsand/or children have been reported, including encephalitis, encephalomyelitis, meningoencephalitis, meningitis and so on. Neurologic complications from respiratory *M. pneumoniae* infection may ultimately result from direct infection of brain tissues as well as secondary destruction of tissuecaused by the generation of autoimmune antibodies.

2) Cardiac: A variety of cardiac complications have been reported, including pericarditis, myocarditis and pericardial effusion with and without cardiac tamponade. In general, cardiac complications are relatively uncommon, occurring in 1% −8.5% of patients with serologic evidence of infection, primarily adults.

3) Renal: Renal diseases such as acute glomerulonephritis and renal failure (sometimes secondary to rhabdomyolysis), tubulointerstitial nephritis, IgA nephropathy, as well as others have been reported sporadically. Attemptsto demonstrate mycoplasma antigen in damaged renal tissue with immunohistochemical techniques have not been uniformly successful, leading to theories that anantibody-mediated pathogenesis and not direct infection maybe responsible for some cases of renal disease.

4) Arthropathies: The difficulty of isolating mycoplasmas from affected joints of patients who fit clinical criteria suggestions that *M. pneumoniae* and other mycoplasmas may be "cofactors" in arthropathies such that direct invasion of joints may not be necessary.

5) Dermatologic: A variety of dermatologic abnormalities have been associated with *M. pneumoniae* infection in up to 25% of patients. Among the more common are erythematous maculopapular and vesicularrashes.

6) Hematologic: Hemolytic anemia has been recognized as a rare but severe complication. Hemolytic anemia has been attributed incold agglutinin disease and autoimmune hemolytic anemiato *M. pneumoniae*-induced cross-reacting antibodies to the Iantigen of human erythrocytes.

8.8.3.6　Laboratory Diagnosis

Clinical laboratory findings are seldom diagnostic. About one-fourthto one-third of persons with lower respiratory tract infections due to *M. pneumoniae* will have leukocytosis and/orelevated erythrocyte sedimentation rate. Moreover, diagnosis of *M. pneumoniae* infections is complicated by the delayed onset of symptoms and the similarity of symptoms to other pulmonary conditions. Often, *M. pneumoniae* infections are diagnosed as other conditions and, occasionally, non-pathogenic mycoplasmas present in the respiratory tract are mistaken for *M. pneumoniae*.

(1) Cultivation

Culture of *M. pneumoniae* from the respiratory tract and other sites is laborious and expensive, requiring serial blind passages, specialized and expensive growth media and incubation periods of up to several weeks. SP4 medium has become the most successful and widely used broth and agar medium for cultivating *M. pneumoniae* for clinical purposes. By MIT or GIT, detection of *M. pneumoniae* is predicated on its characteristic hydrolysis of glucose, with a resultant acidic shift, after 4 days or more of incubation in broth containing a phenol red pH indicator. Initial specimens, as well as broths with color change and blind subcultures, should be transferred to SP4 agar, incubated and examined under a stereomicroscope at regular intervals to look for development of spherical colonies of up to 100 μm in diameter (Figure 8−12).

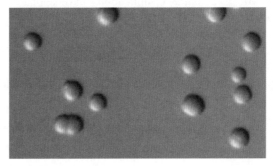

Figure 8−12　Spherical colonies of *M. pneumoniae* growing on SP4 agarat a magnification of ×100

In cubation of *M. pneumoniae* broth cultures under atmospheric conditions at 37 ℃ is satisfactory, but agar plates will yield the best colonial growth if 5% CO_2 is provided and plates are sealed to prevent loss of moisture during prolonged incubation.

(2) Serological and Immunological Diagnostic Methods

Commercial *M. pneumoniae* antibody detection kits which utilize passive (particle) agglutination, indirect immunofluorescence or enzyme-linked immunofluorescent assay (EIA) formats are available for the detection of antibodies to *M. pneumoniae* in human sera. The ImmunoCard® test (Meridian Diagnostics) for IgM is simple and rapid and has proved reliable, especially in children. The Remel enzyme immunoassay detects IgM and IgG simultaneously and is sensitive and specific. A four-fold or greater rise in antibody titre, with apeak at about 3−4 weeks, is indicative of a recent *M. pneumoniae* infection, but because paired sera are not always available or because of the delay in acquiringa second serum, a single antibody titre of 64−128 has been used to institute therapy in a suggestive clinical setting.

Prior to the widespread availability of antibody assaysabove and even before the precise bacteriological characterization of the etiological agent was known, clinicians sometimes used the presence of cold agglutinins to confirm their clinical suspicions of primary atypical pneumonia, also known as "cold agglutinin disease". Cold agglutinins are IgM antibodies produced 1–2 weeks after initial infection in about 50% of *M. pneumoniae* infections, *sometimes persisting for several weeks. It is characterized by the presence of high concentrations of circulating antibodies, usually IgM only bind red blood cells at low body temperatures, typically* 28–31 ℃. However, other infection diseases, such as mumps and influenza virus can course cold agglutinins.

(3) Nucleic Acid Amplification Tests

Serology and culture have largely been supersededby PCR technology, which is specific, sensitive and rapid for detecting *M. pneumoniae*. If an *M. pneumoniae* isolate is required, asensible approach is to test specimens by both the PCR assay and culture and to continue the culture procedure only for those specimens that prove to be PCR positive. The conventional PCR procedure currently used has been adapted using primers derived from the *M. pneumoniae* ATPase gene. Other sequences, primarily the P1 adhesin and conserved regions of 16S rRNA, have also been utilized.

8.8.3.7   Control and Treatment

Antibiotic treatment of *M. pneumoniae* or other mycoplasma-induced infection should start as soon as possible, based on clinical suspicion and a course of at least two weeks is justified. The wait for laboratory confirmation is now less pressing in view of the rapidity of PCR technology. *M. pneumoniae* is sensitive to erythromycin and moderately sensitive to the tetracyclines *in vitro* and the seantibiotics have been used widely in clinical practice. Though they have sometimes proved less effective fortreating pneumonia than in planned trials, it is still worthwhile administering a macrolide or a tetracycline to adults and erythromycin to children and pregnant women. Because of the evidence for an immune component insome cases of *M. pneumoniae* CNS disease and because of the benefits of steroid therapy in many CNS syndromes, steroids are frequently used in combination with antibioticsto treat *M. pneumoniae* CNS infections.

Development of a vaccine also seemed promising in view of the fact that the organism is rather homogeneous antigenically and there appears to be some protection against reinfection. Considering that attachment and initiation of local damage at the cellular and subcellular levels are responsible for *M. pneumoniae* disease, the logical vaccine strategy isto prevent attachment and thereby prevent initiation of disease.

8.8.3.8   Other Human Mycoplasmas

In 1954, Shepard provided the first description of "T-strain" mycoplasmas, later known as ureaplasmas, when he was able to cultivate them *in vitro* from the urethras of men with nongonococcal urethritis (NGU). Also, *M. genitalium* was isolated from the urethras of men with NGU in the early 1980s. *M. fermentans* is an organism which may have a possible pathogenic role both in immunocompetent and immunosuppressed patients. *M. fermentans* has been detected in a small number of immunocompetent adults developing fatalrespiratory distress syndromes. It has also been recovered from the throats of children with pneumonia from whom no other respiratory pathogen was isolated and from bronchoalveolar lavages from AIDS patients with pneumonia. Other organisms such as *M. penetrans* appear to have the potential for being human pathogens, but no conclusive proof demonstrating this has been offered to date. The most recent human mycoplasmal species to be recognized is *M. amphoriforme*, an organism that has been detected in the lower respiratory tract of several immunocompromised persons in association with chronic bronchitis and investigations are now underway todetermine whether a role in human disease can be established with certainty.

U. urealyticum can be found on the mucosal surfaces of the cervix or vagina of 40%–80% of sexually mature a symptomatic women, whereas *M. hominis* may occur in 21%–30%. The incidence of each is somewhat lower in the urethra of males. Colonization is linked to younger age, lower socioeconomic status, sexual activity with multiple partners and oral contraceptive use. There is ample evidence that *M. hominis*, *M. gen-*

italium and *U. urealyticum* play etiological roles in avariety of urogenital diseases of men and women. For some conditions such as NGU for *U. urealyticum* and pelvic inflammatory disease (PID) for *M. hominis*, Koch's postulates have been fulfilled and aportion of clinical cases of these entities are known to becaused by these respective organisms.

Soon after ureaplasmas were first identified and characterized it became apparent that these organisms could besubclassified into several distinct serovars. The number of serovars was eventually expanded to 14. Additional study over several years, using data obtained from 16S rRNA sequencing, led to the breakdown of the 14 serovars into 2 biovars or clusters. Biovar 1, also known as the parvobiovar, contains serovars 1,3,6 and 14, while biovar 2, also known as the T960 biovar, contains serovars 2,4,5,7,8,9,10,11,12 and 13. Recently, the two biovars were designated as distinct species. Biovar 1 became *U. parvum* and biovar 2became *U. urealyticum*. *U. parvum* is the more common of the two biovars isolated from clinical specimens, but both species may occur simultaneously in some people.

8.8.3.9　Pathogenesis and Immunity

Localization and attachment on host cell surfaces are important in the ability of mycoplasmas to colonize and subsequently produce pathological lesions. Like *M. pneumoniae* organisms such as *M. genitalium* also have a flask-shaped morphology and terminal attachment or ganelles. Amajor adhesion protein of *M. hominis*, also known as the variable adherence associated antigen (Vaa) may undergo antigenic variation andassist *M. hominis* in evasion of host immune defenses. The Vaa antigen is expressed *in vivo* during chronic active arthritis and is highly immunogenic in the human host. Besides, the MB antigen of ureaplasmas undergoes a high rate of size variation *in vitro* and is sizevariable on invasive *Ureaplasma* isolates. The MB antigen contains serovar-specific and cross-reactive epitopes and is a predominant antigen recognized during infections. *U. urealyticum* is known to adhere to a variety of human cells including erythrocytes, spermatozoa and urethral epithelial cells.

Arginine metabolism by *M. hominis* and urease activityin *U. urealyticum* have been suggested as potential virulence factors. Release of NH_3 in the urinary tract by *U. urealyticum* can cause elevation of urinary pH and precipitation of magnesium ammonium phosphate, also known as struvite. IgA1 protease, which may facilitate colonizationat mucosal surfaces, was first describedin *U. urealyticum*. Moreover, the presence of phospholipases A and C in *U. urealyticum* has been suggested to be the means by which *U. urealyticum* may initiate preterm labor by liberating arachidonic acid and altering prostaglandin synthesis.

8.8.3.10　Clinical Manifestations

(1) Respiratory Infections

M. hominis has produced sore throats when given orally to adult volunteers. However, it does not seem to cause naturally occurring sore throats in children or adults possibly because the dose encountered issmaller. *M. fermentans* has been associated with adult respiratory distress syndrome with or without systemic disease and with pneumonia in a few children with community-acquired disease. *M. genitalium* has been isolated, together with *M. pneumoniae*, from the respiratory secretions of a few adults but its rolein respiratory disease seems small. *M. hominis* and ureaplasmas, in particular, have been associated with respiratory disease in the newborn.

(2) Urogenital infections

M. hominis and *U. urealyticum* have been isolated most frequently from theurogenital tract. Use of the PCR technique has enabled some mycoplasmas, for example *M. fermentans* and especially *M. genitalium*, to be detected far more often than would otherwise be the case.

1) Urogenital infections in men: Although *M. hominis* may be isolated from about 20% of men with

acute NGU, it has not been incriminated as a cause. There is increasing evidence to implicate *U. urealyticum* in this acute condition. *U. urealyticum* is the most likely specie involved in some chroniccases. *M. genitalium* has been strongly implicated worldwide as a cause of about 25% of cases of acute NGU. It also causes chronic NGU, usually in those who have been treated inadequately. In addition, there is preliminary evidence that *M. genitalium* causes balanoposthitis and it might be involved in some cases of acute epididymitis. Ureaplasmasmay occasionally cause acute epididymitis, but it is very doubtful that they have any role in male infertility. The idea that *M. genitalium* could have a role in infertility is based on the possibility that it might be involved incausing epididymitis and its known ability to adhereto spermatozoa.

2) Reproductive tract disease in women: *M. hominis* is found in the vagina of women who have bacterial vaginosis in much larger numbers than in healthy women. Therefore, they may contribute to the development of the condition. Besides, *M. hominis* has been isolated from the endometrium and fallopian tubes of about 10% of women with PID, toget her with a specific antibody response. Ureaplasmas have also been isolated directly from affected fallopiantubes, but the absence of antibody responses. The pathogenic potential of *M. genitalium* in PID has been associated significantly with endometritis. The part that *M. hominis* is likely to play in infertility in women as a result of tubal damage is small. In contrast, serology has shown a strong association between *M. genitalium* and tubal factor infertility.

(3) Diseaseas Sociated with Pregnancy

M. hominis and ureaplasmas have been isolated from the amniotic fluid of women with severe chorioamnionitis who had preterm labor. Similarly, ureaplasmas have been isolated from spontaneously aborted fetuses and still born or premature infants more frequently than from induced abortions ornormal full-term infants. It suggests that these organisms may have a role in abortion. However, as *M. hominis* and ureaplasmas are part of the extensive microbial flora of bacterial vaginosis, they may act with a multitude of other micro-organisms and not independently.

(4) Urinary Infection and Calculi

M. hominis has been isolated from the upper urinarytract of patients with acute pyelonephritis and may cause a small proportion (possibly about 5%) of such cases. Ureaplasmas do not seem to be involved inpyelonephritis. However, the fact that they produce urease, induce crystallization of struvite and calcium phosphates in urine *in vitro* and calculi experimentally in animal models, raises the question of whether they cause calculi in the human urinary tract. Insupport of this, ureaplasmas are more often found in the urine and calculi of patients with infective-typestones than in those with metabolic stones.

8.8.3.11   Laboratory Detection

(1) Cultivation

Although culture is considered the reference standard for detection of *M. hominis* and *U. urealyticum*, itrequires specialized media and expertise that are not widely available. Confirmed culture results can usually be available within 2−5 days in reference laboratories. Definitive species identification requires additional tests which have historically included growth and metabolic inhibition using homologous antisera (GIT and MIT).

(2) Material

From urethral, cervical or vaginal swabs is added to liquid mycoplasmal medium containing phenol redwith 0.1% glucose, arginine or urea relying on different species. *M. genitalium* metabolizes glucose and changes the color of the mediumfrom red to yellow. *M. fermentans* also metabolizes glucose but also converts arginine to ammonia, as do *M. hominis* and *M. primatum*. Ammonia is also produced when ureaplasmal urease breaks down urea and the color changes from yellow to red. However, kits designed to isolate and identi-

fy M. hominis and *U. urealyticum* and to provide antimicrobial susceptibility profiles, are available commercially.

(3) Nucleic Acid Amplification Tests

The amplification of the 16S rRNA gene of urogenital mycoplasmas and ureaplasmas has been used. DNA primers specific for practically all *Mycoplasma* and *Ureaplasma* species, including *M. fermentans*, *M. genitalium*, *U. urealyticum* and *U. parvum*, have been developed and used for amplification by PCR. This technique is much more sensitive than culture for detecting the two former mycoplasmas and is the only reliable way of determining their presencein clinical specimens.

8.8.3.12　Treatment

Treatment must take into account the fact that several differentspecies may be involved and that a precise microbiological diagnosis may not be attainable. Besides, they are completely resistant to β-lactam or glycopeptide antibiotics.

Patients with NGU should receive an antibiotic that is active against *C. trachomatis*, ureaplasmas and *M. genitalium*. Azithromycin, which is used increasingly for chlamydial infections, is also active against a wide range of mycoplasmas. Some *M. genitalium* strains are resistant to azithromycin and in this circumstance moxifloxacin has been used successfully. A broad-spectrum antibiotic should also be included for the treatment of PID to cover *C. trachomatis*, *M. genitalium* and *M. hominis* as well as various anaerobic bacteria.

Extragenital infections, often in immunocompromised hosts, may be caused by multi-drug-resistant mycoplasmas and ureaplasmas, making guidance of chemotherapy by *in vitro* susceptibility tests is important in clinical setting. Eradication of infection under these circumstances can be extremely difficult, requiring prolonged therapy, even when the organisms are susceptible to the expected antibiotics. Fluoroquinolones such as levofloxacin, moxifloxacin and gatifloxacin tend to have greater *in vitro* activity than older drugs such as ciprofloxacin, but resistant strains have been reported.

8.9　Chlamydia

Chlamydiae were first described in 1907 by Halberstaedter and von Prowazek, who observed cytoplasmic inclusions in conjunctival scrapings taken from children with trachoma and from monkeys inoculated with ocular material from these children. Chlamydiae are obligate intracellular bacterial pathogens of eukaryotic cells with a unique developmental cycle quite distinct from that of other bacteria. Members of Chlamydiae have the following common features:

1) They are Gram-stain-negative bacteria.

2) Unlike most other bacteria, they show an intracellular developmental cycle characterized by morphologically and physiologically distinct stages.

3) They have a proteinaceous cell wall without flagella and peptidogly can.

4) They have ribosomes, but still are "energy parasites" relying on the host cell for synthesis of ATP.

The phylum *Chlamydiae* is based on phylogenetic analysis of 16S rRNA sequences, clearly separating its members (showing>80% 16S rRNA sequence similarity with each other) from all other do main *Bacteria*. The phylum *Chlamydiae* currently comprises a single class, *Chlamydiia*, containing only one order, the *Chlamydiales*. The *Chlamydia* genus (family *Chlamydiaceae*) comprises nine species of which two are primarily human pathogens: *C. trachomatis*, causing ocular and genital infections; and *C. pneumoniae*, causing mainly respiratory diseases. The other species infect animals: *C. psittaci* (chiefly birds), *C. abortus* (sheep), *C. felis* (cats), *C. pecorum* (cattle), *C. suis* (pigs), *C. muridarum* (mice) and *C. caviae* (guineapigs). *C. psittaci*, *C. abortus* and *C. felis* are occasionally transmitted to human. In 1999, it was proposed by Everett (Table 8-16) that a taxonomic reclassification should assign *C. pneumoniae*, *C. psittaci*, *C. abortus*, *C. felis*, *C. pecorum* and *C. pecorum* to a new genus, *Chlamydophila*. However, this new taxonomy has not been generally accepted in the field.

Most human infections are caused by *C. trachomatis*, which was isolated from a patient with lymphogranuloma venereum (LGV) in the 1930s. *C. trachomatis* was first cultured in the yolk sacs of eggs by Chinese Professor Tang Fei-fan in 1957, though they were not yet recognized as bacteria.

Table 8-16 The family *Chlamydiaceae* by Everett

Species	Host	Route of entry
Chlamydia		
Chlamydia trachomatis	Humans	Pharyngeal, ocular, genital, rectal
Chlamydia suis	Pigs	Pharyngeal
Chlamydia muridarum	Mouse, hamster	Pharyngeal, genital
Chlamydophila		
Chlamydophila abortus	Mammals	Oral, genital
Chlamydophila caviae	Guinea pig	Pharyngeal, ocular, genital, urethral
Chlamydophila felis	Cats	Pharyngeal, ocular, genital
Chlamydophila pecorum	Mammals	Oral
Chlamydophila pneumoniae	Humans, frog, koala, horse	Pharyngeal, ocular
Chlamydophila psittaci	Birds	Pharyngeal, ocular, genital

8.9.1 Biological Properties

8.9.1.1 Developmental Cycle

Chlamydiae probably evolved from host-independent, Gram-negative ancestors. The chlamydial envelope possesses bacteria-like inner and outer membranes. They are coccoid, non-motile, obligate intracellular organisms, 0.2-1.5 μm in diameter that parasitize and multiply in the cytoplasm of eukaryotic cells within membrane bound vacuoles, termed inclusions, by a unique developmental cycle. The cycle is characterized by physical changes in the outer membrane and nucleoid structure involving alternation from a metabolically inert, infectious, spore-like elementary body (EB), which can survive in the extracellular environment, to a metabolically active, noninfectious, replicating reticulate body (RB), which cannot survive in the extracellular environment.

Infectious EBs are 0.2-0.4 μm in diameter, have electron-dense DNA condensed with protein and a few ribosomes and are surrounded by rigid trilaminar cell walls. The rigidity of the cell wall is maintained by extensive disulphide linking of the major outer membrane protein, which makes up some 60% of the outer membrane. The EB binds to the host cell and enters by endocytosis. Fusion of the chlamydia-containing endocytic vesicle with lysosomes is inhibited by an unknown mechanism and the EB begins it sunique developmental cycle within the eukaryotic cell. The major outer membrane protein (MOMP) is reduced to amonomeric form and acts as porin, getting nutrients from the host cell. After about 9 h, the EB differentiates into noninfectious RBs which are 0.6−1.5 μm in diameter, have less dense, fibrillar nuclear material, more ribosomes and plastic trilaminar walls ready to divide by binary fission. By 24 h post-infection, a proportion of RBs has begun to reorganize into a new generation of EBs. These reach maturity up to 40 h after entry into the cell and rapidly accumulate within the endocytic vacuole, which may contain more than 1,000 organisms. The developmental cycle is complete>48 h after the start of the cycle when the new EBs release by lysisof the host cell and start a new generation of the cycle(Figure 8−13). In a young inclusion, only EBs are present. However in a mature inclusion, both the forms (EBs and RBs)are present because the developmental cycle is not synchronized.

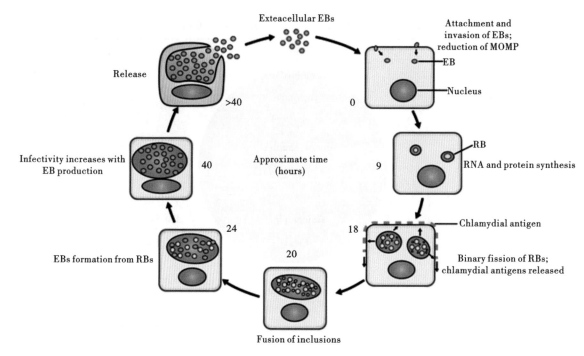

Figure 8−13　The developmental cycle of chlamydiae

EB, elementary body; MOMP, major outer membrane protein; RB, reticulate body

The structural forms of chlamydiae as well as their compositionare highly dependent on the developmental cycle. The properties of the two principal cell forms are summarized in Table 8−17.

Table 8−17　Characteristics of chlamydial elementary and reticulate bodies

Characteristic	Elementary body	Reticulate body
General :		
Diameter (μm)	0.2−0.4	0.6−1.5
Infectivity for new host cells	+	−
Immediate cytotoxicity in cellculture	+	−
Cell wall :		
Rigidity	Rigid	Flexible
Cross-linking of outer membrane	+	−

Continue to Table 8-17

Characteristic	Elementary body	Reticulate body
Susceptibility to :		
Mechanical stress	−	+
Osmotic stress	−	+
Lysis by trypsin	−	+
Synthesis inhibited by penicillin	+	−
Nucleic acids :		
DNA	Compact	Disperse
RNA/DNA ratio	1	3-4
Ribosomes	Scanty	Abundant
Metabolism :		
Net generation of ATP	−	−
ATP-dependent host-free proteinsynthesis	−	+

8.9.1.2　Cultivation

Cultivation of chlamydiae in cell-free mediumhas not been achieved. Thus, they may be propagated in laboratory animals, the yolk sac of chicken eggs or in cell culture. BALB/c or A/Jinbred mice are preferred for isolation. Besides, six-to-seven-day-old fertile chicken eggs can be used to inoculate chlamydia into their yolk sacs and incubate at 35-37 ℃ for 14 days. Negative primary passage may be blind passed again. For isolation of human chlamydial strains, the yolk sac is less sensitive than cell culture. Until recently, culture was considered the gold standard for detection of chlamydiae in specimens because it has a specificity that approaches 100%. All chlamydial strains multiply in a variety of cell cultures, such as HeLa, L434 mouse fibroblasts or McCoy cells in the case of *C. trachomatis* and *C. psittaci*; Buffalo green monkey kidney cells for *C. psittaci* and *C. pecorum*, HeLa or Hep2 cells for *C. pneumoniae*. Enhancement of infection is achieved by pretreating cell monolayers with the use of charged anionic polymers such as Poly-L-lysine or DEAE-dextran, centrifuging the inoculum onto the monolayer and incubating the inoculated cells with medium containing anti-metabolites (cycloheximide, emetine or mitomycin C). Blind passage makes it more credible in diagnostics. *C. pneumoniae* is even more difficult to grow than *C. trachomatis*. *C. psittaci* is a hazard group 3 pathogen and few laboratories attempt to cultivate.

8.9.1.3　Antigenic Structure

All chlamydiae share a similar antigenic framework consisting of common and specific antigenic determinants (Table 8-18). Monoclonal antibodies to the mostimportant chlamydial antigens are commercially available.

The *Chlamydiaceae* are characterized by a common lipopolysaccharide (LPS) antigen. This antigen is heat-stable and is the antigen for complement fixation tests. Antibodies to LPS react strongly to antigens present within inclusions and in the RB membranes. However, reactivity to EBs by immunofluorescence is weak.

All chlamydiae encode a major 60,000 molecular weight heat-shock protein (HSP-60) family member that is associated with sero reactivity in individuals at risk for pathogenic sequelae of infection. Another

60,000 molecular weight protein (OmcB) is cysteine-rich and present in EB outer membranes but not RB outer membranes. This protein is a potent immunogen and useful marker for serological studies of chlamydial infection.

Table 8-18　Structure and function of the major immunoreactiveantigens identified in *Chlamydia*

Molecular weight	Name	Function
≥98,000	Pmp	Unknown. Six Pmp subtypes: A, B, C/D, E/F, G/I and H
75,000	HSP	Chaperone HSP-70 family
60,000	OmcB	Structural, cysteine-rich OMP
60,000	HSP	Chaperone HSP-60 family
40,000	OmpA (MOMP)	Outer-membrane porin. Containingserological determinants of species-, subspecies- and serovar-specificity
40,000	PorB	Outer-membrane porin
12,500	OmcA	Structural lipoprotein, cysteine-rich OMP
−12,000	LPS	Endotoxin, genus antigen

Abbreviations: Pmp, polymorphic membrane protein; HSP, heat shock protein; Crp, cysteine-rich protein (cross linking of disulfide bonds of cysteine-rich proteins give rigidity to the outer membrane of the EB); Omc, outer membrane complex protein; MOMP, major outer membrane protein; LPS, lipopolysaccharide.

A major antigen is the major outer-membrane protein(OmpA or MOMP) that is the quantitatively predominant protein in *Chlamydia* species. This protein is an outer membrane porin and is antigenically complex. For *C. trachomatis* and *C. suis*, four variable sequence (VS) loops are exposed on the surface and accessible to binding of antibodies. *C. trachomatis* serovar-specific antigens have been mapped and are associated with VS1 and VS2; broadly reactive determinants, including a species-specific antigen, are localized with VS4. For *C. trachomatis* and *C. pneumoniae*, some of the OmpA antigenic determinants are conformation dependent. Sequence based antigenic variations of this protein singularly account for the antigenic specificities originally characterized by the micro-immunofluorescence test in which 19 prototype serovars were defined. Antigenic variation is thought to derive from selection by the host immune response to infection.

A new porin, PorB, was discovered following genome sequencing. Like OmpA, PorB is surface-exposed. But PorB is not quantitatively predominant and does not appear significant sequence variation among isolates within a species which is different from OmpA.

An entire multigene family of antigens [polymorphic membrane proteins (Pmps)] was also discovered from genome sequencing including nine representatives in *C. trachomatis* and 21 representatives in *C. pneumoniae* and intermediate numbers of paralogs for other species. The protein sequences are very different, but they are unambiguously related. The functions of these proteins are unknown, but somehave been shown to be surface-exposed outer-membrane proteins and their expression is dependent upon phase variation.

8.9.1.4　Stability and Viability

Chlamydiae are expected to be susceptible to 1% sodium hypochlorite, 70% ethanol, 2% gluta raldehyde and formaldehyde. They can also be inactivated by moist heat (121 ℃ for at least 15 min) and dry heat (160−170 ℃ for at least 1 hour). Chlamydiae are stable in carcass and organs for 1−7 days and water (50 ℃) for about 30 min.

The susceptibility of chlamydiae to antibiotics has been tested in yolk sac of chicken embryos or cell culture. The growth of chlamydiae in culture is inhibited by the tetracyclines, macrolides, azalides, chloramphenicol, rifampin and fluoroquinolones. Chlamydial multiplication is not blocked by aminoglycosides, bacitracin or vancomycin.

8.9.2   Pathogenesis

Chlamydial infection is a complex process involving many factors. The eukaryotic cell becomes infected when chlamydiae adhere to the cytoplasmic membrane. There is evidence that MOMP binds to a heptaransulphate receptor on the host cell. The chlamydiae penetrate into the cell by endocytosis, remaining within avacuole also termed phagosome. In healthy individuals, innate immune cells can fuse with phagosome by lysosomes to destroy invading bacteria. However, chlamydiae avoid this degradative pathway altogether. Chlamydiae modify the inclusion membrane to be undetec Table to lysosomes by MOMP. In addition to remodeling the lipid composition of phagosomes, chlamydiae also modify the proteins on the membrane surface. It has been established that chlamydiae employ a Type Ⅲ Secretion System to deliver chlamydial proteins into the inclusion membrane and the host cytosol. Besides, up-regulation of expression of heat shock protein by chlamydial infection induces production of cytokines such as TNF-α, IL-1β and IL-6 by macrophage to produce inflammations and scars.

Human chlamydial infections are associated with respiratory, ocular and genitourinary disease syndromes (Table 8-19). The syndromes are clinically distinct, but chlamydiae that cause human disease share a number of characteristics, including the propensity to produce ①infections that are frequently long-lasting in the absence of treatment; ②repeated infections following natural clearance or antibiotic treatment of aninitial infection; ③infections that are often a symptomatic or minimally symptomatic; and ④infections that can cause in flammatory and scarring complications in the absence of treatment and often with minimal or no symptoms.

Table 8-19   Disease manifestations of chlamydiae

C. trachomatis			
Trachoma			
Oculogenital diseases			
Adult, male or female:	Adult female:	Adult male:	Infant:
Conjunctivitis	Cervicitis	Urethritis	Conjunctivitis
Proctitis	Salpingitis	Epididymitis	Pneumonia
	Urethral syndrome	Arthritis (Reiter'ssyndrome)	Bronchiolitis
	Postpartumendometritis		Otitis media
Lymphogranuloma venereum			
C. psittaci			
Psittacosis			
C. pneumoniae			
Pneumonia			

8.9.3　Immune Response to Chlamydial Infection

The immune response to chlamydial infection represents acomplex network in which innate immune cells, B cells and T cells act in concert. It can be assumed that a highly regulated balance between different T and B cell subsets decides whether an infection is cleared or develops into a prolonged infection.

Primary infection induces development of antigen-specific immunity. Monocytes/macrophages and dendritic cells participate in the development of antigen-specific cell-mediated immunity by ①acting as antigen presenting cells (APC) and by ②secretion of pro-inflammatory (IL-6, IL-1, IL-12) and anti-inflammatory (IL-10, IL-13) cytokines, which activate other immune cells. Cell-mediated immunity and especially participation of type 1 Th cells are crucial for eradication or limitation of the infection, which are interacting, not directly with the pathogen, but with the infected cell surface. However, chlamydial infections *in vivo* typically result in chronic inflammation characterized by the presence of activated monocytes and macrophages and by the secretion of Th-1/Th-2 cytokines, which is accompanied by delayed hypersensitivity reactions resulting in autoimmune diseases.

Antibodies exhibit aminor effect on the immune protection against infections. Concerning the antibodies responses in chlamydiae infection, IgM response appears 2−3 weeks after the first symptoms of the illness and IgG response after 6−8 weeks. IgA antibodies are only occasionally found during the primary infection but appear frequently in the reinfection. The main antigens triggering an antibody mediated response are LPS and HSP-60.

8.9.4　Major Human Chlamydiae

There are several quite Different disease patterns that result from human infection with chlamydial organisms. Infection with *C. trachomatis* may result in trachoma, a variety of other syndromes that accompany ocular orgenital infection or lymphogranuloma venereum (LGV). *C. psittaci* has one human disease manifestation, psittacosis. *C. pneumoniae* causes respiratory disease and is associated with coronary artery disease.

8.9.4.1　*Chlamydia Trachomatis*

C. trachomatis, is an exclusively human pathogen, with the conjuntival and urogenital tropism. Based on the disease types, *C. trachomatis* has been classified into three biovars: biovar ocular, biovar genital and biovar LGV. The defined 19 *C. trachomatis* serovars (Table 8−20) designated A-K and L1-L3, which differ by the antigenicity of their major outer membrane protein (MOMP), codified by gene *omp*1.

Chlamydiae of biovar ocular exclusively infect the conjunctival mucosal cells and cause trachoma, transmitted by discharge from the inflamed eyes generally in school or family. The primary infection, in the form of follicular conjunctivitis, may heal spontaneously. However, in endemic areas, repeated infections sustain the chronicity of infection and cause scarring of the conjunctiva and cornea. The last stage of the disease is blindness.

Chlamydiae of biovar genital are mainly isolated from the urogenital tract and are associated with sexually transmitted infection (STI), inclusion conjunctivitis or neonatal pneumonitis in infants during vaginal childbirth. The primary infection site is the mucosal membranes of the urogenital tract. The infection may be transferred to the conjunctiva to cause acute follicular conjunctivitis with satisfactory prognosis. Chronic infection of biovar genital is a common cause of infertility in women.

Chlamydiae of biovar LGV are sexually transmitted and cause systemic infection with the major manifestation of lymphadenopathy or swelling of draining lymph nodes. Prognosis is more favorable with early treatment with proper antibiotic.

Table 8-20　The defined biovars and serovars of *C. trachomatis*

Biovar	Serovar	Diseases
Ocular	A,B,Ba,C	trachoma
Genital	D,Da,E,F,G,H,I,Ia,J,Ja,K	STI,conjuntivitis and pneumonitis
LGV	L1,L2,L2a,L3	LGV

8.9.4.2　Clinical Manifestations

（1）Trachoma

Chlamydiae of biovar ocular exclusively infect the conjunctival mucosal cells and cause trachoma, transmitted by discharge from the inflamed eyes generally in school or family. The primary infection, in the form of follicular conjunctivitis with hyperemia, edema and distortion of the vascular pattern of the conjunctiva, may heal spontaneously. Such conjunctival follicles can occur as a response to a number of stimuli, both infectious and toxic. Moreover, in endemic areas, repeated infections sustain the chronicity of infection and heal by scarring of the conjunctiva and cornea. These scars lead to distortion of the lids and inversion of lashes, which increases the trauma to the cornea. Besides, a characteristic feature of trachomais the vascularization of the cornea, which constitutes pannus. This is an important component of trachoma diagnosis.

Collectively, these features of trachoma constitute the acute and chronic conjunctivitis and their blinding sequelae. It is clear in humand isease that the serious sequelae that lead to blindness occuronly as a result of many reinfections or persistent infection and high infectious load.

（2）Inclusion Conjunctivitis

Adult chlamydial ophthalmia commonly results from the accidental transfer of infected genital discharge to the eye. It usually presents as a unilateral follicular conjunctivitis, acute or subacute in onset. About one-third of patients have otitis media with blocked ears and hearing loss. The disease is generally benign and self-limiting. Besides, conjunctivitis appears in 20% –50% of infants exposed to *C. trachomatis* during vaginal childbirth. Amucopurulent discharge and occasionally pseudo membrane formation occur 1–3 weeks later. It usually resolves without visual impairment.

（3）Neonatal Pneumonia

About half of the infants who have conjunctivitis also develop pneumonia. Chlamydial pneumonia usually begins between the fourth and eleventh week of life, preceded by upper respiratory symptoms. Children infected during infancy are at increased risk of obstructive lung disease and asthma.

（4）Genital Infection

The clinical manifestations of genital *C. trachomatis* infection are similar to those of gonorrhoea, but are usually less severe. Many chlamydial infections are asymptomatic. Long term sequelae such as infertility and ectopic pregnancy are generally caused following prolonged or repeated infections and may develop evenin those with few or no symptoms.

1）Infection in men: *C. trachomatis* is detec Table inthe urethra of up to 50% of men with symptomaticnon-gonococcal urethritis (NGU). There is no good evidence that *C. trachomatis* infection leads to male infertility. Both LGV and non-LGV strains of *C. trachomatis* can cause proctitis in those who practice receptive anal intercourse. Non-LGV strains cause a milder disease, which may be asymptomatic or give rise to rectal pain, bleeding and mucopurulent anal discharge.

2) Infection in women: Most infected women have no symptoms. *C. trachomatis* typically infects the columnar epithelial cells of the endocervix. Infection is associated with a mucopurulent discharge from the cervix visible on speculum examination. *C. trachomatis* has been implicated as a cause of the urethral syndrome, such as dysuria, frequency and sterile pyuria. Infection may cause pelvic inflammatory disease, after which the risk of ectopic pregnancy increases 7–10 fold. Moreover, infertility may result from endometritis.

(5) Lymphogranuloma Venereum

The clinical course of LGV can be divided into three stages.

1) Primary stage: After incubation period of 3–30 days, a small, painless papule, which may ulcerate, occurs at the site of inoculation. The primary lesionis self-limiting and may pass unnoticed by the patient.

2) Secondary stage: This occurs some weeks after the primary lesion. It may involve the inguinal lymphnodes or the anus and rectum. The inguinal form is more common in men than women. The main feature of the inguinal form of LGV is painful, usually unilateral, inguinal and/or femoral lymphadenopathy (bubo). Enlarged lymph nodes are usually firm and often accompanied by fever, chills, arthralgia and headache. In women, signs includea hypertrophic suppurative cervicitis, backache and adnexal tenderness.

3) Tertiary stage: This appears after a latent period of several years, but is rare. Chronic untreated LGV leads to fibrosis, which may cause lymphatic obstruction and elephantiasis of the genitalia in either sex or rectal strictures and fistulae. Rarely, it can giverise to the syndrome of esthiomene (Greek: eatingaway) with widespread destruction of the external genitalia.

8.9.4.3 Laboratory Diagnosis

The laboratory diagnosis of chlamydial infection depends on detection of the organisms or their antigens or nucleic acid. In urogenital infection the highest load of *C. trachomatis* is found in the endocervix in women and in the urethra in men. Therefore, a swab is needed for the diagnosis of infection by culture or antigen detection assay.

(1) Cytological Identification

C. trachomatis can be identified in cytological scrapingsor in tissue specimens. Characteristic intracytoplasmic inclusions are recognized by iodine stain or Giemsa stain. The most commonly used stain is iodine, which permits rapid identification.

(2) Cultivation

Cell culture has been the gold standard for detection of *C. trachomatis* due to the extremely high specificity (–100%), although it has a low sensitivity (70%–85%) relative to commercial nucleic acid amplification tests (NAATs). Cells used are McCoy cells, HeLa-229 cell, BHK-21cells or L-929 cells. Cycloheximide-treated McCoy cells are the most widely used cell line at present. They can be examined at 48–96 h after inoculation.

(3) Nucleic Acid Amplification Tests

With the increased ability to sequence DNA, it is now more common to identify genotypes rather than serotypes. The NAAT technology is far more sensitive and specific. The chlamydial genescan be detected in epithelial cell specimens in male and female urines. The potential for widespread use of noninvasive screening tests is an important option offered by this technology.

(4) Serological and Immunological Diagnostic Methods

Although a variety of serological methods have been used in the past, the fluorescent antibody method has been simplified and standardized in an indirect microimmunofluorescence (MIF) test. At present, this is the most commonly used test forevaluation of host response to trachoma or to other *C. trachomatis* strains. For LGV, the complement-fixation(CF) test can be used, although the MIF test remains more sensitive and specific.

8.9.4.4 Control and Prevention

Elimination of trachoma has occurred in a majority of the world following the raised standard of living. However, there is a public health program for the purpose of the ultimate elimination of blinding trachoma by the year 2020. The program is based on what is being called the "SAFE" strategy:

1) Surgical repair of lids already damaged by trachoma to prevent the future development of blindness.

2) Azithromycin for community-wide treatment in trachomaendemic areas.

3) Facial cleanliness to minimize the transmission of *C. trachomatis* after the prevalence of infection has been reduced by antibiotic treatment.

4) Environmental improvements, also aimed at minimizing the transmission of *C. trachomatis* through the provision of latrines (aimedat controlling flies) and safe water supplies.

Current recommendations include treatment of all persons with urethritis (gonococcal or nongonococcal), mucopurulent cervicitis, pelvic inflammatory disease and epididymitis as if they had both gonococcal and chlamydial infection. They should be treated with a penicillin-like antibiotic and a tetracycline antibiotic (or erythromycin in pregnant women). Other individuals recommended for *C. trachomatis* treatment areasymptomatic contacts to patients with established gonococcalor chlamydial infections.

Until nowadays, all vaccine trials have failed, pending further study of the molecular biology of *C. trachomatis* to discover antigenic subunits that might induce a more permanent immunity.

8.9.4.5 *Chlamydophila Pneumoniae*

C. pneumoniae was known as the Taiwan acute respiratory (TWAR) agent from the names of the two original isolates, Taiwan (TW-183) and an acute respiratory isolate designated AR-39. The elementary body of *C. pneumoniae* is pear shaped with alarge periplasmic space, whereas the elementary bodies ofthe other two species (*C. trachomatis*, *C. psittaci*) are round with little or no periplasmic space. The inclusions contain no glycogen, hence stain negative with iodine. Sero-epidemiological studies indicate that 60% – 80% of people worldwide become infected with *C. pneumoniae* during their life. There is no evidence for other than human-to-human (airborne) transmission of *C. pneumoniae* infection.

8.9.4.6 Clinical Manifestations

The pathogenesis of *C. pneumoniae* infections is notunderstood. The most convincing disease association with *C. pneumoniae* is pneumonia, which is relatively mild, often self-limited (in that symptoms resolve without specific antibiotic treatment) and very difficult to distinguish from other forms of pneumonia. It is often cited as one of the causes of "atypical pneumonia", resembling that caused by *M. pneumoniae*.

The limited observations suggest that *C. pneumoniae* causes a range of respiratory disease from pharyngitis and otitis media through bronchitis to pneumonia. On set of illnessis gradual and symptoms are often extended over weeks. There appears to be some tendency for more severe manifestation (asthma) to be seen in some cases of *C. pneumoniae* infection. However, it is apparent that the most of infections are asymptomatic. Reinfection has been documented, even in the same epidemic.

Inflammation is a known element of atherosclerosis and a number of infectious agents, including *C. pneumoniae*, have been proposed to contribute to atherosclerotic disease. The epidemiological data and *in vitro* testing suggest that infection with *C. pneumoniae* is a significant risk factor for development of atherosclerotic plaques and atherosclerosis. However, most current research and data are insufficient and do not define how often *C. pneumoniae* is found in atherosclerotic or normal vascular tissue.

8.9.4.7 Laboratory Diagnosis

A major problem indiagnosis of infection with *C. pneumoniae* is the lack of sensitive, reproducible diagnostic tests. *C. pneumoniae* has been isolated from the yolk sac of chicken eggs and initially from cell culture. However, the isolation and cultivation are relatively difficult.

C. pneumoniae antigen in respiratory tract specimens or isolation systems can be demonstrated with species-specific antibody by MIF which is commercially available. The use and interpretation of the MIF test for diagnosis include obtaining and testing paired serum samples 4 to 8 weeks apart. Acute infection is defined serologically as a single IgM of $\geqslant 1 : 16$ or as a single IgG of $\geqslant 1 : 512$. In primary infections, IgM antibodies appear 2 to 3 weeks and IgG antibodies appear 6 to 8 weeks following infection, so that MIF is not useful in planning treatment. Besides, 50% or more with culture-positive pneumonia have a negative MIF test among children.

There are many NAAT procedures that have been used and none of them have taken the lead as the test of choice.

8.9.4.8 *Chlamydophila Psittaci*

C. psittaci is an important pathogen in a wide range of avian species, all of which are potential reservoirs. *C. psittaci* is shed in nasal secretions and droppings. Nasal secretions contaminate the feathers with highly infectious dusts, in which the *C. psittaci* can survive for months. The route of *C. psittaci* infection is airborne. Human *C. psittaci*-induced disease, typically contracted by inhalation of dried bird feces, is called psittacosis (from psittacine birds) or ornithosis (from non-psittacine birds). The risk of exposureis greatly increased in those occupations in which handling birds is common.

8.9.4.9 Clinical Manifestations

The incubation period is about 10 days and psittacosis is characterized by early in fluenza-like symptomswith general malaise, fever, anorexia, rigors, sore throat, headache and photophobia, followed by severe, sometimes fatal atypical interstitial pneumonia which requires intensive antibiotic and symptomatic therapy.

The illness may resemble bronchopneumonia, but the bronchioles are involved as a secondary event with scanty sputum. *C. psittaci* can disseminate through the body and there may be meningoencephalitis, arthritis, pericarditis or myocarditis or a predominantly typhoidal state with enlarged liver and spleen.

8.9.4.10 Laboratory Diagnosis

C. psittaci can be cultivated in yolk sac of chicken eggs, in mice or in tissue culture system. The bestsource for isolation is bronchial aspirate or sputum. Whole blood may occasionally yield *C. psittaci*. Giemsa staining will permit identification of *C. psittaci* strains in cell cultures. However, *C. psittaci* isolates should be handled only in biosafety level 3 laboratories, since they are likely to result in accidental laboratory infections and in cross-contamination.

Serologically, the CF testis sensitive enough for psittacosis. The usualcriterion is a fourfold increase in titer of paired serum samples, but single titers above $1 : 64$ are highly suggestive. NAATs have been widely used in research on *C. psittaci* infections, but there are no commercially availabletests.

8.9.4.11 Control and Prevention

Control of psittacosis depends on control of avian species with infection. There are import controls to restrict the movement of birds in many countries. Although experimental psittacosis vaccines have been developed in birds, there is no need to develop human vaccine for such an infrequent disease.

8.10　Rickettsia

The pioneering research of Howard Taylor Ricketts, after whom the *Rickettsia rickettsii* is named and others in the early twentieth century demonstrated the rickettsial etiology of Rocky Mountain spotted fever and epidemic typhus. The order *Rickettsiales* includes a diverse group of gram-negative bacteria (0.3–0.5) μm× (0.6–2.0) μm with an obligatory intracellular existence and a mandatory transmission cycle that includes arthropods as hosts, reservoirs and vectors(Figure 8–14). Rickettsias are unable to synthesize certain metabolites and must obtain them from host cells instead. Once inside the host cell, the bacteria multiply primarily in the cytoplasm and continue reproduction. The host cell then bursts and liberates the bacterial cells. Rickettsias do not survive long outside their hosts and this may explain why they must be transmitted from animal to animal by arthropod vectors.

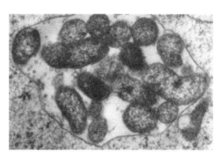

Figure 8 – 14　Electron micrograph of rickettsias, growing inside a vacuole of a blood cell

The order *Rickettsiales* is divided into two families, *Rickettsiaceae* and *Anaplasmataceae*. In general, pathogenicmembers of the *Rickettsiaceae* family, including spotted fever and typhus groups of rickettsia(SFGR and TGR, respectively) and *Orientia tsutsugamushi*, target infection predominantly in endothelial cells in mammals, including humans. In contrast, pathogens in *Anaplasmataceae* have a wider variety of *in vivo* targets, ranging from hematopoietic cells including phagocytes like monocytes, macrophages(*Ehrlichia canis*, *Ehrlichia chaffeensis*, *Ehrlichia muris*, *Ehrlichia ruminantium*, *Anaplasma bovis*, *Neorickettsia helminthoeca*, *Neorickettsia sennetsu*, *Neorickettsia risticii*) and neutrophils (*Anaplasma phagocytophilum*, *Ehrlichia ewingii*); to platelets(*Anaplasma platys*) or erythrocytes (*Anaplasma marginale*, *Anaplasma centrale*); to endothelial cells (*E. ruminantium*) and even intestinal epithelial cells (*N. risticii*). As a consequence of phylogenetic study based onthe 16S rRNA, *Coxiella burnetii* and *Rickettsiella grylli* were reclassified within *Legionellaceae*, *Eperythrozoon* sp. and *Haemobartonella* sp. within *Mycoplasmataceae*.

Few diseases have had a greater impact on the human history than epidemic typhus. *Rickettsia prowazekii*, the etiological agent of epidemic typhus, has caused millions of deaths and much human suffering. Epidemictyphus now occurs mainly in poor populations indeveloping countries, but various other rickettsial diseases are still widely distributed.

8.10.1　Major Human Rickettsias

8.10.1.1　Family *Rickettsiaceae*

There are only two recognized genera in the family *Rickettsiaceae* : *Rickettsia* and *Orientia* responsible for numerous diseases in many parts of the world (Table 8–21). The genus *Rickettsia* has classically been divided into the SFGR (including *R. rickettsii* and *R. akari*) and TGR (*R. prowazekii* and *R. typhi*). *O. tsutsugamushi*, the cause of scrub typhus, is transmitted by mite larvae (chiggers) andis sufficiently unique at the genetic level that itoccupies a distinct clade and genus.

Table 8–21　Human diseases caused by *Rickettsia* and *Orientia* species

Species	Disease	Geographical distribution	Mode oftransmission	Primary vectors	Main vertebrate hosts
Typhus group					
R. prowazekii	Epidemic typhus	Extant foci in Africa, north and southAmerica	Louse faeces	*Pediculus humanus-corporis*	Man, flying squirrels
R. typhi	Murine typhus	Primarily tropics and subtropics	Flea faeces	*Xenopsylla cheopis* andother fleas	Rodents and otherSmallmammals
Spotted fever group					
R. akari	Rickettsialpox	USA, Ukraine, Croatia, Korea, Turkey, Mexico	Bite of mouse mite	*Liponyssoides sanguineus*	House mice; possiblyother rodents
R. australis	Queensland tick typhus	Australia	Bite of tick	*Ixodes holocyclus*	Unknown
R. conorii	Boutonneuse fever	Europe, Africa, Middle East, India	Bite of tick	*Rhipicephalussanguineus*	Unknown
R. japonica	Japanese spotted fever	Japan and northeastern Asia	Bite of tick	*Dermacentor*, *Haemaphysalis*, *Ixodes* spp.	Unknown
R. rickettsii	Rocky Mountainspotted fever	North and southAmerica	Bite of tick	*Dermacentor* spp., *Rh. sanguineus*, *Amblyomma cajennense*	Rodents, opossums, dogs and other smallmammals
R. africae	African tick bite fever	Africa and Westindies	Bite of tick	*A. hebraeum*, *A. variegatum*	Unknown
R. parkeri	American tick bite fever	North and southAmerica	Bite of tick	*A. maculatum*, *A. americanum*, *A. triste*	Unknown
R. sibirica	North Asian tick typhus	Northern Asia	Bite of tick	*Dermacentor*, *Haemaphysalis* spp., etc.	Rodents and other smallmammals
R. honei	Flinders island spottedfever	Australia and southeast Asia	Bite of tick	*Bothriocrotonhydrosauri*	Unknown
R. slovaca	Tick-bornelymphadenopathy	Eurasia	Bite of tick	*Dermacentormarginatum*, *D. reticularis*	Unknown
R. felis	Flea-borne spottedfever	Worldwide	Flea; undeterminedmechanism	*Ctenocephalides felis*	Opossums
Scrub typhus group					
O. tsutsugamushi	Scrub typhus	Asia, Australia, islandsof south-west pacificand Indian oceans	Bite of larval mite	*Leptotrombidium* spp.	Rodents (especially rats)

Rickettsias possess major antigens such as lipopolysaccharide(LPS), 17-kDa lipoprotein, outer membrane proteins of the surface cell antigen (SCA) family and heat shock proteins. The Weil-FelixReaction, initially developed as a diagnostic test for rickettsioses, was based on the antigenic cross-reactions among rickettsial antigens, mostly LPS and antigens of OX (OX_{19}, OX_2 and OX_K) strains of *Proteus vulgaris*. Dilution of patient's serum can be tested against suspensions of the different *Proteus* strains (Table 8-22). Electron microscopic analyses of the rickettsialouter membrane fractions revealed the presence of a 7-to 16-nm-thick external layer, which is termed an S-layer and contains 10 to 15% of the total cellular protein. Such antigens have been characterized, including the OmpB, OmpA (present only in SFGR) and Sca4. Additional 14 genes putatively encoding SCA proteins were identified in sequenced rickettsial genomes, one of which, sca1, was present in all species.

Table 8-22   Weil-Felix reaction

Organism	Weil-Felix reaction		
	OX_{19}	OX_2	OX_K
R. prowazekii	+ + +	+	-
R. typhi	+ + +	+	-
R. rickettsii	+ + +	+ + +	-
O. tsutsugamushi	-	-	+ + +

8.10.1.2   *Rickettsia Prowazekii*

R. prowazekii is the etiologic agent of epidemic typhus (or louse-borne typhus), transmitted by the feces of lice, not the bite. Brazilian doctor, Henrique da Rocha Lima discovered this bacterium in 1916 and named it after his colleague Stanislaus von Prowazek, who had died from typhus in 1915.

(1) Morphology

R. prowazekii is Gram-negative bacterium with a bacilli (rod-shape) structure [(0. 3-0. 5) × (0. 6-2. 0) μm]. However, *R. prowazekii* could not be stained by Gram staining. Using Gimenez staining, *R. prowazekii* would retain basic fuchsine and appear brightred, whereas the background is stained in pale blue with the malachite green counterstain.

(2) Cultivation

As mentioned above, *R. prowazekii* could only grow in association with eukaryotic cells, within which they live free and divide by binary fission in the cytoplasm. As a consequence, *R. prowazekii* must be cultivatedin tissue culture or yolk sac of chicken embryos. L929 and Vero cells are used most frequently. Inoculation into guinea pigs was commonly used in the past.

(3) Genome

The *R. prowazekii* genome is composed of a singular circular chromosome, containing approximately 1 Mb and 834 protein coding genes. Also, 24% of *R. prowazekii* DNA is non-coding the largest amount in any microbial genome. No genes code for anaerobic glycolosis, however, complete coding sequences for the tricarbox ylicacid cycle and respiratory-chain complex are found. Because of lacking genes encoding many essential enzymes, they depend on the host for nutrition.

(4) Stability and Viability

R. prowazekii is expected to be susceptible to 1% sodium hypochlorite, 70% ethanol, 2% peracetic acid, 3% -6% hydrogen peroxide, iodine, glutaraldehyde and formaldehyde, based on the effectiveness of these agents against other Gram negative prokaryotic organisms. *R. prowazekii* can also be inactivated by moist heat (121 ℃ for a minimum of 15 minutes) and dry heat (170 ℃ for a minimum of an hour). *R. prowazekii is stable in lice feces for up to* 100 days and can be viable in a blood sample for several years if kept at-70 ℃. Sulphonamides should not be administered for they exacerbate rickettsial infections.

(5) Epidemiology

Although some mammals, such as flying squirrels, can harbor *R. prowazekii*, humans were considered the only reservoirfor *R. prowazekii*, which is transmitted between people mainly by thehuman body louse (*Pediculus humanus corporis*). Because of this, it primarily shows up in areas of overpopulation and poor economy. However, casesin most countries now typically result from imported or recru descent in fections, rather than from local maintenance of theorganism.

Epidemics occur during timeswhen lice are readily transferred from person to person. Lice become infected when they feed on the blood of an infected person and excrete *R. prowazekii* in their feces after several days. Lice defecate when they feed and *R. prowazekii* from louse feces can enter the body through the bite wound or other abrasions in the skin. Infected licedie prematurely within 7−10 days and *R. prowazekii* does not pass to a new generation in eggs. That is why louse is the vector rather than reservoir. However, for *R. prowazekii* can survive in louse feces for 2−3 months, human could be infected by inhalation probably. Moreover, *R. prowazekii* can establish persistent or latent in fection, so that recru descence at later time would provide an opportunity for transmission to lice and epidemic spread.

(6) Pathogenesis

R. prowazekii could disseminate through the bloodstream, attachto endothelial cells through OmpA, OmpB and other auto-transporter SCAs and enter endothelial cells by induced phagocytosis. Following internalization, *R. prowazekii* resides in thecytosol and is not enclosed in a membrane-bound phagosome. Several proteinsof *R. prowazekii* may be involved in membrane disruption, including phospholipase A2 (PLA2), phospholipase D (PLD) and hemolysins (TlyA and TlyC). Based on the activities of the PLA2, PLD and hemolysins, it was proposed that they may mediate phagosome escape and promote cell lysis latein infection. The pathological manifestations result more from direct injury than from immun opathological mechanisms. After damage of blood vessels, increased vascular permeability and interference with normal circulation can belife-threatening. Although *Rickettsia* does have LPS, it is not endotoxic.

The symptoms often begin suddenly 10−14 days after infection, with nonspecific initial signs including fever, malaise, chills, myalgia (which is often severe) and headache. After a few days after the fever, a pink rash will develop primarily on the extremities and move to the but tocks and stomach in some patients. In more severe cases it may develop hemorrhage, hypotension and renaldys function. Without treated, epidemic typhus will cause death in up to 40% of cases. Besides, the patients who survive a primary infection of *R. prowazekii* may develop a relatively milder reactivation of latent infection years later, referring to as recrudescent typhus or Brill-Zinsser disease.

(7) Immuneresponse to Infection

The data of immune response to *R. prowazekii* infection are quite limited. Most of the understanding of the immune response against *Rickettsia* derives from the mouse model study. The data show that NK cells are activated during the first 2 to 4 days of infection. And IFN-γ and IL-12 are probably the important cytokines involved. Besides, cellular immunity of the Th1 type is fundamental in the host defenses against infection. However, antibody, which can't enter infected cells, does not mediate directly clearance of *R. prowazekii* in the infected cell, but is important in secondary immune responses to the pathogens.

(8) Laboratory Diagnosis

As *R. prowazekii* is dangerous and fastidious to laboratory personnel, identification and cultivation of *R.*

prowazekii is not generally available outside reference laboratories. If necessary, *R. prowazekii* can be cultured in L929 cells. In oculation into guinea pigs or chicken eggs was commonly used in the past.

1)Serological and immunological diagnostic methods：Epidemic typhus is usually diagnosed by serology. Afourfold rise in titer should be documented, usually for retrospective confirmation. A number of serological tests have been described, includin gindirect fluor escence antibody (IFA) tests, various agglutination tests (e. g. ,plate microagglutination, latexagglutination) and enzyme immunoassays such as ELISAs and dot blot assays. Patients with Brill-Zinsser disease usually have elevations in specific IgG rather than IgM. The traditional Weil-Felix reaction is no longer recommended becauseof cross-react with *R. typhi*.

2)Nucleic acid amplification tests：Detection of rickettsial DNA is rapid and specific by PCR, which can distinguish *R. prowazekii* from other rickettsia, including *R. typhi*. A single primer pair that amplifies all or most rickettsias can be designed fromthe genes encoding 16S rRNA.

(9)Control and Treatment

It is actually impossible to eliminate rickettsial infections because of their zoonotic nature. Measures aimed at reducing rodent or *R. prowazekii* populationsmay help to reduce the risk of infection. Besides, there are no commercial vaccines for epidemic typhus. The attenuated E strain of *R. prowazekii* induces protective immunity, but is unsuitable for general use because it could cause a mild typhus in about 10% –15% of those with inoculation and maybe revert to being virulent after animal passage.

The case fatality rate is increased significantly if treatment is delayed for more than 5 days. Thus, empirical tetracycline therapy is necessary and appropriate for patients who have had a fever and a history consistent with the epidemiological features of epidemictyphus. Chloramphenicol is an alternative, but is less effective. β-lactam and aminogly cosideantibiotics are in effective.

8. 10. 1. 3 *Rickettsia Typhi*

Endemic typhus, also known asmurine typhus, is a flea-borne infectious disease caused by *R. typhi* (or *R. mooseri*). Patients infected with this pathogen develop symptoms similar to those of epidemic typhus. However, endemic typhus is much milder thanepidemic typhus. Fatal cases are uncommon but occasionally occur, specifically in the elderly. Nevertheless, it is severe enough to require convalescence of several months after infection. *R. typhi* is another member of the TGR group of rickettsias and resembles *R. prowazekii* in its biologic, genetic and immunologic properties.

(1)Epidemiology

Endemic typhus is found throughout the world, but is most prevalent in warmer countries. The distribution of the disease is associated with the distribution of its hosts and vectors. *R. typhi* is mainly transmitted by the rat flea (*Xenopsylla cheopis*). The flea remain sinfected for life with its lifespan and reproductive activities unaffected.

The primary reservoirs are the various rodents(mainly the rats) , but occasionally other animal sact as hosts. Rats serve not only as simple hosts, but also as amplifying hosts. The humans, infected through fleas, are only accidental hosts in the natural cycleof *R. typhi*. Like transmission of *R. prowazekii*, the flea defecates when it feed on a human host. The *R. typhi*, which is excreted in the flea feces, could be inoculated by fleabite or skin abrasions. *R. typhi* can survive in the flea feces for several years. Hence, *R. typhi* could infect humans by contamination of the conjunctiva orinhalation.

(2)Pathogenesis

The pathogenic substances and process of infection resemble those of *R. prowazekii*. However, murine typhus is often confused with viral illnesses. Most infected people do not realize that they have been bitten by fleas. The symptoms of endemic typhus often begin 8–12 days after infection, including headache, fever, muscle pain, joint pain, nausea and vomiting. 40% –50% of patients will develop a discrete rash 6 days after the onset of above symptoms. Up to 45% will develop neurological signs such as confusion, stupor, seizures or imbalance, but severe cases are not common comparing those of epidemic typhus.

8.10.1.4　Control and Treatment

Like *R. prowazekii*, measures aimed at reducing the risk of infection by avoiding contact with infected fleas, such as keeping rodents and wild animals away from human regions and wearing gloves for handling sick or dead animals. Endemictyphus is highly treatable with antibiotics, including tetracycline, chloramphenicol and doxycycline, when given soon after symptoms begin. The patients can recover fully with less than 1% mortality. There is no commercially available vaccine against endemic typhus.

(1) *Rickettsia Rickettsii*

Spotted fever rickettsiosis, commonly called Rocky Mountain spotted fever (RMSF), was first emerged in the western UnitedStates in 1896. RMSF is caused by *R. rickettsii*, a member of the SFGR group andis transmitted to humans by various ticks, most commonly the dog tick and wood ticks. *R. rickettsii* could be present in the salivary glands of the tick and in the ovaries of female ticks. Humans get infected from the bite of aninfected tick.

Bacteria of *R. rickettsii*, unlike other rickettsias, grow within the nucleus of the host cell as well as in host cell cytoplasm. The symptoms often begin 3–12 days after exposure, including fever and a severe headache. A systemic rash breaks out after a few days, accompanied by gastrointestinal symptoms such as diarrhea and vomiting. The symptoms of RMSFpersist for over 2 weeks if left untreated. Tetracyclineor chloramphenicol generally promotes a prompt recoveryfrom RMSF if administered early and treated patients have less than 1% mortality. Mortality in untreated cases resembles that of typhus, up to 30%. No effective vaccine against RMSF is commercially available.

(2) *Orientia Tsutsugamushi*

O. tsutsugamushi, the causative agent of scrub typhus, is an obligate intracellular bacterium. Scrub typhus is a chigger-borne zoonosis that is of greatest public health importance in tropical rural Asia. Humans are accidental hosts, acquiring *O. tsutsugamushi* during feeding of a larval trombiculid mite, popularly known as chiggers.

(3) Morphology

The bacteria are rods with 0.2–0.5 μm in width and from 0.6 to 3.0 μm in length, slightly larger than typhus and spotted fever group rickettsias. The cell wall of *O. tsutsugamushi* differs notably from that of other rickettsias, contains unique proteins and lacks LPS and peptidoglycan. After Giemsa staining, the bacteria are deep purple and grouped in perinuclear clusters.

(4) Cultivation

O. tsutsugamushi is an obligate intracellular parasite thatinvades host cells by induced phagocytosis and escapes from the phagosome to the cytosol. Once free in the host cytoplasm, the bacteria replicate by transverse binary fission in the perinuclear area. *O. tsutsugamushi* is less stable than other rickettsiasin an extracellular environment and multiplies slowly in culture.

(5) Antigenicstructure

The bacteria have multiple major antigenicproteins with strain-specific and cross-reactive epitopes. Three classical strains (Karp, Gilliam and Kato) and new antigenic types (from Thailand) have been used as prototype strains. One of the major surface protein antigens, 10% to 15% of total protein, is the variable 56-kD aprotein. This protein is an immunodominant antigenand can be recognized by sera from most scrub typhus patients by group-and strain-specific monoclonal antibodies.

（6）Epidemiology

Because of the restricted habitat of the chiggers, transmission often occurs in zones where primaryforest has been cleared and replaced by scrub vegetation, hence the name scrubtyphus. The transmission occurs within a triangular-shaped area of more than 5 million square miles bounded to the north by Siberia and the Kamchatka Peninsula, to the south by Queensland, Australia and to the west by Afghanistan.

The chiggers only feed onmammal tissue fluid once in their lifetime and constitute the reservoir of infection through transovarial transmission. Chiggers are maintained in nature by feeding on a variety of wild rodents. Rodents are important for the population density of chiggers but are not a reservoir of *O. tsutsugamushi*. Humans are accidental hosts, getting infected during feeding of a chigger when they fortuitously encroach on the habitat of the chiggers. Chigger activity is determined by temperature and humidity. Thus, transmission depends on the seasonal activities of both humans and chiggers.

（7）Pathogenesis

Heparansulfate proteoglycans contribute to the attachment of *O. tsutsugamushi* to host cells. The bacteria have been demonstrated in a variety of cells in humans, including monocytes, macrophages, cardiac myocytes, hepatocytes and endothelial cells. Activation of endothelial cell leads to the recruitment of macrophages and chemokines areproduced from macrophages and endothelial cells. *O. tsutsugamushi* can replicate inside macrophages and suppress the production of the inflammatory cytokines TNF-α and IL-6. Besides, scrub typhus bacteria can inhibit apoptosis of macrophages.

Depending on the factors of host and the virulence of the infecting strain, scrub typhus may be mild or fatal. Symptoms develop 7−18 days after exposure and are characterized by sudden onset of fever, headache and myalgia. A maculopapular rash often develops 2−3 days after onset. Especially, apathognomonic eschar is often apparent at the site of the bite with enlargement of local lymph nodes. The eschar begins as a small papule, enlarges, undergoes central necrosis and acquires a blackened crust. Progression of the illness maybe accompanied by interstitial pneumonitis, generalized lymphadenopathy and splenomegaly. Death may result from encephalitis, respiratory failure and circulatory failure. Patients who survive generally become afebrile after 2−3 week sif left untreated.

（8）Immune Response to Infection

Infection with *O. tsutsugamushi* usually results in an acute, self-limiting disease. Antibodies can enhance clearance of the free *O. tsutsugamushi* in the bloodstream. However, immunity to the obligate intracellular *O. tsutsugamushi* is mainly mediated by T cells. Because of heterologous strains, reinfection may occur, but cause a milder disease.

（9）Laboratory Diagnosis

The clinical and laboratory features of scrub typhus are nonspecific. The eschar isthe single most useful diagnostic clue, but eschars appear in only a minority of *O. tsutsugamushi* infections.

1）Cytological identification: *O. tsutsugamushi* can be isolated from blood or tissues of patients. Intra peritoneally in jection into mice with whole blood from patients, the signs of illness or death can be observed. The organisms can be demonstrated in Giemsa-stained smears from the surface of the spleen or peritoneum.

2）Serological and Immunological Diagnostic Methods

For many years, the serodiagnosis of scrub typhus depended on the Weil-Felix reaction, which detects antibodies produced during infection of *O. tsutsugamushi*. However, theWeil-Felix reaction is not sensitive enough (less than 50%). The gold standard confirmatory tests are the indirect immunoperoxidase test and the immunofluorescentassay (IFA), usingthe *O. tsutsugamushi* antigens deriving from cell oryolksac propagation.

3）Nucleic acid amplification techniques：Scrub typhus can be diagnosed by PCR amplification of the 56-kDa protein gene of *O. tsutsugamushi*.

（10）Control and Treatment

Avoiding the contact with chiggers can reduce risk of infection. Applying repellent to boots, socks and legs and not lying directly on the ground could be useful. There sponse of treatment with doxycycline or chloramphenicol is generally rapid and the patients can be afebrile. Thus, if the temperature has not returnedto normal within 48 hours after treatment, infection is not caused by *O. tsutsugamushi*. Currently, there is no commercial vaccine in use.

8. 10. 1. 5　Family *Anaplasmataceae*

There are currently five genera classified within the *Anaplasmataceae* family, including *Ehrlichia*, *Anaplasma*, *Neorickettsia* and *Wolbachia*. Members of this family were first recognized because of veterinary disease, but human diseases are now demonstrated. *E. chaffeensis*, *E. ewingii* and *A. phagocytophilum* emerged as the causes of tick-borne diseases（Table 8-23）.

Table 8-23　Human diseases caused by *Ehrlichia*, *Anaplasma* and *Neorickettsia* species

Species	Disease	Geographical distribution	Means of transmission	Primary vectors
E. chaffeensis	Monocytic ehrlichiosis	North and South America, Africa, Asia	Tick bite	*Amblyomma americanum*
E. ewingii	Ehrlichiosis ewingii	USA	Tick bite	*A. americanum*
A. phagocytophilum	Granulocytic anaplasmosis	USA, Eurasia	Tick bite	*Ixodes spp.*

These organisms are small Gram-negative bacteria. They multiply within membrane-bound cytoplasmic vacuoles and form characteristic microcolonies resembling mulberries. Electron microscopy reveals two morphological forms, larger reticulate cells（replicating forms）and smaller dense-corecells（infectious forms）, in the developmental cycle.

8. 10. 1. 6　Genus *Ehrlichia*

Ehrlichia are the causative agent of ehrlichiosis. *Ehrlichia* survive in phagosomal vacuoles within the host cell. Both of their replicating and infectious formsare capable of binary fission. Phagosomes can contain tens of ehrlichial cells. With staining by Romanowsky-derived dyes, the ehrlichial cells with mulberry-like structure can be seen on peripheral blood smears.

Typically, *Ehrlichia* infect leukocytes in humansand other mammals, in contrast to *Anaplasma*, which infect bone-marrow-derived cells, including erythrocytes, platelets and leukocytes. *E. chaffeensis* and *E. ewingii* are the two major pathogens. *E. chaffeensis* is the cause of human monocytic ehrlichiosis（HME）which presents fever, headache, malaise, myalgia and nausea.

（1）Epidemiology

The infections are tick-borne zoonosis and the pathogens are maintained in nature involving the mammal reservoirs and the arthropod vectors. In arthropods, ehrlichial bacteria are transmitted transstadially（molting from larvae to nymphs and nymphs to adults）, but not transovarially. Therefore, an infected host is needed for maintenance of the life cyclein nature.

Most cases of HME occur in the south-central and southeastern regions of the United States. Reports from other parts of the world also exist. In the United States, the mainarthropod vector is *A. americanum* (the Lone Star tick). The main mammal reservoir for *E. chaffeensis* is *Odocoileus virginianus* (the white-tailed deer). Other reservoirs were also demonstrated, including domestic dogs, opposums, foxes, wolves, raccoons, voles, coyotes and goats.

(2) Pathogenesis

Ehrlichialbacteria enter the body via a tick bite (nymph or adult). The mean incubation time is about 10 days. The bacteria attachto the host cell receptor (E-and L-selectin) through surface-exposed glycoproteins. After internalization, they reside in early endosomes and inhibitfusion of endosomes with lysosomes.

The pathologic lesions in the different organs, such as lungs, liver, spleen and bone marrow, are due to the immune response of the host, leading to perivascular lymphohistiocytic aggregates. Additional pathologic lesions include granulomas inthe bone marrow and liver and interstitial pneumonitis. The interstitial pneumonitis canlead to diffuse alveolar damage. In the central nervous system, *E. chaffeensis* induces the meningoencephalitis with the presence of perivascular lesions. The cellular infiltrates can be seen in the affected organs.

Clinical manifestations of HME range from a mild febrile illness to multisystem organ failure. The most common presentation is fever (almost always>38 ℃), headache and myalgia. Other symptoms and signs include nausea, vomiting, abdominalpain, respiratory and CNS-related manifestations. The skin rash that involves the trunk and extremities occurs in 12% to 36% of patients. The rash is far more common in children within up to 67% of cases. The mortality rate is higher in patients over 60 years old. The overall mortality rate is 2% to 3%.

(3) Laboratory Diagnosis and Treatment

There are four kinds of testing available for diagnosis of HME, including direct visualization of the ehrlichial bacteria on peripheral blood smears or other tissues, cultivation of *E. chaffeensis* in cells, molecular detection of ehrlichial DNA or RNA by nucleic acid amplification techniques and detection of antibodies inserum by immunofluorescence antibody (IFA) or Western blotting. Doxycycline is the preferred antibiotic. Theconsensus of treatment equates to at least 10 days of therapy, till 3 to 5 days after defervescence.

8. 10. 1. 7   Genus *Anaplasma*

All bacteria of this genus are tick-transmitted and have the preference for infecting the bone marrow-derived cells of the host. Human granulocytic anaplasmosis (HGA) is a tick-borne zoonosis caused by *A. phagocytophilum*. Disease includes high fever, headaches, malaise andmyalgia. By Giemsa or Wright-Giemsa staining, bacteriacan be seen on the peripheral blood smear. Like *B. burgdorferi*, *A. phagocytophilum* cycles within hard-bodied ticks. *A. phagocytophilum* primarily infects granulocytes, mostly peripheral blood neutrophils.

(1) Epidemiology

HGA is highly prevalent in both the United States and Europe. Because of the same tick vector, HGA may occasionally occur concurrently with Lymedisease or babesiosis. Deer, canines, rodents anddomestic ruminants are important reservoirs. Immature ticks acquire *A. phagocytophilum* by feeding on the blood of infected animals. And the bacteria are transmitted during asubsequent blood feed. However, the bacteria are maintained transstadially but not transovarially by ticks. Thus, the transmission strongly depends on the seasonal activities of ticks, history oftick bite and distribution of the ticks.

(2) Pathogenesis

Cytokine-associated immunopathological mechanisms are probably important. *A. phagocytophilum* evades the host immunesystem by antigenic variation and by modulating the host immunity. Within phagosomes of phagocytes, *A. phagocytophilum* inhibits the fusion of phagosome with lysosomes. And *A. phagocytophilum* can prevent killing by reactive oxygen species in neutrophils. Besides, *Anaplasma* prolong the lifespan of the host cells by inhibiting apoptosis to accommodate its slow generation time (about 8 h). Moreover, suppression of neutrophil by *A. phagocytophilum* could predispose to other opportunistic infections.

Nevertheless, most symptomatic patients recover in oneto two weeks without any sequelae, even if left untreated. Unlike the reservoirs of *A. phagocytophilum*, infected humans and other animals develop clinical signs. The incubation period is 7-10 days. Clinical signs and symptoms are similarto those of HME, but the disease is less severe and the mortality rate is lessthan 1%. The rash and CNS-related manifestations are rare.

(3) Laboratorydiagnosis

Theisolation of *Anaplasma* species is difficult. HGA is diagnosed mainly by demonstrating the development of specific antibodies during convalescence. However, HGA can be diagnosed by identification in Giemsa-stained peripheral blood neutrophil. Indirect immunofluorescence tests can be used with *A. phagocytophilum* antigens deriving from cell culturepropagation. And *A. phagocytophilum* is detectable by PCR with specific primers.

(4) Controland Treatment

Prevention of HGA is mainly achieved by avoiding tick habitat, by wearing tick-proof clothing and applying insect repellents containing N, N-Diethyl-m-toluamide (DEET). If possible, examine carefully for ticks after hiking in tick habitat and remove any ticks immediately. Vaccines are currently unavailable. Doxycycline can shorten the course of infection and reduces mortality. The use of chloramphenicol is notrecommended.

8.11　Spirochete

Spirochetes are Gram-stain negative, helical or spiral-shaped, motile cells with 0.1-3 μm in diameter and 4-250 μm in length. Most spirochetes possessa unique cellular ultrastructure, endoflagella, which are theinternal organelles of motility (Figure 8-15). The class *Spirochaetia* contains spirochetes in one order, *Spirochaetales*, which is presently comprised of four families, namely *Spirochaetaceae*, *Brachyspiraceae*, *Brevinemataceae* and *Leptospiraceae*.

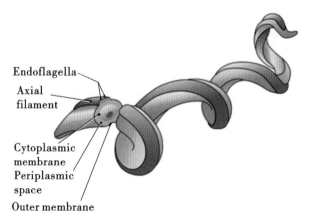

Figure 8-15　Schematic representation of a spirochete

Human diseases caused by these bacteria (Table 8–24) include syphilis, which has been known for thousands of years and infections such as Lyme disease and leptospirosis, the prevalence and geographical distribution of which are still being evaluated.

Table 8–24　Major human diseases caused by spirochaetes

Family	Species	Disease	Distribution	Primary mode of transmission	Animal reservoirs
Spirochaetaceae	T. pallidum	Syphilis	Worldwide	Sexual-congenital	None
	T. pertenue	Yaws	Tropics and subtropics	Direct contact	None
	T. endemicum	Bejel	Arid, subtropical or temperate areas	Mouth-to-mouth via utensils	None
	T. carateum	Pinta	Arid, tropical Americas	Skin-to-skin contact	None
	B. recurrentis	Epidemic relapsing fever	Central, East Africa, South American Andes	Louse bites	None
	Borrelia spp.	Endemic relapsing fever	Worldwide	Tick bites	Yes
	B. burgdorferi	Lyme disease	Worldwide	Tick bites	Yes
Leptospiraceae	L. interrogans	leptospirosis	Tropics and subtropics	Direct or indirect contact with infected urine, tissues or secretions	Yes

8.11.1　Family *Spirochaetaceae*, Genus *Treponema*

By contact with infectious body fluids or by fomites, pathogenic *Treponema* species including the causative agents of venereal syphilis and the nonvenereal treponematosis, disfiguring yaws (caused by *T. pallidum* ssp. *pertenue*), bejel (caused by *T. endemicum*) and pinta (caused by *T. carateum*), cause skin lesions. They show only subtle antigenic differences and are characterized primarily by the clinical syndromes they cause. Other avirulent species form part of the normal bacterial flora of the oral cavity, intestinal tract and genital areas of humans or other mammals.

8.11.1.1　*Treponema Pallidum* Subsp. *Pallidum* (*T. Pallidum*)

T. pallidum (Nichols strain) is a motile spirochete that is generally transmitted by close sexual contact and enters host tissue by breaches in squamous or columnar epithelium. *T. pallidum* is the causative agent of syphilis that, if left untreated, can last for years to decades.

8.11.1.2　Morphology

T. pallidum is a Gram-stain negative bacterium, 6–20 μm in length and 0.1–0.2 μm in width. It has tapered ends with 6 to 14 spiral coils between and the tightly coiled structure is not visible by light microscopy without silver staining (Figure 8–16). In clinical practice, dark field microscopy is used to study the rotatory motion with flexion and back-and-forth squiggle of the virulent *T. pallidum*. This form of motion is suggested to facilitate penetration of *T. pallidum* through tissue. The spiral-shaped body of *T. pallidum* is surrounded by a cytoplasmic membrane, which is enclosed by a loosely associate douter membrane. A thin layer of peptidoglycan between the membranes provides structural stability. Endo flagella organelles that allow for the characteristic corkscrew motility of *T. pallidum*, are located in the axial filament out of the periplasmic space.

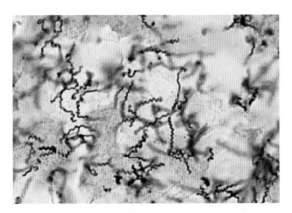

Figure 8 – 16   Silver-stained *T. pallidum* from a syphilitic chancre

8. 11. 1. 3   Cultivation

T. pallidum could be cultivated continuously in artificialmedia with cells. However, *T. pallidum* are highly susceptible to reactive oxygen species. Thus, the cultivation should be carried out under microaerophilic conditions (93.5% N_2, 5% CO_2 and 1.5% O_2). Besides, *T. pallidum* can be propagated through serial intratesticular passage in animals. Rabbits are widely used for experimental infection, although primates, guinea pigs and hamsters can also be infected. *T. pallidum* is highly temperature sensitive, so the rabbits should be maintained at 18–20 ℃ and the skin inoculation sites should be kept free of hair.

8. 11. 1. 4   Antigenicstructure

The *T. pallidum* genomicsequence does not reveal any classical virulence factors accounting for syphilis symptoms. However, the outer envelope of *T. pallidum* contains lipid, protein and carbohydrates and is similar to the outer envelope of Gram-stain negative bacteria. The cell walls contain muramic acid, glucosamine ornithine, glycine and alanine, but lack lipopolysaccharide (LPS). Peptidogly can represents 1% of the dry weight of cells. The *T. pallidum* polypeptides consist of the prefix TpN (for *T. pallidum* Nichols, the reference strain) followed by a consensus relative molecular mass, such as TpN15, TpN33, TpN47 and so on. Several of these, including TpN47, were identified as surface exposed proteins.

8. 11. 1. 5   Genome

The genome of *T. pallidum* subsp. *pallidum* (Nichols strain) was sequenced in 1998. It has one of the smallest bacterial genomes at 1. 138 million base pairs without any recognized extrachromosomal elements, bacteriophage sequences or insertion elements and has limited metabolic capabilities, reflecting its adaptation through genome reduction to the rich environment of mammalian tissue.

8. 11. 1. 6   Stability and Viability

T. pallidum is very sensitive to temperature and drying. Limited heat tolerance, oxygen sensitivity and possibly other asyet-unrecognized factors, may hinder the replication of *T. pallidum* both *in vivo* and *in vitro*. Penicillinremains highly effective in *T. pallidum* infection and the primary and secondary stages of syphilis can typically be cured by a single injection of benzathine penicillin G. However, clinically resistance to macrolides has emerged.

8.11.1.7 Pathogenesis

Several prominent lipoproteins of *T. pallidum* are implicated in the induction of inflammatory mediators via toll-like receptor 2 (TLR-2) recognitionin the host. Without any proved endotoxin and exotoxin, motility is considered as the main virulence factor for *T. pallidum*, which resultin extreme invasiveness, rapid attachment to cell surfaces and penetration of endothelial junctions and tissue layers.

Syphilis is an STI (sexual transmitted infection) caused by *T. pallidum*. The infection is transmitted by sexual contactor through vertical transmission of *T. pallidum* from the infected mother to the baby to cause congenital infection. However, the infection has a great variety of clinical presentations in infected patients that may resemble a variety of other infectiousand autoimmune etiologies.

Syphilis iscontrolled in developed countries following the introduction of open access venereal disease clinics, the availability of penicillin and antenatal serological screening. It still remains a problem in high-risk populations with multiple sexual partners and insome developing countries. Syphilis kills about 100,000 people per year worldwide. According to the WHO data, the median syphilis rate was 25.1 cases per 100,000 adult population among the 55 countries that reported in 2014 (Table 8-25). Untreated syphilis in pregnancy is a major cause of morbidity and mortality, resulting in fetal deaths and stillbirths, preterm or low-birth-weight infants, neonatal death and syphilis infections in infants.

Table 8-25   Syphilis case rates (cases per 100,000 adult population or live births)

WHO region	Median syphilis case rate	Median congenital syphilis rate
African Region	46.6	5.0
Region of the Americas	34.1	33.8
Eastern MediterraneanRegion	2.8	0
European Region	6.2	0.4
South-East Asia Region	5.9	2.3
Western Pacific Region	93.0	6.6
Overall	25.7	4.9

The stages of untreated syphilis can be classified asfollows: primary syphilis (chancre, regional lymphadenopathy), secondary syphilis (disseminated maculopapular eruption, generalized lymphadenopathy), latent syphilis (recurrence of secondary syphilis symptoms) and tertiary syphilis (gummas, cardiovascularsyphilis and late neurological symptoms). A schematicdiagram of untreated syphilis is shown in Figure 8-17.

(1) Primary Infection

This period immediately follows infection with an incubation period of 9 days to one month. In the male, initial infection is usually on the penis; in the female it is most often in the vagina, cervix orperineal region. In about 10% of cases, infection is extragenital, usually in the oral region. The initial lesion is a pain less ulcer, usually in the genital tract, which has arubbery edge and is associated with regionally mphadeno pathy. Serum can be expressed from the ulcer crater. This lesion is known asthe primary chancre, which is frequently overlooked by infected patients because it is temporary and painless. Polymorphonuclear lymphocytes (PMNs) are seen invery early acquired and experimentally induced syphilislesions. In syphilis, the chancre represents a localized, primaryinfection from which the bacteria disseminate.

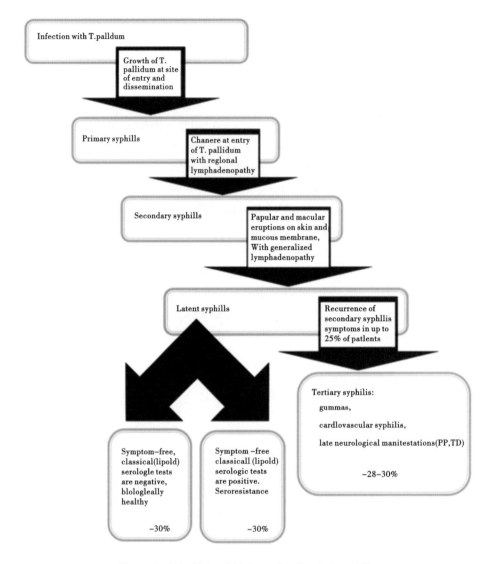

Figure 8-17   Natural history of untreated syphilis

(2) Secondary Phase

The infections of majority patients go on to secondary syphilis six weeks or later. Secondary syphilis results from the dissemination of *T. pallidum* via lymphatics to the bloodstream and formation of lesions at multiple sites in the skin and internalorgans. The enlarged lesions, appearing in warm and moist areas including the perineum and anus, arehighly infectious. Secondary syphilis is characterized by an acute febrileillness with a generalized non-itchy scalingrash, which is also found on the palms andsoles and generalized lymphadenopathy develops. Other symptoms include meningismus, myalgia, weight loss, anorexia and arthralgia. Localized in flammation of the oralcavity, tongue and genital mucous membranes cancause mucous patches. The diverse manifestations of human syphilis demonstrate the invasiveness of *T. pallidum*.

(3) Latent Phase

In the latentstage of syphilis, it seems that *T. pallidum* is clinically silent and only detectable by serological testing. The latent phase may last from five to more than 20 years. During this time, the characteristic granulomatous immune reaction, which is intended to surround and isolate invading *T. pallidum*, has evolved gradually in the host. Late in the latent stage, clinical manifestations are lacking, but serological tests are positive. However, histological evaluation of the lesions of this period reveals typical tissue components of tertiary syphilisalready. At thisstage, the pathogensare no longer transmitted by sexual intercourse.

(4)Tertiary Syphilis

This is the final stage of the disease, which involves other organ systems and may lead to devastating cardiovascular and neurological complications. Within the tissues, *T. pallidum* is of smaller numbers and could be isolated by a granulomatous tissue reaction. However, the patient is non-infective and the pathogensare not detec table in the blood and body fluids.

The clinical symptoms result from various forms of dysfunction. Skin manifestations are the earliest symptoms oftertiary syphilis. However, appearance of these beyond a decade is more usual. Skin lesionsevolve in approximately 15% of untreated patients, including cutaneous nodules and syphilitic gummas. The most typical lesion of cardiovascular manifestation is granulomatous in flammation of the ascending aorta. This syphilitic aortitis follows an asymptomatic course in the majority of patients, while the proportion of symptomatic patients is as low as 10%. Besides, late neurological dysfunctioncan give rise to destruction in the spinal cord, leading to tabesdorsalis, which is characterized by sensory ataxia in the lower extremities, accompanied by gastric pain and vomiting. Destruction of cerebralcortex can beassociated with psychiatric disturbance including delusions and megalomania. A prerequisite to the neurologicalsymptoms is invasion of the CNS by *T. pallidum*. If left untreated, these complications are fatal in syphilitic patients.

(5)Congenital Infection

During pregnancy, the *T. pallidum* could be transmitted from an infected mother to the fetus, resulting in congenital syphilis. Syphilis may contribute to stillbirth, preterm labor and intrauterine growth restriction. The early syndromes of congenital syphilis may be acute with rhinitis, rash, osteochondritis and hepatosplenomegaly or without syndromes. Later complications may arise with neurosyphilis, cranial nerve palsies and the results of the infection on the developing bone and cartilage. A child with congenital syphilis may manifest a range of neurological disorders later in life.

8.11.1.8　Immune Response to Infection

T. pallidum infection evokes cellular and humoral immune responses. The humoral response manifested by production of cardiolipin and treponemal antibodies is the basis for serodiagnosis of syphilis. *T. pallidum* antibodies appear after infection simultaneously with the cardiolipin antibodies. The treponemal antibodies persist in the host even after treatment, whereas the cardiolipin antibodies parallel the dynamics of the infection and are useful in evaluating the therapeutic effect. Besides, autoantibodies to tissue components (e. g. phospholipids), to blood cells and to serum globulins are also produced by syphilitic patients. The existence of such antibodies hints that autoimmunity may play an important role in syphilitic manifestations. Cell-mediated immune responses to *T. pallidum* involve activation of macrophages and consequently the induction of CD^+8 T cells and helper CD^+4 T cells. The various subsets of CD^+4 T cells and the cytokines they produce, play a crucial role in determining the outcome of syphilis in terms of both protective immunity and immunopathology.

8.11.1.9　Laboratory Diagnosis

(1)Cytologicalidentification

T. pallidum has a characteristic corkscrew motility. Darkfield microscopy (DFM)identification of *T. pallidum* with typical motility is a rapid and reliable test. Specimenscollected from active epidermal and mucosal lesions (especially chancres)are most useful. However, mouth lesions cannot be examined by this test for many non-pathogenic treponemesinthis site. Besides, *T. pallidum* can be identified from lesions and in biopsy material by commercial direct fluorescent antibody (DFA). The DFA can be ideally used for specimens from mouth lesions because it will differentiate *T. pallidum* from other treponemes.

(2) Serological and Immunological Diagnostic Methods

Serologicaltests are valuable indiagnosis of syphilis when ulcerative lesions are not available for DFMi-dentification. In primary syphilis, all serologicaltests are less sensitive than direct visualization of *T. pallidum*. Nearlyall serological tests are reactive since syphilis has reached the secondary stage. Examples of results can be found in Table 8–26.

Table 8–26　Diagnosisof syphilis

	VDRL/RPR	TPHA	FTA-ABS	FTA-IgM
Congenital syphilis	+	+	+	+
Primary syphilis	+	−/+	−/+	+
Untreated secondary	+	+	+	+
Treated or late	−	+	+/−	−

VDRL: venereal disease reference laboratorytest; RPR: rapid plasmin reagin-card test; TPHA: *T. pallidum* haemagglutination test; FTA-ABS: fluorescent treponemal antibody-absorption test; FTA-IgM: fluorescent treponemal antibody IgM test.

The diagnostic tests for syphilis can be divided into twogroups: nontreponemal and treponemal. Both groupshave distinctive characteristics and the results are complementary. For the assessment of the patient's status, results of both groups should be taken into consideration.

1) Nontreponemal tests: Nontreponemal tests can quantitatively detectthe anti-lipid IgM and IgGantibodies (reagins). Thesetests include the venereal disease research laboratory (VDRL) and the rapid plasma reagin-card (RPR) tests with similar sensitivities and specificities. The antigen for VDRL is a defined mixtureof cardiolipin, lecithin and cholesterol. Positive results areindicated by flocculation and should be titred. The RPR test, in which the antigenfor VDRL is carried by carbonparticles, is a modification of VDRL. Serum and reagents are mixed on acard and positive results are indicated byagglutination. For VDRL and RPR tests are the most sensitive earlyserological tests, both of them could be used for routine diagnosis and mass screening.

However, these lipid-based tests may be biologicalfalse-positive, because of the existing of other nontreponemal diseases, such as lupus erythematosus, rheumatoid arthritis, lepriasis, measles and parasitosis.

2) Treponemal tests: The antigenused in treponemal tests is derived from Nicholsstrain or Reiterstrain of *T. pallidum*. These tests are more specific and even remain positive after successful therapy. Thus, they could be used to confirm positive nontreponemaltests and toscreen congenital syphilis. However, these tests cannot differentiate between syphilis and the nonvenereal treponematoses (Yaws, Bejel and Pinta), for the almost identical antigens ofthese pathogens.

The *T. pallidum* haemagglutination (TPHA) test is a simple and specific test for routine screening. Its result may be negative in primary infection, but typically remains positive for life even with successful therapy. Fluorescent treponemal antibody-absorption (FTA-ABS) test is an indirect fluorescent antibody test with high specificity, but not specific for the diagnosis of neurosyphilis in cerebrospinal fluid (CSF). Patient serum is mixed with an absorbent (the "ABS" part of the test) containing an extract of Reiter's treponemes to remove the antibodies that are not specific for the syphilis. Then the specificantigen is applied to the pre-adsorbed serum, which is consequently detected by fluorescein-labelled anti-human globulin. Fluorescent treponemal antibody IgM (FTA-IgM) testusually presents in diagnosis of untreatedprimary or secondary syphilis. The positiveresult may reflect persisting antigen. However, interpretation of the FTA-IgM inlate syphilis is less valuable.

3) Nucleicacid amplification techniques: The detection of *T. pallidum* by PCR is theoretically possible from any material, such asswabs, blood, CSF, tissue biopsies and amniotic fluid. The PCR assays demonstrate specificity of 95% –98% for *T. pallidum* and can be used for oral and rectalsamples as well. Therefore, if *T. pallidum* infection is suspected from histological findings or clinical aspects, PCR assays are more sensitive and reliable for thedetection of *T. pallidum*.

4) Diagnosis ofcongenital syphilis: The diagnosis of congenital syphilis depends on acombination of physical, radiographic, serologic findings and efforts to demonstrate the pathogen directly. The diagnosis is proven when it is possible to identify *T. pallidum* by microscopy or PCR in specimens from lesions, placenta, umbilical cord, plasma, CSF orautopsy material.

8. 11. 1. 10   Control and Treatment

Theinterruption of syphilis transmission in its infectiousstagesis extremely important. Building on the finding through routine blood testing, syphilis control programs increasingly emphasized case prevention by aggressive treatmentof sex partners. The exposed sex partners should be identified and then be offered treatment (termed "epidemiological treatment") before they could either spread theinfection and/or develop symptoms. There are no commercialvaccines for syphilis.

All the pathogenic treponemes are sensitive tobenzylpenicillin. Thus, prolonged high-dose therapy with procaine benzylpenicillin has been the traditional method of treatment for primary and secondary syphilis. In late syphilis, aqueous benzylpenicillin is used for neurosyphilis treatment. However, successful elimination of the organism may not result in a clinical curein neurosyphilis.

8. 11. 1. 11   Other Pathogenic *Treponema* Species

The treponemal pathogens were previously divided into four species butrecent DNA homology studies identify aclose relationship between three, which arecurrently classified as subspecies of *T. pallidum*. Therefore, the causative bacterium of syphilis is *T. pallidum* subsp. *pallidum*, of Bejel is *T. pallidum* subsp. *endemicum* and of yaws is *T. pallidum* subsp. *pertenue*. The causative bacterium of pinta, *T. carateum*, retains its previous classification.

8. 11. 1. 12   *T. pallidum* Subsp. *endemicum*

Bejel or endemic syphilis, is a chronic skin and tissue disease caused by infectionof *T. pallidum* subsp. *endemicum*. Bejel is also known by a variety of other names, including endemic syphilis, nonvenereal syphilis or treponematosis-bejel type. Generally, bejelis transmittedby mouth-to-mouth contact or sharing of domestic utensils. It is treatable with penicillin or other antibiotics, resulting in a complete recovery.

8. 11. 1. 13   *T. pallidum* Subsp. *pertenue*

Yawsis mainly prevalent in the tropicsand subtropics, with the infection of the skin, bones and joints caused by *T. pallidum* subsp. *pertenue*. The disease is transmitted by skin-to-skin contact of traumatized skin with exudatefrom yawslesions. Infection is usually acquiredbefore puberty. The incubation period is about 3–5 weeks. The papular lesions usually occur on the legs and then enlarge and erode. This primary stage resolves completely within six months. The secondary stage occurs months to years later and the lesions may involve bones, particularly the fingers, long bones and the jaw, with typically widespread skin lesions characterized by cutaneous plaques andulcers and hyperkeratoticskin on the palmsand soles. The secondarystage does not represent cardiovascular and neurological damage and could heal after six months or later. About 10% of patients develop tertiary yaws within 5 to 10 years, with widespread bone, joint and soft tissue destruction (e. g. gangosa). Available treatmentsinclude intramuscular injection of benzylpenicillin or a course of benzylpenicillin, erythromycin or tetracycline tablets.

8.11.1.14 *T. carateum*

Pinta, caused by *T. carateum*, is endemic in Mexico, Central America and South America. Pinta is thought to be transmitted by skin-to-skin contact (similar to bejel and yaws). Unlike the above treponematoses, the manifestationsof pintaare confined to theskin with non-destructive lesions. Afteran incubation period of one to three weeks, small itching primary lesions develop, commonly on the exposed surface of arms and legs. Local lymph nodes might be enlarged. And the primary lesions may heal with areas of hypopigmentation left. 3–12 months later, further thickened and flat lesions (pintids)appear all over the body and may become dyschromia. However, a proportion of patients will develop latestage pinta, characterized by a mixture of hyperpigmentation and depigmentation. Pinta is treatable with benzylpenicillin, tetracycline, azithromycin or chloramphenicol.

8.11.2 Family *Spirochaetaceae*, Genus *Borrelia*

Allspecies of the genus *Borrelia* are morphologicallysimilar helical rods, 4 – 30 μm long and 0.2 – 0.5 μm indiameter, with 3 to 10 loose spirals. And theborreliaeare actively motile with frequent reversal of the direction of translational movement. The majority of species of genus *Borrelia* are animal or human pathogens. The two major human diseases associated with borreliae are Lyme disease, caused by *Borrelia burgdorferi* and relapsing fever, caused by *Borrelia recurrentis* and several other *Borrelia* species. All *Borrelia* spp. are arthropod borne transmitted by lice, *Pediculus humanus* or ticks of the genus *Ixodes* or *Ornithodorus* during blood feeding. Humans are the only reservoir of louse-bornerelapsing fever (*B. recurrentis*), but the other bacteria are maintained in the naturalcycle between ticks and reservoir hosts (usuallyrodents).

8.11.2.1 *Borrelia burgdorferi*

B. burgdorferi is the major causative agent of the Lyme disease, which was first recognized in Old Lyme, Connecticut and is currently the most prevalent tick-borne disease in the United States. The natural reservoirs of *B. burgdorferi* are wild and domesticated animals, including rodents, deer, birds, sheep, cattle, horses and dogs. For maintaining the populations of tick with *B. burgdorferi*, the rodents and deer are probably important.

8.11.2.2 Morphology

They are flexible helical bacteria with dimension of 0.2–0.3 μm by 4–30 μm consisting of 3–10 coils (Figure 8–18). 7 to 11 end of lagella overlap at the central region of the cell leading to both rotational and translational movements. A multilayered outer membrane surrounds the protoplasmic cylinder, which consists of the peptidoglycan layer, cytoplasmic membrane and the enclosed cytoplasmic contents. The bacteria are Gram-stainnegative and stain well withGiemsa, silver and Warthin-Starry stainings.

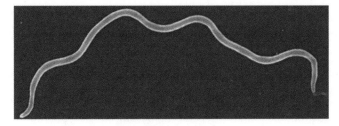

Figure 8–18 Scanning electron micrograph of *B. burgdorferi*

8.11.2.3　Cultivation

B. burgdorferi has proven to be a slow growing bacterium, with a log-phase generation time of 10−12 h at 34−37 ℃. The bacteria are catalase-negativeand microaerophilic with glucose as primary energy source. *B. burgdorferi* can grow well in BSKII medium or its variants supplemented with N-acetylglucosamine and rabbit serum.

8.11.2.4　Antigenicstructure

The outermembrane of *B. burgdorferi* is composed of various unique outer surface proteins (Osps) that have been characterized (OspA through OspF). The Osps are lipoproteins anchored by N-terminally attached fatty acid molecules to the membrane. They are presumed to play a role in virulence, transmission or survival in the tick. OspA promotes the attachment of *B. burgdorferi* to the tick midgut protein (TROSPA), present on tick gut epithelial cells. OspB also has an essential role in the adherence of *B. burgdorferi* to the tick gut. OspC is expressed at high levels in the salivary glands of tick and is necessary for establishment of infectionin mice. Other outer surface proteins are involved in the mammalian inflammatory response, including OspE, OspF and E/F-likeleader peptide.

8.11.2.5　Genome

The genomeof *B. burgdorferi* type strain B31 containsa linear chromosome of 910,724 bp and 21 plasmids (9 circular and 12 linear). The chromosome contains 853 genes encoding a basic set of proteins for DNA replication, transcription, translation, solutetransport and energy metabolism, but no genes for cellular biosynthetic metabolic capacities. There are differential expression ofmajor surface proteins in tick vectors and mammalian hosts.

8.11.2.6　Stabilityandviability

B. burgdorferi is susceptible to 1% sodium hypochlorite, 70% ethanol, heat (60 ℃, 1−3 minutes) and UV. Penicillin, cephalosporin, erythromycin and tetracycline are used for treatment of Lyme disease. Outside the hosts, *B. burgdorferi* can survive up to 48 days at 4 ℃ in human blood and for short periods in urine.

8.11.2.7　Epidemiology

Lyme disease is zoonotic, caused by *B. burgdorferi* via tick vectors (genus *Ixodes*). The primary bridging ticks to humans are *I. scapularis* (deer tick) and *I. pacificus* in North America, *I. ricinus* in Europe and *I. persulcatus* in Asia. With a broad geographic distributionin nature, *B. burgdorferi* circulates between the vertebrate hosts and the ticks in the life cycle. The tick can't pass the *B. burgdorferi* to its progeny. Thus, the larvamustacquire *B. burgdorferi* by blood feeding on the reservoirs. Andthe *B. burgdorferi* survives in the midgut till the larva molts into a nymph. Infected nymphs then transmit *B. burgdorferi* by feeding on another vertebrate to complete the cycle. Deer and rodents are prime mammalian reservoirs of *B. burgdorferi*. Unlike the ticks that carry other tick-borne pathogens, a high percentage of deer ticks carry *B. burgdorferi*. The infected nymphal tick can transmit *B. burg-

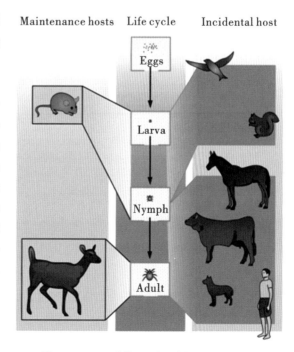

Figure 8−19　Life cycle of *I. scapularis*

dorferi to humansvia its saliva, but humans are definitive hosts, unlikely to continue the life cycle (Figure 8-19).

8.11.2.8 *Pathogenesis*

After *B. burgdorferi* is transmitted, it will acclimate to the host conditions by changing its glycoproteins and proteases on its plasma membrane to facilitate its dissemination throughout the blood. *B. burgdorferi* will express proteins that will interact with endothelial cells, platelets, chondrocytes and the extracellular matrix. Clinical presentations of Lyme disease can range from asymptomatic (about 10% of *B. burgdorferi* infection-slack symptoms) to severe, involving many organs, including the characteristic erythema migrans (Figure 8-20), as well as myocarditis, arthritis, meningitis and neuropathies. The progression of the untreated case-sis typically divided into 3 stages.

Stage 1 affects the area around the bite from an infected tick. Aswelling rash, erythema migrans (also called erythema chronicum migrans), emerges around the center and expands to 15 cm in diameter with a concentric circular fashion. Once the rash starts to subside, symptoms resembling flu may follow. During this stage, antibiotics are most effective to prevent further growth and symptoms.

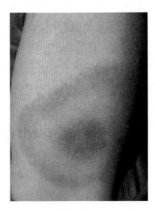

Figure 8-20　Erythema migrans of Lyme disease

Stage 2 occurs after weeks to months. *B. burgdorferi* will spread through the body and induce multiple symptoms, including cardiacand neurological manifestations. The most common cardiac manifestation is heart block that can vary from first degree to complete heart block. Neurologic manifestations may present with either peripheral nervous system or central nervous system involved. Facial paralysis, fatigue and loss of memory are common emerging on this stage. Moreover, the patients may develop encephalitis or meningitis.

Stage 3 ensues months to years later. Because of the prolonged presence of *B. burgdorferi*, the immune system activates responses in the joints. Roughlyone half of those patients will develop arthritis during this stage. Arthritis of Lyme diseaseis characterized by a relapsing form that usually affects the larger joints (mainly the knee joint).

Interestingly, the symptoms of chronic Lyme disease, especially neurological symptoms, resemble those of chronic syphilis. Unlike syphilis, Lyme disease is not spread person to person.

8.11.2.9　Immune Response to Infection

Although no major virulence factors have been identified in *B. burgdorferi*, the pathogen can induce theimmune responses. Specific IgM antibodies to *B. burgdorferi* develop within 4-6 weeks of infection. The earliest response appears to be against the end oflagella and later against outersurface proteins. IgG antibodiesappear 4-6 months after infection and last till the later stage of Lyme disease. However, *B. burgdorferi* has developed certain strategies (e. g. antigenic variation) to escape the host immune system.

8.11.2.10　Laboratory Diagnosis

The characteristic rash and the experiencein an endemic area could be strictly clinical diagnosis of early stage of Lyme disease. Besides, cultivation and PCR can directly detect the presence of *B. burgdorferi* or the DNAfrom tissues or fluids. However, due to the difficulties in using such tests clinically, the vast majority of cases are diagnosed by serologic tests.

Asthe initial test, the sensitivity of enzyme-linked immunosorbent assay (ELISA)approaches 90% with a specificity of 72%. However, ELISA mayhave false-positive results because of the cross-reactivity to other spirochetes (*T. pallidum* or *L. interrogans*), the prior exposure to other borreliae(the group of relapsing fever *Borrelia*) and the autoimmune diseases (e. g. Lupus). Thus, a subsequent Western blot with higher specificity is generally performed in order to exclude these false-positive results. Both Western blot and ELISA can be used for testing IgM and IgG antibodies.

8.11.2.11　Control and Treatment

Asother tick-borne infections, prevention of infection by *B. burgdorferi* is mainly achieved by avoiding tick habitat, by wearing tick-proof clothing and applyinginsect repellents containing N, N-Diethyl-*m*-toluamide (DEET). Another approach to controlling the Lymedisease is the application of acaricide to the mammalianhosts, such as the deer, by placing feeding stations with attractive food (whole kernel corns)in strategic locations. Lyme disease vaccines are available for domestic animals, but there are no commercial vaccines for human.

Treatment of early stage Lyme disease is usually with doxycycline or amoxicillin for 20 to 30 days. For patients with cardiac or neurological symptoms, ceftriaxone can be intravenously administered because ceftriaxone can cross the blood brain barrier.

8.11.2.12　The Group of Relapsing Fever *Borrelia*

Relapsing fevers are characterized clinically by recurrent periods of fever and spirochaetaemia. The group of relapsing fever *Borrelia* includes more than 20 species that are agents of tick-borne or louse-borne relapsing fever.

Tick-borne (orendemic)relapsing fever is a zoonosiscaused by several *Borrelia* species, including *B. duttoni*, *B. hermsii*, *B. parkeri* and *B. turicatae*, which are transmitted to man by soft-bodied ticks(family *Argasidae*), mainly of the genus *Ornithodoros*. The spirochaetes invade the tissues, including the salivary glands, genitalia and excretory system, of the tick. Infection occurs via saliva or excrement during feeding. Transovarial transmission to the tick progeny maintains the spirochaetes in the tick population. The major natural hosts for these species are rodents.

Louse-borne(orepidemic) relapsing fever is more severe than the tick-borne relapsing fever and is causedby *B. recurrentis*, which is an obligate human pathogen transmitted from person to person by the human louse (*Pediculus humanus humanus*). *B. recurrentis* grows in the haemolymph of the human louse but does not invade tissues. Therefore, the louse feces are not infectious and the bacterium is not transferred through eggs to the progeny. Human acquire *B. recurrentis* when the bacteria release from crushed lice and enter the tissues through the skinor mucous membrane.

8.11.2.13　Morphology and Cultivation

The bacteria are 0.3−0.6 μm wide and 10−30 μm inlength and consist of 3−10 coils with 8−10 end of lagella and have been successfully cultivated in BSK IImedium from patients with relapsing fever. The optimal growth temperature is 28−30 ℃, with a generation time of 18 h. However, because of its low yield, cultivation is not useful in diagnosis.

8.11.2.14   Pathogenesis

Inboth forms of relapsing fever, the spirochaetes invade the blood (spirochaetaemia) and inducethe febrile response. Then, the host produces corresponding specific antibodies which can terminate the spirochaetaemia and fever. However, the spirochaetes remain in the tissues and invade the blood again due to the antigenic variation of their outer membrane protein composition. This presentation is responsible forthe relapsing course of infection. The ultimate elimination of the spirochaetes appears to be accomplished due to the antibodies to all the variations.

About one week after infection, characteristic acute symptoms, including high fever, myalgia and hepatosplenomegaly, occur during spirochaetaemia (up to 10^5 spirochaetes/mm^3 of blood). The CNS may be involved in up to 30% of cases. Theprimary febrile symptommay relieve in 3–5 days and terminate suddenly with hypotension and shock. Subsequent high fever maytake place one week later and 3–10 times of relapse may occur. Generally, louse-borne relapsing fever is more severe than the tick-borne variety. The case fatality rate varies from 4% to 40% for louse-borne relapsing fever and from 2% to 5% fortick-borne variety, with myocarditis, cerebral haemorrhage and liver failure.

8.11.2.15   Laboratory Diagnosis

The diagnosis of relapsing fever can becarried on by direct detection of borreliae in peripheral blood samples from febrile stage. By Giemsa or Wright staining, spirochaetes can be seen on the smear by microscopy. Other infections of spirochetes (Lyme disease, syphilis and leptospirosis) do not have the stage of spirochaetaemia.

Althoughthe anti-spirocheteantibodies are produced, the variable nature of antigens makes serological diagnosisdifficult. Falsenegative results can be obtained in the earlystage of infection and cross-reactive antigens may result in false positive results in patients infected by other spirochaetes.

8.11.2.16   Control and Treatment

Prevention of infectionincludes avoidance and elimination of the tick or louse vectors. Insect repellents can be applied to eliminate ticks in human dwellings, but eliminatingticks in the environment is not possible. Prevention of louse-borne infection includes maintenance of personal hygiene and delousing if necessary. There are no commercialvaccines. Treatment of relapsing fever is usually with a one-to two-week-course of antibiotics (tetracycline, penicillin or erythromycin) and most people improve within 24 hours.

8.11.3   Family *Leptospiraceae*, Genus *Leptospira*

Leptospira spp. (leptospires) are long, thin motile spirochetes with fine coils and characteristic hooked ends. The parasitic strains of *L. interrogans* can localize in the kidney of carriers (e. g. rodents and pigs) and be excreted into the environment via urination. Other species, including human beings, may directly or indirectly contact with the urine and acquire leptospirosis. Leptospirosis is a zoonosis and can be sporadic, endemic or epidemic. The highest incidence is found in tropicaland subtropical parts of the world.

8.11.3.1   Morphology

Leptospires are tightly coiled spirochaetes, usually 0. 1 μm ×(6–20) μm. The helical amplitude is approximately 0. 1–0. 15 μm and the wavelength approximately 0. 5 μm. Eitheror both ends of leptospires are usually bent into distinctive hooks (Figure 8–21).

Leptospires possess a double-membrane structure composed of a cytoplasmic membrane, the periplasm and the outer membrane that contains the LPS and many membrane-associated lipoproteins. Between the cell wall and the outer envelope, there are two end of lagella that are wrapped around the cell wall. Leptospires rotate rapidly around their long axis and motion in either direction.

Leptospiresare Gram-negative, butare not readily stained by Gram staining. They can bestained by Giemsa staining, silver deposition and fluorescent antibody methods. Leptospires are so thin that they are usually viewedby darkfield microscopy.

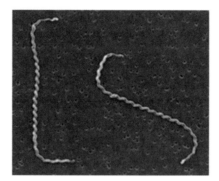

Figure 8 – 21　Scanning electron micrograph of leptospires boundto a 0.2 μm filter

8.11.3.2　Cultivation

All members of the genus *Leptospira* are obligateaerobes or microaerophiles with an optimum growth temperature of 28–30 ℃ and pH from 7.2 to 7.4. They can grow in Korthoff's mediumwith 10% rabbit serum or Ellinghausen-McCullough-Johnson-Harris (EMJH) medium with the generation time of about 8 h. Leptospiras are maintained in semi-solid (0.1% –0.2% agar) media at 30 ℃. Growthin semi-solid media typically results in formation of a dense zone of growth (referred to as a Dinger disk) a few millimeters below the surface of the media. Colonies (1–2 mm in diameter) are visible after 2 weeks on solid medium at 28 ℃.

8.11.3.3　Antigenic Structure

Theserovars ofleptospires are serologically determined on structural heterogeneity of the LPS. And more than 200 different pathogenic serovars are recognized. Protein composition ofthe leptospires outer membrane varies depending on virulenceand growth conditions. Many of the surface lipoproteins such as OMPL1, LipL21, LipL32 (hemolysin), Lk73.5 (sphingomyelinase), LipL41, LipL45 and LipL46 areup-regulated *in vivo*, while others such as LipL36 are down-regulated. Moreover, LigA and LigB, adhesins of leptospires, increase as osmolality rises.

8.11.3.4　Genome

The leptospiral genome is comprised ofone large and one small chromosome, approximately 3,500 – 4,300 kb and 300–350 kb inlength respectively. Leptospires contain variable numbers of rRNA genes with unusual organization, which are dispersed around the larger chromosome. Moreover, many transposable elements, such as insertion sequence (IS), have been identified and found inmany serovars, leading to the conclusion that the genome of leptospires is undergoing IS-mediated genome mutation.

8.11.3.5　Stability and Viability

Pathogenic leptospires can survive in the environment. Leptospiresare stable in soil contaminated with infected urine for many months and in contaminated water for up to 19 days, indicating the potential for long-term exposure to an infection risk.

Leptospirescan be easily killed by drying, by temperatures above 40 ℃ (after about 10 min at 50 ℃ and within 10 s at 60 ℃), by acid conditions (below pH 7.0) or alkaline conditions (above approximately pH 7.8) and by disinfectants such as phenolics, quaternary ammonium derivatives, halogens and aldehydes. Leptospires are susceptible to penicillin, tetracycline and aminoglycoside. Tetracycline hasbeen shown to be superior in a controlled clinical trial and is also effective as a prophylactic agent.

8.11.3.6　Epidemiology

Pathogeni cleptospires are transmitted primarily from the reservoirs by urine. Exposure to the leptospires may be direct, through contact with the urine or tissues of infected animals. However, indirect exposureis more common by contact with humid environment contaminated with the urine. Animals that acquire infection may not develop discernible disease, but become the maintenance hosts. Many rodents are thought to be the main sourcesof infection. Infected rats may carry the bacteria in the kidney. And excretion in urine may intermittently or continuously contain the leptospires. Similarly, cattle, dogs and pigs may becomethe maintenance hosts for their corresponding serovars. For the stability of leptospiresin water, the reisaseasonal pattern of human infections, which peak inthe summer. Infections related to exposure to humid environmenthave shown a significant rise in developed countries. The increase is mainly due to the contact with the surface waters for recreational activities such as fishing, rafting and swimming.

8.11.3.7　Pathogenesis

Leptospirosisis used to describethe infections in both human and animals, regardless of the clinical presentation or strain of *Leptospira* involved. In human, there is no serovar-specific disease, which varies in severity from a mildself-limiting illness to the fatal disease. However, the pathogenesis of leptospirosis is not well understood.

Leptospires generally enter the host through the skin abrasions or mucous membranes. It is possible that entry may occur via the conjunctiva or by inhalation after immersion in contaminated water. Leptospiresthen spreadin the lymphatics and bloodstream with the incubation period of 2 to 21 days. Then, leptospirosis presents with an in fluenza-like illness characterized by the sudden onset of headache, muscular pain, fever and rigors. Conjunctival suffusion and a skin rash may be seen in some cases. After a leptospiraemic phase (lasting 7–8 days) following the onset of symptoms, increasing numbers of leptospires, probably together with immune responses, lead to blood vessel damage, local ischemia and small hemorrhages in most tissues. In some severe cases, renal ischemia occurs and may be precipitated into renal impairment. Other severecases may represent hepatocellular impairment (jaundice), pulmonary hemorrhages (hemoptysis) and myocarditis.

However, the patients may recover with appropriate clinical supports (e.g. dialysis and transfusion) and treatment. Ina few patients, symptoms may persist for many months, but the carrier state occurs rarely in humans.

8.11.3.8　Immune Response to Infection

Specific immunity develops rapidly within 1–2 weeks of clinical or subclinical infection of leptospires. The induced IgG and IgM antibodies can clear the leptospires and lead to rapid phagocytosis of leptospires in the tissues and in the circulation. Moreover, immunity is associated with agglutinating antibodies (opsonin) and a very low level of agglutinating antibody can be protective. Immunity to reinfection is specificfor the same serovar. Cell-mediated responses occur following infection or immunization with vaccines. However, the reappears to be a lower degree of cell-mediated immunity following natural infection.

8.11.3.9　Laboratory Diagnosis

Pathogenic leptospires can be isolated from the blood (or cerebrospinal fluid) of patients during the leptospiraemicphase (7–10 days) or from urine during 2 weeksto months following infection. Andthe leptospires can be enriched by differential centrifugation. Cultivation of primary isolation of leptospires may require incubation of at least 2 weeks with periodic microscopic evaluation.

(1) Cytologicalidentification

Darkfield microscopycan be used to recognize leptospires in cultures. However, direct cytological identification of clinical specimens by dark field microscopy is insensitive and nonspecific. Immuno-histochemical staining has both greater sensitivity and specificity than other staining methods. Besides, leptospires may be visualizedby Giemsa or silver deposition methods.

(2) Serological and Immunological Diagnostic Methods

Both IgM detection by ELISA and detection of agglutinating antibodies by microscopic agglutination test (MAT) are useful for diagnosis. IgM antibodies can mostly be detected 5–7 days after onset of symptoms. Sensitivity of detection is relatively low during the first week, but rapidly risessubsequently. In pigs and cattle, the levels of IgM have been correlated with renal excretion of leptospires.

Early in the illness, detection of IgM is more sensitive than MAT. However, a positive result of IgM should be followed by MAT of acute and convalescent specimens for confirmation. Dilutions of patient's serum can be titrated against the reference serogroups and serovars. 50% agglutination of the leptospiresby the patient's serum indicatedthe titre andthe serogroup or serovar of leptospires. The seraof the convalescent specimensgenerally show a significantly higher titre than that of acute specimens.

(3) Nucleicacid Amplification Techniques

PCR-based methods, relying on 16S rRNA sequences, offer the potential for more rapid diagnosis of leptospirosis and accurate differentiation of *Leptospira* species than the currently serologicalmethods. Reference laboratories can advise on the examination of cerebrospinal fluid or other tissue, including those taken at post-mortem.

8.11.3.10　Control and Treatment

Complete prevention of leptospirosisis actually impossible by eliminating leptospires because of their zoonotic nature and ability to survive for long periodsin the environment. And environmental flooding can increase the risk of infection. Measures aimed atremoval of rodents from thedomestic environment may help to reduce the risk of infection. Besides, measures to reduce leptospire populations in soil, mud or water will reduce the risk of infection to humans. Moreover, extensive immunization of domestic lives tock will prevent disease in the animals. The immunization would also assist in protecting human sindirectly by reducing excretion of leptospires by animals.

Antibiotictherapyis necessary and appropriate for patients as soon as possible. In severe cases, intravenous benzylpenicillinis the antibioticof choice. Erythromycinis an alternative if the patients were allergic to penicillins. And the milder infections can be treated with a 7–10 day course of oral amoxicillin.

8.12　Other Bacteria

8.12.1　Legionella

Legionella has 39 species and 61 serotypes and it is widespread in nature, especially in natural water, man-made hotor cold water system. The primary pathogenic bacterium in this group is *Legionella pneumophila* (*L. pneumophila*).

▶▶ **L. pneumophila**

(1) Biological Structure

It is gram-negative bacillus with width ranging from 0. 5 to 1. 0 μm and length from 2 to 5 μm. It is nonspore-forming and has polar or lateral flagella, pili and microcapsule. It stains poorly with conventional staining method,. Silver impregnation or Giemsa staining is often used. The bacteria appear in red or black brown. *L. pneumophila* is facultative anaerobic and grows well in environment with 2. 5% –5% CO_2 at optimum temperature of 35 ℃. The bacteria demand many nutrients, including many kinds of microelement and amino acids. The most suitable culture medium is BCYE medium. *L. pneumophila* is catalase-positive and oxidase-positive.

(2) Pathogenicity and Immunity

Major pathogenic substances are various kinds of enzymes, toxin, pili, capsule, et al. These substances can cause Legionnaires' disease. Legionnaires' disease is more common in summer and autumn. It spreads by droplets and causes lung infection or systemic disease. Legionnaires' disease includes three types, namely flu-like type, pneumonia type and extrapulmonary infection type. Flu-like type manifests as mild infection, with good prognosis. The pneumonia type is also called Legionnaires' disease, which is a severe infection with 15% –20% mortality rate. The extrapulmonary infection is a kind of secondary infection. The bacteria are one of the hospital-acquired pathogenic bacteria. *L. pneumophila* is a kind of intracellular bacteria and cellular immunity is mainly how the body reacts to it.

(3) Microbiological Examination and Prevention

Bacteria were isolated and cultured from sputum, lung biopsy or pleural effusion. Other identification methods include ELISA and bacteria specific antigen detection through fluorescent antibody labeling. Currently, there is no specific vaccine. Major preventive measures are strengthening water source management and sterilization of man-made water pipe. The medication of choice is erythromycin.

8.12. 2   Haemophilus Influenzae

The bacteria are called Haemophilus because fresh blood or blood derivatives are needed when culturing them. This genus has 21 species, among which the primary pathogenic bacterium is *Haemophilus influenzae* (*H. influenzae*).

▶▶ **H. influenza**

(1) Biological Structure

It is small gram-negative bacillus with width ranging from 0. 3 to 0. 4 μm and length from 1. 0 to 1. 5 μm. It is nonspore-forming and has pili but no flagella. Virulent strains are encapsuled obviously. It is aerobic or facultative anaerobic and grows best at 35–37 ℃. It demands many nutrients and its culture medium requires factor X and factor V. Because factor V in the blood can only be released by erythrocyte after being heated, H. influenza grows well on chocolate blood plate. Besides, because staphylococcus aureus can synthesize factor V while growing, *satellite phenomenon* can be observed while the two bacteria are cultured together. The colonies of *H. influenzae* near staphylococcus aureus are much bigger. This method is used for *H. influenza* identification. *H. influenzae* is sensitive to heat, dryness and common chemical disinfectants. Resistance mutation happens easily in the bacteria.

(2) Pathogenicity and Immunity

It widely exists in the upper respiratory tract of the host. The major pathogenic substance is capsule, pili, endotoxin, et al. The disease it causes divides into primary infection and secondary infection. The immunity formed after contracting the bacteria is mainly humoral immunity.

(3) Microbiological Examination and Prevention

Use nasopharyngeal secretion, pus, etc. as clinical samples for smear microscopy, isolation and culture. And identification is performed based on cultural characteristics, colonial morphology, biochemical reaction and satellite phenomenon. *H. influenzae* type B capsular polysaccharide vaccine shows good immunoprophylaxis efficacy. Because over 25% *H. influenzae* gain resistance from beta-lactamase which is produced through plasmid transfer, medication should be guided by drug sensitivity test during treatment.

8.12.3　Pseudomonas Aeruginosa

The members of pseudomonas are small bacilli which are gram-negative and aerobic. They have capsule and flagella, but no spore formed. They widely occur in soil, air, water, flora and fauna. The genus has various species and the human pathogenic one is *Pseudomonas aeruginosa* (*P. aeruginosa*).

▶▶ **P. aeruginosa**

(1) Biological Structure

It is gram-negative bacillus, with width ranging from 0.5 to 1.0 μm and length from 1.5 to 3.0 μm. It is nonspore-forming and has capsule as well as 1 – 3 flagella at one end, providing active mobility. P. aeruginosa is obligate aerobe and grows best at 35 ℃. It also can grow at 42 ℃. It can produce various kinds of water-soluble pigments, making the culture medium green. Its biochemical reaction is characterized by its strong ability to break down proteins and its positive cytochrome oxidase test.

(2) Pathogenicity and Immunity

It is normal body flora and its major pathogenic substance is endotoxin and exotoxin A. Other pathogenic factors include pili, capsule, extracellular enzyme, et. al. The bacteria can infect any tissue of human body and result in local suppurative inflammation. It is commonly found at damaged skin and mucous membrane, such as wound and burn. The phagocytosis of neutrophile granulocyte plays an important role in the resistance to P. aeruginosa infection.

(3) Microbiological Examination and Prevention

Different samples, such as inflammatory secretion, pus and blood, are taken based on different infection sites, disease types and the purposes of examination. After culture on blood agar plate, the identification is done based on colony characteristics, pigment and biochemical reaction. Methods such as serologic test and phage typing can be applied for further identification. P. aeruginosa causes cross-infections in hospitals by polluting medical equipment and staff. Hospitals should strengthen the sterilization management of diagnostic equipment and overall environment. Its drug resistance is easily formed. Medication should be guided based on drug sensitivity test.

8.12.4　Bordetella

Bordetella mainly includes bordetella pertussis, bordetella parapertussis, bordetella bronchiseptica and bordetella avium. *Bordetella pertussis* (*B. pertussis*) is the major human pathogen. It is also called bacillus pertussis and is the pathogen of pertussis.

▶▶ **B. pertussis**

（1）Biological Structure

It is short gram-negative bacillus with width ranging from 0. 2 to 0. 5 μm and length from 0. 5 to 1. 5 μm. It is nonspore-forming and has flagella. The virulent strains have pili and capsule. It is obligate aerobic and grows best at 35–36 ℃. It requires many nutrients and is usually cultured on Bordet-Gengou agar which contains glycerol, potato extract and blood. With weak resistance, the bacteria can be killed by 1 h direct sunlight plus 30 min heating at 56 ℃.

（2）Pathogenicity and Immunity

The pathogenic substance is capsule, pili, toxin and various bioactivators. Toxin of these bacteria mainly includes pertussis toxin, adenylate cyclase toxin, tracheal cytotoxin and dermotoxin. Pertussis toxin is the main virulence factor. B. pertussis does not invade tissue and blood and mainly causes local tissue damage. The bacteria are transmitted through droplets. Infection source is carriers and patients, especially those with mild and atypical manifestations. The incubation period is 7 to 14 days. Clinical symptoms primarily are paroxysmal and spasmodic cough. The symptom lasts quite long, so it is also called 100-day cough. Children under 5 years old are susceptible to the disease. After infection, various specific antibodies show up in the human body. SIgA, produced in association with local mucosal membranes, can inhibit pathogenic bacteria from adhering to tracheal mucosa. Patients get lasting immunity after recovery.

（3）Microbiological Examination and Prevention

Inoculate nasopharyngeal swabs on Bordet-Gengou agar for culture and isolation, observe and identify typical colonies. Fluorescent antibody method can also be used for quick test. Triple vaccine containing killed vaccine of phase Ⅰ *B. pertussis*, diphtheria toxoid and tetanus toxoid is used for artificial active immunity and the preventive effect is good. B. pertussis is not sensitive to penicillin, so the priority drug is erythromycin, ampicillin, . al.

8. 12. 5　Campylobacter

Campylobacter is a genus of curved gram-negative bacteria, among which the main pathogenic one is *Campylobacter jejuni* (*C. jejuni*).

（1）Biological Structure

It is gram-negative, non-spore forming and has capsule. It appears curved, helical or seagulls-shaped. Both ends are pointed and possess polar flagella. It can rapidly move in straight line or in a spiral course. It is microaerophilic and demands many nutrients. In gaseous environment of 85% N_2, 10% CO_2 and 5% O_2, primary isolation from blood agar plate may include two typical colonies. The first type is anhemolytic, flat, teardrop-shaped, grey and moist with luster. Its edge is irregular and it often grows and spreads along the inoculating line. The second type is also anhemolytic and appears in the form of scattered and single convex colony with neat edge. The colony is translucent with luster. The center is relatively deep. Each single colony grows separately. Biochemical reaction is not active. It is oxidase-positive and hippurate hydrolysis test is positive too. With weak resistance, it is easily killed by dryness, sunlight and weak disinfectants.

（2）Pathogenicity and Immunity

C. jejuni is normally a harmless commensal of poulry as well as many animals, such as cattle, sheep and dog. It can pollute food and water by waste from genital and intestinal tract. People are generally susceptible to it and children under 5 years old have the highest morbidity rate. Its pathogenicity and invasiveness are related to toxin. The bacteria move to the surface of intestinal epithelial cells via flagella invasion. First, it colonizes by pili and then it grows and reproduces to release exotoxin. Bacteria lyse and release endotoxin. It mainly causes gastroenteritis. After contracting the bacteria for 2-4 weeks, specific IgM and IgG antibodies can be produced. The phagocytosis of phagocytes is strengthened by immune regulation and complement activation.

(3) Microbiological Examination and Prevention

Direct smear microscopy: The motility and morphology of campylobacters are sufficiently characteristic for a rapid presumptive diagnosis tobe made by direct microscopy of faeces, either in wet preparations or stained smears. Find out gram-negative curved or seagull-shaped campylobacter and observe its fish-like spiral movement by pendant-drop method.

Isolation and Culture: Use selective medium containing polymyxin B and vancomycin for feces and food samples. Culture the samples in environments with low oxygen for 2 d at 42 ℃ or 37 ℃. Select suspicious colonies and identify them with biochemical reaction such as hippurate hydrolysis test and indoxyl acetate hydrolysis test.

Serological Test: After contracting the disease for one week, antibodies, mainly IgM, will show up in the serum. Specific antibody titer shall be detected through indirect agglutination test and indirect immunofluorescence assay.

Molecular Biological Method: For the *C. jejuni* in feces, blood and other samples, apply a rapid PCR test for its specific DNA. Infected animals are the most vital source of infection. Therefore, to prevent animal feces from contaminating water and food is quite important. *C. jejuni* is moderately resistant to penicillins and most cephalosporins, but sensitive to erythromycin. Erythromycin and aminoglycoside antibiotics can be used for treatment.

8.12.6　Helicobacter

The helicobacter genus contains over 20 species and encompasses two groups: gastric and enterohepatic ones. Among them, *Helicobacter pylori* (*H. pylori*) is the most widely known one.

▶▶ **H. pylori**

(1) Biological Structure

It is gram-negative, helical or curved with width ranging from 0.5 to 1.0 μm and length from 2.5 to 4.0 μm. One end has 2-6 sheathed flagella, which enable active mobility. It is microaerophilic and demands many nutrients. It grows optimally in a gaseous environment of 85% N_2, 10% CO_2 and 5% O_2. Solid medium needs 10% defibrinated sheep bloods and fluid medium needs supplement of 10% newborn calf serum. The colony is translucent and appears in a needle-like shape. *H. pylori* contains urease, which can decompose urea and produce ammonia. Therefore, *H. pylori* is relatively acid-resisting. *H. pylori* is positive to urease, catalase and oxidase, which serves as the main basis for identification.

(2) Pathogenicity and Immunity

H. pylori is the main cause of chronic gastritis and peptic ulcer. The pathogenic substance is invasive factor and toxin. The bacteria related to invasion are composed of urease, flagella, pili, et. al. Urease decomposes the urea oozed by gastric mucosa and produces "ammonia cloud" on the surface of bacteria to neuralize gasric acid. Therefore, a microenvironment which is favorable to the bacteria is formed. Through flagella movement, bacteria are able to penetrate the mucoid lining of the stomach and reach gastric epithelial cells. With the help from pili or adhesin, it colonizes at the cell surface and starts to grow and reproduce. The toxin mainly includes two kinds of exotoxin: VacA and CagA, whose function is to damage gastric epithelial *cells. H. pylori* is regarded as Group 1 Carcinogen. After infection, specific antibodies of IgM, IgG and IgA can be detected in local and the whole body.

(3) Microbiological Examination and Prevention

The detection methods mainly include invasive (includes tissue section staining, rapid urease test, bacterial culture and PCR) and non-invasive tests (includes C^{13} urea breath test, serum immunological detection and HPSA test). Under direct smear microscopy, we can see that the bacteria are gram-negative and appear in curved or S-shape. Rapid urease test is to take a biopsy from the stomach at the time of gastroscopy and place it into a medium containing urea and phenol red as indicator. If the medium changes color from yellow to red (positive), it means the biopsy of mucosa taken from the antrum of the stomach contains live *H. pylori*. Bacterial culture uses selective medium containing vancomycin and amphotericin B. The colony is formed after 3 d culture at 37 ℃ in microaerophilic environment. Identification is performed based on morphological observation and biochemical reaction with oxidase, catalase, urease, et al. Immunological detection is to use ELISA method to test IgG in serum, IgA in sputum or antigen in feces to determine whether one is infected or not. The treatment of *H. pylori* infection usually is "triple therapy" consisting of proton pump inhibitors and the antibiotics clarithromycin and amoxicillin. However, these bacteria have a high recurrence rate and their drug resistance is increasing gradually. Vaccines are in the pipeline.

Chapter 9

Virology

9.1　Respiratory Viruses

Viruses caused 90% –95% of acute respiratory tract infection. The common viruses associated with respiratory infections are influenza virus of Orthomyxoviridae, measles virus, mumps virus, respiratory syscytial virus, parainfluenza virus, coronavirus and adenovirus. Influenza viruses have threatened animals and public health systems continuously. Influenza has been responsible for millions of deaths worldwide each year. Influenza viruses are a major determinant of morbidity and mortality caused by respiratory diseases and outbreaks of infection sometimes occur in worldwide epidemics. Moreover, There are many subtypes of influenza viruses that made the classification and prevention of influenza viruses difficult during influenza outbreak.

9.1.1　Orthomyxoviruses

The family Orthomyxoviruses include influenza A, B and C virus. Influenza A virus can infect a series of different host species, which are known for humans, aquatic birds, pigs, horses and seals. Some of the strains isolated from animals are antigenically similar to strains circulating in the human population. Influenza A virus is antigenically highly variable and is responsible for most cases of epidemic influenza. Influenza B virus may exhibit antigenic changes and sometimes causes epidemics and mainly infect humans. Influenza C virus is antigenically stable and causes only mild illness in immunocompetent individuals.

In 1997, HongKong, a highly lethal H5N1 avian influenza virus was apparently transmitted directly from chickens to humans with no intermediate mammalian host and caused 18 confirmed infections and 6 deaths. H7N7 and H9N2 infection in human also occurred latter. The evidence supports the model that pigs serve as "mixing vessels" for reassortants as their cells contain receptors recognized by both human and avain viruses.

In March 2009, Mexico, the infectious disease monitoring system began registering an increase in influenza (flu) cases. By mid-April, nearly 1000 Mexican cases had been reported, with around 70 deaths. Soon a few cases of this same type of flu cropped up in the United States, primarily in California and Texas. When the Centers for Disease Control and Prevention (CDC) received reports samples from American and Mexican patients to identify the strain of virus. This outbreaks was initially attributed to a "swine flu virus", To allay unfounded fears about acquiring this disease from swine, public health groups urged that it be given the more accurate title of 2009 H1N1 type A Influenza.

9.1.1.1 Biological Characteristics

Influenza virus particle is usually about 100 nm in diameter, although virions may display great variation in size. Each of influenza A and B viruses consist a negative-sense, single-stranded RNA, which is enveloped in a glycolipid membrane (Figure 9-1). Most of the segments code for a single protein. The matrix (M1) protein, which forms a shell underneath the viral lipid envelope, is important in particle morphogenesis. Two virus-encoded glycoproteins, the hemagglutinin (HA) and the neuraminidase (NA), are inserted into the envelope and are exposed as spikes on the surface of the particle. HA is so named because of its ability to agglutinate red cell of some animals. NA is a sialidase that cleaves terminal sialic acid linkages in cell surface glycoconjugates and facilitates an essential step in virus propagation These two surface glycoproteins are the important antigens that determine antigenic variation of influenza viruses and host immunity. The M2 ion channel protein and the NS2 protein are also present in the envelope but at only a few copies per particle. Three large proteins (PB1, PB2 and PA) are bound to the viral RNP and are responsible for RNA transcription and replication. Table 9-1 illustrates the composition of influenza A virus. Antigenic differences exhibited by two of the internal structural proteins, the nucleocapsid (NP) and matrix (M) proteins, are used to divide influenza viruses into types A, B and C. These proteins possess no crossreactivity among the three types. Antigenic variations in the surface glycoproteins, HA and NA, are used to subtype the viruses. Only type A has designated subtypes. Influenza B is somewhat similar but has a unique NB protein instead of M2. Influenza C differs from the others in that it possesses only seven RNA segments and has no neuraminidase. The cleavage that separates HA1 and HA2 is necessary for the virus particle to be infectious and is mediated by cellular proteases. Influenza viruses normally remain confined to the respiratory tract because the protease enzymes that cleave HA are common only at those sites. Examples have been noted of more virulent viruses that have adapted to use a more ubiquitous enzyme, such as plasmid, to cleave HA and promote widespread infection of cells. H5N1 type virus causes infection in this way.

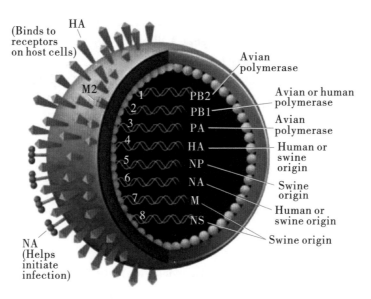

Figure 9-1　Diagram of influenza virus (Wikipedia)

Table 9-1　Influenza virus proteins

Genome segment	Protein	Nucleotides(bp)	Function
1	M1 M2	1027	Major component of virion; lines inside of envelope Integral membrane protein; ion channel
2	HA	1778	Hemagglutinin; envelope glycoprotein; mediate virus attachment to cells
3	NA	1413	Neuraminidase; envelope glycoprotein
4	NP	1565	Associated with RNA and polymerase proteins
5	NS1 NS2	890	Nonstructural protein; inhibits nuclear export of mRNA Minor component of virion
6	PB2	2341	RNA transcriptase components
7	PB1	2341	RNA transcriptase components
8	PA	2233	RNA transcriptase components

Mixtures of parental gene segments may be assembled into progeny virions when a cell is co-infected by two different viruses of a given type. This phenomenon, called genetic reassortment, may result in sudden changes in viral surface antigens (HA and NA)-a property that explains the epidemiologic features of influenza and poses significant problems for vaccine development.

The two surface antigens of influenza undergo antigenic changes because of the segmented nature of the genome. Minorganic antigenic changes in HA or NA, it usually is due to the accumulation of point mutations in the gene, resulting in amino acid changes in the protein are termed antigenic drift. Major antigenic changes in HA or NA, called antigenic shift is most likely to result in an epidemic. Internal proteins of the virus, such as the nucleoprotein (NP), do not undergo antigenic changes.

The steps of influenza viral replication are similar to other virus. Briefly, the NS1 and NP proteins are preferentially synthesized at high rates at early times. Then the two glycoproteins, HA and NA, are modified using the secretory pathway. The influenza virus nonstructural protein NS1 has a posttranscriptional role in regulating viral and cellular gene expression. The NS2 protein interacts with M1 protein and is involved in nuclear export of viral RNPs.

Influenza virus spreads from person to person by contact with contaminated hands or surfaces or by airborne droplets. Influenza viruses have a preference for the respiratory tract and viremia is rarely detected. They multiply in respiratory epithelial cells, leading to functional and structural ciliary abnormalities. Virions are soon produced and spread to adjacent cells, where the replicative cycle is repeated. In the mucous secretions, a few cells of respiratory epithelium are infected if deposited virus particles avoid removal by the cough reflex and escape neutralization by preexisting specific IgA antibodies or inactivation by nonspecific inhibitors. Viral NA lowers the viscosity of the mucous film in the respiratory tract, laying bare the cellular surface receptors and promoting the spread of virus-containing fluid to lower portions of the tract. , many cells in the respiratory tract are infected and eventually killed within a short time.

Immunity to influenza is subtype specific. Antibodies against HA and NA are important in immunity to influenza A virus. Protection correlates with both serum antibodies and secretory IgA antibodies in nasal secretions. The primary role of cell-mediated immune responses in influenza is believed to be clearance of an established infection; cytotoxic T cells lyses infected cells. Immunity can be incomplete, as reinfection with the same virus can occur.

9.1.1.2 Diagnosis and Treatment

Diagnosis of influenza based on isolation of the virus. Traditionally, the chick embryo was the standard host for cultivation of influenza viruses and still used in addition to cell culture by some reference laboratories. Most strains grow in primary monkey kidney cell cultures (MDCK) and viral isolates can be identified by hemagglutination inhibition, a procedure that permits rapid determination of the influenza type and subtype. Identification of viral antigens or viral nucleic acid in the patient's cells (nasopharyngeal and throat swabs) or demonstration of a specific immunologic response by the patient were widely used in the hospital. Rapid diagnosis of infection is possible by direct immunofluorescence or immunoenzymatic detection of viral antigen in epithelial cells or secretions from the respiratory tract. Rapid tests also based on detection of influenza RNA in clinical specimens using polymerase chain reaction. Routine serodiagnostic tests is of considerable help epidemiologically and usually use hemagglutination inhibition (HI), ELISA and PCR method, acute and convalescent sera are necessary for diagnosis.

The best available prevention method (FDA) is by use of killed viral vaccines newly formulated each year to most closely match the influenza A and B antigenic subtypes currently causing infections. Annual influenza vaccination is recommended for high-risk groups of peoples. These include individuals at increased risk of complications associated with influenza infection (those with either chronic heart or lung disease, including children with asthma or metabolic or renal disorders; residents of nursing homes; and those 65 years of age and older) and persons who might transmit influenza to high-risk groups (medical personnel, employees in chronic care facilities, household members). Several approaches to vaccine preparation are being evaluated. A live attenuated, cold-adapted, trivalent influenza virus vaccine administered by nasal spray has proved effective in clinical trials in children. The pandemic threat posed by highly pathogenic H5N1 influenza A viruses has created an urgent need for vaccines to protect against H5 virus infection. Because pathogenic viruses grow poorly in chicken eggs and their virulence poses a biohazard to vaccine producers, a virulent viruses produced by reverse genetics have become the preferred basis for H5N1 vaccine production. Traditional treatment options for influenza infection include broad-spectrum antiviral drugs (ribavirin) and neuraminidase inhibitors (Tamiflu etc.) and antibiotics may reduce secondary bacterial infections. However, there are still many debut about the toxicity of ribavirin and effect of neuraminidase inhibitors (NA).

9.1.2 Paramyxoviridae

Paramyxoviruses are the major respiratory pathogens in children. The paramyxoviruses include the causative agents of two of the most common contagious diseases of childhood (measles and mumps) as well as the most important agents of respiratory infection of infants and young children (respiratory syncytial virus and the parainfluenza viruses). All members of the Paramyxoviridae family initiate infection via the respiratory tract, measles and mumps can disseminated throughout the body and produce generalized disease.

The paramyxoviridae family is divided into subfamilies (Paramyxovirinae and Pneumovirinae) and four generas (paramyxovirus containing Human parainfluenza virus type 1 and 3; rubulavirus containing Human parainfluenza virus type 2, type 4 and mumps virus, Morbillivirus containing Human respiratory syncytial virus). Some properties of paramyxoviridae resemble that of orthomyxoviruses, but the two families differ in many biologic properties.

Paramyxoviruses generally consist of a 15－16 kb molecule of single-stranded RNA of negative polarity, a helical nucleocapsid and an outer lipoprotein envelope. The envelope is covered with spikes, which contain either hemagglutinin, neuraminidase or a fusion protein that causes cell fusion and, in some cases, hemolysis. The genome comprises 6－10 genes separated by conserved noncoding sequences that contain termination, polyadenylation and initiation signals. Most of the gene products are structural proteins found in the virion itself. Spattachecial mention should be made of the two major membrane glycoproteins because they play key roles in the pathogenesis of all paramyxovirus during infection. Cell attachment is mediated via the glycoprotein variously known, for different genera, as H (for hemagglutinating activity) or G (result of carrying neither activity, as result of which hemadsorption cannot be used as a laboratory diagnostic tool for respiratory syncytial virus). This glycoprotein elicits neutralizing, which inhibit adsorption of virus to cell receptors. The other major envelope glycoprotein is known as the fusion protein (F) because it enables the virus to fuse cell together to form the syncytia so characteristic of this family. The F protein is essential for viral penetration of the host cell by fusion of the viral envelope with the plasma membrane and for direct intercellular spread by cell-to-cell fusion, as well as perhaps contributing to the maintenance of persistent infections.

9.1.2.1   Measles Virus

Measles virus is a typical paramyxoviruses containing the genome RNA and nucleocapsid. The measles virus is the cause of measles, an infection of the respiratory system. Symptoms include fever, cough, runny nose red eyes and a generalized, maculopapular, erythematous rash. The virus is highly contagious and is spread by coughing and sneezing via close personal contact or direct contact with secretions. The introduction of an effective live-virus vaccine has dramatically reduced the incidence of this disease in many countries, but measles is still a leading cause of death of young children in many developing countries.

(1) Biological Characteristics

Although monkeys, dogs and mice, can be experimentally infected, humans are the only natural hosts for measles virus. The measles virus has two envelope glycoproteins on the viral surface-hemagglutinin (H) and membrane fusion protein (F). These proteins are responsible for host cell binding and invasion. The virus gains access to the human body via the respiratory tract, where it multiplies locally. The infection then spreads to the regional lymphoid tissue, where further multiplication occurs. Primary viremia disseminates the virus, which then replicates in the reticuloendothelial system. Finally, a secondary viremia seeds the epithelial surfaces of the body, including the skin, respiratory tract and conjunctiva, where focal replication occurs. Multinucleated giant cells with intranuclear inclusions are seen in lymphoid tissues throughout the body (lymphndes, tonsils, appendix).

The incubation period typically lasts 8–12 days but may last up to 3 weeks in adults. During the prodromal phase (2–4 days) and the fist 2–5 days of rash, virus is present in tears, nasal and throat secretions, urine and blood. Infections in non-immune hosts are almost always symptomatic. After an incubation period, the prodromal phase is characterized by fever, sneezing, coughing, running nose, redness of the eyes, Koplik's spots and lymphopenia. The characteristic maculopapular rash appears about day 14th just as circulating antibodies become detectable, the viremia disappears and the fever falls.

There is only one antigenic type of measles virus. Infection confers lifelong immunity, the presence of humoral antibodies indicates immunity. However cellular immunity appears to be essential for recovery and protection. Measles immune responses are involved in disease pathogenesis. Local inflammation causes the prodromal symptoms and specific cell-mediated immunity plays a role in development of the rash. Measles infection causes immune suppression, this is the cause of the serious secondary infections and may persist for months after measles infection (Figure 9–2).

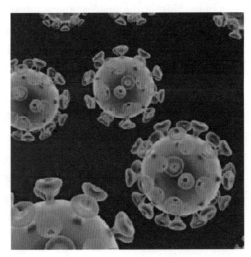

Figure 9-2   Measles virus (Wikipedia)

(2)Diagnosis and Treatment

Blood samples, respiratory secretions, nasopharyngeal swabs and urine collected from a patient during the febrile period are appropriate sources for viral isolation. Monkey or human kidney cells or a lymphoblastoid cell line (B95-a) are optimal for isolation attempts. Measles antigens can be detected directly in epithelial cells of respiratory secretions and urine. Antibodies to the nucleoprotein are useful because that is the most abundant viral protein in infected cells. ELLISA, HI and NT tests all may be used to measure measles antibodies. The major part of the immune response is directed against the viral nucleoprotein. Serologic conformation of measles infection depends on a fourfold rise in antibody titer between acute-phase and convalescent-phase sera or on demonstration of measles specific IgM antibody in a single serum specimen drawn between 1 and 2 weeks after the onset of rash.

Up to now, a highly effective and safe attenuated live measles virus vaccine is available around the world, the antibody titers tend to be lower than after natural infection, but immunity is probably lifelong, The introduction of an effective live-virus vaccine has dramatically reduced the incidence of this disease. Symptomatic care and anticipation of potential complications is important in treatment of measles. Mortality and morbidity has decreased by treatment of Vitamin A in developing countries. Administration of immunoglobulin can be used in treatment of measles. Measles virus is susceptible to inhibition by ribavirin *in vitro*, although clinical benefits have not been proved.

9.1.2.2 Mumps Virus

Mumps virus is the causative agent of mumps, a well-known common childhood disease characterised by swelling of the parotid glands, salivary glands and other epithelial tissues, causing high morbidity and in some cases more serious complications such as deafness. Mumps is transmissible by direct contact with saliva or by droplet spread. Mumps virus mostly causes a mild childhood disease, but meningitis and orchitis are fairly common, more than one-third of all mumps infections are asymptomatic.

(1)Biological Characteristics

Humans are the only natural hosts for mumps virus. Primary replication occurs in epithelial cells of nasal or upper respiratory tract. Virus is shed in the saliva from about-2 days to +9 days after the onset of salivary gland swelling. Viremia then disseminates the virus to the salivary glands and other major organ systems. About one-third of infected individuals do not exhibit obvious symptoms (in-apparent infections) but are equally capable of transmitting infection.

The incubation period is typically about 16−18 days but may range from 2 weeks to 4 weeks. Central nervous system involvement is common. Mumps causes aseptic meningitis. The most characteristic feature of symptomatic cases is swelling of the salivary glands, which occurs in about 50% of patients. A prodromal period of malaise and anorexia is followed by rapid enlargement of parotid glands as well as other salivary glands. Gland enlargement is associated with pain.

There is only one antigenic type of mumps virus and it does not exhibit significant antigenic variation, so immunity is permanent after a single infection. In natural infection, antibodies to the HN glycoprotein, the F glycoprotein and the internal nucleocapsid protein develop in serum followed by a cell-mediated immune response.

(2) Diagnosis and Treatment

An isolate can be confirmed as mumps virus by hemadsorption inhibition using mumps-specific antiserum. For rapid diagnosis, immunofluorescence using mumps-specific antiserum can detect mumps virus antigens as early as 2−3 days after the inoculation of cell cultures in shell vials. Antibody rise can be detected using paired sera by ELLISA or HI test.

It is considered a vaccine-preventable disease, although significant outbreaks have occurred in recent years in developed countries such as America, in areas of poor vaccine uptake. Still immunization with attenuated live mumps virus vaccine is the best approach to reducing mumps-associated morbidity and mortality rates. Attempts to minimize viral spread during an outbreak by using isolation procedures are futile because of the high incidence of the high incidence of asymptomatic cases and the degree of viral shedding before clinical symptoms appear.

9.1.2.3   Respiratory Syncytial Virus

Respiratory syncytial virus (RSV) is the leading cause of lower respiratory tract infections in infants and young children, being responsible for about half of all cases of bronchiolitis and a quarter of all cases of pneumonia before three years of children.

(1) Biological Characteristics

Respiratory syncytial virus replication occurs initially in epithelial cells of the nasopharynx. Virus may spread into the lower respiratory tract and cause bronchiolitis and pneumonia. There is lymphocyte migration, resulting in peribronchiolar infiltration; submucosal tissues become edematous; and plugs consisting of mucus, cellular debris and fibrin occlude the smaller bronchioles.

The incubation period between exposure and onset of illness is 3−7 days. The spectrum of respiratory illness caused by respiratory syncytial virus ranges from unapparent infection or the common cold through pneumonia in infants to bronchiolitis in very young babies. Bronchiolitis is the distinct clinical syndrome associated with this virus. About one-third of primary respiratory tract severely enough to require medical attention. Reinfection is common in both children and adults. Although reinfections tend to be symptomatic, the illness is usually limited to the upper respiratory tract, resembling a cold, in healthy individuals.

High levels of neutralizing antibody that is maternally transmitted and present during the first several months of life are believed to be critical in protective immunity against lower respiratory tract illness. Severe respiratory syncytial disease begins to occur in infants at 2−4 months of age, when maternal antibody levels are falling. However, primary infection and reinfection can occur in the presence of viral antibodies. Serum neutralizing antibody appears be strongly correlated with immunity against disease of the lower respiratory tract but not of the upper respiratory tract. Both serum antibodies are made in response to respiratory syncytial virus infection. Primary infection with one subgroup induces cross-reactive antibodies to virus of the other subgroup. Cellular immunity is important in recovery from infection. A n association has been noted between virus-specific IgE antibody and severity of disease.

(2) Diagnosis and Treatment

Respiratory syncytial virus can be isolated from nasal secretions. Human heteroploid cell, HeLa and HEp-2 are the most sensitive cell lines for viral isolation. The presence of respiratory syncytial virus can usually be recognized by development of giant cells and syncytial virus differs from other paramyxoviruses in that it does not have a hemagglutinin, therefore, diagnostic methods cannot use hemagglutination or henadsorption assays. Immunofluorescence on exfoliated cells or ELLISA on nasopharyngeal secretions are commonly used. Direct identification of viral antigens in clinical samples is rapid and sensitive. Serum antibodies can be assayed in a variety of ways, immunofluorescence, ELISA and Nt tests are all used. Polymerase chain reaction assays are useful for subtyping respiratory syncytial virus isolates and for the analysis of genetic variation in outbreaks.

At present, the only approved chemical for respiratory syncytial virus infection is ribavirin, but it is strictly used in infants with severe illness. Paliduzumab is used for passive immunization of RSV infections, but is expensive and difficult to use clinically. Much research effort has been expended in an attempt to develop a respiratory syncytial virus vaccine which poses a special problems: the target group-newborns, would have to immunized soon after birth to afford protection at the time of greatest risk of serious respiratory syncytial virus infection and eliciting a protective immune response is difficult in the presence of maternal antibody at this early age. A strategy being tested is maternal immunization with a vaccine. The aim is to ensure transfer of protective levels of virus-specific neutralizing antibody to infants that would persist for 3−5 months, the period of greatest vulnerability of newborns to severe respiratory syncytial virus disease. Because there is no effective medicinal treatment, syncytial virus vaccine has stood in the way of vaccine development.

9.1.2.4 Parainfluenza Viruses

Parainfluenza viruses are common respiratory pathogen closely associated with both human and veterinary disease. Virions are approximately 150−250 nm in size and contain negative senseRNA with a genome encompassing-15,000 nucleotides. Generally speaking, they produce relatively harmless upper respiratory tract infection, but they are also the commonest cause of more serious condition in young children known as "croup" and occasionally cause pneumonia. Of the four serotypes of parainfluenza viruses able to infect humans, only the first three are associated with severe disease.

(1) Biological Characteristics

Primary infections in young children usually result in rhinitis and pharyngitis, often with fever and some bronchitis. However, children with primary infections caused by parainfluenza virus type 1,2 or 3 may have serious illness, ranging from laryngotracheitis and croup (particularly with types 1 and 2) to bronchiolitis and pneumonia (particularly with type 3). The severe illness associated with type 3 occurs mainly in infants under the age of 6 month; croup or laryngotracheobronchitis is more likely to occur in older children, between ages 6 months and 18 months. Parainfluenza virus type 4 does not cause serious disease, even on first infection. The most common complication of parainfluenza virus infection is otitis media.

Most infants have maternal antibodies to the virus in serum, yet these antibodies do not prevent infection or disease. Reinfection of older children and adults also occurs in the presence of antibodies elicited by an earlier infection. However, those antibodies modify the disease, as such reinfections usually present simply as non-febrile upper respiratory infections (colds). Natural infection stimulates appearance of IgA antibody in nasal secretions and concomitant resistance to reinfection, but it disappear within a few months. The immune response to the initial parainfluenza virus infection in life is type-specific. However, with repeated infections the response becomes less specific and cross reactions extend even to mumps virus.

(2) Diagnosis and Treatment

Antigen detection methods are useful ways for rapid diagnosis. Antigens may be detected in exfoliated nasopharyngeal cells by direct or indirect immunofluorescence tests. These methods are rapid but less sensitive than viral isolation and must be carefully controlled. Definitive diagnosis relies on viral isolation from appropriate specimens. Primary monkey kidney cells are the most sensitive for isolation of parainfluenza viruses, but such cells are difficult to obtain. A continuous monkey kidney cell line, LLC-MK2, is a suitable alternative. Parainfluenza viruses grow slowly and produce very little cytopathic effect. Another way to detect the presence of virus is to perform hemadsorption using guinea pig erythrocytes. Serodiagnosis should be based on paired sera. Antibody responses can be measured using Nt, HI or ELISA tests. Polymerase chain reaction assays are not commonly used at this time because of difficulties of RNA detection in respiratory secretion. Sequence analyses are useful in molecular epidemiology studies of parainfluenza virus infections.

Contact isolation precautions are necessary to manage nosocomial outbreaks of parainfluenza virus. These include restriction of visitors, isolation of infected patients and gowning and hand washing by medical personnel. Both subunit vaccines and a live attenuated type 3 virus vaccine to be administered intranasally are being tested. The antiviral drug ribavirin and IFN have been used with some benefit in treatment of immuno-compromised patients with lower respiratory tract disease.

9.1.3   Other Respiratory Viruses

9.1.3.1   Coronaviruses

Coronaviruses are species of virus belonging to the subfamily Coronavirinae in the family Coronaviridae, in the order Nidovirales. Coronaviruses are widespread in nature, infect a range of hosts with variable tissue tropisms and highly species specific. Animal coronaviruses cause diseases of economic losses in domestic animals. Persistent coronaviruses infections were established in their natural hosts of some animals. The human coronaviruses cause common colds and have been implicated in gastroenteritis in infants. A novel coronavirus was identified because of a worldwide outbreak of a severe acute respiratory syndrome (SARS) in 2003. SARS coronavirus causes severe respiratory disease. The incubation period averages about 6 days. Common early symptoms include fever, malaise, chills, headache, dizziness, cough and sore throat, followed a few days later by shortness of breath. Many patients have abnormal chest radiographs. Some cases progress rapidly to acute respiratory distress, requiring ventilatory support. Death from progressive respiratory failure occurs in almost 10% of cases, with the death rate highest among the elderly. Clinical features of coronavirus-associated enteritis have not been clearly described.

(1) Biological Characteristics

Coronaviruses are enveloped viruses with a positive-sense single-stranded RNA genome and with a nucleocapsid of helical symmetry. The genomic size of coronaviruses ranges from approximately 26 to 32 kilobases, the largest for an RNA virus. The viral structural proteins include nucleocapsid and the spike glycoprotein that makes up the petal-shaped peplomers (Figure 9-3). Some viruses, including human coronavirus OC43, contain a third glycoprotein (HE) that causes hemagglutination and has acetylesterase activity. Several open reading frames encoding nonstructural proteins and the HE protein differ in number and gene order among coronaviruses.

The human coronaviruses produce "cold", usually a febrile, in adults. The symptoms are similar to those produced by rhinoviruses, typified by nasal discharge and malaise. The incubation period is from 2 days to 5 days and symptoms usually last about 1 week. The lower respiratory tract is seldom involved, although pneumonia in military recruits has been attributed to coronavirus infection. Asthmatic children may suffer wheezing attacks and chronic pulmonary disease in adults may exacerbate respiratory symptoms.

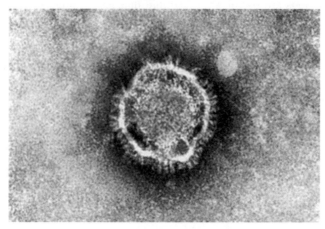

Figure 9-3 **Human Coronavirus.**
Note the characteristic large, widely spaced spike that form a "corona" around virion (150,000×)(Wikipedia)

Replication of Coronavirus begins with entry to the cell which takes place in the cytoplasm in a membrane-protected microenvironment. Upon entry to the cell the virus particle is uncoated and the RNA genome is deposited into the cytoplasm. The virus attaches to receptors on target cells by the glycoprotein spikes on the viral envelope (either by S or HE). The particle is then internalized, probably by absorptive endocytosis. The S glycoprotein may cause fusion of the viral envelope with the cell membrane. The first event after uncoating is translation of the viral genomic RNA to produce a virus-specific RNA dependent RNA polymerase. The viral polymerase transcribes a full-length complementary (minus-strand) RNA that serves as the template for a nested set of five to seven subgenomic mRNAs. The genomic RNA encodes a large polyprotein that gets processed to yield the viral RNA polymerase. Newly synthesized genomic RNA molecules interact in the cytoplasm with the nucleocapsid protein to form helical nucleocapsids bud through membranes of the rough endoplasmic reticulum and the Golgi apparatus in areas that contain the viral glycoproteins. Mature virions may then be transported in vesicles to the cell dies to be released.

There are two genera in the Coronaviridae family: Coronavirus and Torovirus. The toroviruses are widespread in ungulates and appear to be associated with diarrheas. There seem to be two serogroups of human coronaviruses, represented by strains 229E and OC43. Coronaviruses of domestic animals and rodents are included in these two groups. There is a third distinct antigenic group, which contains the avian infections bronchitis virus of chickens. There appears to be significant antigenic heterogeneity among viral strains within a major antigenic group (ie, 229E-like). Cross-reactions occur between some human and some animal strains.

Coronaviruses tend to be highly species-specific. Most of the known animal coronaviruses display a tropism for epithelial cells of the respiratory or gastrointestinal tract. Coronavirus infections may be disseminated *in vivo*, such as with mouse hepatitis virus. In contrast, the outbreak of SARS in 2003 was characterized by serious respiratory illness, including pneumonia and pneumonia and progressive respiratory failure. In all likelihood, the SARS virus originated in a nonhuman host and acquired the ability to infect humans. In rural regions of southern China, where the outbreak began, people, pigs and domestic fowl live close together and there is widespread use of wild species for food and traditional medicine-conditions that promote the emergence of new viral strains. Coronaviruses are suspected of causing some gastroenteritis in humans, but the agents have not been isolated. The novel coronavirus recovered in 2003 from patients with Severe Acute Respiratory Syndrome (SARS) appears to represent a new (fourth) group of viruses and the genome differ in many part compared with the other coronavirus strains because it causes both upper and lower respiratory tract infections.

Immunity against the surface projection antigen is probably most important for protection. Resistance to reinfection may last several years, but reinfections with similar strains are common. Most patients (>95%) with SARS developed an antibody response to viral antigens detectable by a fluorescent antibody test or ELISA.

(2) Diagnosis and Treatment

Polymerase chain reaction assays are useful to detect coronavirus nucleic acid in respiratory secretions and in samples. Isolation of human coronavirus in cell culture has been difficult. However, the SARS virus was recovered from or pharyngeal specimens using acute and convalescent sera is the practical means of confirming coronavirus infections. ELISA and hemagglutination tests may be used. Coronavirus antigens in cells in respiratory secretions may be detected using the ELISA test if a high-quality antiserum is available.

There is no proven treatment for coronavirus infection and the vaccine has stood in the way of development. Control measures that were effective in stopping the spread of SARS included isolation of patients, quarantine of those who had been exposed and travel restrictions, as well as the use of gloves, gowns, goggles and respirators by health care workers.

9.1.3.2 Adenovirus

Adenoviruses (members of the family Adenoviridae) are medium-sized, nonenveloped (without an outer lipid bilayer) viruses (Figure 9-4) with an icosahedral nucleocapsid containing a double stranded DNA genome. Their name derives from their initial isolation from human adenoids in 1953. It has many sera types, it can replicate and produce disease in the eye and in the respiratory, gastrointestinal and urinary tracts. Of the almost 100 different serotypes of adenovirus, 49 are known to affect humans. Adenovirus can cause pharyngoconjunctival fever, pneumonia, acute hemorrhagic cystitis and gastroenteritis. Many adenovirus infections are subclinical and virus may persist in the host for months. A few types serve as models for cancer induction in animals. Adenovirus are especially valuable systems for molecular and biochemical studies of eukaryotic cell processes.

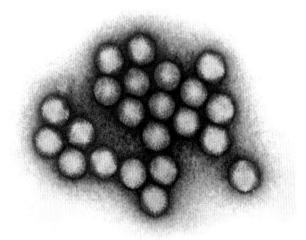

Figure 9-4   Electron micrograph of adenovirus (17, 500×) (Wikipedia)

(1) Biological Characteristic

The adenovirus genome is linear, non-segmented double-stranded (ds) DNA that is between 26 and 48 kbp. Replication and assembly occurs in the nucleus, are able to replicate in the nucleus of vertebrate cells using the host's replication machinery. All adenovirus share a common group-specific, complement-fixing antigen associated with the hexon component of the viral capsid. Adenoviruses are characterized by their ubiquity and persistence in host tissues for periods ranging from a few days to several years. Adenovirus replicative cycle is sharply divided into early and late events.

Inhalation of droplet nuclei and the oral route are the ways of the adenovirus enters the host. Direct inoculation onto nasal or conjunctival mucosa by hands, contaminated towels or ophthalmic medications. Cell necrosis and inflammation are produced when virus replicates in epithelial cells. Viremia sometimes occurs and can result in spread to distant sites, such as the kidney, liver, bladder, lymphoid tissue. Integration of adenoviral DNA into the host cell genome has been shown to occur.

Symptoms include fever, rhinitis, cough, pharyngitis and conjunctivitis. Adenoviruses are also common causes of non-streptococcal exudative pharyngitis, particularly among children less than 3 years old. The acute respiratory syndromes vary in both clinical manifestations and severity. Acute and occasionally chronic, conjunctivitis and keratoconjunctivitis have been associated with several serotypes. More severe disease, such as laryngitis, croup, bronchiolitis and pneumonia, may also occur. A syndrome of pharyngitis and conjunctivitis (pharyngoconjunctival fever) is classically associated with adenovirus infection. Adenovirus also can cause acute hemorrhagic cystitis, in which hematuria and dysuria are prominent findings. Some serotypes are significant causes of gastroenteritis. The diversity of major syndromes and serotypes commonly associated with adenoviruses are summarized in Table 9-2.

Immunity after infection is serotype specific and usually long lasting. In addition to type-specific immunity, group-specific complement-fixing antibodies appear in response to infection.

Table 9-2 Disease associated with adenovirus serotype

Disease	Associated serotype	Clinical feature
Acute respiratory disease	3,7,14,21	Common in infants and young children
Pneumonia	3,7	Cause pneumonia in children
Pharyngoconjunctival fever	3,7,14,21	The contamination of water in the reason of outbreaks
Epidemic keratoconjunctivitis	8,19,37	Common in adults, easy to transmit
Haemorrhagic cystitis	11,7,21,35	Common in infants and young children
Diarrhoea and vomiting	40,41	Common in infants

(2) Diagnosis and Treatment

Samples should be collected early from affected sites to isolate virus. Virus isolation in a cell culture requires human cells and primary human embryonic kidney cells are most susceptible but usually unavailable. Established human epithelial cell lines, such as Hep-2, Hela and KB are sensitive. The development of characteristic cytopathic reeffects-rounding and clustering of swollen cells, indicates the presence of adenovirus in inoculated cultures. Serologic testing of acute and convalescent sera may be necessary to confirm the relationship between the virus and the illness.

In the past, US military recruits were vaccinated against two serotypes of adenovirus, with a corresponding decrease in illnesses caused by those serotypes. That vaccine is no longer manufactured. The viruses are released into the small intestine, where they produce an asymptomatic, non-transmissible infection. This vaccine has been found effective but is neither available nor recommended for civilian groups. In addition to vaccination, other methods of prevention and control are available. However, there are no proven antiviral drugs to treat adenoviral infections, so treatment is largely directed at the symptoms (such as acetaminophen for fever). The antiviral drug cidofovir has helped certain of those patients who had severe cases of illness; the number helped and to what degree and the particular complications or symptoms it helped with and when and where this happened, were not given in the source. A doctor may give antibiotic eyedrops for conjunctivitis, while awaiting results of bacterial cultures and to help prevent secondary bacterial infections.

9.2 Enterovirus

Enteroviruses are members of the picornavirus family, a large and diverse group of small RNA viruses characterized by a single positive-strand genomic RNA. Enterovirusws are transient inhabitants in human alimentary tract and can be isolated from the throat or lower gastrointestinal tract, which are the primary sites for the replication of enteroviruses, although enteroviruses do not cause obvious diseases in the gastrointestinal tract. Enterovirus infections are usually asymptomatic but can range from cold-like symptoms to paralytic disease. Differences in pathogenesis for the enteroviruses mainly result from differences in tissue tropism and cytolytic capacity of the virus. Human enterovirus mainly include the following four viruses: poliovirus, coxsackievirus, echovirus and new enteroviruses. The four viruses have a number of features in common:

1) They all replicate in the intestinal tract.

2) They commonly cause asymptomatic immunizing infections which protect against future infections with the same virus.

3) They can give rise to viraemia.

4) They occasionally cause infection of the central nervous system.

5) They are commoner in children than adults.

6) In temperate climates they cause infections usually in the summer and autumn.

9.2.1 Polioviruses

Poliovirus is the causative agent of poliomyelitis. Poliomyelitis is an acute infectious disease that in its serious form affects the central nervous system. The destruction of motor neurons in the spinal cord results in flaccid paralysis. Most poliovirus infections are subclinical.

9.2.1.1 Biological Properties

Poliovirus particles are typical enteroviruses. The virion of enteroviruses consists of a capsid shell of sixty subunit, each of four proteins (VP1-VP4) arranged with icosahedral symmetry around a genome made up of a single strand of positive sense RNA. There are three types of poliovirus, identified by neutralization tests, their RNA molecules differing by 50% in hybridization studies. The prototype strains are: type 1, the Brunhilde and Mahoney strains; type 2, which includes the rodent-adapted strains, the Lansing and MEFI strains; and type 3, the Leon and Saukett strains. The three types are antigenically distinct, but overlap occurs in neutralization tests. Type 1 is the common epidemic type, type 2 is usually associated with endemic infections, but type 3 has caused recent epidemics. The size, chemical and physical properties and the resistance of the three types areal identical and so their antigenic properties provide one of the main methods of differentiating them.

9.2.1.2 Pathogenesis and Pathology

The mouth is the portal of entry of the virus and primary virus replication takes place in the oropharynx or intestine. The virus is regularly present in the throat and in the faeces before the onset of illness. The virus may be found in the blood of patients with nonparalytic poliomyelitis and in orally infected monkeys in the preparalytic phase of the disease. Antibody to the virus appear early in the disease, usually before paralysis occurs. It is convinced that the virus first replicated in the tonsils, the lymph nodes of the neck, Peyer's patches and the small intestine. The central nervous system may then be invaded by way of the circulating blood. Poliovirus can spread along axons of peripheral nerves to the central nervous system, where it continues to progress along the fibers to the lower motor neurons to increasingly involve the spinal cord or the brain. Poliovirus invades certain types of nerve cells and in the process of its intracellular multiplication it may damage or completely destroy these cells. The anterior horn cells of the spinal cord are most prominently involved, but in severe cases the intermediate gray ganglia and even the posterior horn and dorsal root ganglia are often involved. Poliovirus does not replicate in muscle in vivo. The changes that occur in peripheral nerves and voluntary muscles are secondary to the destruction of nerve cells. Some cells that lose their function may recover completely. Inflammation occurs secondary to the attack on the nerve cells.

9.2.1.3 Clinical Syndromes

When an individual susceptible to infection is exposed to the virus, the response ranges from inapparent infection without symptoms, to a mild febrile illness, to severe and permanent paralysis. Most infection are subclinical; only about 1% of infections result in clinical illness. The incubation period is usually seven to fourteen days, but it may range from three to thirty-five days.

Asymptomatic illness results if the virus is limited to infection of the oropharynx and the gut. At least 90% of poliovirus infections are of the asymptomatic type.

Abortive poliomyelitis, the minor illness, is a nonspecific febrile illness occurring the approximately 5% of infected individuals. Symptoms of fever, headache, malaise, sore throat and vomiting occur within three to four days of exposure.

Nonparalytic poliomyelitis or aseptic meningitis occurs in 1% to 2% of patients with poliovirus infections. The virus progress into the central nervous system and the meninges, causing back pain and muscle spasms in addition the symptoms of minor illness.

Paralytic polio, the major illness, occurs in 0.1% to 2.0% of persons with poliovirus infections and is the most sever outcome. Major illness follow three to four days after minor illness has subsides, thereby producing a biphasic illness. In this disease the virus spreads from the blood the anterior horn cells of the spinal cord and the motor cortex of the brain. The severity of the paralysis is determined by the extent of the neuronal infection and the neurons affected. Spinal paralysis may involve one or more limbs, whereas bulbar paralysis may involve a combination of cranial nerves and even the medullary respiratory center.

Paralytic poliomyelitis is characterized by an asymmetric flaccid paralysis with no sensory loss. Poliovirus type 1 affects 85% of patients with paralytic disease. Type 2 or 3 may cause vaccine-associated disease because of reversion from attenuated virus to virulence. The degree of paralysis may vary from involving only a few muscle groups (e.g., one leg) to complete flaccid paralysis of all four extremities. The paralysis may progress over the first few days and result in complete recovery, residual paralysis or death. Most recoveries occur within six month, but as long as 2 years may be required for complete remission.

Bulbar poliomyelitis can be more severe and may involve the muscles of the pharynx, vocal cords and respiration and result in death in 75% of patients. Iron lungs, chambers providing external respiratory compression, were used to assist the breathing of polio patients during the 1950s. Before vaccinations programs, iron lungs filled the wards of children's hospiatals.

Post-polio syndrome is a sequelae of poliomyelitis that may occur much later in life (30 to 40 years) for 20% to 80% of the originally affected muscles. Poliovirus is not present, but the syndrome is believed to be due to a loss of neurons in the initially affected nerves.

9.2.1.4 Immunity

Immunity is permanent to the type causing the infection. There may be a low degree of heterotypic resistance induced by infection, especially between type 1 and type 2 polioviruses. Passive immunity is transferred from mother to offspring. The maternal antibodies gradually disappear during the first 6 months of life. Passively administered antibody lasts only 3−5 weeks. Virus-neutralizing antibody forms soon after exposure to the virus, often before the onset of illness and apparently persists for life. Its formation early in the disease implies that viral replication occurs in the body before the invasion of the nervous system. As the virus in the brain and spinal cord is not influenced by high titers of antibodies in the blood, immunization is of value only if it precedes the onset of symptoms referable to the nervous system.

9.2.1.5 Laboratory Diagnosis

Virus isolation is the most useful method for establishing a diagnosis. Examination of cerebrospinal fluid is an essential part of the laboratory diagnosis of meningitis. The sample is directly inoculated into cell culture. Faecal samples should also be submitted, although isolation can be made from rectal and throat swabs. Since virus excretion can be intermittent, two specimens should be collected on successive days, as early as possible in the illness, ideally within 5 days of the onset. Virus is detected by the development of a cytopathic effect usually within a few days; the virus is confirmed by neutralization tests with type-specific antisera.

In paralytic poliomyelitis, the virus can be found in the faeces for a few days preceding the onset of acute symptoms and is present in over 80% of cases in the faeces during the first 4 days. After 3 weeks some 50% of patients still excrete the virus and 25% at 5−6 weeks. Only a few cases continue to excrete the virus after the 12th week. No permanent carriers are known but prolonged excretion is recognized in immunocompromised hosts. The virus can be isolated from the oropharynx of many cases for a few days before and after the onset of the illness. Isolation of from the cerebrospinal fluid is seldom successful in cases of paralytic poliomyelitis.

Paired serum specimens are required to show a rise in antibody titer during the course of the disease. Only first infection with poliovirus produces type-specific responses. Subsequent infections with heterotypic polioviruses induce antibodies against the heat-stable group antigen share by all three types. Neutralizing antibodies appear early.

9.2.1.6 Treatment, Prevention & Control

No specific antiviral therapy is available for polioviruses infections. Supportive therapy is important for patients with paralytic disease to assist in their potential recovery. The prevention of paralytic poliomyelitis is one of the triumphs of modern medicine. Infection with wild type poliovirus disappeared from the United States in 1979. However, health care delivery systems are not sufficient to provide adequate vaccine administration in undeveloped countries and wild type virus disease still exits in Africa, the Middle East and Asia.

Both live-virus and killed-virus vaccines are available. Formalinized vaccine (Salk) is prepared from virus grown in monkey kidney cultures. At least four inoculations over a period of 1−2 year years have been recommended in the primary series. Periodic booster immunizations have been necessary to maintain immunity. Killed-virus vaccine induces humoral antibodies, but does not induce local intestinal immunity so that virus is still able to replicate in the gut. Oral vaccines contain live attenuated virus grown in primary monkey or human diploid cell cultures. The vaccine can be stabilized by magnesium chloride so that it can be kept without losing potency for a year at 4 ℃ and for weeks at moderate room temperature (about 25 ℃). Nonstabilized vaccine must be kept frozen until used.

A major campaign is under way by the World Health Organization to eradicate poliovirus from the world as was done for smallpox virus. The Americas were certified as free from wild poliovirus in 1994. Progress is being made globally, but thousands of cases of polio still occur each year, principally in Africa and the Indian subcontinent.

9.2.2 Coxsachievirus and Echoviruses

Coxsackievirus, a large subgroup of the enteroviruses, are divided into two group, A and B, having different pathogenic potentials for mice. They produce a variety of illnesses in humans. Herpangina (vesicular pharyngitis), hand-foot-mouth disease and acute hemorrhagic conjunctivitis are caused by certain coxsackievirus group A serotypes. Pleurodynia (epidemic myalgis), myocarditis, pericarditis, meningoencephalitis and severe generalized disease of infants are caused by some group B coxsackieviruses. Echoviruses were identified by cell culture of faeces of patients suffering from paralytic and non-paralytic illness. There are over 30 serotypes of the enteric cytopathic human orphan viruses and, true to their name, there is still no clear association of all types with specific disease.

9.2.2.1 Biological Properties

Coxsackieviruses are highly infective for newborn mice. Certain strains (B1-6, A7, 9, 16 and 24) also grow in monkey kidney cell culture. At least 29 different immunologic types of coxsackieviruses are recognized; 23 are listed as group A and 6 as group B types. Most of the echovirus types have been associated with sporadic cases of aseptic meningitis or one of the other disease patterns already mentioned. A number of types, notabley 4, 6, 9, 16, 20, 28 and 30, have considerable epidemic potential and the clinical features are very varied.

9.2.2.2 Pathogenesis and Pathology

Virus has been recovered from the blood in the early stages of natural infection in humans and of experimental infection in chimpanzees. Virus is also found in the throat for a few days early in the infection and in the stools for up to 5–6 weeks. Virus distribution is similar to that of the other enteroviruses.

9.2.2.3 Clinical Syndromes

Several clinical syndromes may be caused by either coxsackievirus or echovirus, but certain illnesses are especially associated with coxsackievirus. For example, coxsackie A viruses are highly associated with herpangina, whereas myocarditis and pleurodynia are most frequently caused by coxsackie B serotypes. These viruses can slso cause polio-like paralytic disease. The most common results of infection are no symptoms, mild upper respiratory or "flu-like" disease.

Herpangina is inappropriately named because it has no relation to herpesvirus. Rather, it is caused by several types of coxsackie A virus. Fever, sore throat, pain on swallowing, anorexia and vomiting characterize herpangina. The classic finding is vesicular ulcerated lesions around the soft palate and uvula. The virus can be recovered from the lesions or from feces. The disease is self-limited and requires only symptomatic management.

Pleurodynia (Bornholm disease) is an acute illness in which patients have sudden onset of fever and unilateral low thoracic, pleuritic, chest pain, which may be excruciating. Abdominal pain and even vomiting may also occur, Muscles on the involved side may be extremely tender. Pleurodynia lasts an average of 4 days but may relapse after the patient has been asymptomatic for several days. Coxsackie B virus is the causative agent.

Viral or aseptic, meningitis is an acute febrile illness accompanied by headache and signs of meningeal irritation. Perechiae or skin rash may occur in patients with enteroviral meningitis. Recovery is usually uneventful except if associated with encephalitis or in infants younger than one year old. Outbreaks of picornavirus meningitis occur each year during the summer and autumn.

Fever and rash may occur in patients infected with either echoviruses or coxsackieviruses. The eruption are usually maculopapular but occasionally may appear as petechial or even vesicular eruptions. The petechial type or eruption must be differentiated from that of meningococcemia. The child with enteroviral in not as ill or as toxic and has a lesser degree of leukocytosis than the child with meningococcemia.

Hand-foot-and-mouth disease is a vesicular exanthem caused by an enterovirus, usually coxsackievirus A16. The colorful name is descriptive, since the main features of this infection are vesicular lesions of the hands, feet, mouth and tongue. The patient is mildly febrile and the illness subsides in a few days.

Mycocardial and pericardial infections caused by coxsackie B virus occur sporadically to older children and adults but are most threatening in newborns. Neonates with these infections have febrile illness and sudden unexplained onset of heart failure. Cyanosis, tachycardial, cardiomegaly and hepatomegaly occur. Electrocardiographic changes are found in patients with myocarditis. Mortality is high and autopsy reveals other involved organ systems, including brain, liver and pancreas. Acute benign pericarditis affects young adults but may be seen in older individuals with symptoms resembling myocardial infarction but with more sever fever.

9.2.2.4　Laboratory Diagnosis

(1) Clinical Chemistry

Cerebrospinal fluid (CSF) from poliovirus or enterovirus aseptic meningitis reveals a predominantly lymphocytic plepcutosis (presence of 25 to 500 cells). In contrast to bacterial meningitis, the CSF glucose level is usually normal or slightly low. CSF protein level is normal to slightly elevated. The CSF is rarely positive for the virus.

(2) Culture

Coxsackieviruses and echoviruses can usually be isolated from the throat and stool during infection and often from CSF in patients with meningitis. Virus is rarely isolated in myocarditis, since the symptoms occur several weeks after the initial infection. The coxsackie B viruses can be grown on primary monkey or human embryo kidney cells. Many coxsackie A virus strains do not grow in tissue culture and must still be grown in suckling mice. The specific enterovirus type can be determined only by using specific antibody and assays (e. g. , neutralization, immunofluorescence).

(3) Serology

Serology confirmation of enterovirus infection can be made by detection of specific IgM or a fourfold increase in antibody titer between acute illness and convalescence. The many serotypes of echovirus and coxsackievirus make this approach difficult, but it may be useful in documenting poliovirus infection.

9.2.2.5　Treatment, Prevention & Control

No specific antiviral therapy is available for coxsackieviruses or echoviruses infections. Supportive therapy is extremely important for patients to assist in their potential recovery. No vaccines exist for coxsackieviruses or echoviruses. Transmission can presumably be reduced by improvements in hygiene and living conditions.

9.2.3 New types of Enteroviruses:Enterovirus 71

At least four new type enteroviruses (types 68 – 172) grow in monkey kidney cultures and three of them cause human disease. Enterovirus 68 has been isolated from the respiratory tracts of children with bronchiolitis or pneumonia. Enterovirus 70 is the chief cause of acute of hemorrhagic conjunctivitis. Acute hemorrhagic conjunctivitis has a sudden onset of subconjunctival hemorrhage ranging from small petechial to large blotches covering the bulbar conjunctiva. The disease is most common in adult, with an incubation period of 1 day and a duration of 8–10 days. Complete recovery is the rule. Enterovirus 71 (EV71) has been isolated from patients with meningitis, encephalitis and paralysis resembling poliomyelitis. It is one of the main causes of central nervous system disease, sometimes fatal, around the world. In some areas, the virus has caused outbreaks of hand-foot-and-mouth disease and herpangina. Enterovirus 72 is the hepatitis virus A. Infections of enterovirus 70 and 71 have been associated with severe central nervous system disease. A particular acute form of extremely contagious hemorrhagic conjunctivitis has also been associated with enterovirus 70.

The first isolation of EV71 was in fecal matter of a baby with encephalitis in California in 1969. In 1973, EV71 was first recognized as causing epidemics of HFMD in Japan. Also in the 1970s, two large epidemics of EV71 occurred in Europe which were recognized from the virus causing HFMD or other symptoms. The first outbreak in Europe was in Bulgaria. EV71 was the causative agent in 77% of the children with non-specific febrile illness and neurological disease. Of the 451 children with the disease, approximately 10% died. In the second epidemic in Hungary, symptoms were aseptic meningitis and encephalitis. Small sporadic outbreaks continued to break out in the 1980s in Hong Kong and Australia. By the late 1990s, large outbreaks occurred in the Asia-Pacific region. The death rate was less than 1 percent of the patients. This outbreak had 1.5 million infections, 405 severe cases and 78 deaths. The latest outbreak was in China in 2008, when 490,000 infections were reported with 126 deaths. In many areas in the Asia-Pacific region, cyclical epidemics have occurred every 2 to 3 years. Fatality rates from these outbreaks have been as high as 14%, with the majority of these having complications such as encephalitis. Thus far, outbreaks of EV71 arise at a low level in the Africa, Europe and the US.

9.2.3.1 Pathogenesis

Transmission of EV71 is through direct contact of discharge from the nose, throat, saliva and blisters or stools of infected persons. The infection is most contagious during the first week of the illness, but fecal matter can continue to contain viral particles for up to 11 weeks. After direct contact with EV71, the virus must be able to replicate itself to reach an infectious dose. EV71 can remain viable at room temperature for several days. Initial replication begins in the intestinal tract. The virus then spreads into the bloodstream by the third day of infection. The virus then spreads to organ systems, causing a second viral infection episode on days 3–7. The infection can further progress to the central nervous system in more severe infections.

9.2.3.2 Symptoms

EV71 infections can cause a wide range of symptoms and is most common in children under the age of 5. The most common feature is hand-foot-and-mouth disease (HFMD). HFMD usually occurs in children and is generally mild. It consists of a papulovesicular rash on the palms and soles as well as multiple oral ulcers (also known as herpangina). In children under the age of two, atypical rashes are frequently seen. Other symptoms that can occur from EV71 are upper respiratory infections, fever, gastroenteritis, bronchiolitis and pneumonia. EV71 infections can also cause neurological and systemic complications such as aseptic meningitis, acute flaccid paralysis and encephalitis (usually in the brainstem). These symptoms are usually successive to or in conjunction with HFMD. Only a small portion of infected children develop these complications, which can be severe and even fatal. Children can develop these symptoms in a matter of hours to days.

9.2.3.3   Diagnosis, Treatment & Prevention

For diagnosis of EV71 infections, many different tests can be performed, depending on the manifestations of the disease. The most efficient approach for diagnosis is throat swabs and swabs from at least two vesicles or from the rectum for patients with no vesicles. Other approaches for diagnosis is the use of EV71-specific primers to perform PCR directly on samples. This allows for faster diagnosis than virus cultures, but this only tests for EV71. DNA microarray is a tool used as well and it has been reported to be 90% accurate in diagnosis of EV71 infections, however it is an expensive tool. In cases that have central nervous system involvement, lumbar punctures are essential for diagnosis.

For mild infections of EV71 which typically include hand-foot-and-mouth disease, there is no particular treatment. Symptoms typically clear up within seven to 10 days from the day of infection. To relieve pain from mouth sores that develop, an oral anesthetic can be used. The treatment of the general pain associated with the disease can be treated with over the counter drugs such as ibuprofen and acetaminophen. Antiviral agents and intravenous immunoglobulin have both been used as an attempt to treat the EV71. The antiviral drug, Pleconaril, has been used in clinical trials of aseptic meningitis, however it's not effective against EV71. Other capsid-function inhibitors have been studied, some of which have promising activities against EV71. Intravenous immunoglobulin has been used in the large outbreaks of EV71 in Asia. It was thought to neutralize the virus and have non-specific anti-inflammatory properties. When comparing those who received intravenous immunoglobulin to those who did not, recipients seemed to benefit from the treatment if it was given during early onset of the infection.

To prevent EV71 outbreaks, good hygiene and improved sanitation are important. Since transmission is through the fecal-oral route, it is important to frequently wash one's hands, disinfect contaminated surfaces and wash soiled clothing. EV71 is resistant to many cleaning products, thus it is important to use disinfectants that are chlorinated or iodized. A vaccine for EV71 is currently under research. Two research groups has made the inactivated alum-adjuvent EV71 vaccine, but it is currently in a phase III trial. This vaccine has thus far had high efficacy and sustained immunogenicity. Virus-like particle (VLP) vaccines have also been studied. The studies have shown that a VLP with yeast is a potential vaccine for EV71.

9.3   Gastroenteritis-related Viruses

Gastroenteritis-related viruses are viruses with distinct infectious route of gastrointestinal tract besides enterovirus. Acute gastroenteritis is one of the most common diseases caused by acute gastroenteritis viruses in humans worldwide. Gastroenteritis, also known as infectious diarrhea, is inflammation of the gastrointestinal tract that involves the stomach and small intestine. Symptoms may include diarrhea, vomiting and abdominal pain. Fever, lack of energy and dehydration may also occur. This typically lasts less than two weeks. It is not related to influenza though it has been called the "stomach flu".

Rotavirus, enteric adenoviruses, astrovirus and calicivirus, are known to cause viral gastroenteritis. Rotavirus is the most common cause of gastroenteritis in children and produces similar rates in both the developed and developing world. Viruses cause about 70% of episodes of infectious diarrhea in the pediatric age group. Rotavirus is a less common cause in adults due to acquired immunity. Calicivirus is the cause in about 18% of all cases. Calicivirus is the leading cause of gastroenteritis among adults in America, causing greater than 90% of outbreaks. These localized epidemics typically occur when groups of people spend time in close physical proximity to each other, such as on cruise ships, in hospitals or in restaurants. People may remain infectious even after their diarrhea has ended. Calicivirus is the cause of about 10% of cases in children.

9.3.1 Rotaviruses

Rotaviruses are the main viral acute gastro-enteritis in infants and young children and although the infection is usually mild it has a high mortality in developing countries. Rotaviruses also cause diarrhoea in the young of a wide variety of mammals and birds. Rotavirus is transmitted by the faecal-oral route, via contact with contaminated hands, surfaces and objects and possibly by the respiratory route. Viral diarrhoea is highly contagious.

9.3.1.1 Classification and Antigenic Properties

Rotaviruses are members of the Reoviridae family and are characterized by their nonenveloped icosahedral structure and 70-nm diameter. The capsid consists of a double protein layer; the outer capsid is composed of the structural proteins VP7 and VP4 and the inner capsid mainly of VP6. The core is found inside the inner capsid and encloses the rotavirus genome, composed of 11 segments of double-stranded RNA. Given the segmented nature of the RNA genome, co-infection of cells with two different stains of rotavirus may result in reassortant virus, with RNA segments from each of the progenitos.

Rotaviruses possess common antigens located on most, if not all, the structural proteins. These can be detected by immunofluorescence, ELISA and immune electron microscopy (IEM). Three major antigenic subgroups of human rotaviruses have been identified. Outer capsid proteins VP4 and VP7 carry epitopes important in neutralizing activity, though VP7 glycoprotein seems to be the predominant antigen. These type-specific antigens differentiate among rotaviruses and are demonstrable by Nt tests. At least nine serotypes have been identified among animal isolates. Some animal and human rotaviruses share serotype specificity. For example, monkey virus SA11 is antigenically very similar to human serotype 3.

There are six viral proteins (VPs) that form the virus particle (virion). These structural proteins are called VP1, VP2, VP3, VP4, VP6 and VP7. In addition to the VPs, there are six nonstructural proteins (Nsps), that are only produced in cells infected by rotavirus. These are called Nsp1, Nsp2, Nsp3, Nsp4, Nsp5 and Nsp6. At least six of the twelve proteins encoded by the rotavirus genome bind RNA. The role of these proteins play in rotavirus replication is not entirely understood; their functions are thought to be related to RNA synthesis and packaging in the virion, mRNA transport to the site of genome replication and mRNA translation and regulation of gene expression.

There are eight species of rotavirus, referred to as groups A, B, C, D, E, F, G and H. Humans are primarily infected by species A, B and C, most commonly by species A. A-E species cause disease in other animals, species E and H in pigs and D, F and G in birds. Within rotavirus A there are different strains, calledserotypes. As with influenza virus, a dual classification system is used based on two proteins on the surface of the virus. The glycoproteinVP7 defines the G serotypes and the protease-sensitive protein VP4 defines P serotypes. Because the two genes that determine G-types and P-types can be passed on separately to progeny viruses, different combinations are found. A whole genome genotyping system has been established for group A rotaviruses, which has been used to determine the origin of atypical strains. The prevalence of rotavirus the individual G-types and P-types varies between and within, countries and years. The viruses usually associated with human gastroenteritis are classified as group A rotavirus, but antigenically distinct rotaviruses have also caused diarrheal outbreaks, primarily in adults. Molecular epidemiologic studies have analyzed isolates based on differences in the migration of the 11 genome segments following electrophoresis of the RNA in polyacrylamide gels. Extensive genome heterogeneity has been demonstrated in numerous studies. These differences in electropherotypes cannot be used to predict serotypes; however, electropherotyping can be useful epidemiologic tool to monitor viral transmission.

9.3.1.2 Pathogenesis

Rotaviruses replicate exclusively in the differentiated epithelial cells at the tips of the small intestine. New virus is produced after 10–12 h. Progeny virus is released in large numbers into the intestinal lumen ready to infect other cells. Biopsies show atrophy of the villi with reactive crypt hyperplasia and lymphocytic infiltrates in the lamina propria. The cellular damage leads to malabsorption of nutrients, eletrolytes and water and the crypt hyperplasia to hypersecretion. An osmotic and secretory disrrhoea with vomiting and dehydration results. It has been established that the product of RNA 4, VP4, holds a central position for replication, spread and pathogenicity of rotaviruses, but that product of other RNA segments also contribute to the development of disease. The infection is followed by a local, humoral and cell-mediated immune response and is normally overcome within a week. IgA in the gut is the best know correlate of protection. Infection with one serotype seems to provide homotypic protection. In the immunodeficient host, however, a persistent infection can occur with severe chronic diarrhoea.

9.3.1.3 Epidemiology

Rotavirus infections occur world-wide. Most symptomatic infections are seen in children under 2 years of age; by the age of 3 years, more than 90% of children have been infected by most of the major serotypes. In family outbreaks there may be evidence of subclinical infection in older children and adults who may be the source for infection of young children in family or nursery outbreaks. The release of enormous numbers of virions during the acute stage contributes to the easy transmission of the virus. Only a few virus particles are sufficient to cause disease in the susceptible host. Longer-lasting outbreaks may be maintained by the ability of the virus to survive outside the body for some time. In temperate climates there is a pronounced seasonal incidence, with peaks in the winter months occurring with 'clockwise precision'. In tropical areas, on the other hand infections occur evenly throughout the year. Various surveys in different parts of the world have shown that at any time there is co-circulation of genomically and serologically different rotaviruses.

At the molecular level, several factors have been identified which an explain the genomic and antigenic variability of co-circulating rotavirus strains:

1) Like the genomes of other viruses that depend on virion-associated RNA-dependent RNA polymerases for their replication, rotavirus genomes undergo frequent point mutations which accumulate in time.

2) Rotavirus, like other segmented RNA viruses, undergo extensive reassortment events in doubly infected cells. This has been shown to occur both in vitro and in vivo. If RNA segments coding for subgroup-and serotype-specific proteins are involved, antigenic shift can occur in reassortants.

3) Rotavirus may be introduced into humans from animal species and this may contribute to the genomic variability. Human group A rotavirus isolates have been described, the genome of which is very closely related to that of cat and cattle rotaviruses. The group B ADRVs may have been derived recently from animals. Human group C rotaviruses are significantly different from animal group C rotaviruses.

4) Rotaviruses establishing chronic infections in immunodeficient hosts undergo various forms of genome rearrangements, resulting in highly atypical RNA profiles. Evidence is now emerging that such rearrangements may occur more frequently than originally thought.

5) Various combinations of these factors may occur, e. g. reassortment of viruses with rearranged ge-

nomes or point mutations combined with reassortment.

9.3.1.4 Clinical Features

The onset of symptom is abrupt after a short incubation period of $1-2$ days. Diarrhoea and vomiting are seen in the majority of infected children and last for $2-6$ days. Although symptoms of respiratory tract infection are frequently observed at the time of rotavirus infection, there is no evidence that rotaviruses replicate in the respiratory tract. The clinical symptoms can range from mild to very severe, in part depending on the rotavirus strain. Asymptomatic infections of neonates with 'nursery trains' are not uncommon. It has been estimated that about half of all gastro-enteritis cases requiring admission to hospital are caused by rotaviruses. Infection has been detected in older children and adults, but these are usually asymptomatic. Only in the elderly have rotavirus diarrhoea outbreaks been observed. The disease is especially grave and protracted in immunodeficient children, If children are already malnourished, rotavirus infection can be life-threatening. Five million children under the age of 2 years die each year from disrrhoeal disease in developing countries; rotavirus infections contribute to these deaths to the extent of about 20%.

9.3.1.5 Laboratory Diagnosis

At the peak of the disease as many as 10^{11} virus particles per millilitre of faeces are present. Therefore, the diagnosis is not difficult. Agglutination tests using latex particles coated with rotavirus-specific antibody and different forms of enzyme-linked immunosorbent assay (ELISA) are most commonly used. Electron microscopy, when routinely applied to diagnosis of viral diarrhoea in infants and young children, will easily detect the characteristic virus particles. Group, subgroup and G and P serotypes of rotavirus are determined by ELISA with monoclonal antibodies and, more recently, by reverse-transcription polymerase chain reaction with gene-and type-specific subgroup II, serotype G1P8 or G4P8 or of subgroup 1 serotype G2P4. In the majority of cases there are sufficient numbers of virions in faeces to allow identification of RNA profiles by PAGE. Although fastidious, it is possible to continuous monkey kidney cells. To ensure success it is necessary to incorporate trypsin in the culture medium.

9.3.1.6 Treatment and Control

Therapy consists mainly of oral, sometimes intravenous, rehydration with fluid of the appropriate electrolyte and glucose composition. As with any infectious agent transmitted by the faecal-oral route, attention to hygienic measures such as handwashing and disinfection of contaminated surfaces and faeces is very important. For a variety of reasons, rotavirus infections have so far resisted prevention by widespread vaccination. Furthermore, it is not fully clear to what extent vaccination with one rotavirus serotype cross-protects against other serotypes. However, polyvalent 'cocktail' vaccines containing two or more different serotypes have been shown to have a significant effect on preventing severe disease. A number of candidate vaccines of live attenuated rotavirus of bovine or simian origin and of bovine and simian rotavirus reassortants carrying human VP7 genes of different serotypes are currently being rotavirus vaccines will be available in the near future.

9.3.2 Enteric Adenoviruses

Human adenoviruses are classified into 47 serotypes and six subgenera (A-F) with different tropisms. Human adenoviruses belong to the Adenoviridae family and, within the genus, the majority of enteric adenoviruses reported to date belong to subgenus F. They are DNA viruses without an envelope, 70 nm in diameter and with icosahedric symmetry. The protein capsid is composed of 252 capsomers—240 hexones and 12 pentones—and structures called fibers that protrude to the outside. The hexones contain proteins II, IV, VIII and IX, which participate in the stability and assembly of the viral particle. The pentone proteins (III and III a) have the function of cellular penetration and the fibers are hemagglutinins and are responsible for binding the virus to receptors. There are at least eight proteins making up the core; these maintain the integrity of the genome and participate in enzymatic activity. The genome consists of a linear molecule of double-stranded DNA that represents 15% of the viral mass.

The enteric serotypes that are most frequently associated with gastroenteritis caused by adenovirus are 40 and 41, which belong to subgenus F. More rarely, serotypes 31, 12 and 18 of subgenus A and serotypes 1, 2, 5 and 6 of subgenus C have been involved in the etiology of acute diarrhea.

In the same way as in gastroenteritis produced by rotavirus, the lesions produced by serotypes 40 and 41 in the enterocytes lead to atrophy of the villi and compensatory hyperplasia in the crypts, with subsequent malabsorption and loss of fluids. After the infection, specific antibodies develop in most cases and non-neutralizing antibodies are useful for measuring the immune response. The specific type-neutralizing antibodies can provide protection both in the current illness and in reinfections by the same serotype, although patients may continue to eliminate the virus in their feces for months after an effective humoral response.

9.3.3   Astroviruses

In 1993, the Astroviridae family was established with a single genus, the astrovirus, which encompasses human and animal viruses. Astrovirus has been reported as small round viruses of 28 nm with an appearance like that of a five-or six-pointed star by direct visualization with electron microscopy. The name stems from the Greek *astron*, meaning star. However, it has recently been verified that this virus has a different morphology, with an icosahedric appearance, a diameter of 41 nm and well defined spikes. When these viruses are subjected to a high pH, they transform and present the typical morphology of the initially described star. The genome of human astroviruses is composed of single-stranded, positive-sense RNA which contains three 'open reading frames' (ORFs). ORF1a and ORF1b encode viral protease and polymerase, respectively. ORF2 encodes protein capsid precursor and is found at the 3'-terminus of the genome. The protein structure of astrovirus is not well known at present. However, it seems that the precursor of the capsid proteins, an 87-kDa polyprotein, gives rise to the structural capsid proteins VP32, VP29 and VP26. Trials with monoclonal antibodies against human astrovirus suggest that VP26 and/or VP29 may be important in the neutralization, heterotypic immunity and binding of the virus to the target cells. These proteins, especially VP26, seem to be responsible for the antigenic variation observed among the different serotypes.

Astroviruses are classified into serotypes based on the reactivity of the capsid proteins with polyclonal sera and monoclonal antibodies. To date, there have been reports of four neutralizing monoclonal antibodies, developed by Sanchez-Fauquier et al. against serotype 2 human astrovirus and by Bass and Upadhyayula against serotype 1 astrovirus. They all react with the VP26 capsid protein, involved in the neutralization of human astroviruses. Astroviruses can also be classified into genotypes on the basis of the nucleotide sequence of a 348-bp region of the ORF2 and there is a good correlation with the serotypes. There are seven established genotypes, which correspond with seven serotypes. The existence of an eighth genotype has been suggested, due to the sequence of a putative serotype 8. Serotype 1 is predominant in most studies, followed by 2, 3, 4 and 5. Serotypes 6, 7 and 8 are rarely detected.

The pathogenesis of the disease induced by astrovirus has not yet been established, although it has been suggested that viral replication occurs in intestinal tissue. Studies in adult volunteers have not clarified the pathogenic mechanisms. In animal studies, atrophy of the intestinal villi is observed, as well as inflammatory infiltrates in the lamina propria, leading to osmotic diarrhea. Symptomatic astrovirus infection occurs mainly in small children and the elderly, which suggests a reduction in antibodies in recent years, but the determinants of immunity are not well known. Studies in adult volunteers indicate that people with detectable levels of antibodies do not develop the illness.

9.3.4 Human Caliciviruses

Human caliciviruses are members of the Caliciviridae family and two genera have been described, the Norwalk-like viruses (NLVs) and Sapporo-like viruses (SLVs). The virions are composed of a single structural capsid protein, with icosahedric symmetry. This protein, composed of 180 molecules, folds into 90 dimers, which form a continuous shell with protrusions in the shape of an arch. A key characteristic is the existence of 32 cup-shaped depressions, situated on the axes of the icosahedron, from whose Latin designation, *calyx*, the virus derives its name. The genome of the NLVs consists of positive-sense, single-stranded RNA organized into three ORFs. ORF1 encodes the non-structural proteins, such as RNA-dependent RNA polymerase and helicase, ORF2 encodes the structural protein of the capsid and ORF3 encodes for a small protein whose function is unknown. The genome of the SLVs differs from the NLV genome in that the ORF1 encodes the non-structural proteins as well as the structural protein of the capsid. ORF2 encodes a small protein of unknown function and the significance of ORF3 is still uncertain.

The human caliciviruses genera (NLVs and SLVs) can be further divided into genetic clusters. The NLVs include Norwalk virus (the type species), Desert Storm virus, Southampton virus, Snow Mountain agent, Hawaii virus, Toronto virus, Bristol virus and Jena virus. The SLVs includes Sapporo virus (the type species), Parkville virus and London virus.

In studies carried out on volunteers, infection by calicivirus was observed to produce an expansion of the villi of the proximal small intestine. The epithelial cells remain intact and there is shortening of the microvilli. The mechanism by which diarrhea is produced is unknown, although it has been suggested that the delay in gastric emptying observed in Norwalk virus gastroenteritis may play a role. Infection by the Norwalk virus induces a specific IgG, IgA and IgM serum antibody response, even if there has been previous exposure. Two weeks after infection by the Norwalk virus, an increase in jejunal synthesis has been demonstrated for IgA and most patients are resistant to reinfection for 4–6 months. Nevertheless, a lack of long-term protection has been observed.

9.3.5 Other Agents of Viral Gastroenteritis

9.3.5.1 Torovirus

Torovirus is a genus within the Coronaviridae family. Torovirus was detected for the first time in the feces of patients with gastroenteritis in 1984. These viruses have an envelope of 100–140 nm, with a capsid of helicoidal symmetry and a single-stranded RNA genome of positive sense. They are associated with persistent and acute diarrhea in children and may represent an important cause of nosocomial diarrhea.

9.3.5.2 Coronavirus

Included in the Coronaviridae family, these viruses are between 60 and 220 nm, with helicoidal symmetry and a spiculated envelope that gives them the appearance of a crown. The genome is composed of positive monocatenary RNA. Coronavirus was linked with diarrhea in humans for the first time in 1975, but studies have not yet been able to establish a definite etiologic role.

9.3.5.3 Picobirnaviruses

These are small viruses, without an envelope, 30–40 nm in diameter, with a capsid of icosahedric symmetry and a genome made up of two or three segments of bicatenary RNA. They were identified for the first time by Pereira et al. in 1988. Since then, they have been found in a wide variety of animal species and in both children and adults with diarrhea, including immunodepressed patients. In a recent publication, however, this virus was not found in HIV-infected children with diarrhea.

9.4   Hepatitis Virus

Viral hepatitis occurs worldwide and is considered to be one of the major global public health problems. Viral hepatitis is a liver infection that can be caused by one or more of the five known hepatotropic viruses (Table 9-3): hepatitis A virus (HAV), hepatitis B virus (HBV), hepatitis C virus (HCV), hepatitis D virus (HDV) and hepatitis E virus (HEV). In addition, hepatitis G virus (GBV-C/HGV), may be present at low or undetectable levels in the liver of infected hosts, but since it is more readily detected in circulating lymphocytes, it is usually considered to be lymphotropic rather than hepatotropic. Viral hepatitis is a legal group B infectious disease, which is highly contagious, has a complicated route of transmission, affects a wide range of population and has a high incidence rate. Its pathological features include hepatocellular degeneration, necrosis, inflammation, nausea, vomiting, tired of oil, fatigue, loss of appetite, hepatomegaly and abnormal liver function. Some patients may have jaundice, some may have no symptoms of infection or self-limited latent infection, some may also manifest as chronic hepatitis or liver failure. The characteristics of the six known hepatitis viruses are shown in Table 9-3.

Table 9-3   The six known hepatitis viruses

Virus	Classification	Envelope	Genome	Genome size	Spread	Prevalence
HAV	Picornaviridae, genus Hepatovirus	No	ssRNA	7.5kb	Fecal-oral	High
HBV	Hepadnaviridae	Yes(HBsAg)	dsDNA	3.2kb	Parenteral	High
HCV	Flaviviridae, genus Hepacivirus	Yes	ssRNA	9.4kb	Parenteral	Moderate
HDV	Unclasssified	Yes(HBsAg)	ssRNA	1.7kb	Parenteral	Low, regional
HEV	Caliciviridae, genus proposed	No	ssRNA	7.6kb	Fecal-oral	Regional
HGV	Flaviviridae	Yes	ssRNA	9.4kb	Blood and sexual contact	Common

9.4.1   Hepatitis A Virus

Hepatitis A virus (HAV) is usually transmitted by the faecal-oral route, either through person-to-person contact or ingestion of contaminated food or water. Certain sex practices can also spread HAV. Infections are in many cases mild, with most people making a full recovery and remaining immune from further HAV infections. However, HAV infections can also be severe and life threatening. Its incidence tends to decrease with improvements in hygiene conditions but at the same time its severity increases. Most people in areas of the world with poor sanitation have been infected with this virus. Safe and effective vaccines are available to prevent HAV infection.

9.4.1.1 Biological Properties

HAV is a unique member of the family of picornaviruses, a genus of Hepadnavirus. HAV is a three-dimensional symmetrical spherical particle of 27 – 32 nm, containing a linear single stranded RNA genome with a size of 7.5 kb. Although the first temporary classification is enterovirus 72, HAV's nucleotide and amino acid sequence are sufficient to assign it to the new RNA virus. Only one serotype is known. HBV or other hepatitis viruses do not have antigenic cross-reactivity. The genome sequence analysis of a variable region involving 1D gene and 2A gene was divided into 7 genotypes.

HAV has a strong resistance, it is able to tolerate 56 ℃ for 30 minutes, room temperature for a week. In dry excrement at 25 ℃ to survive 30 days in shellfish, sewage, fresh water, seawater, soil can survive for several months. This stability is very beneficial to HAV spread through water and food. High-pressure steam (121 ℃ for 20 minutes), boiling for 5 minutes, UV irradiation, formalin (1 : 4,000, 37 ℃ for 72 hours), potassium permanganate (30 mg/L for 5 minutes), iodine (5 minutes), chlorine (free chlorine 2.0 – 2.5 mg/L, 15 minutes), 70% alcohol at 25 ℃ for 3 minutes can effectively inactivate HAV. Heat the food to over 85 ℃ for 1 minute, disinfection surface with sodium hypochlorite (the latter diluted chlorine bleach) is a necessary condition of active HAV. HAV emphasis on relative resistance of disinfection process in the treatment of patients with hepatitis and its products need extra precautions. HAV initially in the feces by liver preparation of sensitivity and specificity of immune electron microscopy examination polymerase chain reaction (PCR) method already can detect the HAV in feces and other samples and measurement of specific antibody in the serum. Although fresh virus isolates are difficult to adapt and grow, various primate cell lines will support the growth of HAV. The effect of no cell lesion is obvious. Mutations in the viral genome were selected during adaptation to tissue culture.

9.4.1.2 Detection

HAV was first visualized after aggregation of fecal material with serum containing specific homologous antibodies. The fecal material was collected from Joliet prison volunteers inoculated with the MS-1 strain of hepatitis virus characterized by Krugman and colleagues. The technique of immune electron microscopy of stool was then used to assay for specific anti-HAV antibodies in convalescent-phase sera after episodes of naturally occurring hepatitis and to investigate the transmission of virus. HAV can now be detected by a variety of immunologic and molecular techniques, including radioimmunoassay (RIA), DNA-RNA hybridization and reverse transcriptase PCR (RT-PCR) amplification. RT-PCR amplification was used to identify specific viral strains implicated in parenteral transmission of virus.

9.4.1.3 Prevention, Control & Treatment

Inactivated HAV vaccines have been available since the early 1990s and provide long-lasting immunity against hepatitis A infection. The immunity is largely related to the induction of high titers of specific antibodies. Thanks to the existence of a single serotype of HAV, these vaccines are highly efficacious. They consist of viruses grown in cell culture, purified, inactivated with formalin and adsorbed into an aluminum hydroxide adjuvant, making their financial cost relatively high. The effectiveness of pediatric mass vaccination programs in reducing the incidence of hepatitis A has been evidenced in several countries. As a general rule, in low-and inter-mediate endemic regions, where, paradoxically, the severity of the disease is high, vaccination against hepatitis A should be recommended in at least high-risk groups, including travelers to high endemic areas, MSM, drug users and patients receiving blood products. In addition, the inclusion of hepatitis A vaccines in mass vaccination programs in those countries receiving high numbers of immigrants from endemic countries is also recommended.

The aim of the control measures is to prevent individual faeces from contaminating food, water or other sources. Heating foods to over 85 ℃ for one minute, use of a 1 : 100 solution of household bleach, hand-washing and avoiding contact with uncooked foods, are all techniques that may reasonably decrease the likelihood of hepatitis A transmission.

Management of HAV includes supportive therapy. Closely observe the elderly, pregnancy, postoperative or immunocompromised patients with the condition, if the condition turns heavy, should be promptly treated as severe hepatitis. In the early stages of acute hepatitis, patients should be hospitalized or treated locally for isolation and bed rest and activities should be gradually increased during the recovery period. However, they should avoid overwork and facilitate recovery. Chronic hepatitis activity should be properly rest, improve the condition should be noted that the combination of static and dynamic should not be too tired. By acute hepatitis or chronic hepatitis should be bed rest and hospitalization.

Patients with viral hepatitis should eat high-protein, low-fat, high-vitamin foods, carbohydrate intake should be appropriate, not too much, in order to avoid the occurrence of fatty liver. During the recovery period it's advised to avoid over eating. Absolute forbidden alcohol, do not drink alcohol-containing beverages, nutrition products and medicines. Patients with various types of hepatitis have significant loss of appetite, frequent vomiting and jaundice, in addition to rest and nutrition, intravenous infusion of 10% –20% glucose solution and vitamin C and so on. According to different conditions, the patients can be treated with the correspondent Chinese and Western medicine.

9.4.2 Hepatitis B Virus

Hepatitis B virus (HBV) has an overwhelming distribution in the world and causes important human health problems. It has infected one-third of the global population and more than 350 million people are chronic carriers. HBV can cause transient and chronic infections of the liver. Transient infections run a course of several months and chronic infections are often lifelong. Chronic infections can lead to liver failure with cirrhosis and hepatocellular carcinoma.

9.4.2.1 Biological Characteristics

The stability of HBsAg does not always coincide with that of the infectious agent. However, both are stable at 20 ℃ for over 20 years and stable to repeated freezing and thawing. The virus also is stable at 37 ℃ for 60 minutes and remains viable after being dried and stored at 25 ℃ for at least 1 week. HBV (but not HBsAg) is sensitive to higher temperatures (100 ℃ for 1 minute) or to longer incubation periods (60 ℃ for 10 hours). HBsAg is stable at pH 2. 4 for up to 6 hours, but HBV infectivity is lost. Sodium hypochlorite, 0. 5% (e. g. 1 : 10 chlorine bleach), destroys antigenicity within 3 minutes at low protein concentrations, but undiluted serum specimens require higher concentrations (5%). HBsAg is not destroyed by ultraviolet irradiation of plasma or other blood products and viral infectivity may also resist such treatment.

Three types ofHBV viral particles are visualized in infectious serum by electron microscopy. The most common are spherical particles with a diameter of 22 nm. These small particles consist entirely of HBsAg-like tubular or filamentous forms, they have the same diameter, but may be longer than 200 nm and are caused by the excessive production of HBsAg. Larger 42nm spherical virus particles (originally referred to as Dane particles) are less observed. The outer surface or envelope contains HBsAg and surrounds the 27nm internal nucleocapsid core containing HBcAg(Figure 9–5). The variable length of the single-stranded region of the circular DNA genome results in genetically heterogeneous particles with multiple buoyant densities. The structure of Hepatitis B Virus and schematic representation of three hepatitis B surface antigen

(HBsAg) are shown in Figure 9-5.

The HBV virion genome is circular and approximately 3.2 kb in size and consists of DNA that is mostly double stranded. Different HBV isolates share 90%–98% nucleotide sequence homology. It has compact organization, with four overlapping reading frames running in one direction and no noncoding regions. The minus strand is unit length and has a protein covalently attached to the 5' end. The other strand, the plus strand, is variable in length, but has less than unit length and has an RNA oligonulceotide at its 5' end. The four overlapping open reading frames (ORFs) in the genome are responsible for the transcription and expression of seven different hepatitis B proteins. These include structural proteins of the virion surface and core, a small transcriptional transactivator(X) and a large polymerase (P) protein that includes DNA polymerase, reverse transcriptase and RNase H activities. The transcription and translation of these proteins is through the use of multiple in-frame start codons. The HBV genome also contains parts that regulate transcription, determine the site of polyadenylation and a specific transcript for encapsidation into the nucleocapsid. The particles containing HBsAg are antigenically complex. HBsAg have four phenotypes: adw, ayw, adr and ayr. In the United States, adw is the predominant subtype. These virus-specific markers are useful in epidemiologic investigations, as secondary cases have the same subtype as the index case.

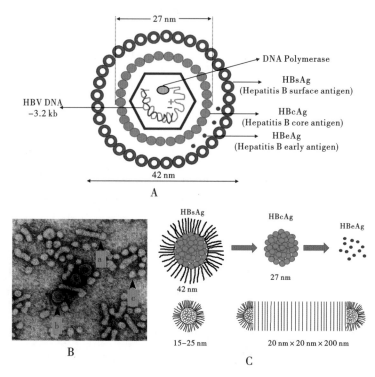

Figure 9-5   Structure of Hepatitis B Virus

A: Structure of Hepatitis B Virus particle. B: Three types of Hepatitis B surface antigen (HBsAg) are visualized in infectious serum by electron microscopy. a: tubular particles (22 nm in diameter); b: Dane particles (42 nm in diameter); c: small spherical particles (20 nm in diameter). C: Schematic representation of three hepatitis B surface antigen (HBsAg). The 42 nm spherical Dane particle can be disrupted by nonionic detergents to release the 27 nm core that contains the partially double-stranded viral DNA genome. Hepatitis B early antigen (HBeAg) is a soluble antigen and it may be released from core particles (hepatitis B core antigen, HBcAg) by treatment with strong detergent

Replication of the HBV genome can broadly divided into three phases (Figure 9-6): ①Infectious virions contain a genome in their internal icosahedral core, which is a partially double-stranded, circular but non-covalently closed DNA of approximately 3.2 kb in length (relaxed circular or RC-DNA); ②After infection, the RC-DNA is transformed into a plasmid-like covalently closed circular DNA (cccDNA) inside the host cell nucleus; ③ from the cccDNA, several genomic and subgenomic RNAs are transcribed by cellular RNA polymerase Ⅱ; of these, the pregenomic RNA (pgRNA) is selectively packaged into progeny capsids and is reverse transcribed by the co-packaged P protein into new RC-DNA genomes. Matured RC-DNA containingnucleocapsids can be used for intracellular cccDNA amplification or be enveloped and released from the cell as progeny virions.

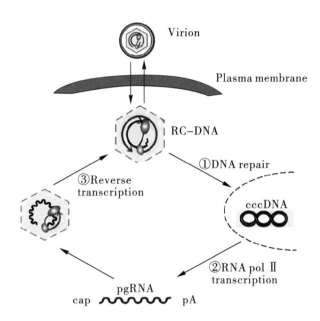

Figure 9-6   Replication cycle of the HBV genome

Enveloped virions infect the cell, RC-DNA containing nucleocapsids are released into the cytoplasm. ① RC-DNA is transported to the nucleus and repaired to form cccDNA. ② Transcription of cccDNA by RNA polymerase Ⅱ produces pgRNA, amongst other transcripts. ③ pgRNA is encapsidated, together with P protein and reverse transcribed inside the nucleocapsid. (+) strand DNA synthesis from the (−) strand DNA template generates a new molecule of RC-DNA. New cycles cause intracellular cccDNA amplification; alternatively, the RC-DNA containing nucleocapsids are enveloped and released as virions

9.4.2.2   Pathogenesis & Pathology

Three mechanisms seem to be involved in liver cell injury during HBV infections. The first is an HLA class Ⅰ restricted cytotoxic T-cell (CTL) response directed at HBcAg/HBeAg on HBV-infected hepatocytes. A second possible mechanism is a direct cytopathic effect of HBcAg expression in infected hepatocytes. A third possible mechanism is high-level expression and inefficient secretion of HBsAg.

In the acute stage there are signs of inflammation in the portal tracts; the infiltrate is mainly lymphocytic. In the liver parenchyma, infected hepatocytes show ballooning and form acidophilic (Councilman) bodies as they die. In chronic hepatitis, damage extends out from the portal tracts, giving a piecemeal necrosis appearance. Some lobular inflammation is also seen. As the disease progresses, fibrosis and, eventually, cirrhosis develops. Chronic liver damage results from continuing, immune-mediated destruction of hepatocytes expressing viral antigens. In addition, autoimmune reactions may contribute to the damage as immune responses are induced to various liver-specific antigens.

The infected hepatocytes are characteristically enlarged and their cytoplasm has a ground glass appearance. HBsAg is found associated with the endoplasmic reticulum and the cell nuclei has core particles containing HBcAg. It has been postulated that liver injury may result from immune mechanism due to larger antigenic load present in hepatocytes and in the serum. Necrosis of hepatocytes results in scattered focal inflammatory response with macrophage and lymphocyte infiltrations together with portal inflammation and endophlebitis of the central veins. In severe cases, lines of necrosis extends from the portal tracts to the central veins and this often precedes chronic hepatitis and cirrhosis. Asymptomatic carriers may either have normal liver histology or may show chronic liver inflammation that is recognized as chronic persistent hepatitis. This normally resolves within months or years of acute infection. Some may develop chronic periportal hepatitis which correlates clinically with chronic active hepatitis and continuing patchy necrosis with fibrosis likely to lead to major disruption in liver architecture characteristic of cirrhosis. It takes around 4−5 years for cirrhosis to develop. Some carriers may go on to develop hepatocellular carcinoma.

9.4.2.3　Virus Transmitting

Hepatitis B virus (HBV) is transmitted through exposure to infectious blood, semen and other body fluids. HBV can be transmitted from infected mothers to infants at the time of birth or from family members to infants in early childhood. Transmission may also occur through unsafe sexual intercourse, transfusions of HBV-infected blood and blood products, contaminated injections during medical procedures and sharing of needles and syringes among injecting drug users. HBV also poses a risk to healthcare workers who sustain accidental needle-stick injuries while caring for HBV-infected people.

9.4.2.4　Laboratory Diagnosis

HBV diagnosis is accomplished by testing for a series of serological markers of HBV and by additional testing to exclude alternative etiological agents such as hepatitis A and C viruses. Serological tests are used to distinguish acute, self-limited infections from chronic HBV infections and to monitor vaccine-induced immunity. Liver biopsy permits a tissue diagnosis of hepatitis. Tests for abnormal liver function, such as serum alanine aminotransferase (ALT) and bilirubin, supplement the clinical, pathologic and epidemiologic findings.

The laboratory can test for a wide range of HBV antigens and antibodies, using immunoassays based on enzyme reactivity (EIA) or chemiluminescence (CLIA) and ELISA. HBV DNA can be quantified in serum or plasma using real time polymerase chain reaction (PCR) assays. Acute HBV infection is characterized by the presence of HBsAg and immunoglobulin M (IgM) antibody to the core antigen, HBcAg. During the initial phase of infection, patients are also seropositive for hepatitis B e antigen (HBeAg). HBeAg is usually a marker of high levels of replication of the virus. The presence of HBeAg indicates that the blood and body fluids of the infected individual are highly contagious. Chronic infection is characterized by the persistence of HBsAg for at least 6 months (with or without concurrent HBeAg). Persistence of HBsAg is the principal marker of risk for developing chronic liver disease and liver cancer (hepatocellular carcinoma) later in life.

9.4.2.5　Prevention, Control & Treatment

Prevention of hepatitis B should be carried out by cutting off the main route of transmission through comprehensive measures. Hepatitis B patients and carriers of blood, secretions and utensils should be strictly sterilized; strict selection of blood donors to prevent the spread of blood; promote the use of disposable syringes and infusion sets; where the operation, the use of exposure to blood and other medical equipment. Must also be strictly disinfected, to prevent the mutual transmission of patients and medical staff; for high-risk groups to carry out specific prevention, active immunization of hepatitis B vaccine is the most effective preventive measures. A safe and effective vaccine is available to prevent HBV infection.

As a comprehensive public health strategy, HBV vaccine is the most effective measure to prevent HBV and to eliminate HBV transmission in the world. WHO recommends that all infants receive the hepatitis B vaccine as soon as possible after birth, preferably within 24 HBV vaccine is recommended for routine screening of all pregnant women for HBsAg, postexposure immunoprophylaxis of infants born to HBsAg-positive mothers and vaccination of unvaccinated adults at increased risk for infection.

Prevention and treatment of Hepatitis B virus infection is international problems. According to WHO estimates, at least 350 million people worldwide carry HBV, 300 million have cirrhosis and HBV infection and HBV has been derived from more than 90% of infants after about 40 years of infection For cirrhosis, 50 years of development of liver cancer, 25% –40% of those infected died because of this, as WHO was ranked as the ninth cause of death. Therefore, domestic and foreign medical scientists devoted great energy and financial resources, mainly through interfering with viral replication and regulation of immune and promote host cell toxicity in two active protection and exploration and development of new antiviral measures, which greatly enriched the therapeutic content of hepatitis B.

Acute hepatitis B is clinically divided into two types of jaundice, its clinical manifestations are basically the same, so the treatment principles and methods are basically similar. The early course of acute symptoms are obvious, severe liver damage, bed rest, nutritional supplements, supplemented by appropriate drugs to control symptoms and promote the recovery of liver disease, prevent the progression of the disease and change to chronic. Severe can be given hypertonic glucose, vitamin C, creatinine, magnesium aspartate and potassium. Stable or into the recovery period, according to the combination of movement, adjust the diet to meet the nutritional needs. The course of acute hepatitis B more than 2 months or hepatitis B virus replication indicators continued non-negative, can be adjusted immune function, combined with appropriate antiviral therapy.

Chronic hepatitis B virus infection is a serious clinical problem. More than 5% of the world's population have had HBV infection. The carrying rate of HBV in China is about 10% and that of chronic hepatitis B is about 30 million. Chronic hepatitis should pay attention to antiviral therapy. During the activity should be appropriate bed rest, after the condition improved, should pay attention to the combination of movement. To rest can engage in light work. Symptoms disappear, liver function returned to normal for 3 months or more, can resume normal work, but should avoid overwork and must be regularly reviewed. Should enter the high protein diet. Heat intake should not be too high, to prevent fatty liver. Also should not eat too much sugar, so as not to cause diabetes. With antiviral drugs, this purpose is to inhibit viral replication, reduce contagion, improve liver function, reduce liver disease, improve quality of life, reduce or prevent the occurrence of cirrhosis and primary hepatocellular carcinoma. Chronic hepatitis B patients often have some degree of immune dysfunction. Long-term HBV infection can lead to cellular immune dysfunction in patients and sometimes can trigger autoimmunity, causing autoimmune diseases. Therefore, the treatment of immunomodulation is very important. Specific immune ribonucleic acid can transmit specific cellular immunity and humoral immunity. Specific transfer factor enhances specific cellular immunity. Common transfer factor can enhance cellular immune function and regulate immune function. Thymosin is an immune enhancer, can improve the body immunity and enhance anti-virus ability.

The goal of treatment for chronic hepatitis B is to suppress HBV replication, prevent the progression of liver disease and thereby the development of cirrhosis, liver failure and HCC. Interferon alpha (α-IFN) is the first-line treatment option for patients without cirrhosis. Interferon has antiviral, anti-proliferative and immuno-modulatory effects. At a dose of 100 mg daily, lamivudine leads to a marked reduction or elimination of detectable HBV DNA in plasma in about 40% of HBeAg positive and 60% –70% of HBeAg negative patients.

9.4.3 Hepatitis C Virus

Hepatitis C virus (HCV) is a major health burden that affects more than 170 million people around the world. Unfortunately, most patients who are infected with Hepatitis C infection cannot clear the virus and progress to the chronic infection. This rate is higher in human immunodeficiency virus (HIV) infected patients and lower in women and children. Cirrhosis, portal hypertension, hepatic decompensation and hepatocellular carcinoma have been reported as results of chronic HCV infection and it is estimated that more than 300,000 deaths have occurred annually due to HCV infection. More than 50% of hepatocellular carcinoma cases in endemic population have happened due to chronic HCV infection and consisted of more than 6% of cirrhosis causes around the world.

9.4.3.1 Biological Characteristics

The hepatitis C virus particle consists of a core of genetic material (RNA), surrounded by an icosahedral protective shell of protein and further encased in a lipid (fatty) envelope of cellular origin. Hepatitis C virus is a linear and a positive one-chain structure with around 9,600 nucleotides. Hepatitis C virion has a diameter of around 55–56 μm and its genome consists of one long open reading frame (ORF), which end in the two untranslated regions at 5' and 3'. The genome size is 9.4 kb and encoding around 3015 amino acids. The precursor is cleaved into at least 10 different proteins: the structural proteins Core, E1, E2 and p7, as well as the non-structural proteins NS2, NS3, NS4A, NS4B, NS5A and NS5B (Figure 9–7). Hepatitis C is not a DNA virus, thus it cannot enter into the host genome and it does not proliferate with DNA; its half-life is around 2.5 hours. Although Hepatitis C is a hepatotropic virus, it can be proliferated in extrahepatic tissues, including peripheral blood mononuclear cell (PBMC).

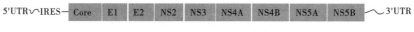

Figure 9–7　Genetic organization of the HCV genome

Hepatitis C virus is divided into the seven main genotypes and more than 100 different subtypes. Genotypes have more than 30% differences in their nucleotide sequences; in most similar species (Quasi-species) differences between nucleotide sequences is 20% –25%. Subtypes 1a and 1b are found worldwide and cause 60% of all cases. The virus undergoes sequence variation during chronic infection. This complex virus population in hosts is called "quasi-species". Although there is a difference in response to anti-viral therapy depending on the genotype of the virus, this genetic diversity is not associated with any difference in clinical disease.

9.4.3.2 Pathogenesis

HCV is a non-cytopathic virus that enters the liver cell and undergoes replication simultaneously causing cell necrosis by several mechanisms including immune-mediated cytolysis in addition to various other phenomena such as hepatic steatosis, oxidative stress and insulin resistance. HCV cannot directly enter into the genome of host cells; it can attack to immune system and infected hepatocytes and lead to cellular inflammation and necrosis and finally fibrosis and hepatocellular carcinoma. In patients with coinfection of Hepatitis C and HIV, hepatic fibrosis progression is more rapid in infection with each of them separately.

HCV interferes with defense mechanisms and interferon signaling pathways.

9.4.3.3   Laboratory Diagnosis

Diagnosis of HCV infection was performed by direct and indirect methods. In indirect methods, antibodies such as Anti-HCV IgM for recent infection and Anti-HCV IgG for old infection, in which secretions against Hepatitis viruses were measured. In the direct method, virus antigens were purified and detected by nucleoid acid. Overall, rapid immunoassay tests were used for screening and recombinant immunoblot tests in order to confirm HCV infection. The HCV-RNA test is positive in patients with at least 50 international units of HCV and HCV-RNA can diagnose infection at one to two weeks after HCV exposure. Laboratory assessments were used for the diagnosis and follow-up of HCV infection among patients. Serological assays, which detect anti-HCV antibodies in the patient after seroconversion, are used for initial HCV diagnosis. Enzyme immunoassay (EIA) detects HCV antibodies, but does not distinguish between acute, chronic or infection. Alanine aminotransferase (ALT) and aspartate aminotransferase (AST) are used to assess of liver condition. Suspected patients for HCV infection must assess with anti HCV with EIA antibodies and HCV-RNA with sensitive test. Among patients with clinical and biological symptoms of chronic Hepatitis C, both of anti-HCV antibody and HCV-RNA were needed for diagnosis of HCV infection. Enzymatic immunoassay screening included rapid diagnosis tests and recombinant immunoblot assay (RIBA) was confirmatory laboratory tests. Quantity and quality of Hepatitis C virus were checked by recognition of viral RNA according to nucleic and amplification tests (NATs). Viral core antigens as laboratory diagnosis and genotyping with serologic and molecular methods are other diagnostic methods for Hepatitis C infection.

Qualitative and quantitative molecular assays are used to confirm initial diagnosis, determine viral load and genotype the dominant strain. Viral load and genotype information are used to guide appropriate treatment. Various other biomarker assays are performed to assess liver function and enable disease staging. Most of these diagnostic methods are mature and routinely used in high-resource countries with well-developed laboratory infrastructure. Few technologies, however, are available that address the needs of low-resource areas with high HCV prevalence, such as Africa and Southeast Asia.

9.4.3.4   Prevention, Control & Treatment

There is no vaccine against HCV. Control measures focus on preventive activities to reduce the risk of HCV infection. Hepatitis C virus (HCV) is mostly transmitted through exposure to infectious blood. This may happen through transfusions of HCV-infected blood and blood products, contaminated injections during medical procedures and sharing of needles and syringes among injecting drug users. Sexual or interfamilial transmission is also possible, but is much less common. Screening blood donors is currently the main measure to prevent HCV infection. In addition, HCV contamination of blood products is also an important source of infection, especially gamma globulin, should be strictly screened.

In general, patients infected with HCV genotypes 1, 4 and 6 require more aggressive treatment for longer periods of time, while HCV genotypes 2 and 3 are more favorable for treatment response. Traditionally, patients have been treated with a combination of peginterferon alfa and ribavirin. Peginterferon must be injected, can cause significant side effects and has low efficacy as monotherapy, especially for HCV genotype 1. The efficacy of ribavirin has been compromised by increasing viral resistance. Thus, treatment can be enhanced with second-line drugs such as telaprevir and boceprevir, which target viral non-structural proteins 3 and 4 (NS3 and NS4). Miravirsen is a microRNA that blocks viral replication and is being used as a new second-line drug for the treatment of HCV infection in clinical trials.

Interferon therapy should be applied early for acute hepatitis C infection and this can reduce the chronic. The main problem with the treatment of chronic HCV infection is relapse after withdrawal. Interferon 6 months after the course of treatment,50% of patients relapse. Relapse again with interferon treatment is generally still valid. The treatment of chronic hepatitis can be combined with interferon and ribavirin (ribavirin),the infectious agent plus ribavirin,especially long-acting interferon (such as pegylated interferon) and ribavirin combined application is one of the most effective treatment options.

9.4.4 Hepatitis D,E and G Viruses

Hepatitis D virus (HDV) infections occur exclusively in persons infected with HBV. The dual infection of HDV and HBV can result in more serious disease and worse outcomes. The hepatitis B vaccine provides protection from HDV infection. Hepatitis E virus (HEV),like HAV,is transmitted through consumption of contaminated water or food. HEV is a common cause of hepatitis outbreaks in the developing world and is increasingly recognized as an important cause of disease in developed countries. HEV infection is associated with increased morbidity and mortality in pregnant women and newborns. A safe and effective vaccine against HEV was licensed in January 2012 but is not yet widely available. Hepatitis G virus (HGV, also termed GBV-C) was recently discovered and resembles HCV,but more closely,the flaviviruses;the virus and its effects are under investigation and its role in causing disease in humans is unclear.

9.4.4.1 Biological Characteristics

Hepatitis delta virus (HDV),firstly identified in 1977,is a defective virus which uses hepatitis B virus (HBV) envelope proteins for successful infection of hepatocytes. The HDV virion is composed of an outer coat containing HBV envelope proteins and host lipids surrounding an inner nucleocapsid that consists of small and large hepatitis delta antigens (HDAg) and a single-stranded circular RNA of 1679 nucleotides with a diameter of 36 nm. HDV has a particle size of 26–37 nm and a buoyant density of 1.24–1.25 g/ml in CsCl. The HDV RNA genome is capable of self-cleavage through a ribozyme and encodes only one structural protein,the hepatitis delta antigen (HDAg),from the antigenomic RNA. There are two forms of HDAg,a shorter (S;22 kDa) and a longer (L;24 kDa) form. Currently,HDV has eight genotypes (HDV1–8) recognized with distinct geographic distributions.

The HEV viruswas first identified in 1983. It causes sporadic cases of hepatitis or outbreaks and the disease is generally self-limited although it may cause fulminant hepatitis in pregnant women,elderly,those with underlying chronic hepatitis,immunosuppressed and transplant recipients. The HEV genome is a non-enveloped single stranded RNA virus in the genus *Hepevirus* and the family Hepeviridae. It has four genotypes. Genotypes 1 and 2 cause disease in humans while genotypes 3 and 4 cause diseases both in humans and animals especially in pigs. It is possible for the virus to spread from animals to humans. According to World Health Organization (WHO),20 million HEV infections develop every year,15% of them being symptomatic.

HGV,an RNA virus in the Flaviviridae family,has a genome very similar to that of hepatitis C virus (HCV),coding for structural and nonstructural proteins. The name HGV denotes two independent viruses: HGV and GBV-C. HGV replicates in peripheral blood cells,while replication in liver cells has not been observed till date. HGV has five major genotypes: type 1 predominates in West Africa,type 2 in Europe and the United States,type 3 in parts of Asia,type 4 in Southeast Asia and type 5 in South Africa.

9.4.4.2 Laboratory Diagnosis

The first step in the diagnosis of hepatitis delta virus (HDV) infection is testing HBsAg-positive individuals for the antibody to the HD antigen (anti-HD). In anti-HD-positive patients,the next step is testing for HDV RNA in serum to determine whether the antibody reflects an ongoing active HDV infection (HDV-RNA-positive) or represents a serologic scar to past HDV infection (HDV-RNA-negative). In the HDV-positive individual with liver disease, it is critical to distinguish acute HDV/hepatitis B virus (HBV) coinfection from chronic HDV superinfection in HBsAg carriers; the course, prognosis and management of the two conditions are different. The differential diagnosis can be achieved through the scrutiny of the battery of HDV and HBV markers, which combine in patterns characteristic for each condition.

The laboratory diagnosis of HEV infection depends on the detection of HEV antigen, HEV RNA and serum antibodiesagainst HEV (immunoglobulin [IgA, IgM and IgG). Anti-HEV IgM antibodies can be detected during the acute phase of the illness and can last approximately 4 or 5 months, representing recent exposure, whereas anti-HEV IgG antibodies can last more than 10 years, representing remote exposure. Thus, the diagnosis of acute infection is based on the presence of anti-HEV IgM, HEV antigen and HEV RNA, while epidemiological investigations are mainly based on anti-HEV IgG.

Diagnosis of HGV infection is mainly by use of polymerase chain reaction (PCR), as serological techniques are still being developed.

9.4.4.3   Prevention, Control & Treatment

HDV infection is an important cause of chronic hepatitis B and progressive development. Although the rate of HDV infection is relatively low, it can affect thousands of HBsAg carriers and patients with chronic HBV infection. Therefore, the prevention and treatment of HDV has important significance.

Prevention of HDV Infection: Hepatitis B vaccine not only prevents HBV infection, but also prevents HDV infection. However, in HDsAg carriers or HBsAg-positive chronic hepatitis, how to prevent overlapping HDV infectionit is an important issue. HDV virus transmission methods and ways and HBV prevention of HBV transmission measures, are applicable to HDV. In particular, the control of iatrogenic infection, to prevent the spread of HBV and HDV is of great significance.

Treatment of HDV infection: interferon treatment seems to inhibit the replication of HDV, but long-term efficacy is not sure, often relapse after stopping.

Hepatitis E is treated in the same way as Hepatitis A Treatment of hepatitis E pregnant women, with special emphasis on early diagnosis and early treatment. Patients with severe hepatitis should strengthen supportive therapy, the application of albumin and lose new blood, prevent cerebral edema and hepatorenal syndrome. Late pregnancy patients should prevent postpartum hemorrhage. HEV preventionis the same as hepatitis A.

Chronic carriage of HGV is possible, but does not result in chronic hepatitis.   Although GBV-C is detected in many patients with chro-nic hepatitis, it does not appear to cause liver disease. In addition, it does not appear to mo-dulate the course response to treatment of chronic HCV or hepatitis B virus infections.

9.5   Arbovirus

Arboviruses (arthropod-borne viruses) were defined by the World Health Organization Scientific Group as viruses that are principally maintained in nature or to an important extent, through biological transmission between susceptible vertebrate host by hematophagous arthropods or through transovarian and possible venereal transmission in arthropods; the virus multiply and produce viremia in the vertebrates, multiply in the tissues of arthropods and are passed on to new vertebrates by the bites of arthropods after a period of extrinsic incubation. Thus, arboviruses represent ecologic groupings of viruses with complex transmission cycles involving arthropods.

Arboviruses use arthropod vectors as their main transmission route and are therefore defined as arthropod-borne viruses. Mosquitoes, ticks, midges and sandflies are known virus transmitting arthropods. The majority of arboviruses belong to the Flaviviridae, Bunyaviridae or Togaviridae families, but a small number are member of the Reoviridae and Orthomyxoviridae families.

Of the over 545 suspected arbovirus species more than 150 are documented to cause disease in humans and the majority are zoonotic. They are sustained in a transmission cycle between arthropods as vectors and vertebrate animal reservoirs as main amplifying hosts (Table 9-4). Humans are infected in spill-over events and are often dead-end hosts, as they do not develop the high viremias needed to infect arthropods. Only a few viruses like yellow fever, chikungunya and dengue virus have expanded their host range to include humans as an amplifying host. They can lead to mosquito-borne disease outbreaks, often in urban settings, without the need of an animal reservoir. This urban transmission cycle in part explains the "success" of these viruses. Based on the pattern of occurrence the individual viruses in Table 9-4 were labeled as endemic (reflecting stable presence in a reservoir), sporadic (reflecting isolated infections) or epidemic (reflecting occurrence during seasons with increased disease activity or outbreaks). Large epidemics can occur for example because of climate variations, like extraordinary rainfall or movement of large populations or viruses into new areas. Arboviruses may also be transmitted through blood from viremic patients, which is a particular concern for the blood supply in endemic areas and when taking care of patients with hemorrhagic fever. Cases of human-to-human transmission of West Nile virus through blood transfusions and organ transplantation have been reported, but all arboviruses that produce viremia in humans are thought to be a potential risk.

Summary of taxonomy and essential ecology of medically important travel-related arboviruses.

Table 9-4　Summary of taxonomy and essential ecology of medically important travel-related arboviruses

Family genus	Serogroup	Virus	Vector	Host	Geographical distribution
Bunyaviridae Nairovirus	Crimean-Congo hemorrhagic fever	Crimean-Congo hemorrhagic fever virus	Tick	Domestic and wild animals, birds, small mammals	South-East and Eastern Europe, Africa, Asia
Orthobunya-virus	Bwamba	Bwamba virus	Mosquito	Unknown	Sub-SaharanAfrica
	Bunyamwera	Bunyamwera	Mosquito	Possibly rodents	Sub-SaharanAfrica
		Ilesha virus	Mosquito	Unknown	Sub-SaharanAfrica
		Ngari virus	Mosquito	Unknown	Sub-SaharanAfrica
	California encephalitis	La Cross virus	Mosquito	Small mammals	North America
		Guaroa virus	Mosquito	Unknown	Central andSouth America
		Tahyna virus	Mosquito	Hares, rabbits, hedgehogs, small mammals	Europe, Asia, Africa

Continue to Table 9-4

Family genus	Serogroup	Virus	Vector	Host	Geographical distribution
	Simbu	Oropouche virus	Midge	Humans, Sloths (maybe primates, birds)	Central andSouth America
Phlebovirus	Phlebovirus fever	Toscana virus	Sandfly	Humans, bats	Southern Europe
		Sandfly fever other	Sandfly	Human, rodents	Southern Europe, Northern Africa, Asia
Flaviviridea Flavivirus	Dengue virus	Dengue virus	Mosquito	Primates, humans	Asia, Africa, Americas
	Japanese encephalitis	Japanese encephalitis virus	Mosquito	Ardeid birds, pigs	South and South-East Asia, Oceania
		West Nile virus	Mosquito	Birds	North and South America, South and Eastern Europe, South-East Asia, Oceania
	Ntaya virus	Ilheus virus	Mosquito	Birds	Central andSouth America
	Yellow fever	Yellowfever virus	Mosquito	Primates, humans	Sub-Saharan Africa andSouth America
Reoviridae Coltivirus	Colorado tick fever	Colorado Tick fever virus	Tick	Small mammals	North America

China conducted a systematic and in-depth study on the biological characteristics, epidemiological features, disease status, transmission medium, prevention and control of these viruses and achieved outstanding results in some aspects, which played an important role in the prevention and control of these diseases in China.

9.5.1 Japanese Encephalitis Virus

Japanese encephalitis (JE), caused by Japanese encephalitis virus (JEV) infection, is the most important viral encephalitis in the world. Approximately 35,000-50,000 people suffer from JE every year, with a mortality rate of 10,000-15,000 people per year. JEV mainlyaffects children due to imperfect immunity in children, especially the blood-brain barrier is not fully developed, making it easy for the virus to invade the brain tissue and being protected by a variety of antibodies from the mother, the baby before being born has a strong immunity. The age characteristics of JE are not static. In recent years, the prevalence of children has been eased due to the widespread immunization of children and adolescents with the JE vaccine and the proportion of JE patients in both adults and the elderly is much greater. Although the safety and efficacy of JE vaccines (inactivated and attenuated) have been demonstrated, China still accounts for 50% of the reported JE cases worldwide.

9.5.1.1   Biological Characteristic

Japanese encephalitis virus is a member of the Flaviviridae family and is a single-strand positive chain RNA virus. The viruses are spherical, enveloped, with a diameter of 45-50 nm. The genome is approximately 11 kb and contains one ORF encoding the polyprotein. The entire genome encodes three structural proteins (C, M, E) and seven nonstructural proteins (NS1, NS2a, NS2b, NS3, NS4a, NS4b, NS5). Noncoding regions (5' and 3') can be found on both sides of the ORF. JEV structural proteins consist of the glycosylated envelope protein (E) and the membrane protein (M), which forms the icosahedron nucleocapsid embedded in the phospholipid bilayer. E protein is involved in many important biological processes, including hemagglutination, virus neutralization and viral particle assembly. The nonstructural viral proteins provide functional regulatory enzymes for JEV replication. JEV can be divided into five genotypes according to the E gene and genomic sequences.

JEV is susceptible to ether, chloroform, bile and deoxycholates due to the envelopes. The virus is fragile to heat and can be inactivated at 56 ℃ for 30 min or 100 ℃ for 2 min. The virus is sensitive to dryness, U. V. rays or formaldehydes as well. JE virus at-20 ℃ can survive for months and glycerol or serum preservation can increase the stability and it can be stored for several years at −80 ℃.

9.5.1.2   Cultivation of Virus

Japanese encephalitis virus has typical neurotropic properties. Inoculation of mice, golden hamsters, monkeys, horses, sheep, goats and other animals can cause typical neurological symptoms. Primary cells such as C6/36, BHK21 and Vero and golden hamster kidney, porcine kidney, dog kidney and chicken embryo are all sensitive to Japanese encephalitis virus and have typical cytopathic effect. Typical cytopathic effects (CPE) appear 3 to 5 days post-infection in cultured cells, with characteristics of increased granulation, cell shrink, fall-off from culture flask and breakage or even vacuolization followed by cell fusion in C6/36. Suckling and grown-up mice are frequently used experimental animals. Under the cover of agarose, chicken embryo, hamster kidney, Vero and other cells can form plaque. Can agglutinate a variety of animal red blood cells, such as geese, chicken embryos, pigeons, chickens, sheep, HI experiments generally use goose red blood cells. The virus is continuously passaged in the brain of cells and mice to reduce its virulence. The Chinese encephalitis attenuated strains 14-2 and 2-8 were obtained by successive passage and selection of the SA14 strain on hamster kidney cells.

9.5.1.3   Epidemiology

Japanese encephalitis is mainly distributed in Asia. Countries with more incidence are Japan, China, North Korea, the Philippines, Malaysia, Indonesia and so on. In Southeast Asian countries, cases of Japanese encephalitis occur all year round due to the humid climate, hot and mosquito populations. Japanese encephalitis is strictly seasonal in other parts of the world except in the tropical areas. In 80% −90% of cases, cases are concentrated in the three months of July, August and September. Climate and rainfall are also closely related to the prevalence of this disease, mainly due to the nature of mosquitoes. China is in temperate natural conditions, during summer and autumn-the most suitable seasons for mosquitoes, people have more opportunities to get Japanese encephalitis, while mosquito bites in winter and spring, will not result in JE infection. Due to the different geographical environment, the popular season is also slightly different. The highest peak in South China is in June-July, North China from July to August, while the northeast as August-September.

People are mostly latent infection with Japanese encephalitis virus and are highly sporadic. It is very rare that two patients in the same family have both at the same time. Sex has nothing to do with the incidence, but generally more men than women. Japanese encephalitis can occur at any age, but the incidence is mainly for children under 10 years of age, the highest incidence of children aged 2–6, infants under the age of infrequent incidence. This is mainly due to imperfect immunity in children, especially the blood-brain barrier is not fully developed, easy to make the virus invade the brain tissue and the baby because of the mother before the birth of a variety of antibodies, has a strong immunity. The age characteristics of JE are not static. In recent years, the prevalence of children has been eased due to the widespread immunization of children and adolescents with the JE vaccine and the proportion of JE patients in both adults and the elderly is much greater.

9.5.1.4 Laboratory Diagnosis

The diagnosis of JE should be based on epidemiological and clinical symptoms and laboratory tests to be diagnosed. Japanese encephalitis has obvious seasonal epidemic, more common in July-September, the main violation of school-age children, high fever, headache, vomiting, disturbance of consciousness and nervous system infection positive signs. Confirmed need to rely on laboratory tests. Diagnosis of the virus infections depends on the isolation of virus, detection specific RNA from serum, spinal fluid or tissues and serological tests.

The viruses are usually able to grow in common cell lines, such as Vero, BHK, HeLa and MRC-5. *Aedes albopictus* C6/36 mosquito cells are useful. Infection can be detected through the use of cytopathologic studies, immunofluorescence and the hemadsorption of avian erythrocytes. Intracerebral inoculation of suckling mice or hamsters may also be used for virus isolation. Antigen detection and reverse transcription-polymerase chain reaction (RT-PCR) are available for direct detection of viral proteins or RNA in clinical specimens, respectively.

Various serological methods are available for the diagnosis of infections, including specific IgM antibody tests, hemagglutination inhibition (HI), neutralization tests (NT) and complement fixation experiments.

(1)Specific IgM Antibody Assay

ELISA or indirect immunofluorescence can be used to detect specific IgM antibodies in serum or cerebrospinal fluid of patients, the positive is of early diagnostic significance. Specific IgM antibodies typically appear 4 days after infection and individual patients can be detected even on the first day of onset. The first week when the positive rate of 80% or more, 2–3 weeks reached a peak, the positive rate of up to 90%.

(2)HI experiment

Double copies of blood need to be collected from Patients, with interval of 1–2 weeks for two blood sampling, 4 times higher antibodies can be diagnosed, single serum antibody titer of 1 ∶ 320 has diagnostic significance.

(3)Neutralization Test

One week after the onset of neutralization antibody positive, the general double antibody titer increased more than 4 times can be diagnosed and more for retrospective diagnosis.

(4)Complement Binding Experiments

With high specificity, but antibodies appear late, after 2 weeks of onset. Double serum antibody titer increased more than 4 times or more than a single serum antibody titer greater than 1 ∶ 32 can be diagnosed. In addition there are indirect hemagglutination test, specific inhibition test of leukocyte adhesion assay.

9.5.1.5 Prevention& Treatment

JE prevention mainly adopts two measures, mosquito control and vaccination. Three Culex tritaeniorhynchus habits. Adult mosquitoes have a wide range of activities, habitat in the wild, partial to animal blood. It mainly breeds in paddy fields and other shallow waters and therefore the elimination of the JE media must be closely integrated with agricultural production. Protecting the susceptible population is an effective measure. At present, there are mainly two kinds of Japanese encephalitis vaccines that are mainly used in the world, namely Japan mouse brain purified inactivated vaccine and Chinese hamster kidney cell inactivated vaccine. Vaccination of the main target for the popular area of more than 6 months of children under 10 years of age. Because JE inactivated vaccine inoculation, about 40 days before the emergence of immunity, it should be vaccinated in the first month before the epidemic, the first vaccination need to be injected twice, the first subcutaneous injection, an interval of seven to ten days after multiple inoculation, after Strengthen the injection once a year. Two to three weeks after vaccination in vivo produce protective antibodies, usually for four to six months.

The main source of infection of JE is domestic animals, especially young pigs that have not passed the epidemic season. Therefore, it is necessary to strengthen the management of zoonotic sources and improve the sanitation of livestock and livestock sheds. In recent years, vaccines are used to immunize young pigs to reduce viremia in swine herds, thereby controlling the prevalence of Japanese encephalitis in the population.

Currently, there is no particularly effective treatment for JE. J encephalitis acute onset, rapid change, serious illness, we should pay attention to early detection of patients, timely rescue, seriously high fever, convulsions, respiratory failure in these three. In the early stages of disease using integrated Chinese and Western methods of active treatment, can save the lives of most patients, but also can minimize sequelae. Treatment of Japanese encephalitis there is no effective drugs, future research should be to strengthen the treatment of drugs. Although the existing inactivated and attenuated live vaccines are effective, they all contain the viral genome and are difficult to achieve 100% safety. Therefore, the researches on recombinant vaccines and peptide vaccines will be of great concern.

9.5.2 Dengue Virus

Dengue virus is an emerging human pathogen that poses a huge public health burden by infecting annually about 390 million individuals of which a quarter report with clinical manifestations. Dengue is prevalent in 128 countries and more than 2.5 billion individuals are in danger each year of contracting dengue virus worldwide. According to some estimates, almost 400 million individuals are infected annually. About 2.5% of all diseased people die.

9.5.2.1 Biological Characteristics

The virus belongs to the genus Flavivirus within the family of the Flaviviridae. Four distinct serotypes have been identified, called DEN-1, DEN-2, DEN-3 and DEN-4. There are 60% –80% homology among the four serotypes. Morphologically, dengue virus is similar in several respects to JEV and has a spherical shape with an envelope of 45–55 nm in diameter. The genome of Dengue virus is a positive-sense, single-stranded RNA of approximately 11 kb, encoding three structural proteins (capsid (C), membrane (M) and envelope (E)) and seven non-structural proteins (NS1, NS2A, NS2B, NS3, NS4A, NS4B and NS5). Envelope proteins are involved in the major biological functions of the virus. They bind to receptors on host cells and are associated with red blood cell agglutination, induced neutralizing antibodies and protective immune responses and NS1 contains genes and type-specific determinants and are also responsible for the induction of high titers of protective antibodies.

Dengue virus can multiply in Aedes albopictus C6/36 mosquito cells, Vero, baby hamster kidney

(BHK). Typical CPE is seen in infected cells. Sucking mice is sensitive to dengue virus. Dengue virus resistance is weak. Normal disinfectants, lipid solvents, 56 ℃ for 30 minutes and many proteases can inactivate the virus. Dengue virus prone to mutation. Nucleotide sequence analysis revealed that the nucleotide variation among different isolates in the same serotype virus was 10% , while the nucleotide variation among different serotypes was 30% . And according to the degree of homology of the virus oligonucleotide fingerprinting, different strains of the same virus can be divided into different topological types. New dengue virus strains formed after the virus mutation can often cause an outbreak of endemic dengue. The resistance virus is heat sensitive and can be inactivated at 56 ℃ for 30 minutes. Chloroform, acetone and other lipid solvents, lipase or sodium deoxycholate can inactivate Dengue virus by disrupting the virus envelope. The viral nucleic acid released by the virus after detergent treatment can be quickly degraded by the nuclease. The virus is sensitive to stomach acid, bile and protease. It's also UV, γ-ray sensitive. Dengue virus can be inactivated by disinfectants such as alcohol, 1% iodine, 2% glutaraldehyde, 2% –3% hydrogen peroxide and 3% –8% formaldehyde.

Natural hosts for dengue virus infections include humans, lower primates and mosquitoes. The main vectors of DENV are Aedes aegypti, mainly found in tropical areas and Aedes albopictus, more common in subtropical areas. Once infected, these mosquitoes remain a living reservoir that efficiently transmit the virus. The expanded distribution of these vector species, due to global warming and, for example, international trade in used tires; the failure to control the vectors; and the ongoing urbanization are largely responsible for the dramatic increase of dengue cases worldwide during the last few decades.

9.5.2.2　Immunity&Pathogenesis

Human dengue virus infections cause a range of diseases, including dengue fever of unknown cause, dengue haemorrhagic fever (DHF) and dengue shock syndrome (DSS). The body immunity formed by dengue virus infection is mainly humoral immunity. The same type of virus-specific antibodies produced after dengue virus infection can remain lifelong, but at the same time acquired immunity to other serotypes (abnormal immunity) lasts only 6 months to 9 months. Re-infection with other types 3 virus may cause DHF/ DSS. The activated T lymphocytes after virus re-infection can react with the homotype or other viruses and the released cytokines may be involved in the occurrence of DHF/DSS.

Dengue virus infection is generally encountered in older children and adults. But pregnant women seem to be more likely to present more severe forms of dengue infection than general population, easy causing premature birth, low birth weight and miscarriage. Dengue has some symptoms, such as sudden fever, various non-specific signs and other symptoms, including frontal headache, general aches, retro-orbital pain, joint pain, nausea and vomiting, weakness and rashes. Viremia when fever, sustainable 3−5 days. DHF is a serious syndrome that individuals (usually children) with passively acquired or pre-existing non-neutralizing dengue antibodies may be present due to previous infection with different viral serotypes. With high fever, bleeding, circulatory failure and so on, DSS is a more serious disease characterized by shock and blood concentration. Case fatality rate for severe dengueis from 0.2% to 5% , mainly caused by severe bleeding and plasma leakage that leads respiratory distress and multi-organ impairment.

WHO classifies any severe involvement of organs such as liver, heart and central nervous system as one of the case definition for severe dengue. Neurological involvement in dengue can be further classified into dengue encephalopathy immune-mediated syndromes, encephalitis, neuromuscular or dengue muscle dysfunction and neuro-ophthalmic involvement. Most of these occur acutely during acute illness but immune-mediated syndromes typically occur following resolution of dengue fever.

9.5.2.3 Laboratory Diagnosis

Specific diagnosis of dengue virus depend on the isolation of virus from the positive serum, dengue virus RNA is detected by RT-PCR and serological tests.

Dengue viruses are most likely to be isolated from acute serum samples obtained within 5 days after the onset of illness. The early patient blood was taken and inoculated in Aede albopictus cell lines (C6/36). After isolation of the virus, specific neutralization tests or hemagglutination inhibition tests were required to identify them. The use of ELISA to detect specific IgM antibodies in the patient's serum is positive and contributes to the early diagnosis of dengue fever. If dengue virus antigen is detected in the patient's serum, it can also serve as a definitive diagnosis. Detection of dengue virus RNA in the patient's serum is more sensitive than virus isolation and can be used for early rapid diagnosis and serotype identification, but the technical requirements are high.

9.5.2.4 Prevention& Treatment

Controlling the media to prevent mosquito bites is an important measure to prevent and control dengue virus infection. Mosquito control has been used to disinfect mosquito breeding sites with pesticides. However, due to the resistance of insecticides and other reasons, mosquito control is mainly controlled by removing mosquito breeding places, conducting publicity and education, enhancing residents' awareness of mosquito breeding grounds and improving sanitation conditions.

At present, there is no safe and effective dengue virus vaccine. Live attenuated vaccine strains DEN1 – 4 have some immunogenic effects; however, the stability of attenuated strains is poor, which may cause clinical symptoms and cause DHF and DSS caused by ADE. It is generally believed that non-structural protein NS1 cannot induce ADE effect, so the recombinant DNA technology to construct non-structural protein NS1 subunit vaccine or genetic engineering vaccine may obtain satisfactory immune effect. No specific treatment has been found for dengue.

9.6 Hemorrhagic Fever Virus

In the 1920s and 1930s, a type of natural disease named "hemorrhagic fever" was discovered in the world and collectively referred to as viral hemorrhagic fevers (VHFs) because they are caused by RNA viruses belonging to the families Arenaviridae, Bunyaviridae, Filoviridae and Flaviviridae (Table 9–5). These viruses naturally occur in carriers of animal hosts or arthropods. Arthropod ticks and mosquitoes are vectors for certain diseases. After transmission from their reservoir host or vector to humans, these viruses cause an acute infection. All types of VHF are characterized by fever and bleeding disorders and all can progress to high fever, shock and death in many cases. Important viruses of hemorrhagic fever in China include Hantavirus, Crimean-Congo haemorrhagic fever virus and dengue virus.

Table 9–5 Relevant VHF viruses

Family	Virus	Host or vector	Disease	Endemic region
Arenaviridae	Lassa virus	Rodents	Lassa fever	West Africa
	Sabia virus	Rodents	Brazil hemorrhagic fever	Brazil
	Junin virus	Rodents	Argentina fever hemorrhagic fever	Northwest ofArgentina

Continue to Table 9–5

Family	Virus	Host or vector	Disease	Endemic region
	Machupo virus	Rodents	Bolivia hemorrhagic fever	Northeast ofBolivia
	Guanarito virus	Rodents	Venezuela hemorrhagic fever	Venezuela
Bunyaviridae	Hantavirus	Rodents	Hemorrhagic fever with renal syndrome	Asia (China, Korea) , Europe
	Crimean-Congo haemorrhagic fever virus	Hyalomma ticks	Crimean-Congo hemorrhagic fever	Africa and Near-, Middle-, Far East (Pakistan, Afghanistan, China)
	Rift Valley fever virus	Mosquitoes	Rift Valley fever	Sub-Saharan Africa, Egypt, first outbreak outside Africa in 2000 in Yemen and Saudi Arabia
Flaviviridae	Dengue virus	Mosquitoes	Dengue fever, dengue hemorrhagic fever, dengue shock syndrome	Tropical and subtropical areas world-wide (increasing incidence in Latin America andAsia)
	Yellow fever virus	Mosquitoes	Yellow fever	Tropical Africa and Central-/South America (Asia is still free of yellow fever)
	Kyasanur Forest fever virus	Tick	Kyasanur Forest fever	India
	Omsk hemorrhagic fever virus	Tick	Omsk hemorrhagic fever	Siberia
Filoviridae	Ebola virus	Unknown	Ebola hemorrhagic fever	Africa, Asia (Philippines)
	Marburg virus	Unknown	Marburg hemorrhagic fever	Africa, Europe

At the 1982 WHO Working Conference on Haemorrhagic Fever inTokyo, it was suggested that the world's hemorrhagic fever with renal syndrome associated with Hantaan virus and related viruses be referred to as HFRS uniformly. The distribution of cases of hemorrhagic fever with renal syndrome in more than 30 countries around the world, outbreak distribution in more than 70 countries on five continents, has become the world's public health issues.

9.6.1   Hantavirus

Hantavirusesare distributed worldwide and cause two serious and often fatal human diseases: haemorrhagic fever with renal syndrome (HFRS) and hantavirus cardiopulmonary syndrome (HCPS) caused by Old World and New World hantaviruses, respectively. China, the world's most affected country by HFRS, registers 50,000 to 100,000 HFRS patients each year, with a mortality rate of 5% to 10% over the past decade.

9.6.1.1   Biological Characteristics

Hantaviruses are classified in the family Bunyaviridae, genus *Hantavirus*. There are currently 24 recognized serotypes/genotypes, each associated with a specific rodent host. The mature Hantavirus particles are round or oval and the morphology of Hantavirus is polymorphic compared with other Bunyaviruses. The virus is an icosahedral enveloped virus, 80–120 nm in diameter. The hantavirus genome consists of three segments, designated large(L), middle(M) and small(S) (Figure 9–8). The L segment encodes an RNA-dependent RNA polymerase; the M segment encodes a glycoprotein precursor that is further processed to produce G1 and G2 transmembrane glycoproteins; and the S segment encodes a nucleocapsid protein. Both G1 and G2 have neutralizing sites and hemagglutination points. N protein is responsible for inducing humoral and cellular immunity in infected cells.

Hantavirus is easily destroyed by heat, detergents organic solvents and hypochlorite solutions. It can also be inactive by 56 ℃ for 30 minutes or UV (50cm) for 1h. Hantavirus has been shown to survive in the environment for 2–3 days at normal room temperature.

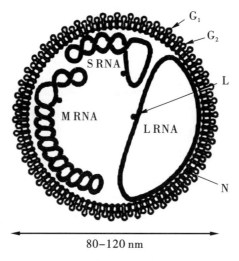

80–120 nm

Figure 9–8　Structure of Hantavirus

Hantaviruses are usually cultured in Vero E6 cells and it can also grow in other cell lines including major human umbilical vein endothelial cells, major hamster kidney cells, chicken embryo fibroblasts, major murine macrophages and a large number of human continuous cell lines Kidney cells and more. In Hantavirus infected cells, a larger number inclusion of different forms can be seen, inclusions may be filiform, granular, vesicular and so on. Immuno-electron microscopy proved that the inclusion body consists mainly of the viral nucleoprotein.

9.6.1.2　Epidemiology &Pathogenesis

In 1978, hantaviruses were first described as the etiological agent of hemorrhagic fever with renal syndrome (HFRS) inKorea. Since 1993, Pathogenic hantaviruses, in nature carried by a specific rodent host species, can cause severe disease in humans with mortality rates from 12% (HFRS) to 40% (HCPS). Both diseases are acute febrile infections, Humans do not belong to the natural host range of hantaviruses and infection generally occurs accidentally by inhalation of virus-containing aerosols from rodent excretions such as urine, faeces and saliva.

Hence HFRS cases are reported in Europe and Asia, while HCPS has only been described in the Americas, with different hantaviruses being found where their hosts predominate. HERS has obvious seasonal characteristics, that is, cyclical in a certain number of monthly epidemic peak peaked at the same time, but at the same time showed the sporadic, distributed throughout the year, the disease has emerged. However, HFRS is not exactly the same in different age and epidemic types of different epidemic areas. Although the periodicity of HFRS epidemic is not very obvious, it still has periodic characteristics. According to Chinese data, HFRS shows a national epidemic peak in 8 years on average and one epidemic peak occurs in 3 – 5 years in county-level epidemic area Common and cyclical causes are primarily associated with cyclical changes in density and viral load in the main host animals and also with the immune status of susceptible populations and the chance of exposure to HFRS.

The pathogenesis of hantavirus disease is not yet fully understood. Hantavirus infections, HCPS and HFRS, are characterized by sudden onset with flu-like symptoms, such as fever, headache, abdominal pain and nausea, followed by a hypotensive phase with often severe thrombocytopenia and increased vascular permeability, leukocytosis, elevated levels of lactate dehydrogenase and C-reactive protein. After this phase, the infection manifests in different organs. HCPS is a predominantly cardiopulmonary disease in which renal symptoms may be observed as well. In contrast, in most cases, HFRS affects predominantly kidney function. Laboratory findings in HFRS and NE demonstrate high-serum creatinine and low-serum albumin and urinalysis shows hematuria and albuminuria. This oliguric phase with acute renal failure is followed by the diuretic phase in which renal function improves and the convalescent phase during which patients recover completely. Acute renal failure is observed in 90% – 95% of infections with Old World hantaviruses. Although case fatality rate for HFRS ranges from 5 to 15% and up to 50% for HCPS. The major histopathologic findings of fatal cases of HFRS were renal medulla necrosis, extensive tubular degeneration. In HCPS, the major histopathological changes include interstitial pneumonia, hyperemia, edema and monocyte infiltration and the formation of clear membrane areas, as well as intact respiratory epithelium. Cardiogenic shock due to respiratory failure is responsible for the often fatal outcome of HCPS. Death due to HFRS maybe because of several complications: renal insufficiency, edema and hemorrhages, encephalopathy or shock. Signs and symptoms of hantavirus infection may present differently and can affect different organs.

The incubation period for HFRS is about two weeks. The classic course of HFRS can be considered five well-recognized stages: fever, hypotension, oliguria, diuresis and recovery. Fever usually starts abruptly without prodromal symptoms, with headache and myalgia lasting 3 – 7 days. Then there is the stage of hypotension, thrombocytopenia, petechia and proteinuria. Hypotension phase lasts hours or days. This phase begins when blood pressure returns to normal start. It lasts for 3 – 7 days until urine output increases. This diuretic period can last for several weeks and the patient excretes several liters of urine daily. Full recovery can take weeks or months. The death rate is 3% – 20%.

9.6.1.3　Laboratory Diagnosis

Laboratory diagnosis of hantavirus infection is based on four primary categories of tests: serology, immunochemistry, reverse transcription (RT)-PCR and virus culture. The most practical approach for the laboratory diagnosis of hantavirus infection is based on serologic tests. The most commonly used serological tests are indirect IgM and IgG ELISA as well as IgM capture ELISAs, which have higher specificity than indirect ELISAs. Indirect immunofluorescence assays are also regularly used for diagnostics but have lower specificity. The detection of IgG or IgM antibodies to hantavirus using ELISA is the method most commonly used in the diagnosis given that the majority of HPS cases show IgM antibodies during the acute period of the illness and they remain detectable for 6 – 8 months. The appearance of specific IgG can occur during or shortly after the appearance of IgM antibodies, they can remain at high levels for several years.

The use of RT-PCR allows the detection of viral RNA in whole blood, clot or tissues obtained in the first 10 days of the disease. The method is also useful for detecting viral RNA in tissues of infected rodents. Hantavirus can be isolated in cultured cells, but the primary isolation takes weeks without CPE, so this method is not diagnosable.

9.6.1.4 Prevention, Control& Treatment

HFRS epidemic prevention and control to take anti-rodent-based comprehensive measures to multiple high-incidence areas and other affected areas at high risk of vaccination. Conscientiously do a good job of environmental sanitation rodent habitat removal activities, adhere to the combination of anti-rodent control. Before entering large-scale field work sites such as water conservancy, agriculture, minerals, national defense, bridges and railways, epidemiological surveillance and epidemic-site surveillance should be carried out. Organizations and publicity campaigns must be strengthened so that rodent control and rodent prevention are well done in construction and camping sites. Vaccination of HFRS inactivated vaccines against medical, nursing, testing and immunization personnel (high-risk groups) should be based on occupations or occupations where there is a high number of young adults and other endemic areas with high exposure to rodents and wild foci. The type of affected area choose the appropriate type of vaccine. Vaccination should be completed within one month before the peak season begins. One year after the first immunization should be strengthened vaccination. Strengthen personal protection, try to avoid contact with rodents and their feces (urine, excrement) or secretions (saliva), rodent control should pay special attention to personal protection. When entering the field of operation and stay overnight, we must strengthen personal protection to prevent contact with infection.

A variety of vaccines have been developed using kill viruses and recombinant DNA technology. Formaldehyde-inactivated vaccines (SEO and HTN) have been shown to produce neutralizing antibodies. The formalin-inactivated HTN vaccine used in the South Korean trial showed a 75% neutralizing antibody response rate. There are three specific vaccines, an inactivated vaccine (Hantaan type) extracted from the brain of an infected mouse, a monovalent vaccine (Hantaan or Seoul type) that is inactivated from cell culture and a cell derived from Hantaan or Seoul types. Inactivated bivalent vaccine has been developed in China and HFRS confrontation. Any of the three vaccines on a large scale indicates that the vaccine stimulates an effective immunization against HFRS. The development of DNA vaccines and recombinant vaccines against HPS and HFRS is currently underway.

At present, we still need to adopt a comprehensive treatment. First of all should pay close attention to the "three early and one on" (early detection, early rest, flat treatment and the nearest treatment), for the various stages of pathophysiological changes to take prophylactic treatment and prevention and treatment of complications of treatment, in particular, early should do a good job Virus treatment and liquid therapy. Severe patients should pay close attention to anti-shock, prevention of bleeding and renal failure treatment.

Antivirals Ribavirin is commonly used in the treatment of Hantaan virus in China and clinical trials have shown that ribavirin treatment significantly reduces HFRS mortality within 5 days of onset. Current Hantavirus pulmonary syndrome treatment includes maintaining adequate oxygenation and supporting hemodynamic function.

In the treatment of fever, the principle of anti-virus, anti-seepage, anti-bleeding. Prevent hypotension and renal failure. Early bed rest, given high calorie, multi-vitamin, digestible diet. Due to vomiting can not eat, should be balanced intravenous salt and glucose solution. In the hypotensive period of treatment, it is mainly to actively supplement the blood volume and to prevent microcirculation dysfunction, acidosis, cardiac insufficiency, etc. Strive to restore blood pressure as soon as possible and maintain stability. Supplementary blood volume should be early, fast, appropriate amount. In the treatment of oliguria, urine output in the 500−1,000 ml oliguria tend to oliguria less than 500 ml/day, 50 ml/day for the closed urine. The current treatment principle is to stabilize the body environment, promote renal function recovery, prevent complications. In the polyuria treatment, daily urine output increased to 500−2,000 ml, oliguria to polyuria stage of migration, more than 2,000 ml, to enter the polyuria, urine output of more than 3,000 ml for polyuria. Polyuria early treatment of oliguria according to principles. The number of urine after treatment according to the current principles of the current regulation of water and electrolyte balance. Strengthen supportive therapy. In the recovery period of treatment, continue to pay attention to rest and gradually increase the amount of activity. Strengthen nutrition, to high sugar, high protein, multi-fiber diet. After discharge, according to the condition recovery, rest 1 to 3 months, heavy cases may be extended.

9.6.2   Crimean-Congo Hemorrhagic Fever Virus

Crimean-Congo haemorrhagic fever (CCHF) is an acute viral disease caused by the Crimean-Congo hemorrhagic fever virus (CCHFV). Among the tick-borne viruses, Crimean-Congo haemorrhagic fever (CCHFV) is the most important cause of severe and fatal human hemorrhagic disease. The range of clinical cases and reports of CCHFV in ticks extends over large regions of Africa and Eurasia (including the Mediterranean region) and from the Middle East to India. Ticks of the family Ixodidae are the acknowledged vectors of CCHFV transmission to humans. Hyalomma marginatum has the most prominent role globally in the natural history of CCHF in the Mediterranean basin and Middle Asia.

9.6.2.1   Biological Characteristics

CCHFV belongs to the Nairovirus genus of Bunyaviridae family. Like other Bunyaviridae, CCHFV is a packaged minus-strand RNA virus. The genome of CCHFV contains three negative segments, large (L), medium (M) and small (S) segments, which encode the polymerase proteins, glycoprotein and viral nucleocapsid, respectively. These viruses are sensitive to heat, formaldehyde, detergents and low-pH inactivation.

9.6.2.2   Epidemiology &Pathogenesis

CCHF is a natural animal disease. Ixodid (hard) ticks, especially the genus Hyalomma, are the host and vector for CCHFV. Many wild animals and domestic animals, such as cows, sheep, goats and rabbits, are hosts of the virus. The virus is transmitted by infected tick bites or direct contact with CCHF-infected and infected animal products. CCHF is usually easily infected by humans. CCHF was found in Eastern Europe, especially in the former Soviet Union. It is also distributed in the Mediterranean, Central Asia, Southern Europe, Africa, the Middle East and the Indian subcontinent. The prevalence of CCHF is regional and seasonal. In China, Xinjiang and Yunnan are major affected areas.

CCHF is a serious human disease with a high mortality rate. Reported mortality rates vary widely from 2% to 30 % across studies and endemic countries. The incubation period is about 7 days. The disease suddenly begins to have a high grade fever, headache, fatigue, myalgia, abdominal pain, nausea, vomiting, diarrhoea, thrombocytopenia and rash, to haemorrhages from various body sites, shock and death in severe cases. With the development of the disease, a large area of severe bruising, severe nosebleed and uncontrolled bleeding at the injection site can be seen. Severe patients may experience hypotension and pulmonary failure. The pathogenesis has not been clarified yet. Direct virus damage and immune damage mechanisms may play an important role in the disease.

9.6.2.3   Laboratory Diagnosis

Such as the patient's blood early inoculation of isolated pathogens, complement fixation test, indirect hemagglutination test or indirect fluorescent antibody test was positive, you can confirm. The blood routine examination significantly reduced white blood cells and sometimes reduced to $1 \times 10^9/L$, thrombocytopenia. Urine routine examination and more proteinuria and hematuria. Early onset may be mild liver dysfunction, some patients with elevated serum bilirubin. It is suspected that the diagnosis of CCHF was carried out in a specially equipped high biosafety level laboratory. IgG and IgM antibodies can be detected in serum, starting on day 6 of the disease. IgM can detect 4 months, IgG levels decreased, but can be detected for 5 years. Recently, RT-PCR for detecting viral genomes has been successfully applied to diagnosis.

9.6.2.4 Prevention& Treatment

Prevention of tick bites and direct contact with the patient's blood, animal blood or viscera is an effective protective measure. Although an inactivated murine brain-derived vaccine for CCHF has been developed and used in small-scale in Eastern Europe, no safe and effective vaccine is widely used in humans. In China, an inactivated vaccine against CCHF has also been developed and the main results of small-scale use in pastoral areas show safety efficiencies. Currently, CCHF does not have a specific antiviral drug. Supportive treatment is the main force of treatment. Strict isolation of patients, less family visits to avoid contact with patients and virus contaminants. Prevent patients from spreading the virus to health care workers and eliminate any chance of causing a nosocomial infection. Diet should be light, eat more fruits and vegetables, with a reasonable diet, pay attention to adequate nutrition, would like to comply with the doctor's advice.

9.6.3 Ebola Virus

Ebola virus was first identified in Africa, in 1976. Ebola virus causes Ebola haemorrhagic fever (EHF) that is one of the most virulent viral disease known to humankind, with a mortality rate of 50% to 90%.

9.6.3.1 Biological Characteristics

The Ebola virus belongs to the Filoviridae family. The two known filoviruses, marburg virus and Ebola virus, are different in antigenicity and are divided into different genera. Filoviruses are enveloped, single-stranded, negative-sense RNA viruses. They vary in length from 800 nm to 1,400 nm. The infectivity of Filovirus is destroyed by heating 60 ℃ for 30 minutes, by ultraviolet rays and gamma irradiation, by lipid solvent and by bleach and phenolic disinfectant.

The current research shows that chimpanzees, monkeys, bats and other animals may be the natural EBV host and source of infection. In natural conditions, humans and chimpanzees, monkeys can be infected and died, the virus has been isolated from the rhesus monkey. EBHF is transmitted mainly through multiple routes of contact with the virus carriers such as blood, body fluids and contaminants. Seven weeks after clinical recovery, the patient's semen can still transmit the virus. In nature there is low virulence or nonpathogenic EBV. In some parts of Africa, residents antibody positive rate reaches 30% or more and no one pathogenic. In the Guinea-Congo Basin tropical rain forest region and the Sudan dry grassland region, the highest positive rates of serum EBV antibodies occurred mainly in ethnic groups that settled in rain-prone forests.

The incubation period for Ebola haemorrhagic fever is 2 to 21 days. Sudden onset fever, headache, sore throat and muscle pain, followed by abdominal pain, abdominal pain, diarrhea, rashes, internal and external bleeding, often resulting in shock and death. The virus is oriented towards macrophages, hepatocytes and endothelial cells. There are very high levels of virus in many tissues, including the liver, spleen, lungs and kidneys, as well as blood and other fluids.

9.6.3.2 Diagnosis

The Ebola virus is highly contagious and should be promptly isolated and treated and preliminary diagnosis should be made as soon as possible based on the epidemiological exposure history and clinical manifestations of suspicious patients and the patients should be treated in isolation in time. At the same time the relevant laboratory tests to confirm its diagnosis are required as soon as possible.

Clinical routine tests: early may have proteinuria, elevated transaminases, AST> ALT; leukocytosis, thrombocytopenia.

Experimental diagnosis: ① Electron microscopy: Can be directly detected in patients with blood, urine and sweat gland skin tissue in the virus particles, the results faster. Patients can also be vaccinated early serum or urine Vero cell culture, cultured with glutaraldehyde fixed, ultra-thin sections of the virus particles. ② Serological diagnosis: Common methods for indirect immunofluorescence and ELISA, check IgM and IgG antibodies. However, due to the high content of virus in the patient's hematuria, the examination of the antigen is more conducive to early diagnosis. ③ RT-PCR technology: Specificity, but also for the diagnosis of the disease.

9.6.3.3   Prevention & Treatment

Preventive measures: ① Health Education Extensively carry out health education to publicize the basic knowledge of the disease, highly contagious and dangerous, as well as the route of transmission and prevention and treatment of the disease. Let the masses grasp the scientific knowledge of the disease, improve their vigilance without panic, improve self-care awareness and actively participate in the prevention and treatment of this disease. ② Strengthening training mainly focuses on the training of frontier quarantine departments, quarantine departments of the port and relevant medical and testing personnel so that they can gain a thorough understanding of the systematic knowledge of the disease and related international quarantine diseases and be familiar with the relevant quarantine laws and regulations and quarantine technologies and keep an eye on international on the disease outbreak status. ③ There is no vaccine for immunization. Some progress has been made in the development of inactivated vaccines and genetically engineered vaccines abroad.

Clinical treatment: There is no effective drugs for treatment, mainly by symptomatic treatment, triazole drugs on the disease is invalid. Recovery of patient serum and animal antisera prepared immunoglobulin has a better therapeutic effect, in case of emergency (laboratory infection and emergency rescue) can be used. Early application of delayed onset and prevent the occurrence of symptoms of hemorrhagic fever. Progress has also been made in the development of human-specific monoclonal antibodies and it is expected that special treatment drugs will be obtained.

9.7   Herpes Viruses

9.7.1   Herpes Simplex Virus(HSV)

Herpes simplex virus is a typical herpes virus, is a herpes virus subfamily HSV-1 and HSV-2 two serotypes. The main feature is a wide range of host, can infect people and a variety of animals, such as rabbits, mice and so on. Proliferative replication cycle is short, strong ability to cause cytopathic, the formation of latent infection in the sensory ganglion. The earliest human herpes virus was HSV. Late 19th century virus isolation using cell culture in vitro technology, according to the characteristics of cytopathic lesions of pox virus and herpes zoster. At the beginning of the 20th century, HSV and its related diseases were identified. However, it was not until the 1960s that two serotypes of HSV were found. At the beginning of this century, sequencing of HSV-1 and HSV-2 genes was completed and the sequence of HSV genome, Gene products, virus replication and gene regulation system has a new understanding.

1)Shape and structure: HSV has the typical herpesvirus morphological characteristics, with envelopes, virosomes spherical, diameter 120−150 nm, viral nucleic acid linear dsDNA, about 150 kb, encoding at least more than 70 kinds of proteins. Among them, the virus-encoded ribonucleotide reductase, thymidine kinase can promote the synthesis of nucleotides; DNA enzymes catalyze viral DNA replication. The specific catalytic effect of the viral enzyme on the matrix can serve as a target for antiviral drugs.

2) HSV glycoprotein: At least 11 kinds of HSV envelope glycoproteins play an important role in the proliferation, replication and pathogenicity of the virus and are also the main antigens for inducing the body's immune response. The currently recognized and officially named HSV envelope glycoproteins are gB, gC, gD, gE, gG, gH, gI, gJ, gL, gK and gM, respectively; they play different roles either independently or in complex form. Among them, gB, gD and gH are necessary for HSV to produce infectious progeny. GB and gD have the function of adsorbing and assisting to penetrate into cells and are related to virus infection. GD is also the most immunogenic neutralizing antigen and can be induced the body produces neutralizing antibodies that have been used to develop subunit vaccines; gH has the function of fusion into cells and release of the virus. gC, gE and gI as structural glycoproteins, with immune escape function. In addition, gC is a receptor for complement C3 and gE/gI complex is a receptor for IgGFc, which prevents the antiviral effect of the antibody. gG is a type-specific glycoprotein divided into gG-1 and gG-2 to distinguish HSV-1 and HSV-2 serotypes.

3) Serotype: There are two serotypes of HSV, HSV-1 and HSV-2, also known as HHV-1 and HHV2. HSV-1 often causes mucous membranes and damaged skin (such as mouth, eyes, lips) and nervous system infections above the waist. HSV-2 mainly causes infections below the waist (such as genitalia). HSV-1 and HSV-2 commonly used gG type specific unit anti-binding assay typing, but also based on cell-selective experiments, vinyl ethylene deoxyuridine resistance and viral DNA restriction endonuclease mapping.

4) Cultivate characteristics: HSV can multiply in a variety of cells, producing a clear viral cytopathic effect (CPE). Common human embryo lung, human embryonic kidney cells, hamster kidney or primary rabbit kidney and other cells isolated and cultured virus. After the virus infects the cells, CPE occurs in 48 hours, which is characterized by cell swelling, rounding and fusion and eosinophilic inclusion bodies appear in the nucleus, followed by rapidly falling off and disintegration.

The extent of HSV infection in animals   Host a wider range. Commonly used laboratory animals are mice, guinea pigs and rabbits. Different routes of vaccination can produce different infections, such as herpes keratitis caused by rabbit corneal inoculation, vaccination in the brain or intraperitoneal injection in mice causes herpetic encephalitis and genital vaccination can cause genital herpes.

9.7.1.1 Pathogenicity and Immunity

HSV infection in the crowd is very common. After the first HSV infection, no obvious clinical symptoms, recessive infection accounts for about 80% to 90%, dominant infection accounted for only a minority. Patients and virus carriers are two sources of infection. HSV-1 and HSV-2 are different not only the routes of transmission but also the clinical characteristics of both types of virus infection. The virus enters the body through the mucosa and the damaged skin. Most of the cells are characterized by lytic infection. The typical pathological injury is skin and mucous membrane blisters. The serum is filled with virus particles and cellular debris. HSV-1 is transmitted primarily through direct or indirect contact. The virus infect the human oral cavity, mucocutaneous, conjunctival and central nervous system, causing stomatitis, cold sores, pharyngitis, keratoconjunctivitis and herpes encephalitis; HSV-2 is usually sexually transmitted, genital and genital mucosal violations, causing Genital herpes. The virus can also be transmitted vertically through the placenta or birth canal, pregnant women genital herpes can be transmitted to the newborn during labor.

(1) Primary Infection

The main clinical manifestations of HSV-1 primary infection are skin and mucosal herpes zoster, which occur mostly in infants and young children between 6 months and 2 years of age. About 10% to 15% of primary infections are manifest as dominant infections. Common herpetic gingivostomatitis in the oral cavity and gingival mucosa appear herpes herpes, herpes rupture after the formation of ulcers, the lesion contains a large number of viruses. In addition, can also cause herpes keratitis, herpes zoster eczema or herpes zoster encephalitis. Primary infection with HSV-2 occurs mostly after sexual activity and causes mainly genital herpes-borne (STD) sexually transmitted diseases (STDs). Primary genital herpes more serious, manifested as skin and mucosal vesicular ulcers, severe pain. 80% of primary genital herpes is caused by HSV-2 and only a few are caused by HSV-1.

Latent and reactivation of infection HSV primary infection, the body quickly produce specific immunity, most of the virus can be removed and the symptoms disappear. However, a small number of viruses can lurk in nerve cells in the ganglia for long periods of time, do not show clinical symptoms and are in a relatively balanced state with the body. The latent sites for HSV-1 are the trigeminal ganglia and the superior cervical ganglia, while HSV-2 lurks in the sacral ganglia. When the body is subject to a variety of non-specific stimulation, such as fever, cold, sun, menstruation, emotional stress or some bacteria, virus infection or the use of renal cortex hormones, the latent virus is activated re-proliferation of proliferating virus Feel the axonal nerve fiber down to the end of the dominant epithelial cells continue to proliferate, causing recurrent herpes. HSV reactivation of the virus led to recurrence of the disease is more common, the infection is often in the same place with the primary infection. For example, the primary disease is herpetic keratitis and the site of recurrence is the cornea. Recurrent keratitis lesions can lead to corneal ulcers, scars, is one of the main causes of blindness.

(2) Congenital Infection

There are three ways of intrauterine, birth and postpartum contact infection, of which the birth canal infection is the most common. Pregnant women suffering from acute genital herpes may be infected during delivery through the birth of the fetus, can cause neonatal skin, eyes and mouth exposed parts of the local rash, severe cases of children with herpes zoster or disseminated infection. Pregnant women due to primary infection or latent HSV or micro-live, the virus can be placenta or cervical retrograde infection of the fetus, causing miscarriage, premature birth, stillbirth or congenital malformations. Neonates can also become infected after they have been exposed to HSV infection or from the external environment.

In the past, the causal relationshipis still not enough evidence not only HSV and malignant tumor but also the HSV-2 dye and cervical cancer, HSV-2 infection may have synergistic effects.

In anti-HSV infection, cellular immunity is more important than humoral immunity, cellular immunity involves CTL. TH multiple T-cell subsets, as well as activated giant cells, NK cells and other latent HSV reactivation of infection caused by disease recurrence, serum in the Antibody and the rapid rebound, play a neutralizing antibody to eliminate the role of free virus. Prevent the spread of the virus in the body, but can not effectively prevent the virus to the nerve tissue migration, the virus lurking in ganglion cells without neutralization. When stimuli appear again later, they will trigger the persistence of virus that reactivates latent infection.

9.7.1.2   HSV and Gene Therapy

HSV-1 can be transformed into an effective vector for the introduction of foreign genes and may be applied to gene therapy of CNS diseases by utilizing the characteristics of latent infection in HSV-1 neurons. In addition, the herpes simplex virus thymidine kinase (HSV-TK) gene as the most studied suicide gene, commonly used in cancer gene therapy research.

9.7.1.3 Microbial Examination Method

Virus isolation and identification   Samples often take blister fluid, sleep solution, corneal swab or corneal scraping, vaginal swab and cerebrospinal fluid and other specimens were routinely treated after inoculation of rabbit kidney cells and human embryonic kidney cells and other susceptible cells for isolation and culture. Virus proliferation quickly, one in 2−3 days after the emergence of CPE, the disease characterized by cell swelling, rounded, the formation of fused cells, which can be initially determined. Then neutralization test, DNase electrophoresis analysis and HSV-1 and HSV-2 monoclonal antibody rabbit fluorescence test were further identified.

Quick diagnosis   The early diagnosis of HSV infection is of great importance to timely anti-virus treatment, especially for herpes encephalitis and herpes keratitis patients. Commonly used immunofluorescence technology, immune enzyme technology to detect intracellular HSV-specific antigen; nucleic acid hybridization or PCR can also be used to detect the presence or absence of virus-specific nucleic acids in the specimen.

Please learn to diagnose blood   Commonly used in clinical enzyme-linked immunosorbent assay and indirect immunofluorescence detection of HSV-specific antibodies. Specific M antibodies suggest a sense of seizure and detection of specific IgG antibodies is used in epidemiological investigations.

9.7.1.4 Prevention and Control Principles

Currently no specific prevention measures for HSV infection. Care should be taken to avoid intimate contact with the patient and to cut off the route of transmission. If pregnant women have HSV-2 birth canal, cesarean section can be carried out to prevent neonatal infection. Severe neonatal HSV infection should be given effective anti-viral drug treatment. Acycline guanosine and gonadotropin have been used for the treatment of genital herpes and herpes keratitis, etc. , can shorten the detoxification time and promote the healing of the lesion; also intravenous drug treatment of systemic herpes or herpes encephalitis, the treatment effect Better, but not prevent the recurrence of latent infection. Interferon can also be used for the treatment of herpes.

HSV glycoprotein subunit vaccine is being developed.

9.7.2 Varricella-zoster Virus

Varicella-zoster virus is the causative agent of both chickenpox and shingles. In children with primary infection caused by chickenpox, after the virus lurking in the body, a small number of people in adolescence or adult latent virus reactivation caused by recurrent infections caused by shingles, it is called varicella-zoster virus.

9.7.2.1 Biological Characteristics

VZV is HHV-3, only one serotype. Biological traits are mostly similar to HSV. These include: ①latent infection in the sensory ganglia; ②cellular immune responses play an important role in disease control; ③thymidine kinase is also expressed, which is sensitive to anti-viral drugs; ④skin lesions are predominantly vesicular and so on. But unlike HSV, VZV is transmitted through the respiratory tract and the virus affects the skin through systemic infections after local lymphoid tissue proliferation.

VZV genome in HHV the smallest, isabout 120−130 kb, encoding about 70 different egg stomatal. In vitro cultured human or monkey fibroblasts or human epithelial cells proliferation, CPE appeared more slowly; observed infected cells can be seen in the nucleus of eosinophilic inclusion bodies and the formation of multinucleated giant cells. General experimental animals and chicken embryo are insensitive to the disease.

9.7.2.2   Pathogenicity and Immunity

Man is the only host of VZV, the skin is the main target cell of the virus. VZV highly infectious, the main source of infection in patients, In patients with chickenpox acute blister contents and upper respiratory secretions or blister patients blister contents contain high titer virus. Children are generally predisposed to morbidity in susceptible populations as high as 90%.

Initial infection of infants with VZV disease called chickenpox, good hair age 3−9 years old, mostly in winter and spring epidemic, the virus mainly by respiratory droplets spread or contact transmission. Invade the virus first local (oropharyngeal) lymph node proliferation, into the blood flow to the mononuclear phagocyte system a large number of proliferation, the virus re-enter the blood to form a second viremia, with the bloodstream spread to the body and ultimately located in the skin. About 2−3 weeks after the incubation period of systemic skin pimples, blisters and can develop impetigo. Rash distribution was mainly concentric, to drive more, often accompanied by fever.

Children with chicken pox generally mild condition, is a benign, self-limiting disease, incidental complications such as viral encephalitis or pneumonia. However, children with cellular immunodeficiency, leukemia or long-term use of immunosuppressive agents can present as critically ill, life-threatening. Adult chickenpox-when the stock is heavier, 20% −30% concurrent pneumonia, mortality is also high. Pregnant women suffering from chickenpox performance is also more serious and may lead to fetal malformations, abortion or stillbirth. Chickenpox infection in newborns is often disseminated, the mortality rate is higher, varicella-encephalitis survivors may have permanent sequel.

Shingles occur only in patients with a history of varicella in the past, more common in adults and the elderly, the incidence increased with age. A small amount of virus can be latent in the sensory ganglia of the dorsal root ganglia or cranial nerves of the spinal cord after childhood recovery from chickenpox. After the decline in immunity in the body by some factors (such as cold, heat, drugs, X-rays organ transplantation, etc.), the latent virus is activated, the virus reaches the innervation of the axon along the skin cell proliferation Herpes occurs.

Herpes along the nerve distribution was banded, so called zoster. Bands often occur in one side of the body to the trunk line for the community, the site of a good chest, abdomen, severe pain.

Such as violations of the trigeminal nerve branch, can affect the cornea can cause corneal ulcers or even blindness. Occasionally occur encephalitis. The incidence of shingles was sporadic, people of all ages have occurred, but mostly in the elderly over the age of 60, most of the disease after the onset of life no longer occur, the recurrence rate was only about 4%. The contents of the herpes zoster in patients with the disease contain the virus and thus go to become a source of infection of children's chickenpox.

Children suffering from chicken pox, the body produces long-lasting specific cellular immunity and humoral immunity, minimal risk of chickenpox. However, the virus produced in the body neutralizing antibodies, can not effectively remove the virus in the ganglia, it can not stop the occurrence of shingles.

9.7.2.3   Microbiological Examination Method

According to the clinical manifestations can make a diagnosis. If necessary, desirable lesion skin blisters basal specimens, skin scraping, blister fluid biopsy tissue HE staining done, check the nuclear eosinophilic inclusion bodies and multinucleated giant cells. VZV antigens can also be detected by monoclonal antibody immunofluorescent staining for rapid diagnosis as well as VZV-specific IgM antibodies by FAMA, ELISA, indirect immunofluorescence and micro-neutralization assays, which are reduced to several weeks after the rash subsides Unable to level. Therefore, the detection of specific IgM antibodies have diagnostic significance for VZV infection. VZV DNA can also be detected by PCR. Microscopic observation of the virus particles used electron microscope. To isolate human embryo fibroblasts, neutralization test and immunological techniques are available to make its specific identification.

9.7.2.4 Prevention and Control Principles

Vaccination of large numbers of live attenuated VZV vaccines has been successfully used for specific prophylaxis and vaccinated populations are susceptible children over the age of 1 who are uninfected with VZV. Shingles immunoglobulin can be injected immunosuppressed patients, to prevent or reduce VZV infection with a certain effect.

Normal children with chicken pox generally do not need antiviral treatment. Antiviral drugs are mainly used for the treatment of immunocompromised children with chicken pox, adult chicken pox and shingles. Effective antiviral drugs for VZV include acyclovir and interferon.

9.7.3 Human Cytomegalovirus

Cytomegalovirus beta herpes virus subfamily, HHV-5, is the causative agent of giant cell inclusion body disease. The virus is prevalent in nature and includes human cytomegalovirus, human, mouse, horse, cow and pig, human disease human cytomegalovirus. HCME was first isolated from the salivary gland of a 19-years-old CID infant. The typical cytopathic effect caused by this virus is that the cell volume is significantly enlarged. Inclusion bodies appear in the nucleus and in the plasma. In 1960, the virus was named as giant cells virus. In 1973 the International Virus Commission herpes virus research group officially named the virus as human herpesvirus 5 (HHV5). HCMV infection in the crowd is very common, the concern is that HCMV is one of the important pathogens causing congenital malformations; in the body immune dysfunction, prone to dominant infection; also immunosuppressed patients (such as organ transplantation, cancer and AIDS patients Etc.) an important cause of death.

9.7.3.1 Biological Traits

Form and structure. With the typical morphological structure of herpesvirus, there is a homogeneous membrane structure with a uniform virus particle diameter of about 180−250 nm between the envelope and the capsid. The outermost layer of the virion is a lipid envelope that contains multiple glycoproteins (eg, gB, glycoprotein B). HCMV there are still some different morphological characteristics of other herpes viruses. Observe the infectious compact particles and coated particles under electron microscope. A large number of dense particles present in infected cells, no capsid and viral DNA, composed of cortex protein pp65, surrounded by a coating envelope. The number of non-infectious enveloped particles is very small, with the difference between the virion is virus capsid and envelope, but no viral DNA.

Genome and expression products. HCMV genome has the largest capacity in herpesvirus, about 240 kb. It is a linear dsDNA molecule encoding 165 genes. As early as 1990, the entire genomic sequencing of HCMV AD169 strain has been completed (EMBL gene database entry number X17403). Like HSV, HCMV DNA is also composed of UL and US and the two fragments are arranged in different orientations at the interconnections, upside down, causing the DNA to form four isoforms. The virus replicates in the host cell and has a clear temporal appearance, that is, immediate early antigen, early antigen and late antigen. IEA is a virally encoded regulatory protein that activates the expression of certain genes of the virus's early genes and host cells. The main function of EA is to turn off the replication of host cell DNA and to synthesize viral DNA polymerase to induce viral proliferation. Both IEA and EA emerge rapidly after infection, so IEA and EA can be used for rapid diagnosis with the corresponding antibodies. LA is mainly a viral structural protein, whose expression is regulated by IEA and EA. LA can cause the response of neutralizing antibody. The viral protein antigens appearing on the cell membrane after virus infection can be recognized by the host cell's immune system and eventually lead to cell destruction, which is the key to eradicate the virus.

Cultivate characteristics. HCMV can infect a variety of cells in the human body, such as fibroblasts, endothelial cells, epithelial cells and nerve cells, but only in vitro proliferation of human fibroblasts. The virus replicates slowly in cultured cells and typically takes 7 – 12 days to develop a characteristic CPE that is characterized by rounded, swollen cells, enlarged nuclei and the formation of giant cells, hence the name of the virus. If at this time after the observation with HE staining, there can be seen around the nucleus surrounded by a "halo" of large eosinophilic inclusion bodies.

HCMV is sensitive to lipid solvents and can inactivate the virus under various physical and chemical factors such as heating (56 ℃ for 30 minutes), acidic environment, ultraviolet light and repeated freezing and thawing. Virus species require high storage conditions, 4 ℃ can only save a few days, –196 ℃ and vacuum freeze-drying can be long-term preservation.

9.7.3.2 Pathogenicity and Immunity

HCMV infection rate in the population is very high, our country adult HCMV antibody positive rate of 90%. Primary infection occurs mostly in patients under 2 years of age usually hidden infection, only a few people have clinical symptoms, under certain conditions, the virus can invade multiple organs and systems to produce serious diseases. After infection most of the population can become infected with latent infection long-term. Latent infection sites mainly in the salivary gland, breast, kidney and peripheral blood mononuclear cells and lymphocytes. Latent viruses can be re-activated resulting in recurrent infections.

Patients and asymptomatic carriers are the main sources of infection with HCMV. The virus can be continuously or intermittently discharged from saliva, milk, urine and other cervical secretions. The virus can be spread vertically or horizontally: ①mother to child transmission: the fetus can be transmitted through the placenta (congenital infection), but also through the birth canal or breast milk (perinatal infection); ②contact transmission: through human and human Close contact between, such as a mouth or hand spread. HCMV exposure among kindergartens is high in kindergarten; ③Sexually transmitted: transmitted through sexual contact; ④iatrogenic transmission: including transfusions or organ transplants.

(1) Congenital Infection

HCMV is the most common cause of congenital infection of the virus. In women with primary infection or latent infection reactivation during the first trimester (within 3 months), HCMV can infect the fetus through the placenta or via the cervix, causing an internal infection. Congenital infection rate of about 0.5% –2.5%, of which 5% –10% of newborns clinical symptoms, known as giant cell inclusion disease (CID). CID is an acute infection caused by HCMV, the performance of children with hepatosplenomegaly, jaundice, thrombocytopenic purpura and hemolytic anemia; a few were congenital malformations, such as microcephaly, mental retardation; severe cases can cause miscarriage or stillbirth. Some children may be months or years after birth out of clinical symptoms, manifested as mental retardation and congenital sensory nerve deafness.

(2) Perinatal Infection

Neonates give birth to the virus through the birth canal or from the mother's milk during childbirth. Infected children, generally no obvious clinical symptoms, but from the urine and pharyngeal secretions can continue to release a large number of viruses, is an important source of infection, a few can also be manifested as short-term interstitial pneumonia, hepatomegaly mild swelling Large and jaundiced, most children with good prognosis.

(3) Post-natal Infection

After the primary infection of HCMV, most people are infected with latent infection for a long period of time without any clinical symptoms. Affected by certain incentives, such as therapeutic immunosuppression, virus reactivation caused by latent infection recurrence. Clinical manifestations of mononucleosis; rare complications of pneumonia, hepatitis and so on. Infection is mostly self-limiting, but virus discharge lasts longer. The normal population can also be infected by transfusion of HCMV, enter a large number of HCMV-containing blood can occur mononucleosis and hepatitis, fever, fatigue, myalgia, liver dysfunction and other symptoms.

(4)Infection in Immunocompromised Populations

Immunocompromised patients (such as organ transplant, leukemia, lymphoma and ADS patients) are at high risk of HCMV infection and the prognosis is poor. Regardless of the primary infection or the reactivation of latent HCMV in vivo, the recurrent infection can cause more serious diseases and often cause systemic infections such as HCMV pneumonia and hepatitis, with high mortality rate. Numerous investigations have shown that HCMV is one of the most common opportunistic infections in AIDS patients.

It is generally accepted that HCMV has oncogenic potential and HCMV DNA has been detected in a variety of human tumors such as cervical cancer, prostate cancer, colon cancer and Kaposi's, although there is currently no direct evidence.

HCMV infection can induce the body to produce the corresponding humoral and cellular immunity. HCMV envelope glycoproteins gB and gD are important antigens that elicit neutralizing antibodies. However, the body fluid of rabies against HCMV infection has only a protective effect. Because studies have shown that specific neutralizing antibodies can not prevent the reactivation of latent virus, the mother's specific antibodies can not reduce intrauterine or perinatal HCMV infection, but can reduce the symptoms. HCMV primary infection common in serum antibody-positive organ transplant recipients and the disease is often serious. Cellular immunity plays an important role in limiting the spread of HCMV and the reactivation of latent viruses. Cellular immune-mediated clearance of the virus is mainly associated with the role of CD8$^+$ CTL. Patients with deficient cellular immune function are at high risk for HCMV infection. HCMV infection can also cause damage to immune function or lead to immunosuppression.

9.7.3.3 Microbiological Examination Method

Cytology. Tissue samples or urine samples (sediment after centrifugation) smears, Giemsa staining or HE staining microscopic examination of macrophages and nuclear eosinophilic inclusion bodies. The method is simple and rapid, can be used to aid diagnosis, but the detection rate is not high Virus separation. The most commonly used specimens were middle morning urine, blood, pharynx or cervical secretions and were seeded on human embryonic lung fibroblasts. After 4−6 weeks of culture, the characteristic CPE was observed. Can also be carried out on a glass slide 2−4 days after the period of incubation and then immunofluorescence or immune enzyme technology to detect infected cells in the antigen, commonly used in clinical laboratory diagnosis. Positive virus isolation is the current clinical diagnosis of "gold standard".

Virus antigen detection. The use of specific monoclonal antibodies such as anti-pp65 monoclonal antibodies, rapid detection of HCMV early antigen (eg, pp65) in specimens such as leukocytes by ELISA, immunofluorescence staining, etc. , provides rapid diagnosis with high sensitivity and specificity. If the clinical use of pp65 antigenemia test is a more reliable method for rapid diagnosis.

Serological examination. Currently used in serum ELISA, IgM and IgA specific. IgG test can be used to understand the rate of population infection, the use of double serum can be used for clinical diagnosis. Detection of specific IgM and IgA antibodies can help diagnose active HCMV infection. In addition, since IgM can not pass from the mother to the fetus through the placenta, if the HCMV IgM antibody is detected from the neonatal serum, the fetus has an intrauterine infection.

Detection of viral nucleic acid Detection of HCMV genomic DNA in tissue sections by in situ hybridization can also be used to detect viral DNA in samples by nucleic acid hybridization or quantitative PCR. The positive rate of nucleic acid detection, latent infection can also be detected.

9.7.3.4 Prevention and Control Principles

There is no safe and effective vaccine for HCMV. The live attenuated vaccine can be used in high-risk groups and has certain protective effect. However, it has not yet solved the problem of latent infection and carcinogenic potential and has not been applied clinically. Development of a subunit vaccine that contains no viral DNA is the current research direction. Severe HCMV infection in patients with immunosuppressed can be treated with ganciclovir and valganciclovir that inhibit viral DNA polymerases and are particularly useful in the prophylactic treatment of HCMV infection in patients with kidney and bone marrow transplants as well as in AIDS patients. High titer of anti-HCMV Ig also has some therapeutic effect.

9.7.4 EB Virus

EB virus HHV-4, is a subfamily of the herpes virus. In 1964, Epstein and Barr et al. used a modified tissue culture technique to detect a new human herpesvirus from African pediatric malignant lymphoma cell cultures. The morphological structure of the virus was observed by electron microscopy to be similar to other herpesviruses, but antigenicity different and has the characteristics of addicted B lymphocytes, named EBV. In 1983, the complete genomic sequence of EBV prototype strain (strain B95.8) was determined by Barr. Humans are the only natural hosts of EBV and are associated with a variety of diseases. EBV is the infectious agent of mononucleosis syndrome pathogens, Burkitt lymphoma and nasopharyngeal carcinoma and other malignancies occur in patients with EBV infection is a human important oncology virus.

9.7.4.1 Biological Characteristics

Form and structure. EBV morphological structure is similar to other herpes viruses. The complete virion is round in shape with a diameter of 180 m and contains a core-like linear dsDNA of about 173 kb in length. The capsid consists of 162 capsid grains and is icosahedrally symmetric. Glycoprotein spikes on the surface of the envelope, unlike HSV, , EBV genome is larger, there are multiple repeats, UL and US without inverted arrangement, so no isomers. Different strains of green plants different number of repeats, can be used for identification.

EBV is in the intracellular latent state, the genome from linear into a ring, ring-like appendages force-free existence. In proliferative infections, the circular viral genome is re-linearized with DNA, the virus multiplies, lyses cells and releases progeny virus particles.

At present, EBV can not be cultured in vitro by conventional methods. Generally, human umbilical cord blood is used to culture EBV cells or lymphoblasts containing EBV genomes.

Based on the genetic polymorphism of the virus, the prevalence of EBV in the population can be divided into two subtypes. Type 1 (type A) viruses are more capable of transforming B lymphocytes than type 2 (type B) viruses in vitro in cell culture. Our country is mainly type 1 virus.

Specific antigen Currently known EBV genome has 84 open reading frame (ORF), encoding at least 80 kinds of virus protein, which gp350/gp220 adhesion protein, gp85 fusion glycoprotein. Epstein-Barr virus (EBV) is a disease-causing B-cell surface and mainly infects B cells. One of the reasons for this is that there is a CD21 molecule on the B cell. The gp350/gp20 of the virus binds to the receptor and causes infection. In the human body, the virus can also infect the nasopharynx, the parotid duct and the cervical epithelium. The virus under different infection status of protein expression, their detection has clinical significance.

(1) Proliferative Infection Expressed Antigen

1) Early antigen: is a non-structural protein of the virus, divided into EA/R and EA/D two types, which have EBV-specific DNA polymerase activity. The advent of EA signals that EBV proliferates actively and infects cells into the lysis cycle. EA antibodies appear in the early stages of infection, patients with NPC are resistant to EA-D antibodies and patients with malignant lymphoma in African children have anti-EA-R antibodies.

2) capsid antigen: a late-synthesized virus structural protein, present in the cytoplasm and nucleus. Specific VCA-IgM antibodies appear early, disappear fast; and VCA-lgG appeared late, long duration.

3) Membrane antigen: It exists on the surface of virus envelope and the surface of infected cell membrane. Glycoprotein gp350/220 can induce EBV to adsorb on and off of susceptible cell surface receptor and induce the production of neutralizing antibody. gp350-specific CTL may play an important role in the control of acute EBV infection, so gp350/220 is one of the candidate antigens designed for the EBV subunit vaccine. Detection of specific MA-IgM for early diagnosis and MA-IgG can exist in the body long-term.

(2) Latent Infection Expressed Antigen

In the Herpesvirus family, EBV expression of the latency gene is more clearly understood. EBV in B memory cells due to the immune surveillance of T cells, the performance of latent infection. In the process of latent infection, infected cells contain a small amount of circular, plasmid-like EBV genome, allowing only a small part of the virus due to transcription, in order to maintain the latent state. B cells with the EBV genome can gain the ability to maintain long-term growth and proliferation in cell culture, called "transformation" or "immortalization". When the cell divides, under the action of the cellular DNA polymerase, part of EBV gene is caused to be transcribed and the EBV latent antigen is selectively expressed. There are two main categories:

1) EBV nuclear antigen: DNA-binding protein in infected B cell nuclei. Currently, there issix kinds. Among them EBNA-1 is the only EBV protein expressed in various latent infection states. Its main function is to stabilize the viral circular adduct, to inhibit the function of cell processing and antigen presentation, so as to keep the EBV genome present in infected cells and not to be lost during cell division. EBNA-2 plays a key role in immortalization. EBNA antibodies appear late in infection.

2) Latent membrane egg: expressed in B cell membrane, including LMP1, LMP2A, LMP2B three. LMP1, an activated growth factor receptor, is an oncogenic protein that converts not only B lymphocytes in vitro but also rodent passages and tumorigenesis. LMP1 plays an important role in the formation of epithelial-derived tumors such as nasopharyngeal carcinoma and has various biological activities such as transformation of cells and inhibition of apoptosis. The main role of LMP2A is to prevent the latent infection from turning into a function that reactivates the infection.

9.7.4.2 Pathogenicity and Immunity

EBV infection in the crowd is very common in China around 3-year-old children EBV antibody positive rate as high as 90%. Most children with no obvious symptoms after the initial infection and some cause mild pharyngitis and upper respiratory tract infection, latent virus in vivo and even lifelong virulent adolescent and adult infection, can be characterized as typical infectious mononucleosis.

The source of infection of EBV infection is in patients and latent infections, the main route of transmission of infection through saliva (such as kissing, etc.), but also through sexual contact.

EBV infection host cell pathogenesis: EBV by saliva into the oropharyngeal epithelial cell proliferation, the release of virus infection in local lymphoid B cells, B cells into the blood lead to systemic EBV infection. Activated B cells secreting specific gliadin EBV is also B cell mitogen, polyclonal activation of B cells, produce heterophile antibodies, infected B cells can stimulate T cell proliferation, the formation of atypical lymphocytes, mainly cells T-cells and NK cells, the peripheral blood mononuclear cells was significantly higher. Atypical lymphocytes also have cytotoxic effects that kill EBV-infected cells.

The EBV gene expression of IL-10 analogue (BCRF-1) inhibits Th1 cells, prevents the release of IFN-γ and the immune response of T cells to the virus but promotes B cell growth. The continuous proliferation of B cells and other synergistic factors act together with other synergistic factors to induce lymphoma. In addition, EBV infection is associated with the development of tumors in immunosuppressed patients.

EBV infection caused by the disease are:

1) Infectious mononucleosis syndrome. Is a sexual all-lymphoproliferative disease. In the first adolescent infection when a larger number of EBV onset. The incubation period is about 40 days. The typical manifestations after onset are fever, pharyngitis, cervical lymphocyticitis, swollen liver, blood mononuclear cells and abnormal lymphocytes. The duration of the disease can last for several weeks and the prognosis is good. A large number of virus proliferating and multiplying in epithelial cells of oral mucosa of acute patients, the virus can be discharged from saliva for 6 months. Children with severe immunodeficiency, AIDS patients and organ transplant recipients have a higher case fatality rate.

2) Burkitt lymphoma. Is a less differentiated monoclonal B-cell lymphoma that occurs in endemic areas in Central and South Africa, New Guinea and some temperate regions of South America. It is endemic and is more common in children aged about 6 years. The predilection sites are facial, Palate. Serological epidemiological findings show that before the onset of Burkitt's lymphoma in children infected with EBV, all patients with positive serum antibodies to EBV and more than 80% of the antibody titers higher than normal, found in the tumor tissue EBV genome, it is believed that EBV and Burkitt lymphoma are closely related.

3) Nasopharyngeal cancer. Mainly occurred in Southeast Asia, North Africa and Eskimo regions, China's Guangdong, Guangxi, Fujian, Hunan. Jiangxi, Zhejiang and Taiwan provinces (regions) as a high incidence area, occurred in more than 40 years of age. The relationship between EBV and NPC is very close. The main basis is that: ①EBV markers (viral nucleic acid and viral antigens) are found from NPC biopsies; ②antibody titer of EBV-related antigens (EA, VCA, MA, EBNA) Higher than normal, some patients have detected these antibodies before the lesions of the nasopharyngeal mucosa. NPC is only high in certain areas and specific populations, so EBV can not be considered the only risk factor for NPC.

Hodgkin's disease is a malignant lymphoma. EBV is associated with 50% of Hodgkin's disease and contains EBV DNA, EBNA and LMP in Hodgkin's disease cells.

After primary infection, the body produces specific neutralizing antibodies and cellular immunity. EBV VCA antibodies and MA antibodies appear first, followed by EA antibodies. The body produces EBNA antibodies as infected cells are lysed and recovered. Thus, the appearance of EBNA antibodies indicates that the body has established cellular immunity and the infection is controlled to prevent exogenous reinfection but not to completely eliminate latent EBV in the cells. In the body of latent virus and the host to maintain a relatively balanced state, a small amount of EBV continued to occur in the mouth of low-titer proliferative infection, this persistent infection can be maintained for life.

9.7.4.3   Microbiological Examination Method

1) Virus isolation and culture. Saliva, pharyngeal fluid, external blood cells and tumor tissue were used as standard vehicles and inoculated into fresh human B cells or cord blood lymphocyte cultures. After 4 weeks, the virus was identified by immunofluorescence examination of EBV antigen.

2) Virus antigen and nucleic acid detection. Direct detection of antigen or viral DNA in specimens is an important experimental method. EBV DNA in specimens can be detected by in situ nucleic acid hybrid-

ization or PCR or EBV antigen can be examined by immunofluorescence.

3) Serological diagnosis. Includes both specific and nonspecific antibody assays. Detection of EBV-specific antibodies was used by Enzyme-linked immunosorbent assay or immunofluorescence to detect VCA or EA-specific antibodies. The titer of VCA-IgM antibody in serum of patients was increased, which showed the existence of EBV primary infection. The titer of EA-IgA and VCA-IgA antibody continued to increase, which has the diagnostic value for nasopharyngeal carcinoma.

4) Heterophile antibody testing is mainly used to assist in the diagnosis of infectious mononucleosis. Allo-acid antibodies are antibodies that appear to nonspecifically aggregate sheep red blood cells in the early stages of the disease. The antibody titers peak in the 3−4 weeks of onset, the recovery period decreased, will soon disappear.

9.7.4.4　Prevention and Control Principles

Most patients with infectious mononucleosis (about 95%) can recover, only a small number of patients with splenic rupture, therefore, should limit the acute phase of patients with severe activity. Determination of EBV EA-IgA, VCA-IgA antibody is conducive to the early diagnosis of nasopharyngeal carcinoma. EBV vaccine developed in foreign countries, can be used to prevent infectious mononucleosis and consider immunoprophylaxis for malignant lymphoma and nasopharyngeal carcinoma in African children. The immune protection effect of the domestic-built genetic engineering vaccine is under observation.

9.8　Retroviruses

General feature of Retroviridae: Retroviridae is a group of RNA viruses containing reverse transcriptase, spherical, enveloped, the surface of glycoproteinprotrusions. The genome is two identical single-stranded positive-stranded RNAs have three structural genes, gag, pol and env and a number of regulatory genes ranging in number. Retroviral replication by reverse transcription, integration process, integrated into the host cell chromosome DNA called provirus. Retrovirus is divided into 7 genera, only lentivirus kill cells, the rest are non-cytomegalovirus. The main cause of human disease is human immunodeficiency virus and human T-cell virus. Human immunodeficiency virus is the causative agent of acquired immunodeficiency syndrome (AIDS).

Retroviridae is a group of RNA viruses that contain reverse transcriptase (RT), which is divided into 7 genera and is mainly human immunodeficiency virus and human T-cell virus.

Retroviruses are found in almost every vertebrate species, most of them infected only with one species of animal, although there are also natural inter-species infections. The source of homologous host retroviruses, the core protein group specific antigenic determinants.

Sharp and structure: Retroviral size of about 100 mm, spherical, internal spiral-symmetric ribonucleoprotein, icosahedral icosahedral outer side of the capsid protein, a capsule, the surface glycoprotein protrusions.

The virus core contains two identical single-stranded positive-stranded RNAs, about 5 to 11 kb in length, joined by partial base complementation at the 5 'end to form linear diploids. Each of the retroviral genomes was similar in structure and sequence and all three structural genes (gag, pol, nev) were similar in sequence and were all in the sequence of 5'gag-pol-env-3 ', of which gag encoding core protein Antigen), pol encodes reverse transcriptase and protease and env encodes glycoprotein protrusions (either type or subtype specific antigens) on the envelope. Retroviruses also contain a number of regulatory genes that encode non-structural proteins that alter the gene transcription and expression of the virus. The genomes of α, β, γ retroviruses are simple and have only structural genes, while δ, ε retroviruses, lentiviruses and foamy viruses contain a number of regulatory genes ranging from structural genes to structural genes. Lentiviruses regulate more genes.

copy. Retroviral replication through a unique process of reverse transcription, the viral genomic RNA first reverse transcribed into double-stranded DNA and then integrated into the cell chromosomal DNA.

pol encodes reverse transcriptase, protease, RNase H and integrase. After the virus is adsorbed, the viral RNA enters the cell after it is penetrated and the reverse transcriptase uses RNA as a template to synthesize DNA. After a complicated process, the viral RNA is transcribed into DNA and the terminal U5, U3 ends are swapped to the opposite ends of the DNA, forming long terminal repeats, with the LTR appearing only in the viral DNA.

The newly synthesized viral DNA is integrated into the host cell chromosome, which is called the provirus at this time. The structure of the provirus remains stable, but the integration sites can be different, with the end-specific sequence of the LTR responsible. The progeny virus genome is transcribed from the proviral genome. The U3 sequence of LTR contains promoters and enhancers and is transcribed by the RNA polymerase II of the cell. The provirus, like a set of genes in a cell whose expression is regulated by the cellular genome, The integration of the virus and the presence or absence of cellular transcription factors, to a large extent determine whether the viral genes can activate expression.

The full-length transcripts will assemble as a viral genome into the progeny virus. Other transcripts are spliced and used as mRNA for translation of the precursor protein. The precursor protein is digested and modified to become a viral protein. The progeny virus is released by sprouting. The viral protease cleaves GAG and POL to polymerize the precursor protein, eventually forming an infectious offspring virus, preparing for the next infection.

Host and spread. Retroviral host range depends on whether there are suitable receptors on the cell surface. According to the host range, reverse

Viruses can be divided into: ①ecotropic virus: only infected with the same species of cells, causing toxic infections; ②amphotropic virus: can produce heterologous cells toxic infection, because it recognizes a wide range of receptors; ③Heterotrophic virus: A toxigenic infection occurs only on xenogeneic cells but only in the presence of an antiviral agent in its original host cell.

According to the mode of transmission, retrovirus can be divided into two types of endogenous and exogenous viruses. Endogenous viruses are heterotropic viruses that, by vertical transmission, are present in all germ cells and somatic cells of the host and the viral DNA becomes a constant genetic component of the host. Many vertebrates, including humans, have an endogenous RNA virus multiple copies of the sequence. The integration of the endogenous virus is controlled by the host cell's genetic material and internal or external (chemical) factors can induce the replication of the endogenous virus. Endogenous viruses are usually not pathogenic to the host and do not cause transformation of cultured cells. Exogenous viruses are transmitted horizontally and exist only in infected cells and pathogenic retroviruses are exogenous. Exogenous viruses are also often long-term latent in the cells.

Infection and cancer. In retroviruses, only lentivirus kill cells, the rest are non-cytomegalovirus. Non-cytocidal disease-causing retroviruses cause tumors primarily.

Some retroviruses have a complete retroviral genetic construct that replicates independently, such as HIV, HTLV and MMTV. Such retroviral genomes contain no oncogenes. However, some retroviruses contain oncogenes. For example, RSV contains src, Mo-MSV contains mos and Ab-MLV contains abl. These viruses are all defective viruses (except RSV). The viral oncogene is derived from the host cell and the gene on the cell is called the proto-oncogene. Wave activation and expression of the gene can lead to the transformation of the cell. During the long evolutionary process of biology, the virus captured the gene in some way and integrated it into their genes, the oncogenes. Retroviruses containing oncogenes are highly carcinogenic and can cause tumors in vivo only after a short incubation period and rapidly induce cell morphological transformation in vitro. The reason for tumorigenesis is that oncogenes are activated and expressed at high levels. The original Oncogenes are usually precisely controlled within the cell, expressed only at low levels.

Retroviruses without oncogenes are much less carcinogenic and do not cause cell transformation in vitro, but they may have the ability to transform blood stem cells in vivo and generally require a long incubation period, either as a promoter or enhancer of the virus Was inserted into the vicinity of the protooncogene of the cell, resulting in the expression of the gene in large quantities.

9.8.1 Human Immunodeficiency Virus

Human immunodeficiency virus (HIV) is the causative agent of acquired immunodeficiency syndrome (AlDS) and is a member of the lentivirus family of retroviruses.

9.8.1.1 Biological Traits

Structure and composition. Structure and composition Spherical, diameter 100–120 mm, with envelope, glycoprotein spikes on the surface, each spike formed by the gp120 and gp41 trimer. Inside the envelope consists of p17 intima. The core consists of two identical + ssRNA, reverse transcriptase, integrase, protease and RNase H. The p24 is surrounded by a capsid that forms a cylindrical nucleocapsid together with the p24 capsid.

The HV genome RNA is about 9.2 kb in length. The proviral DNA has an additional LTR sequence outside the DNA, 9.8 kb in length. The HIV gene structure is more complex than other retroviruses and contains three structural genes (gag, pol, env) and six regulatory genes (tat, nef, vif, rev, vpr, vpu), HIV-2 has no vpu and instead is the vpx gene. The mRNAs encoded by gag, pol, env, vpr, vpu, vif and so on require REV protein to help the cytoplasm to localize and express. They are late genes. The expression of tat, rev, nef and so on are independent of REV protein and are early genes. HIV found no oncogene sequence.

HIV structural proteins are cut from the precursor protein surface to: ①gag encoding a relative molecular mass of about 55×10^3 GAG protein p55, so gag also known as the p55 gene. P55 is translated from full-length mRNA and synthesized to connect with the cell membrane. Two genomic RNA molecules and other proteins are recruited to form buds, which are then cleaved by the virally-encoded protease 4 into the matrix proteins P17 (matrix), capsid P24 (CA), nucleocapsid (P7) nucleoprotein (NC), P6 four mature structural proteins; ②pol encoded POL protein. The GAG-POL precursor protein (P160) is usually translated from the full-length mRNA and the POL peptide is cleaved from the GAG-POL by a viral protease upon further maturation of the virus and further cleaved into protease (PR), integrase P32 IN), RNase H (P15) and reverse transcriptase P51. Due to incomplete fragmentation, about 50% of the RT protein and RNase H are still linked together to form P66, called P66/p51, which has a dual enzyme activity. Enzymatic activity of RT includes RNA-dependent DNA polymerase (ie, reverse transcriptase) and DNA-dependent DNA polymerase activity. RT does not have reading-proof and has a high incidence of mismatches at transcription. Protease P11 is an asparaginase that exists as a dimer and is responsible for the cleavage of GAG and GAG-POL aggregates and is a key enzyme necessary for HIV replication. The integrase P32 helps to insert the HIV provirus DNA into the genome of the infected cells. The integrase has three enzyme activities: DNA exonuclease, double-strand endonuclease and ligase. ③Env coding 160 kDa glycoprotein (gp160) After synthesis, it is transferred to the Golgi and glycosylated, which is then cleaved by host cell proteases into gp41 and gp120. gp41 is a transmembrane glycoprotein (TM), gph20 is an envelope glycoprotein (SU) on the surface of the envelope, gp41 and gp120 are polymerized into trimers, which are non-covalently linked to form spikes that infect cell membranes and viral envelope surfaces.

Six regulatory genes control viral gene expression and play an important role in pathogenicity: ①TAT encodes TAT protein (P14), which is an RNA-binding protein that is required for HIV replication and which transactivates transcription upon binding to LTR REV protein (P19), also an RNA-binding protein, functions to transport intact viral transcripts from the nucleus, reversing HIV from early gene expression to late gene expression. ②REV is required for HV replication The lack of REV is still active transcription of the former virus is still active but the virus late genes can not be expressed, can not produce progeny virosomes; ③nef, vpr, vpu and vif encoded in vitro experiments confirmed that virus replication is not necessary, but in vivo Affect the virus virulence. NEF is the first HIV protein that can be detected after HIV infection. It induces chemokine expression and activates T cells. NEF also down-regulates the expression of CD4 and MHC class I molecules. VPR protein promotes the pre-integration of the virus complex from the cytoplasm to the nucleus, but also the cell cycle stays in the G2 phase. VIF protein inhibits the expression of human cells inhibitory proteins, thereby increasing the virus's infectivity.

Viral receptor. The process of HIV replication is similar to that of other retroviruses, which first attach to host cells. All primate lentiviruses have CD4 molecules as receptors, CD4 molecules are predominantly expressed on T lymphocytes and also on the surface of monocytes-macrophages and other cells. In addition to the CD4 receptor, HIV-1 also needs a co-receptor to enter the cell. The envelope glycoprotein gp120 of the virus first binds to CD4 and subsequently binds to a co-receptor, resulting in altered envelope conformation of the virus, activation of the gp41 fusion polypeptide, triggering membrane fusion.

In vitro cultured cell lines found that 12 chemokine receptors can cause HIV co-receptor role, CXCR4, CCR5, CCR2 and CCR3, but only in vivo CCR5 and CXCR4 can be used as a co-receptor. CXCR4, a chemokine receptor for SDF-1, is a cofactor for thymus-specific HIV; CCR5, a chemokine receptor for RANTES, MIP-1α and MIP1-β, is a costimulatory receptor for macrophage-like HIV. There are also amphibious viruses, co-receptors can be both CCR5 and CXCR4. CCR5 and CXCR4 are found in lymphocytes, macrophages, thymocytes, neurons, rectum and cervical cells. Early HIV infection is mainly phagocytic HIV strains, later gradually to T-cell HIV-based strains, resulting in massive destruction of CD4 T cells.

The CCR5 gene can mutate and affect HIV-1 infection. Approximately 13% of Caucasian CCR5 alleles have a 32bp deletion, resulting in CCR5 being unable to express on the cell surface and are known as CCR5-delta-32 mutations. Approximately 1%–2% of Caucasians are mutant pure Zygote, can completely resist HIV infection. The CCR5 gene promoter can also mutate and cause a delay in HIAV infection. Co-receptors are also targets of anti-HIV drugs. Enfuvirtide and Malawi are both acting on this link to block viral envelope-cell fusion.

Type and variation. There are two types of HIV: HIV-1, HIV-2. Typing is based on the gene sequence and evolutionary relationships with other primate lentiviruses. Two types of nucleic acid sequence difference of more than 40%. HIV causes a global epidemic, with HIV-2 predominantly circulating in West Africa.

The HIV genome frequently mutates and there are a number of HIV strains with the same genetic variation in the same infection. These variants are called quasi-strains and are the result of highly mismatched reverse transcriptase transcripts. The mutation of env was the most frequent with a mutation rate of about 1‰, similar to the mutation rate of influenza virus. The env-encoded gp120 contains a site that binds to both the CD4 molecule and the co-receptor and determines the HIV-tropic and macrophage cell-tropic properties as well as neutralizing epitopes. gp120 has 5 variable regions, all located on the surface, of which V3 is an important neutralizing epitope. Variability in the envelope protein makes it difficult for HIV vaccines to stabilize. There are 12 subtypes of HIV-1 subtype M (main), O (Outlier) and N (new) according to the env sequence. The M subgroup includes 9 subtypes (A-K, with E and I) O and N groups each one subtype; HIV-2 has six subtypes (A-F). There is no correspondence between genotypes and serotypes and neutralizing antibodies and there is no evidence that different gene subtypes differ in their biological phenotype and pathogenicity. There are mainly M group HIV-1 in the world, but subtype distribution is different. America, Europe and Australia are B subtype and Asia includes China as C, E and B.

Cultivate characteristics. HIV only infects cells with CD4 molecules on its surface and can only undergo toxic infections in activated cells. Therefore, peripheral blood T lymphocytes, commonly used in laboratories, are activated by mitogens (such as PHA) and mixed with HIV-infected lymphocytes, Cultured 2 to 4 weeks to separate the virus.

resistance. HIV is less resistant to physical and chemical factors. Commonly used disinfectants 0.5% sodium hypochlorite, 10% bleach, 50% ethanol, 35% isopropanol, 0.3% hydrogen peroxide, 0.5% paraformaldehyde, 5% Live HIV. Heat 56 ℃ for 10 minutes to inactivate HIV in liquid or 10% serum. Freeze-dried blood products must be heated at 68 ℃ for 72 hours to completely inactivate HIV.

Detection of antibodies. Antibodies can be detected for a long time after the production of antibodies. This conversion is called seroconversion and the average time from HIV infection to seroconversion is 3 to 4 weeks. Most infected people in 6 to 12 weeks.

9.8.1.2 Pathogenicity and Immunity

(1) Sources of Infection and Routes of Transmission

Lentivirus is a complete exogenous virus, only by exposure to foreign viruses. HIV carriers and AIDS patients are sources of HIV infection. HIV can be isolated from HIV, semen, prostatic fluid, vaginal secretions, cerebrospinal fluid, saliva, tears and milk, spinal cord and central nervous tissue specimens. Sexual transmission, blood transmission and vertical transmission are the main routes of transmission of HIV infection.

Sexual transmission. Sexual transmission is the main mode of transmission of HIV, AIDS is an important sexually transmitted disease. Although homosexuality is considered to be a major risk factor for AIDS, the main mode of transmission worldwide in areas of high HIV prevalence (Africa and South-East Asia) is heterosexual contact, which is about 70% of all sexually transmitted, The number of partners increases proportionately. The presence of other STDs such as syphilis, gonorrhea and HSV-2 infections can increase the risk of sexually transmitted HIV a hundredfold because inflammation and ulceration caused by these infections facilitate HIV breakthrough in the mucosal barrier.

(2) Blood Transmission

HIV infection occurs when people take HIV-containing blood, blood products (such as factor VIII) organs or tissue grafts, etc. or use HIV-contaminated syringes and needles, artificial insemination with HIV-containing semen. Epidemiological data show that HIV infection due to intravenous drug sharing injection device accounted for about 38% of the cases detected in our country, intravenous drug use was the main route of transmission of HIV in our country, but the latest survey shows that sexual transmission is becoming HIV transmission in our country The main route, the HIV epidemic is spreading from high-risk groups to the general population. 3. Vertical transmission. Vertical transmission includes the placenta, birth canal or breastfeeding and other means of transmission. In seropositive women without antiretroviral therapy, the risk of mother-to-child transmission is from 13% to 40% and the risk of breast-feeding is higher than that of placenta transmission. With antiretroviral treatment, vertical transmission opportunities can be reduced by more than 50%.

Blood, sexual and vertical transmission can cover almost any HIV infection. Daily contact with people living with HIV, insect bites and other media are not transmitted, there is no supporting evidence.

Clinical manifestations. Typical HIV infection processes include primary infection, spread of the virus in the body, clinical latency, increased HIV expression, clinical disease (AIDS) and death. The untreated HIV infection lasts about ten years and dies most of the year after entering AIDS.

During the acute phase of primary infection, the period from exposure to HIV to the production of antibodies generally lasts for 1 to 2 weeks and manifests as nonspecific symptoms such as fatigue, rash and mononucleosis.

Clinical latency usually lasted 5 to 15 years, an average of 10 years, HIV continued replication, CD4 T cells decreased by an annual average of 50 to 90 cells/μL rate decreased, clinical manifestations of fever, chronic diarrhea, generalized lymph nodes and other symptoms. When the number of CD4/CD8 T cells is inverted and the CD4 T cell count is less than 200 cells/μL, the immunocompromised patients have clinical manifestations of severe immunosuppression, opportunistic infections and malignancies entering the AIDS stage. Common opportunistic infections are pneumococcal pneumonia (PCP), thrush (Candida albicans infection), Cryptosporidium diarrhea and so on. Common tumors are Kaposi sarcoma, malignant lymphoma and so on. Kaposi's sarcoma is a vascular tumor that can be seen in the skin, mucous membranes, lymph nodes, internal organs, etc. and is caused by herpes virus type 8 (HHV8), which is extremely rare in healthy people. The risk of developing Kaposi's sarcoma in AIDS patients is 20,000 times higher than in the general population. AIDS patients also have a higher incidence of malignant lymphoma 1,000 times higher than the general population. In addition, 40% to 90% of AIDS patients are also neurological symptoms, including aseptic meningitis, subacute encephalitis, vacuolar myelopathy, AIDS dementia syndrome. Neonatal response to HIV infection and adults are different, because the immune system is still imperfect, the role of neonatal destruction of HIV is particularly sensitive perinatal HV infection in children without treatment, usually 2 years of age symptoms and in 2 years dead.

Pathogenesis. After HIV infection enters the incubation period, the virus continues to replicate at high levels, producing about 10 billion viruses every day and removing it. The average life cycle of HIV (from infected cells to progeny virus) was 2.6 days, similar to the rate of CD4 T lymphocyte renewal. The half-life of T-cells producing toxic infections is about 1.6 days. Due to the large number of copies and reverse transcriptase inherent mismatch rate, the virus is mutated every day, the late infection of the virus usually virulent strains than the initial infection to the AIDS stage, usually to T lymphocyte strains for the the Lord.

CD4 T lymphocytes and memory cells The most important feature of HIV infection is the depletion of CD4 T helper cells (Th). HIV destroys CD4 T cells by a variety of mechanisms: ①the direct killing of CTL by HIV antigens on the cell surface or the destruction of HIV-carrying CD4 T cells by anti-HIV antibody-mediated ADCC; ②T lymphocyte HIV infection CD4 T cells usually induce cell fusion, forming multinucleated giant cells, leading to cell death; ③HIV replication and non-integrated viral DNA accumulation in large numbers of cells, inhibition of normal cell biosynthesis; ④embedded in the cell membrane gp120 and CD4 molecules self-fusion, Disrupt cell integrity and permeability; ⑤induced apoptosis of CD4 T cells; ⑥gp41 and MHC class II molecules on the cell membrane homology, induced cross-reaction of autoantibodies, resulting in T cell injury.

A small fraction of HIV-infected CD4 T cells can be returned as resting memory cells, with no or only very low viral gene expression in these cells. Memory cells decay very slowly with a half-life of about 43 months, constituting a consistent pool of HIV viruses. When exposed to HIV antigens again, memory cells are activated and the progeny virus is released. If there are one million HIV-infected memory cells in the body, it will take about 70 years to clear the cell bank, so HIV can not be completely removed once infected.

Monocytes-macrophages in addition to Th cells express CD4 molecules, but also other small cell surface expression of CD4 molecules such as monocytes-macrophages, dendritic cells, glial cells (mainly microglia Cells), intestinal mucosa of the cup, columnar epithelial cells and chromaffin cells, HIV can also infect these cells. Monocyte-macrophage surface receptor is CCR5, unlike CD4 T cells, monocytes-macrophages have a strong resistance to the cytopathic effects of HIV and HIV can lurk in these cells and subsequently spread to the body, And produces long-term toxin, therefore, monocyte-macrophage is another in vivo HIV virus pool.

Mononuclear macrophages play an important role in the pathogenesis of HIV. Alveolar macrophage infection leads to interstitial pneumonia in AIDS patients. HIV seldom infects nervous system cells such as neurons, oligodendrocytes and astrocytes. The advanced nervous system diseases of AIDS are mainly caused by HIV-infected monocytes and macrophages. HIV-infected monocytes enter the central nervous system and release cytokines and chemokines. These cytokines are toxic to neurons and chemokines cause brain inflammatory cell infiltration.

(3) Lymphatic Organs

Lymphatic organs play a central role in HIV infection. 98% of human lymphocytes gathered in the lymphatic vessels, only 2% distributed in the peripheral blood. Specific immune responses are also formed in lymphoid organs. The microenvironment of the lymph nodes is well suited for HIV infection and dissemination and lymph nodes have a large population of CD4 T cells that are highly susceptible to HIV. As HIV infection progresses to the advanced stage, the tissue structure of lymph nodes is also destroyed.

The body's immune response to HV. Infected with HIV, both cellular and humoral immunity respond to HIV. CTL, NK clearance and ADCC are the main mechanisms of anti-HIV in the body.

1) Cellular immunity. The cellular immune response is directed against HIV proteins. CTLs recognize the encoded products of env, pol, gag and other genes that are mediated by MHC-restricted CD3-CD8 lymphocytes. CTL through a variety of mechanisms to clear HIV: CTL and HLA-binding peptide binding by perforin in the cell membrane perforation and then destroy cells; CTL expression of FasL and infected cells on the surface of the Fas (CD95) to induce apoptosis; ③CTL expression of chemokines such as MIP-1α, MlP-1β and TRANTES, these molecules can bind and block CCR5, prevent HIV penetration target cells; CTL cells also secrete IFN-γ and other anti-viral factors, so that the adjacent cells into the anti-Virus infection status. In the early stage of HIV infection, CTL response rapidly appeared, HIV blood load decreased temporarily and CTL response intensity was positively correlated with the ability of the body to control HIV infection. However, HIV could avoid CTL killing by mutating surface antigen and down-regulating the expression of MHC effect. NK cells also have HIV-1 gp120 activity. Cellular immune response can be seen in all HIV-infected people, but with the development of the disease will be weakened.

2) Humoral immunity. HIV antibodies 1 to 3 months after the body can detect HIV antibodies, including anti-gp120 neutralizing antibodies. Although neutralizing antibodies have a protective effect, they can only neutralize the virus in the serum or act on the infected cells that express the viral antigens and are ineffective against the proviral that is integrated in the cells. Due to the continuous variation of HIV envelope or due to the highly glycosylated lead to the occlusion of antigenic determinants, neutralizing antibodies can not play a long-term stable role.

The humoral immune system of HIV-infected persons has the contradiction of highly activated and low immunoreactivity. The hyperactivities are marked with polyclonal hyperproteinemia, bone marrow plasmacytoidosis, high expression of active molecules of B lymphocytes in circulating blood, Auto-reactive antibodies and autoimmune symptoms. Low immunoreactivity is manifested as a decrease in the responsiveness of B cells to antigenic stimulation, which is often not the case for HIV-infected individuals after immunization with protein or polysaccharide vaccines.

9.8.1.3　Microbiological Examination Method

Evidence of HIV infection includes: ①serology (antibodies); ②viral nucleic acids or proteins; ③virus isolation.

Detection of antibodies. The HIV antigen can be detected in the serum after infection and the antibody is undetectable for an extended period of time after antibody production. This conversion is called seroconversion and the mean time between HIV infection and seroconversion is 3 to 4 weeks. Most infected Antibodies were detected within 6–12 weeks and all were positive after 6 months. More clinical was use of enzyme-linked immunosorbent (ELA) detection of HIV antibodies, the sensitivity of more than 98%. Since HIV and other retroviruses have cross-over antigens, EIA can only be used for screening for HIV infection. Positives must be independently tested to rule out the possible false positives of EIA. Commonly used confirmation test is Western blot, this method can detect the specific molecular weight of HIV antibodies corresponding anti-p24, anti-gp41, gp120, gp160 and so on.

As the infection progresses, the pattern of antibody response can change. Antibodies to the anti-envelope glycoproteins (gp41, gp120, gp160) persist, but antibodies to the GAG proteins (p17, p24, p55) are reduced later in life, with reduced levels of anti-p24 antibodies generally being a precursor to clinical signs.

Antigen detection. Commonly used ELISA tests for capsid protein p24. The p24 antigen can be detected in plasma soon after infection. Once the antibody is produced, p24 is usually undetectable since p24 and anti-p24 form a complex. However, the p24 antigen can be re-detected later in the infection, which means poor prognosis. Therefore, p24 positive either early HIV infection or has been developed to AIDS.

Detect nucleic acids. Common methods include nucleic acid hybridization, PCR, RT-PCR and so on. Nucleic acid hybridization, PCR can be used to detect cells in the provirus DNA. RT-PCR method for HIV RNA detection of blood samples, currently used quantitative RT-PCR method for the detection of HIV RNA in plasma samples, currently used quantitative RT-PCR detection of plasma viral RNA copy number, also known as viral load to Log/mL, used to monitor the development of HIV-infected patients and evaluate the efficacy.

HIV and RNA tests can be used for the early diagnosis of HIV infection in newborns, because of neonatal maternal antibodies in vivo, serological test results with great uncertainty.

Virus isolation and identification. HIV can be cultured using peripheral blood lymphocytes and it takes around 4–6 weeks to separate HIV from patient samples, much for research. The method is to sample cells mixed with mitogen-stimulated peripheral blood mononuclear cells. Normal lymphocytes (or passaged T cell lines H9 and CEM) were first isolated and stimulated with PHA and cultured for 3 to 4 days. Mononuclear cells, bone marrow cells, plasma or cerebrospinal fluid of patients were inoculated, Plus PHA activation of normal human lymphocytes, cultured 2 to 4 weeks, such as the emergence of varying degrees of lesions, especially multinucleated giant cells, then the virus proliferation. Further quantitative by the following methods: ①reverse transcriptase activity test; ②indirect immunofluorescence assay p24, calculate the percentage of infected cells; ③RT-PCR determination of HIV nucleic acid.

Drug resistance test. Due to frequent gene mutations, HIV generally produces drug resistance, antiretroviral therapy need to rely on drug resistance testing to select sensitive drugs, there are two methods of genetic testing and phenotypic testing. Genetic testing is the identification of coding mutations in the HIV viral reverse transcriptase and protease genes and then predicting the drug resistance of the strain by database alignment. Phenotypic testing is similar to the bacterial drug sensitivity assay, in which virus nucleic acids are seeded in cells and serial dilutions of anti-retroviral drugs are included in the culture to detect the virus's infection of the cells. Genotype detection convenient, fast, clinical more commonly used.

9.8.1.4　Prevention and Control Principles

There is currently no clinically effective HIV vaccine. Many candidate vaccines are under development and testing. These HIV-based glycoprotein-based recombinant vaccines are not effective in clinical trials. HIV vaccines are difficult to develop because: ①frequent HIV mutations; ②not all of the HIV in the cell expression, replication; ③the body's immune response can not completely remove the virus; ④there is no suitable animal model. Chimpanzees are the only HIV-susceptible animals, but chimpanzees are from a lack of sources and produce only viremia and antibodies after HIV infection without immunodeficiency.

Precaution. Since there is no HIV vaccine, the primary response to prevent HIV infection is to stay clean, maintain good living habits and minimize the risk of HIV infection. Policy measures to prevent and control HIV infection include: ①A wide range of AIDS prevention education campaigns; this is the most important and effective measure at this stage and the stable control of the outbreak in developed countries is related to this. ②Safe sex: Preventing the HIV epidemic of the key measures, epidemiological surveys show that the use of condoms to prevent HIV infection rate of 69%; ③ban prostitutes to combat drug abuse behavior; ④voluntary blood donation system: According to WHO survey, voluntary blood donors than paid blood donors. Blood collection should be done HIV antibody testing to ensure the safety of blood transfusion and blood products, prohibit the import of blood products; ⑤global and regional HIV infection monitoring network to keep track of epidemic spread, quarantine border.

Medical treatement. The current antiretroviral drugs target the following four aspects of the HIV replication cycle:

1) Inhibit reverse transcriptase. There are two types of drugs: ①nucleoside reverse transcriptase inhibitors such as azidothymidine (AZT) , 2', 3'-dideoxyinosine (ddI) , 2', 3'-dideoxycytiddC) and lamivudine, etc. ; ②non-nucleoside reverse transcriptase inhibitors, such as delavirdine and resistant Nevirapine. These drugs can interfere with viral DNA synthesis and inhibit the virus's proliferation in the body.

2) Inhibit the protease. Saquinavir, ritonavir, Indinavir and Nefnavir inhibit HIV protease so that the precursor protein can not be cleaved into mature protein, affecting the virus's maturity.

3) Inhibit virus and cell membrane. Fusion inhibitors such as Enfuvirtide (ie, Fuzeon, T-20) bind to gp41, blocking HIV envelope-cell fusion.

4) Inhibit integrase. Raltegravir acts on HIV integrase and inhibits the integration of the viral genome into the chromosome of the cell and was approved for clinical use in 2007.

Due to frequent HIV mutations, its reverse transcriptase, protease easily mutated clinically antiretroviral drugs can not be used alone can easily lead to drug-resistant strains. Highly active antiretroviral therapy (HAART), commonly used in combination with multiple drugs, is usually triple therapy with two reverse transcriptase inhibitors and one protease inhibitor, reducing the plasma viral load to low At a detectable level, the body's immune system is restored. HAART should be considered when the number of CD4 T cells is less than 350 μL. Opportunistic infections occur when the number of CD4 T cells is less than 200 μL. HAART must be performed immediately. However, HAART can not eradicate HIV infection because HIV persists in resting memory CD4 T cells and monocyte-macrophages and the viral load rebounds rapidly after stopping HAART.

9.8.2 Human T-cell Virus

Human T-cell virus (HTLV) is the first human retrovirus to be discovered. Immediately thereafter, a second human retrovirus was isolated from the peripheral blood of a patient with hairy cell leukemia. The two were 65% homologous in genome, so the former was named HTLV-1 and the latter was HTLV-2.

Biological Charactristics: Belongs to the delta retrovirus, about 100 nm in diameter. Encapsulated glycoprotein spikes on the surface, with the target cell surface CD4 molecules, capsid contains P24, P19 and P15 three proteins. The genome is about 9.0 kb in length and has LTRs on both ends. It contains three structural genes (gag, pol, env) and two taxons (rex). The genome has no oncogene sequences. The precursor protein encoded by the gag gene is proteolytically cleaved into P24, P19, P15, which makes up the capsid or nucleocapsid of the virus. All three proteins have antigenicity and corresponding antibodies can appear in the sera of infected persons. Env encodes two glycoproteins, gp46 and gp21, of which gp46 is located on the cell surface and p21 is a transmembrane protein.

The two regulatory genes are related to the pathogenicity of HTLV. Tax-based gene encoding TAX (P40) distributed in the infected nucleus, Bing has two activities: ①activation of the LTR, transactivation of viral DNA transcription and promote viral mRNA synthesis; ②permeability of NF-κB expression, NF-Further stimulating IL-2 receptor (IL-2r) and IL-2 expression. The rex gene encodes P27, a phosphorylated protein that is located in the nucleus and determines which mRNAs located in the nucleus are transported outward to the cytoplasm for the synthesis of proteins, which are closely related to the cell's expression.

Pathogenicity and immunity: HTLV-1 and HTLV-2 are retroviruses that cause tumors in humans and are all exogenous viruses. The source of infection of HTLV is in patients and HTLV infected persons. HTLV-1 infection is mainly transmitted sexually, transfused and injected horizontally and transmitted vertically through placenta, birth canal and breast-feeding. The prevalence of HTLV-1 is clearly regional, with high positive rates being detectable in Kyushu, some parts of Africa and some islands in the Caribbean; while the seroprevalence is extremely low in the rest of the world and is characterized by the spread of infection.

HTLV-1 is the causative agent of adult T-cell leukemia (ATL). ATL occurs in adults over the age of 40. HTLV infection incubation period is long, no clinical symptoms, about 1/20 infected with acute and chronic adult T-cell leukemia. Acute ATL mainly as leukocytosis, lymph nodes and hepatosplenomegaly; and erythema, rash and other skin and nervous system damage and other symptoms, the prognosis is poor. Chronic ATL in addition to an increase in white blood cell count and skin symptoms only a few cases of lymph nodes, hepatosplenomegaly symptoms. In addition, clinical sub-occult and lymphoma type. HTLV-1 also causes HTLV-1 related myelopathy (HTLV-1, HAM) and tropical spastic paraplegia (TSP). Mostly female patients, the main symptoms of chronic progressive may be disorders and dysuria, sometimes accompanied by sensory disturbances. The pathogenesis of HTLV-2 has no definite conclusion.

The mechanism of HTLV-induced leukemia Unlike other acute RNA tumor viruses (such as Rous sarcoma virus), HTLV has no oncogene and its pathogenesis is related to two regulatory proteins TAX and REX: ①When HTLV enters CD4 T cells, TAX activates NF-κB, Which in turn activates the IL-2 receptor gene so that the IL-2 receptor appears on the cell membrane of CD4 T cells. Activation of the IL-2 gene by TAX-activated pro-HTLV-1 virus leads to overexpression of IL-2. IL-2 and IL-2 receptor binding, leading to a large number of CD4 T cell proliferation; ②TAX can also activate the protooncogene to express the transformed protein to further promote cell transformation and proliferation; ③HTLV provirus integration into the cell chromosome may lead to cell genes mutation.

After the body is infected with HTLV-1, HTLV-1 antibodies such as anti-P24, P21 and gp46 antibodies may appear in the serum. However, the expression of the virus antigen is reduced after the antibody is detected, affecting the cellular immunity to clear the infected cells.

Microbiological examination: The detection of HTLV-specific antibodies is the main method of laboratory diagnosis of HTLV infection. The serum cross-reactivity of HTLV-1 and HTLV2 is strong, which can not be distinguished by conventional serological methods. Often method: ①ELISA: HTLV-1 virus lysate or lysate/recombinant P21 protein as antigen and patient serum to detect HTLV1/2 antibodies; ②indirect immunofluorescence; HTLV-1/2 infected T. The cell lines were made into cell smears of target cell antigens and then fluorescently labeled anti-human IgG fluorescence microscopy was used to observe the fluorescence positive cells after adding the patients serum reaction. Positive sera need to be confirmed by Western blotting. Serological testing of HTLV did not cross-react with HIV serology.

PCR is used to detect proviral DNA in peripheral blood mononuclear cells and to diagnose the type of HTLV with the highest sensitivity.

Virus isolation can be activated peripheral blood lymphocytes after PHA, IL-2-containing nutrient solution was added to culture for 3−6 weeks to detect cell culture supernatant reverse transcriptase activity, the positive specimen electron microscopy of cells in the C-virus particles, And anti-HTLV rabbit serum or monoclonal antibody for virus identification.

Prevention principle. At present there is no specific prevention and treatment of HTLV infection, IFN-α and reverse transcriptase inhibitors and other drugs can be used for treatment.

Prospect: Since the AIDS epidemic was discovered for nearly thirty years, remarkable progress has been made in the control and research of HIV infection. However, the epidemic is still endemic in the world at a rapid rate, posing a serious threat to human health. There are still a great deal of problems to be solved.

Retrovirus and HIV discovery process. In 1908 Danish scholar Vilhelm Ellerman and Oluf Bang found that chicken erythroleukemia was acellular filtrate, but did not cause concern. In 1910, American scholar Peyton Rous transplanted the chicken-shaped tumor to healthy chickens. The sarcomas also appeared in the grafts of the grafts. The sarcomas were ground and filtered through a bacterial filter. The chickens could still develop sarcomas after inoculation of healthy chickens. Virus(RSV). Rous also found several other avian tumor viruses, confirming that the virus is one of the causes of the tumor and won the 1966 Nobel Prize in Physiology and Medicine.

A 1961 study confirmed that the RSV virus genome consists of RNA. In 1964, American study Howard Temin observed that actinomycin D inhibits RSV replication, but radiotensin D inhibits DNA synthesis. Temin proposed the reverse transcription theory, saying that RSV a certain group first reverse transcribed into DNA and then integrated into the host Cell chromosomes become provirus. David Baltimore also found a similar phenomenon. Temin and Baltimore won the 1975 Nobel Prize in Physiology and Medicine. The mechanism of RSV induced tumors has led to the discovery of oncogenes (v-src) and proto-oncogenes (c-src).

Human retroviruses were found late. US group scholar Robert Gallo found that interleukin-2 (IL-2), which stimulates T cell growth, can stimulate T cells by stimulating T cells with IL-2 in vitro cultured for a long time, to isolate the virus infected T cells lay the foundation. In 1981, Gallo et al. Isolated the first human retrovirus, human T cell leukemia virus (HTLV), from the blood of leukemia patients and named it human T-lymphotropic virus type 1 (HTLV-1).

In 1981, the American scholar Michael Gottlieb et al reported that 5 patients with unexplained fever oral leukoplakia and pneumonia were both male homosexuals. Pulmonary biopsy confirmed pneumocystis carinii pneumonia. The blood test showed that the CD4 T cell count was very low, which is AlDS The first report. 1983 France Pasteur Luc Montagnier, Francoise Barre-Senoussi, etc. from a lymphatic gland disease patients to obtain lymph node biopsy tissue and lymphocytes isolated from a retrovirus, later confirmed to be the AIDS pathogen, named Human immunodeficiency virus (HIV). 2008 Montagnier and Barre-Sinoussi won the Nobel Prize in Physiology and Medicine.

The origin and spread of HIV. Many lentiviruses are isolated from primates other than humans and these lentiviruses can be grouped into five major clades. The genomic structure of primate (human, monkey) lentiviruses is very similar, with vps gene being carried by both HIV-1 and SIVcpz infected with chimpanzees while vpx gene is carried by HIV-2 and most SIVs. It is presently believed that SIVsm and HIV-2 of black and white eyebrows infected with West Africa are a variant of the same strain whereas SIVcpz and HIV-1 from chimpanzees are a variant of another strain. HIV therefore originates in SIV in Africa and is infected by human exposure to SIV-infected primates.

Using molecular detection technique to retrospectively study the autopsy specimens of previous cases, the sequence evolution analysis obtained showed that SIVcpz infect humans in the 1930s and further developed into HIV-1. In the 1960s, SIVsm infected humans and varieties in West Africa For HIV-2. HIV infection was originally confined to Africa. The specific economic and social conditions of the mid-20th century provided an opportunity for HIV proliferation to reach the scale of the global epidemic.

HIV/AIDS epidemic. The epidemic of HIV/AIDS is characterized by a wide geographical area and high speed, involving all countries in the world. According to UNAIDS's 2009 annual report, as of the end of 2008, an estimated 33.4 million people worldwide were infected with HIV, of which 2.7 million were newly infected in 2008 and 2 million died of AIDS. The number of new infections tends to stabilize, but the total number of HIV-infected persons in the world is still on the rise due to antiviral treatment to prolong the life span of HIV-infected people. Southern Africa is a hardest hit by HIV/AIDS. In 2008, 37% of newly infected cases and 38% of AIDS deaths occurred in the region, especially in sub-Saharan Africa. 67% of the global HIV-infected people live in this area HIV prevalence in countries as high as 15% –28% About half of HIV infections worldwide are women, 60% of them in sub-Saharan countries.

There are currently about 5 million HIV/AIDS cases in Asia and the most serious are Southeast Asian countries. By the end of 2008, there were about 276,000 AIDS-related AIDS cases in our country, including 82,000 AIDS cases and 38,000 deaths. In 2008, there were 46,000 cases of HIV infection, about 15,000 cases of AIDS, nearly 10,000 deaths and infections The male to female ratio is about 2 : 1. The prevalence of HIV in our country is characterized by: ①the epidemic is still on the rise but the rate of increase has slowed down; ②sexual transmission has gradually become the main route of transmission; ③the distribution of the HIV/AIDS epidemic is very different and the epidemic is serious in some areas; ④Not yet effectively controlled.

HIV/AIDS treatment. Currently more than 20 kinds of antiretroviral drugs, drug resistance is the main reason for the failure of HAART treatment. Due to the frequent mutation of HIV gene, the drug targeting HIV protein has the problem of drug-target mutation. In recent years, a research and development direction has been to select the host cell protein as a drug target to avoid drug resistance problems caused by mutation of the virus. For example, Malawi, a recently approved CCR5 antagonist, competes with HIV for binding to CCR5 co-receptor Prevent HIV from entering host cells. In contrast, the fusion inhibitor enfuvirtide binds to gp41 and inhibits the fusion of HIV with the cell membrane, possibly resulting from resistance to gp41 mutations.

HIV vaccine. HIV vaccine research is currently in a dilemma. Multiple HIV-based glycoprotein gene recombinant vaccines have failed in clinical trials. The HIV vaccine MRKAd5 (v520), which was tested in Phase IIb trials, failed in September 2007 and the previous vaccine for recombinant gp120 failed in phase III clinical trials. MRKAd5 is a vaccine that uses adenovirus type 5 (Ad5) as a carrier, a trivalent vaccine composed of a recombinant Ad5 expressing HIVgag, pol and nef genes. The immunization schedule is that after one month of primary inoculation, In December 2004, a total of 1,500 HIV-negative high-risk groups were tested in North America, South America, the Caribbean and Australia. By September 2007, 49 of those vaccinated were infected with HIV, even higher than those who received placebo.

These vaccines enter the in vivo test after they have been tested in vitro. The results of the in vivo tests indicate that there is disconnect between the in vitro studies and the simulated in vivo environment. The problem is that so far no animal model of HIV infection has been established. Primates (such as chimpanzees) HIV, but does not cause AIDS, is not conducive to the observation and evaluation of HIV vaccine effect.

At present, perhaps basic research on HIV should be stepped up. Only after more in-depth understanding of HIV can vaccine development be possible. The only available retrovirus vaccine, Equine Infectious Anemia Virus (EIAV) vaccine, was established in our country and is effective in blocking the ELAV transmission in horses. Before the establishment of molecular technology, the EIAV vaccine established live attenuated vaccines by classical virological methods (mainly host variation and virulence variation). The current role of EIAV vaccines remains unclear. For safety reasons, attenuated live attenuated retroviruses and inactivated vaccines can not be applied to humans, but exploring the mechanism of action of the EIAV vaccine will be a good reference for the development of HIV vaccines.

9.9 Prion and Prion Diseases

9.9.1 Introduction to Prion and Prion Diseases

In this chapter we will talk about various aspects of the biology of prions and focus on what is currently known about the mammalian PrP prion protein. Also we will briefly describe the prions of yeast and other fungi.

9.9.1.1 Prions

Prions are infectious proteins behaving like genes, i. e. proteins that not only contain genetic information in its tertiary structure, but are also able to transmit and replicate in a manner analogous to genes through different mechanisms. The term prion is derived from "proteinaceous infectious particle" and arose from the Prusiner hypothesis that the infectious agent of certain neurodegenerative diseases was only in a protein, without the participation of nucleic acids. Currently there are several known types of prion, in addition to the originally described, which are pathogens of mammals and they have been found in yeast and other fungi too. Prion proteins are ubiquitous and not always detrimental to their hosts. This vision of the prion as a causative agent of disease is changing, finding more and more evidence that could have important roles in cells and contribute to the phenotypic plasticity of organisms through the mechanisms of evolution.

9.9.1.2 Properties of PrP Isoforms

Normal form of the protein, PrPC, is a 35 kDa cell surface glycoprotein that is anchored to specific areas of the membrane (caveolae or lipid rafts) by a glycosyl phosphatidyl inositol (GPI) lipid linker-it may have a role in cell adhesion or signaling processes-half-life on the cell surface is 5 h, after which protein is internalized by a caveolae-dependent mechanism (conversion to PrPSc likely occurs during this internalization)-the acidic pH of the endosomal compartment may facilitate the conformational change-normal PrP is soluble in detergents and readily digested by proteases

Compared to monomeric, soluble and protease sensitive PrPC, PrPSc is multimeric, water insoluble and protease insensitive. And the beta sheet ratio increased significantly for PrPSc.

9.9.1.3　Prion Diseases

Prion diseases are incurable neurodegenerative conditions affecting both animals and humans. They may be sporadic, infectious or inherited in origin. Human prion diseases include Creutzfeldt-Jakob desease (CJD), Gerstmann-Straussler-Scheinker disease, kuru and fatal familial insomnia. The appearance of variant CJD and the demonstration that is caused by strains indistinguishable from bovine spongiform encephalopathy (BSE) in cattle, has led to the threat of a major epidemic of human prion disease in the UK and other countries where widespread dietary exposure to bovine prions has occurred. This chapter summarizes the history and epidemiology of these diseases and then focuses on important areas of current research in human prion disorders.

9.9.2　Background and Research History of Prions

About one hundred years ago, sheep diseases characterized by trembling were described in French sheep and as itching disease or trotting disease in Germany (McGowan, 1922). This disease is generally called "scrapie" now, a phrase that portraits the behavior of affected animals trying to relieve the itching by scraping their body against hard objects. The serious effects of this epidemic on the Scottish and English herbs were huge enough for the Government to set up grants for scrapie research, which was mainly performed at the Royal Veterinary College in London from 1910. For many years, from the 1940s to 1950s, many countries restricted the imports of sheep from Britain until proved scrapie-free.

In the 1920s, Creutzfeldt (1920) and Jakob (1921) described first cases of progressive mental, motor and neurological deficits in young patients. Later in 1922, 'Creutzfeldt-Jakob disease' (CJD) was first used to describe degenerative CNS diseases. Spielmeyer introduced the term "CJD" to describe this human neurological disease with rapidly progressive myoclonus, ataxia and dementia, drawing from earlier case reports by Creutzfeldt and Jakob. Modern diagnostic criteria for CJD are quite different from the conditions this term described back at that time. CJD meant to refer to a wide range of conditions not necessarily the "CJD" today.

Australian people started to adventure the Papua New Guinea highlands in the 1950s and this place had been governed by the United Nations. A new disease, kuru was discovered after travelling into this isolated area. This novel disease was investigated and doctors found that it was characterized by truncal ataxia and tremor, with inevitable and relentless progression to dementia or even death. Environment and genetic etiology were the focus of research about this disease back then. Scientists eventually found that the disease was contagious and transmissible and shared the same characters as scrapie and CJD on histology. The pioneering finding that these "TSEs" (transmissible spongiform encephalopathies) had an transmissible character led to Dr Carleton Gajdusek's winning of the 1970's Nobel Prize for medicine (Gajdusek et al, 1966).

The revealing of transmissibility made it possible to develop examination to identify CJD and every single case should be categorized based on their transmissibility or no transmissibility. In 1987, Beck and Daniel proposed the following diagnostic criteria for prion diseases, the histological combination of spongiform vacuolation in any part of brain grey matter in the cerebral area, neuronal loss and astroglial proliferation, amyloid plaques positive or negative and it's believed to be a universal discovery for prion diseases of both human and animal.

Although the transmissible character of the disease was found, the nature of the pathogen still has no answer. People believe it to be a virus because it's able to pass through tiny pore sized filters. Compared to other transmissible diseases, the incubation time of those diseases was much longer (for kuru, up to 5 decades) and the nick name "slow virus" was given for this phenomenon. Based on further research of the material of the infectious pathogen, it was found to be not containing DNA.

This heretical suggestion arose because infectivity was not affected by treatments that would usually inactivate nucleic acids (such as ultraviolet [UV] light and nucleases) (Alper et al, 1966, 1967). Also, unlike viral infections, these diseases fail to elicit an immune response; and importantly, no virus has ever been consistently demonstrated in association with the disease.

Griffith suggested in 1967 that the infectious agent might be a protein and a protease-resistant sialoglycoprotein was isolated by Bolton et al in 1982, using progressive enrichment of brain homogenates for infectivity. This protein was shown to accumulate in affected brains and to be the major constituent of infective brain fractions (Griffith, 1967; Bolton et al, 1982; Prusiner et al, 1982). In 1982, Prusiner coined the term prion (from proteinaceous infectious particles) to distinguish these infectious particles from viruses or viroids. The protein component of these particles was then designated the prion protein (PrP) (Prusiner, 1982) (work for which he was later awarded the Nobel Prize). More recent X-ray crystallography studies on prions suggest that even if nucleic acids are present in association with prion protein, this would be at a size too small to encode phenotypic diversity (Alper, 1993), further strengthening the protein-only prion hypothesis.

9.9.3 Prion Disease Related Epidems and Public Health Problems

TSE refers to transmissible spongiform encephalopathy and human TSEs can be categorized into 3 types, sporadic (80%), inherited (15%) and infectious (5%). Though research of transmissible prion diseases for instance kuru and recently atypical variant CJD (vCJD), has promote large progress in the research of these diseases, the majority of human patients are infected by sporadic CJD.

Every year, Sporadic CJD cases are reported at a rate of 1 to 2 per two million population; this incidence is observed worldwide and till recently has been stable. It is believed to arise from a conformational rearrangement in one prion molecule as a rare stochastic event in an otherwise healthy human. Alternatively, it is thought that the primary misfolded prion proteins are generated after a somatic mutation in the corresponding gene in one neuron.

Mutations in the prion protein, which is located on human chromosome 20p, accounts to approximately 15% of human TSEs. More than 30 disease causing mutations have already been studied; all resulting in autosomal dominantly inherited disorders. Those different mutations display wide range of phenotypic alleles, even within infected families with the same mutation.

GSS (Gerstmann-Straussler-Scheinker syndrome) is the most commonly observed familial TSE. Usually this happens in the 30 s or 40 s of life and mainly shows as a chronic cerebellar ataxia with pyramidal characters. Dementia appears later than in CJD, with lethal usually taking effect five years since diagnosis. In 1989, the mutation generating GSS was initially discovered by Hsiao as being P102L, but some other permutations in the prion gene have been found to lead to the infection (Hsiao et al, 1989). Some other TSEs include incidents that show symptoms similar as CJD and GSS and also have cases lacking either the general phenomena or the usual histological patterns of TSEs, though immuno-histo-chemistry for abnormal PrP is generally positive (Collinge et al, 1992). A variety of cerebellar ataxia, progressive dementia, extrapyramidal features, pyramidal signs, myoclonus, pseudobulbar signs, seizures, chorea and amyotrophic characters are seen. The disease is diagnosed by DNA sequencing of the prion protein gene.

In 1986, the human TSE spectra were further enriched by inclusion of FFI (fatal familial insomnia), this disease shows progressive autonomic dysfunction and untreatable insomnia (Lugaresi et al, 1986). Though patients with FFI show moderate leveled cortical astrocytosis, medial-dorsal thalamic nuclei and atrophy of the anterior-ventral is consistently observed. Two FFI sufferers have been shown to have a periodic electroencephalogram (EEG) and widespread spongiosis; both patients were lately described to bare mutations at codon 178 in the prion protein gene (Medori et al, 1992a, 1992b; Gambetti et al, 1993), a mutation that had been characterized previously in CJD sufferers. Since then, laboratory animals have been infected by FFI (Collinge et al, 1995; Tateishi et al, 1995). The discovery that the time spongiform encephalopathies happen from mutations in the prion protein gene (Medori et al, 1992; Kretzschmar et al, 1995; Mastrianni et al, 1996) the secondary prions are still infectious strongly supports the idea that the prion protein is the main and only pathogen of the disorder. This discovery also leads to TSEs being unique among human disorders as they might happen naturally, due to mutation in genes or caused by transmissible route.

Nowadays, the lowest cases of TSEs every year are those resulted from either iatrogenic or contaminated food. Many documented cases of iatrogenic prion infection are available, happening from cross exposure via surgical facilities (Gibbs et al, 1994), intake of hormones produced from gathered cadaveric pituitary glands (Rappaport and Graham, 1987), corneal transplantation (Kennedy et al, 2001; Gottesdiener, 1989) and xenograft of cadaveric dura mater organ or tissue (Clavel and Clavel, 1996). Elevated awareness of the dangers of possible infection of TSEs via these pasages has caused changes in clinical practices, with pituitary hormones now produced by recombinant protein preparation and deeper examination of cadaveric volunteers for transplanted grafts. This examination is carried out by looking for a history of familial TSEs or of probable exposure to TSE infection by use of cadaveric growth hormone or dura mater transplantation. Because there is still no fast examination available, this examination process, although not infallible, is helpful.

In the 1990s, the transmission of BSE (bovine spongiform encephalopathy) to humans in the UK attracted the world's attention (Hill et al, 1997a; Collinge et al, 1996). The source of BSE will possibly always kept unknown but it is thought that a case of "sporadic BSE" appeared in one cow, by conformational rearrangement in one prion molecule or by mutation of a single prion protein, very similar to the way that sporadic typed CJD is thought to happen in mankind. This thing may have happened as a rare case for centuries. However, in the 1980s, routines in animal industry changed, leading to parts of cattle carcases entering the cow food chain again. This promoted the transmistion of other cows with BSE and over time, generated a BSE epidemic in cattles and then beef entered the british food chain as well as other people with imported british beef on a grand scale.

So far, 119 people have died from vCJD, after the transmission of BSE to humans (Hill et al, 1997a), which gives rise to a vast public problem (National CJD Surveillance Unit, 2002). This is only a small portion of the cases of familial and sporadic TSEs annually, but the size of population in Britain currently carrying the virus is still unclear (Ghani et al, 1999; Hilton et al, 2000). It is reported from the research of kuru that the average incubation time of these disorders is in the order of decades and the fact that vCJD involves bovine prions crossing a "transmission barrier" will further make this incubation period longer (see below). Indications for epidemiological models include these models need to be interpreted with caution, because average incubation time is correlated to the later epidemic seriousness. A disturbing discovery is about an elevation in the cases of sporadic CJD in Britain over the two decades This was believed to show better case confirmation, but recent study has given the possibility that these incidents of sporadic CJD may constitute of people who have actually got the disorger from eating beef with BSE-virus, but showing an alternative features to that generally observed with vCJD (Asante et al, 2002).

Significant danger would arise, because atypical carriers will pass the virus on through donated blood, surgical facilities or cadaveric tissue transplantation and also because the long incubation period of vCJD means that the disease could hibernate. Though math and statistical research show that vCJD will probably not become a problem in the UK people (Risk evaluation for infection of vCJD via operational facilities: a simulation method and numerical situation. UK Department of Health, 2001), but it keeps to be a rare chance. The situation of those chances is showed by earlier transmissions from operational facilities (Gibbs et al, 1994), if we don't have more results on the quantity of asymptomatic carriers, their amplitude will keep to be hard to measure(Hilton et al, 2002; Ghani, 2002).

9.9.4   Prion Protein 3-dimentional Structure

Prion protein is a Glycoprotein with about 250 amino acids, it associated with Membrane through a C-terminal glycosyphosphatidylinositol (GPI) linkage. Prion protein's Role in membrane trafficing has been proposed, it possibly involved in some endocytic pathways. Knockout mice develop and behave normally, but perhaps prone to seizures. Prion protein Interacts with laminin, which plays a role in cell adhesion and neurite formation. Also, Prion protein interacts with the laminin receptor resulting in internalization of membrane-bound PrPC. Prion protein Binds Cu^{2+}, it may have an antioxidant function that promotes neuron survival. Prion protein is Abundant in brain and it is also detected in spleen, lymph node, lung, heart, kidney, skeletal muscle, uterus, adrenal gland, parotid gland, intestine, proventriculus, abomasum and mammary gland.

The aberrantconformation of the prion protein (PrP) is the universal character of the prion diseases, ant it stays in at two metabolism conformations with distinct chemical and physic characters. The usual state of the normal protein, called PrP^C, is generally a well preserved cell membrane-surface protein anchored through a glycophosphatidyl inositol. The protein is observed in a variety kind of cells and especially in neurons. The molecular mass of PrP^C is 33–35 kDa, it's a glycol-protein, with secondary structure a lot of α-helix that is prone to protease digestion and soluble in surfactants. The isoform that's disorder related, called PrP^{Sc}, which is observed merely in diseased brains as polymerized insolubles, is partially immune to protease digestion and not soluble in surfactants and secondary structure contains a lot of beta-sheet. Just like what we mentioned above, prions do not seem to carry large quantity of DNA/RNA and this hypothesis is supported by the examinations of Kellings and colleagues, they showed that no family of similar nucleic acid sequences constantly purified together with PrP^{Sc}(Kellings et al, 1994). Therefore, a new method to show how prions multiply is required. Prusiner modified the only-protein idea suggested by Griffith in the 1967 and he demonstrate a hypothesis of transmission that depends on a ill-folded "scrapie" state of the usual protein, one PrP^{Sc} prion molecule being capable of inducing the conformational change of the carrier's natural PrPc prion molecule in the cell to follow its abnormal folding state(Figure 9–9). This prion (proteinaceous infectious particle) could code dissimilarities in disorder mechanisms by varying its folding state, make it possible to infect different "alleles" without the presence of DNA/RNA (Prusiner, 1982).

The idea that an infectious agent could be capable of producing diseases with different phenotypes without the presence of DNA (or RNA) to encode this informationbecame the greatest objection to the prion hypothesis. One of the powers of this hypothesis is that it gives an explanation about how TSEs can come out through hereditary, infectious or spontaneous routes (Figure 9–10).

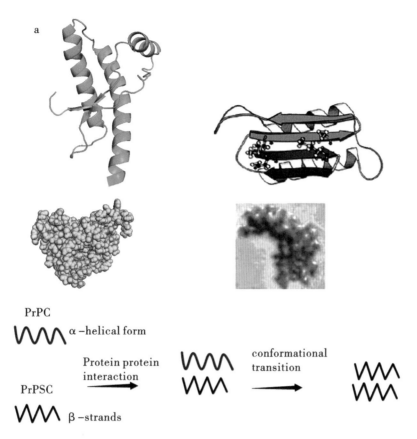

Figure 9-9　a. Structure of prion protein (top left, 1QLX. pdb, contains 40% a-helix and little β-sheet) , top right is a proposed abnormal conformer of prion protein. And shape of prion protein (bottom left normal form and right an abnormal conformer).
b. The "Prion Hypothesis" suggests that an abnormal conformer (PrP^{Sc}) of the cellular prion protein (PrP^c) is capable of inducing PrP^c to undergo a change of conformation into PrP^{Sc}

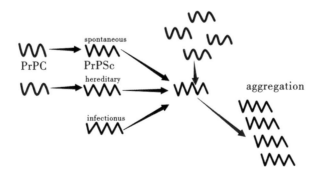

Figure 9-10　The abnormally folded PrP^{Sc} forms of the prion protein may arise either spontaneously or in patients carrying a mutation that makes misfolding more likely or from an exogenous infective source. Once a misfolded form has arisen, other PrP^c molecules are converted, propagating the disease in a form of a chain reaction

　　A lot of research show that dissimilar types of scrapie would produce distinct alleles and even if the contagious reagent is transmited from one species to another, these alleles are kept. These results indicate that they aren't coded by the primary sequence of an organism's prion protein molecule (Bruce et al, 1994; Bessen and Marsh, 1992, 1994).

Weissmannhypothesized an alternative mechanism in 1991 (Weissmann, 1991). The hypothesis says that the protein content of a prion (called the apoprion) could result in disorder by itself, but a small carrier-obtained DNA/RNA (named the coprion) could bind with it. The conjugation of the two (the holo-prion) could cause a host modified type of disorder. According to this model, we could forsee that deletion of co-prion will lead to the loss of isoform-specific characters and replacement of co-prions from a different isoform would result in a correlated transform in isoform characters. Also, transmitability is immune to experiments that make DNA/RNA inactive, while isoform-specific characters is not. Those ideas have not been supported by published Experiments yet and illustration that PrP^{Sc} is capable of acquiring isoform-specific characters outside of cells did not support it, but prion molecule protein conformation mediats strain diversity support it (Bessen et al, 1995).

9.9.5 Different Strain of Prions

A major problem for the "protein-only" hypothesis has been how to explain the existence of multiple isolates or strains, of prions, different strains are distinguished by their biological properties. They produce distinct incubation periods and patterns of neuropathological targeting (so-called lesion profiles). Conventionally, distinct strains of a pathogen like viruses are explained by differences in DNA sequence (i. e. HIV). Some postulate that strain characteristics can be encoded by small nucleic acids or "coprions". This coprion, however, should be sensitive to UV, but no tests to prove this have been done. When Western blot is performed, PrP showd three different bands, this is corresponding to the modification of two, one or no sugar group at the two glycosylation area of the prion molecule (see Figure 9–11). Digestion of infected brain sections with the proteinase K-a protease at specific environments breaks down PrP^{c} thoroughly, with PrP^{Sc} sort of unchanged (Figure 9–11). Proteinase K digestion of prion protein PrP^{Sc} do cut about 70 residues from the N-terminal of the protein, leaving it a lower molecular weight band on the gel (Figure 9–11).

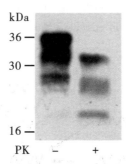

Figure 9–11 PrP^{C} is seen to result in three bands, with masses between 16 and 36 kDa, on Western blot. Treatment with proteinase K (PK) under defined conditions degrades the more numerous PrP^{C} molecules, revealing PrP^{Sc}. Proteinase K cleaves some residues from PrP^{Sc}, causing an apparent decrease in its molecular weight (figure courtesy of Dr Andy Hill)

After the controlled proteolysis, different types of strain generate diistinct migration features on SDS-PAGE (poly-acrylamide gels), indicating that these protein have conformations different from one another. Also, the percentage of diglycosylated, mono-glycosylated and un-glycosylated forms is also not the same. The phenomenone has made the difference of ratios of the viral prion protein in distinct types to be utilized as indicater of prion strain "isoform," with the discovery that specific prion strain isoforms of protein results in variant CJD or sporadic in homo sapiens (Figure 9–13) (and will be discussed later) (Wadsworth et al,

1999).

Transmission of human prions and bovine prions to wild-type mice also results in murine PrP^{Sc} with fragment sizes and glycoform ratios that correspond to the original inoculum (Collinge et al, 1996). If the encoded strain type diversity and is dependent on conformation of prion proteins and their biochemical characters, the conformation and biochemical features will be kept after infection of both cases, to lab animals the same or another organism. Research have showed that this is the case, with isolated CJD as experimental materials. The research have shown that both glycosylation percentage and digested PrP^{Sc} pieces size were retained after transmission in genic modified mice with mankind PrP expressed. Infection of mankind prion virus and cow prion virus to wildtype rate also lead to murine PrPSc that have the same glycosylation percentage and digested PrP^{Sc} pieces size as the source virion (Collinge et al, 1996). vCJD is related to the sugar ratio of PrPSc, which is different from classic CJD but similar to mad cow disease, either in cattle or when it spreads to some other species (Collinge et al, 1996). Hill et al, 1997), both in cows and after transmitted to a lot of other organisms (Collinge et al, 1996; Hill et al, 1997). These results suggest that strain variation is encoded by a combined effect of PrP isoform types and glycosylation states, which firmly support the "only protein" theory of transmission. Since PrP glycosylation happens before transformation to PrPSc, distinct glycosylation percentages might corresponds to distinct conformation of PrPSc for the selection of Since PrP glycosylation occurs before transformation to PrPSc, different glycosylation ratios may represent different conformation of PrPSc for the selection of specific PrPC glycosylation. specific PrPC glycosylation state. We could conclude from this theory that, PrP protein isoform (conformation) or strain typing would be the essential criteria for the classification of strain type and glycoform will be related as a downstream step. People have always know that protein glycosylation type and from are dependent on the cell types, glycoform features of PrP^{Sc} may caused by the distinct neuro-pathological alleles that tell distinc prion protein strains apart (Collinge et al, 1996). Specific PrP^{Sc} glycosylation might multiply more favorably and quickly in neuron type cells with PrP glycosylation like this incorporated on the cell membrane. This targeting would as well suggest the incubation time length observed in distinc strains, targeting more essential brain areas or areas with a strong expression of PrP protein, to produce significantly less incubation time.

9.9.6   Genotype of Organisms with Prion Disease

Since the first unveiling of this disease, more than 30 disease-generating aberrations have been reported in the prion protein (Figure 9-12). TSEs are not normal for having both family related features and contagious nature. Non-pathogenic features are also reported (Figure 9-12) and the most significant of the findings is the valine/ methionine variation at codon 129 (51% MV, 38% MM, 11% VV in the UK people). A research project of 22 sporadic CJD incidents showed that nearly all (21 out of 22) was not heterozygous at position 129 for either valine or methionine (Palmer et al, 1991). Subsequently, this research is now repeated in the UK (Windl et al, published) and abroad at larger scale. (Windl et al, in press) (Laplanche et al, 1994; Salvatore et al, 1994). The genotype of 7 CJD sufferers who received pituitary hormone therapy also represented an obvious overdose of valine homozygote at position 129 (Collinge et al, 1991), a finding that was later reproduced in the United States (Brown et al, 1994) and France (Laplanche et al, 1994). In addition, all incidents of vCJD reports till now have happened in people who are not heterozygous for Met at this 129 codon (Ironside et al, 2000). These observations indicate that the absence of homozygosity at position 129 gives secure from prion virus infection probably by decreasing the prion virus's capability to perform conformation change into the state required to multiply CJD virus. However, it is not yet clear would this safeguarding be thorough full protection or be in part, the reason is that transmission from outer source prion virus might still happen in homozygous ones of position 129 and the difference is with more incubation tme. The phenomenon has a lot of indications for evaluation of the epidemic scale and grandness of the vCJD disease.

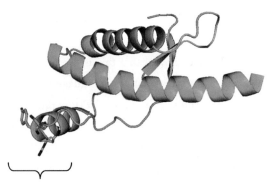

Figure 9-12　Some of the important residues and the region in defining the species barrier are shown on the structure of the prion protein

9.9.7　Transmission of Prion Diseases Between Different Mammalian Species

On primary passage of prions from species A to species B, not all inoculated animals of species B develop disease; those that do have much longer incubation periods. On second passage of infectivity to species B animals, transmission parameters resemble within-species transmission. "Species barrier" restricts transmission of prion strains between species and this has been known for many years (Pattison, 1965). This is showed by lengthened incubation time and a reduction in the ratio of herds suffering to the disorder, when prion viruses from one organism are transmitted into a different one ("first passage"). When those herds are found to all fall ill, with obviously consistent incubation time length, which contrasts with the circumstance when prion proteins are transfered into herds of the same organisms. If after transmission into another organism contagious tissue is extracted from the suffered mamal that do fall ill and infected to more other animals ("second transmission"), the infectious pattern is similar to that of the first organism, with a relatively less and similar length of incubation time (Figure 9-13) compared to most (if not all of them). This barrier to transmission between organisms can be measured quntatively by differences in latency and infection rates between the first and second channel of transmissions. ID50 can also be more precisely quantified by inoculation with 10-fold series diluents and by measuring the infectious dilution of 50% of animal deaths.

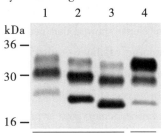

Figure 9-13　Different strains of CJD are seen on gel electrophoresis to have differences in both molecular weight and the percentage of diglycosylation, monoglycosylation and unglycosylated forms. These features can be used as a biochemical indicator of "Strain Type". For PrP^{sc} type, 1-3 classical CJD and 4 vCJD

When mice that aregenerally resistant to hamster prion virus at normal conditions are modified to encode hamster PrP proteins, they become very sensitive to Sc237 hamster prion viruss (Prusiner et al, Rubin et al, Stanton et al, 1990). It was originally showed that this organism barrier was caused by the PrP amino acid sequence and structure differences between the source species and the infected animals. The discovery of sporadic and infected CJD in sufferers with prion virus protein at 129-codon valine methionine polymorphisms homozygote also indicates that transmission and infection is most likely to happen very easily if the PrPc original amino acid sequence and structure is in line with or the same as the functional contagious PrP-Sc for prion multiplication and transmission(Figure 9–14, Figure 9–15) (Palmer et al, 1991. Collinge et al, 1991).

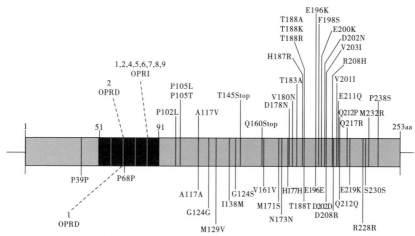

Figure 9–14   **Human prion protein polymorphisms and Pathogenic mutations**

The pathogenic mutations related to human prion disease are shown on top of the PrP coding scheme. These consist of 1,2 or 4–9 octapeptide repeat insertions within the octarepeat region between codons 51 and 91, a deletion of 2 octapeptide repeats and various point mutations causing missense amino acid substitutions. Point mutations are designated by the wild-type amino acid preceding the codon number, followed by the mutant residue, using single letter amino acid conventions. Polymorphic variants are shown below the PrP coding sequence. Deletion of one octapeptide repeat is not associated with disease

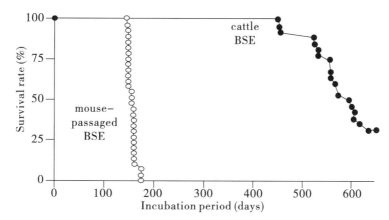

Figure 9–15   **Decrease in incubation period with second passage**

Initial transmissoin of mice with prions obtained from a cattle origin (cattle BSE) results in less that 100% of mice succumbing to infection. Additionally, those mice that succumb do so after prolonged and variable incubation periods. If homogenate is prepared from mice that did succumb following initial BSE inoculation, then transmission of this "mouse-passaged" BSE ("second passage") results in a much more uniform and rapid incubation of disease, with approximately 100% clinical infection (figure from Journal of NeuroVirology, 9: 183–193, 2003 by Edward McKintosh, Sarah J Tabrizi and John Collinge)

BSE prion viral proteins can effectively spread to a broad spectrum of organisms, but their infection features can be maintained even after transmitted through intermediate organisms with distinct original amino acid sequence and prion protein structures of PrP (Bruce et al, 1994). Sporadic CJD prion viral proteins are not easily transmitted to wildtype mice, but genetic modified mice with mankind prion protein encoding genes are easily infected and easiness could be shown by having a similar less incubation time and will not be changed by the second generation, so they are similar to be lacking of organism barrier (Hill et al, 1997). On the other hand, vCJD prion viral proteins (also defined by the same major protein amino acid sequence and structure) are more easily transmitted to wildtype mice, but less effectively transmitted to genetic modified mice (Hill et al, 1997). These observations indicate that both primary peptide sequence/protein structure and conformation state of the prion protein are the controlling factors of the organism barrier. Therefore, the phrase "transmission obstacle barrier" is considered to be a more appropriate phrase (Collinge, 1999). Initially, evaluation of infection barriers depended on herds showing clinical disorders. By utilizing this evaluation technique, the very efficient barriers do exist to limit the spread of hamster prion viruses to mice (Kimberlin and walker, 1979; Scott et al, 1989). Although mice with with hamster Sc237 prion viral proteins taken lived similar time length as mice that were simulated without taking the virus and showed no signs of clinical disorders, tests on their brain tissues over a long period of time after taking the virus showed that their PrPSc and/or infectivity was high and strong (Hill et al, 2000). The observation indicates that transmission barriers disorders happens not only in the multiplication of contagious prion viral proteins, but also in the following neuro-degeneration results from the gradual gathering of the prion viral proteins.

9.9.8　Function of Pr P^C

The primary role of sufferer organism's PrP^C for prion viral protein multiplication and disease causing ability is showed by the obervations that PrP gene distroyed mice　(called Prnp0/0) are immune to scrapie transmission (Bueler et al, 1993; Manson et al, 1994), but genetic transformation of the murine PrP^C gene into the mice lead to sensitivity to infection coming back (Fischer et al, 1996). A primary aim of scientific study into TSEs is trying to grasp the part of the host usual standard functional prion protein plays and the reason why PrP^{Sc} aggregation is associated with neuronal disease such as neuron degeneration.

To understand the usual typical role PrP^C plays, mice with Prnp$^{0/0}$ have been investigated as well. Two strains were produced with genes targeted at Prnp0 = 0 were normal in development and seemed to have no major obvious mulfunctions (Manson et al, 1994; Bueler et al, 1992). The relative well being of those PrP null mouse were believed to generated from naturally effective selected adjustment in the process of growing up. But, results from Prnp controlled knockout mouse indicate otherwise (Mallucci et al, 2002); those mice experience abnormality of viral PrP protein infection in neurons at about two month time (nine weeks). The mice are still healthy showing no sign of neuro-degeneration or an obvious clinical diagnostics, illustrating that sudden deletion of PrP from neurons after growing up is adapted and that the prion pathogen's physiology of disease disease causing properties is not usually to be caused by removal of PrP usual standard function (Mallucci et al, 2002).

The prionviral particle is a cell-surface sialoglyco-protein which readily binds copper (Hornshaw et al, 1995; Brown et al, 1997; St¨ockel et al, 1998) and shows SOD (superoxide dismutase) activity in the reaction tube after renatured with the company of $CuCl_2$ at a concentrations high than the threshold (Brown et al, 1999). Prion viral particle is detected in the major proportion of adult body (Manson et al, 1992) and prion protein is observed at a peak amount in the CNS (central nervous system) and immune defense circle (Dodelet and Cashman, 1998). Freshly produced PrP^c is transferred to the cell plasma membrane and was then recycled quickly through a vesicle trafficking involved system and the transition time is about one hour if transported from the plasma membrane to the early endosomes (Shyng et al,1994). The biophysical and biochemical steps are observed together with plasma membrane receptors and this phenomenon indicates that PrP^c might be similar. ' the very strong binding to Cu metal indicates that cuprum metabolism or transportation might actually be its real responsibility (Jackson et al,2001).

9.9.9　Therapeutics Combating Prion Disease

Drugs that have interactions with PrP^{Sc} constituts of Congo red (Ingrosso et al,1995),pentosan polysulphate,dextran sulfphate,anthracycline (Tagliavani et al,1997) and some different polyanions (Ehlers and Diringer,1984;Farquhar and Dickinson,1986;Kimberlin and Walker,1986) and beta-strand insertion sequences (Soto et al,2000). Unluckily,major proportion of those drugs are merely helpful if given well ahead of the appearance of clinical symptoms and usually presents either elevated serious toxicity,decreased/reduced concentrations of bio-availability or sometimes both. Although the capability to associate with PrPS^{c,} and protect PrP^c from being converted to aberrant forms,gives a meaning approach to hindering or protecting the body from the disease advancement,it is not easy to achieve a full recovery after therapy for prion viral infection. We are in search of a better understanding of the function of PrPc protein and progress in examination and diagnosis ahead of time to develop therapies that will secure a full recovery(Figure 9-16).

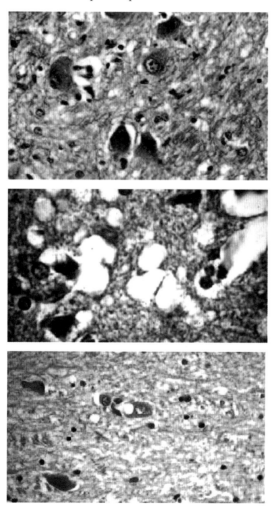

Figure 9-16　Histology of normal brain (top),Spongiform Encephalopathy (kuru,middle) and Creutzfeldt-Jakob desease (CJD,bottom)

UK and USA nowadays are carrying out clinical trials by using chlorpromazine and quinacrine treatment in CJD and vCJD sufferers, but the data are not publicly released yet. It has proved the obstacles to transfer in vitro results to the clinical trials, because there has not been any data that supports those compounds to be useful on combating prion viral infection in living organisms and these days quinacrine administration in a mammalian animal of CJD showed to be not effictive (Collins et al, 2002). However, public requirement for any therapy that will combat or stop the rigorous advancement of those dangerously fatal disorders is considerably huge. A legal problem these days has demand a United Kindom health area related officer to give in vein pentosan polysulphate to two sufferers, therefore this experimental theray largely still in the lab will forward proceedingly highlights the strong demand of searching for a helpful prion curing therapy.

9.9.10   Diagnostic Examination and Prion Detection Technology

Early diagnosis well ahead of huge neurological damage has taken place is vital to a successful therapy for prion viral infection. Human Prion Diseases, including Transmissible spongiform encephalopathies (TSE) and Creutzfeldt-Jakob disease (CJD) have the following symptoms. In sporadic cases: rapidly progressive dementia, visual disturbances, cerebellar dysfunction, pyramidal and extra pyramidal dysfunction and myoclonus. In variant cases: behavioral changes (psychosis, depression), painful sensory symptoms and delayed neurologic signs.

Host cells, especially neurons, express PrPC and PrPC become PrPSc after an infection. PrPC has functions including anti-oxidative stress regulation, Ca and Cu homeostasis, circadian rhythms, learning, memory and synapse formation. So, the study of prion detection technology is important. Cows could be checked for BSE by using the method as follows: a homogenate is prepared from the brain and digested with PK (proteinase K). The digested sample is applied to a plate for detection by anti-PrP antibody. If it showd Prp positive, ELISA (enzyme-linked immunosorbent assay) is performed repeatedly. If a positive result is obtained again, Western blotting and immunohistochemistry (IHC) are performed. Western blotting uses a membrane to absorb PK-digested peptides separated by SDS-PAGE (sodium dodecyl sulfate polyacrylamide gel electrophoresis). Western blotting provides information on both prion infections and the mobility of digested peptides, which is influenced by the host genotype and prion strains. The IHC is based on representative pathological features of prion diseases including neuronal cell loss, vacuolation, astrocytosis and amyloid plaques. IHC analysis means examination of brain sections by light microscopy, the accumulation of PrP amyloid plaques, neuronal cell loss (or vacuolation) and astrocytosis. Although vacuolation is also used as an index of prion infection, various combinations of prion strains with host species result in the accumulation of PrP without vacuolation in brain sections. Recently, the protein misfolding cyclic amplification (PMCA) method has been developed, which enables *in vitro* amplification of PrPres from a small quantity of PrPSc as seed by sequential cycles of incubation and sonication. Interestingly, levels of PrPres amplified by this method correlated with the prion infectivity titer. Furthermore, PMCA could detect prions in blood. In addition, it could be used to diagnose not only terminally diseased hamsters but also prion-infected pre-symptomatic hamsters. This method has the highest sensitivity of any method for detecting PrPres reported so far. To date, its application to sheep, goat, cattle, hamster scrapie and mouse scrapie has been reported. PMCA will show the mechanism of conformational change of PrP. So far, several factors such as RNA and metals have been found to be involved in the conformational change.

The observation of spongiform alteration and amyloid-plaque accumulation on histology could be diagnosed as symptoms of TSEs. The exist of contagious prion viral proteins could merely be showed by transfering brain homogenate to animals that could show typical symptoms, a very expensive and time consuming process. Spongiform alteration and gliosis are utilized for histological diagnosis, no matter it's from experimental mammals, herds or mankinds. The generation of particular PrP antibodies has given immune-histochemist to analyze the histological phenomenon, progressing and elevating the accuracy of the early diagnosis, this is even more helpful when plaques are not large enough or there is uncertainty about another disease that could also produce spongiform alteration. Besides the advantage of being highly susceptible, protein immuno analysis, this increased diagnostic sensitivity and specificity (Wadsworth et al, 2001). Although the generation of particular PrP antibodies has resulted in histological progress, most TSEs diagnosis still asks for brain graft and therefore requires a brain sample through biopsy.

Spongiformalteration and amyloid plaques were not observed in lymphoid organ sample but histological illustration of the existance of prion viral protein is likely to happen with antibodies particular for PrP. In vCJD lymphotropism appears to be a major feature of the disease, this is unusual. Histological pieces are usually steriled with HCOOH, depriving of PrPc, unfolding the prion viral protein to allow antibody association with PrPSc.. This permits vCJD to be reliably confirmed from tonsil samples, making the requirement for a more damaging brain sample extraction not necessary in these sufferers (Hill et al, 1997b; Wadsworth et al, 2001; Hill et al, 1999). Immuno-histo-chemistry and Western blotting diagnosis were performed on tonsillar biopsies of suspected vCJD sufferers and this combination provided a 100% sensitivity and specificity diagnostic test in a recent incident series of fourty three incidents (19 negative and 24 positive).

Although prion diseases are confirmed by taking a sample of brain tissue during a biopsy or after death, healthcare providers can do a number of tests before to help diagnose prion diseases such as CJD or to rule out other diseases with similar symptoms. Prion diseases should be considered in all people with rapidly progressive dementia.

Theclinical tests include: MRI (magnetic resonance imaging) scans of the brain, Samples of fluid from the spinal cord (spinal tap, also called lumbar puncture), Electroencephalogram, which analyzes brain waves; this painless test requires placing electrodes on the scalp, Blood tests, Neurologic and visual exams to check for nerve damage and vision loss.

9.9.11　Further Discussion

Statistics has suggested recently that diseases of human TSEs might have happened for many centuries (S Mead, paper submitted); and the appearance of TSEs in United Kindom mammal herds has had society results for several dozen of years. Despite those findings, it is this putative danger of an outburst of vCJD disease in the Britain people that has given an elevated concern to try to work out this new diseases never described before. Herds TSEs are now regarded to happen across all nations only with the exception of New Zealand and Australia and to appear not just as scrapie in sheep population, but as BSE in zoo animals, cows, domestic cats and transmissible mink encephalopathy and as chronic wasting disorder in American deer and elk herds. Transmissible diseases are not understood for their readiness to be restricted within national borders; BSE has already spread into many European areas and vCJD may therefore also do the same. Our comprehension of the etiology and pathology of prion viral protein caused diseases has improved greatly over the past few years, but we still face huge scientific challenges for research if we are to avoid major epidemics of vCJD and find appropriate therapies. The most important of these is to demonstrate the real nature of this new contagious pathogen, further illustration of the function of PrP^c and the discovery and development of clinically available therapies.

9.10   Other Viruses

9.10.1   Parvoviruses

Parvoviruses are small viruses (about 20 nm) with a single stranded DNA genome and need a helper virus or totally depend on host cells for replication. Parvoviruses are host specific and belongs to familyParvoviridae and genus Erythrovirus. Parvovirus B19, which was the first (and until 2005 the only) one known human virus in this family Parvoviridae and genus *Erythrovirus* was originally discovered from the blood of symptomless blood donors. A new virus in this family, named Bocavirus has been characterized recently, after isolation from the respiratory tract of children presented with acute respiratory disease.

9.10.2   Parvovirus B19

Parvovirus B19 is present world wide causing infections only in human and acquired predominantly in childhood and is often asymptomatic. About two out of 10 people who get infected with this virus will have no symptoms, others may have only mild, rash illness. The virus was discovered by chance in 1975 by Australian virologist YvonneCossart. It gained its name because it was discovered in well B19 of a large series of microtiter plates(Figure 9-17).

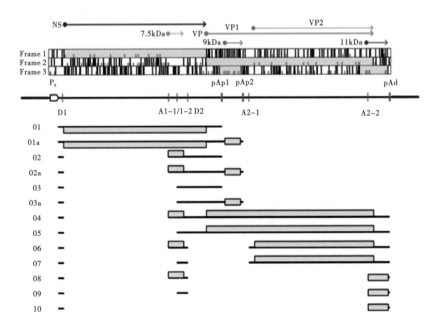

Figure 9-17   Schematic representation of B19V genome organization and functional mapping

  Top: open reading frames identified in the positive strand of genome; arrows indicate the coding regions for viral proteins positioned on the ORF map. Center: genome organization, with distinct representation of the terminal and internal regions and indication of the positions of promoter (P6), splice donor (D1, D2), splice acceptor (A1-1/2, A2-2/2) and cleavage-polyadenylation (pAp1, pAp2 andpAd) sites. Bottom: viral mRNAs species; black boxes indicate the exon composition and light boxes indicate the ORFs contained within mRNAs

Parvovirus B19 is a non-enveloped, icosahedral virus that contains a single-stranded linear DNA genome. The infectious particles may contain either positive or negative strands of DNA. The icosahedral capsid consists of two structural proteins, VP1 (83 kDa) and VP2 (58 kDa), which are identical except for 227 amino acids at the amino-terminal of the VP1-protein, the so-called VP1-unique region. Each capsid consists of a total of 60 capsomers: VP2 is the major capsid protein and comprises approximately 95% of the total virus particle. VP1-proteins are incorporated into the capsid structure in a non-stochiometrical relation based on antibody-binding analysis and X-ray structural analysis the VP1-unique region is assumed to be exposed at the surface of the virus particle. At each end of the DNA molecule there are palindromic sequences which form "hairpin" loops. The hairpin at the 3' end serves as a primer for the DNA polymerase. It is classified as erythrovirus because of its capability to invade red blood cell precursors in the bone marrow. Three genotypes (with subtypes) have been recognized. VP2 codons were found to be under purifying selection. In contrast VP1 codons in the unique part of the gene were found to be under diversifying selection. This diversifying selection is consistent with persistent infection as this part of the VP1 protein contains epitopes recognized by the immune system. Like other non-enveloped DNA viruses, pathogenicity of parvovirus B19 rely on host cells. In humans the P antigen (also known as globoside) acts as the cellular receptor for parvovirus B19.

Parvovirus B19 usually presents as a respiratory infection, with an erythematous maculopapular rash and arthralgia. It spreads from person to person, just like a cold, often through respiratory secretions and hand-to-hand contact and is considered as a highly contagious virus infection. Parvovirus B19 can also spreads through other secretions, such as saliva, sputum or nasal mucus, when an infected person coughs or sneezes. Parvovirus B19 can also spread through blood or blood products and also congenitally. In parts of the world with changing seasons, people tend to get infected with parvovirus B19 more often in late winter, spring and early summer. Mini-outbreaks of parvovirus B19 infection occur about every 3 to 4 years.

Clinically (erythemainfectiosum), symptomatic infection starts with prominent erythema of the cheeks (slapped cheek disease), spreading to the trunk and limbs, followed by lymphadenopathy and arthralgia. Most commonly, disease is seen in children of 5 to 10 years old and has been called the Fifth disease, because, historically, it was one of five common childhood illnesses characterized by a rash. Parvovirus B19 induces aplastic crisis in children with chronic hemolytic anemia caused by lysis of early erythroid precursors. Once infected, patients usually develop the illness after an incubation period of four to fourteen days.

The disease commences with high grade fever and malaise, when the virus is most abundant in the bloodstream and patients are usually no longer infectious once the characteristic rash of this disease has appeared. After a brief prodromal symptom with fever, headache, nausea, diarrhea, a red rash forms on the cheeks, with relative pallor around the mouth ("slapped cheek rash"), sparing the nasolabial folds, forehead and mouth. It is followed by "Lace-like, (reticular)" red rash on trunk or extremities. Infection in adults usually only involves the reticular rash, predominating with multiple joint pain and exacerbation of rash by sunlight, heat, stress. Teenagers or young adults infected with Parvovirus B19 may develop the so-called "Papular Purpuric Gloves and Socks Syndrome".

Parvovirus infection in pregnant women during the second or third trimester of pregnancy may result in non-immune hydrops fetalis due to severe fetal anemia, sometimes leading to miscarriage or stillbirth. The risk of fetal loss is about 10% if infection occurs before 20 weeks of pregnancy (especially between weeks 14 and 20), but minimal there after. As infection leads to virus replication in the throat and viremia, a strong antibody response will be elicited in infected persons. Individuals with B19 IgG antibodies are generally considered immune to recurrent infection, but reinfection is possible in a minority of cases. About half of adults are B19-immune due to a past infection.

Parvovirus infection can also trigger severe anemia in people who have compromised immune systems, which may result from HIV infection, cancer treatments and anti-rejection drugs used after organ transplants. Parvovirus B19 is a cause of chronic anemia in individuals who have AIDS. It is frequently overlooked. Treatment with intravenous immunoglobulin usually resolves the anemia although relapse can occur. Arthralgias and arthritis are commonly reported in association with parvovirus B19 infection in adults whereas erythema infectiosum is the main symptom observed in children. The occurrence of arthralgia coincides with the initial detection of circulating IgM-and IgG-antibodies against the viral structural proteins VP1 and VP2. Parvovirus B19 infection may affect the development of arthritis.

At the moment, there are no effective vaccine or treatments that directly target Parvovirus B19 virus. Intravenous immunoglobulin therapy (IVIG) therapy has been a popular alternative. Preventive measures include the general measures to reduce chances of infection or spreading infection by washing your hands often with soap and water, covering mouth and nose when cough or sneeze, not touching eyes, nose or mouth, avoiding close contact with people who are sick by and staying home when sick.

Clinical Pictures(Figure 9-18, Figure 9-19):

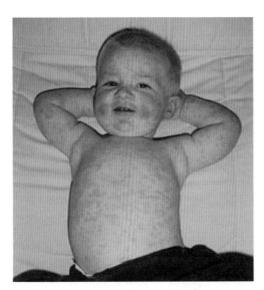

Figure 9-18 Child showing signs of erythemainfectiosum, also known as fifth disease

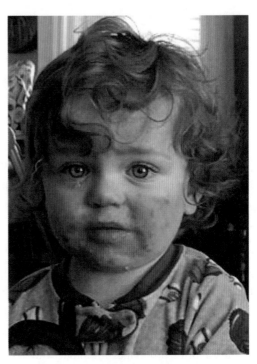

Figure 9-19 The "slapped cheek" appearance typical of fifth disease

9.10.3　Human Papillomavirus (HPV)

Human papillomavirus (HPV) belongs to the genus Papillomavirus of thePapillomaviridae family and mainly causes proliferative lesions of human skin and mucous membranes. Cervical cancer and other malignant tumors are closely related to high-risk HPV (type 16, type 18, etc.) and genital warts to the low-risk HPV(Figure 9-20) (type 6, type 11, etc.).

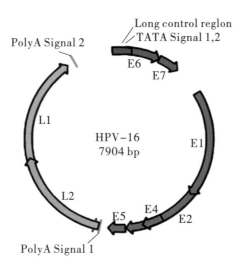

Figure 9-20　Genomil structure of HPV-16

9.10.3.1　The Biological Characteristics

HPV is 52 – 55 nm, spherical non-enveloped virus with icosahedral three-dimensional symmetry. The viral genome is a supercoiled, double-stranded circular DNA of about 8 kb divided into late (LR) and non-coding (NCR) regions of the early region of NCR, also known as long control region (LCR) or upstream regulatory region (URR).

LR includes two ORFs (L1 and L2, which encode the viral primary capsid protein L1 and the secondary capsid protein L2, respectively. The genetically engineered L1 and L1 + L2 proteins have self-assembling properties that can be assembled in eukaryotic cells. Virus-like particle (VLP) contains no viral nucleic acid and its conformation and antigenicity are similar to that of natural HPV particles, which can induce the body to produce neutralizing antibodies. The E region contains 7 early ORFs (E1-E7), proteins involved in viral replication, transcriptional regulation, translation and cell transformation. The E1 and E2 proteins are the basis of viral replication and are involved in transcriptional regulation. The E2 protein enhances the regulation of LCR and the transcription of early genes (E6, E7). E5, E6, E7 are transformants and the encoded proteins can bind to p53 and pRB proteins. E1 and E4 can degrade keratin and cause the collapse of cytoskeleton and cell transformation. According to the different nucleotide sequences of the virus, it has been found that HPV has more than 200 types based on the DNA homology between the various types.

HPV has high tropism for skin and mucosal epithelial cells. The proliferating virus can only be found in the nucleus of the upper layer of the skin. Only low copies of the viral nucleic acid are found in the basal layer cells. The early gene is located in the spinous cell layer. The late gene expression (capsid protein) is defined as the uppermost layer of epithelial cells. The viral DNA replication occurs mainly in the epidermal-spongiosa and granulosa layers and induces epithelial proliferation, epidermal thickening, accompanied by spike cell proliferation and epidermal keratosis. Epithelial proliferation forms papillomas, also known as warts. An episome of the viral DNA can often be inserted anywhere in the host chromosome, leading to cell transformation. Because HPV replication needs to rely on epithelial cytokines closely related to the stage of cell differentiation and so on, so far it can not be cultured in conventional tissue cells.

9.10.3.2　Pathogenicity

According to different tissue tropism, HPV infection can be divided into two types, those infecting skin and those addicted to skin mucosa and there is a certain overlap between these two categories. Skin damage caused by UV or X-ray radiation and skin and mucous membrane damage caused by other physical and chemical factors can create similar conditions for HPV infection. Spread occurs mainly through direct contact with infected parts of the lesion or indirect contact with the virus contaminated items. Genital tract infections are closely related to recent sexual behaviors. The infectivity rate of HPV is positively correlated with the number of sexual partners. Therefore, HPV is the causative agent of sexually transmitted diseases and causes genital tract infections, which are categorized as sexually transmitted diseases (STD). Mothers with genital tract HPV infection can cause neonatal infection through vertical transmission between mother and child during childbirth.

Due to the large number of types of HPVs, it causes infections in different parts of the body, including skin warts, plantar warts, genital warts and laryngeal papilloma, other than infections related to STD including cervical cancer. Skin warts, including both common wart (serotype 2&4) and plantar warts (serotype 1), are mostly self-limiting and cause transient damages and the virus persists in only localized skin and mucous membranes, producing no viremia. Types 1, 2, 3 and 4 mainly cause epithelial cell infection of the hands and feet keratosis, causing common warts, more commonly in adolescence. Type 7 usually infects the butcher's and butcher's hand's skin, causing the warty eruptions. Flat warts are often caused by type 3 and type 10, which are more common in adolescent's face, back and forearm.

Condyloma acuminatum is mainly caused by genital warts (HPW) infected with HPV-6 and HPV-11. It belongs to sexually transmitted diseases and its incidence rate has been increasing year by year. Female infection is mainly on vaginal labia and cervix, whereas in males it is more common in the external genitalia, perianal and other parts. Condyloma rarely leads to carcinogenesis, so HPV-6 and HPV-11 are a low-risk HPVs. HPV-6 and HPV-11 types can also cause laryngeal papillomas in infants, which is considered although a benign tumor, but can also be serious due to obstruction of the airways and life-threatening complications.

Cervical cancer and other reproductive tract cancer are mainly associated with multiple types of high-risk HPV infections of the cervix, vulva, penis and other reproductive tract. Intraepithelial neoplasia, on long-term development can become a malignant tumor, the most common is cervical cancer. The most relevant types that causes cervical cancer are HPV types 16 and 18, followed by types 31, 45, 33, 35, 39, 51, 52 and 56. HPV-57b cause nasal benign and malignant tumor, HPV-12, 32 types may lead to oral cancer.

At present, it is considered that HPV infection is normal in cervical squamous epithelium and is the initiating factor of cervical cancer. After a latent period of HPV infection, the expression of E6 and E7 genes are increased and they are combined with p53 andpRB protein respectively to promote the degradation and block p53 and pRB. Negative regulation of the cell cycle induces cell immortalization to transform infected cells. Of course, HPV infection is not the only factor of cervical cancer occurrence, such as host gene mutation during infection or wild-type p53 gene mutation or other factors in the environment affect the occurrence and development of cervical cancer. Human papillomavirus transform by the same mechanisms as employed by other DNA viruses: inactivation of tumor suppressor proteins.

9.10.3.3 Microbiological Examination

HPV infection with typical clinical damage can be quickly diagnosed based on clinical manifestations or presence ofkoilocytic cells in Pap smears, but subclinical infection is required for tissue immunology and molecular biology laboratory testing.

(1)Nucleic Acid Testing

HPV typing and laboratory diagnosis is done by DNA hybridization, typically using HPV consensus or type-specific probes that can detect about 50 copies of HP genome in tissue; and in situ hybridization on tissue sections could detect each group of cells having a minimum of 10−15 copies of the viral gene. HPV DNA-specific conservative regions were designed for PCR amplification of various types of primers. The use of specific probe hybridization in detection of amplification products of HPV infection is a rapid diagnostic method with high specificity and sensitivity.

(2)Serological Test

The VP-ELSA method was designed by using the synthetic antigenic epitope of the viral protein or the genetically engineered HPV-like particle as the antigen. The antibody in the patient's serum can be detected by the Western blotting using the expressed fusion protein as an antigen.

9.10.3.4 Prevention and Control Measures

Local drug treatment (salicylic acid) or freezing, electrocautery, laser, surgery and other therapies can effectively removemucocutaneous common warts and genital warts. Human papillomavirus virus-like particle vaccine (HPV-VLP Vaccines), including bivalent (HPV-16,18) and tetravalent (HPV-6,11,16,18) vaccines, have a prophylactic effect on cervical cancer and genital warts. A recombinant vaccine is now available containing antigens from HPV 6,11,16 and 18 which is indicated in adolescents and young adult women, but contraindicated in pregnancy. They are recommended for women who are 9 to 25 year old and have not been exposed to HPV. However, since it is unlikely that a woman will have already contracted all four viruses and because HPV is primarily sexually transmitted, the U. S. Centers for Disease Control and Prevention has recommended vaccination for women up to 26 years of age. Since the vaccine only covers some high-risk types of HPV, cervical cancer screening by routine Pap smears beginning at age 21 is recommended even after vaccination. Additional vaccine candidate research is occurring for next generation products to extend protection against additional HPV types. The protection against HPV 16 and 18 has lasted at least 8 years after vaccination for Gardasil and more than 9 years for Cervarix. It is thought that booster vaccines will not be necessary.

9.10.4 Poxvirus

The poxvirus belongs to the Poxviridae family and causes natural infection in humans and many vertebrates. They are distinguished by their large size, complex morphology and cytoplasmic site of replication. Among them, Variola virus and Molluscum contagiosum virus (MCV), Monkeypox virus, Cowpox virus and other animal poxviruses can cause human infection.

9.10.4.1 Structure

Poxvirus is the largest virus and its structure is the most complex. It is brick-shaped or oval-shaped [(300−450) nm × 260 nm × 170 nm]. The protein capsid composed of more than 30 kinds of structural proteins and is in a compound symmetrical form. The virus core consists of Double-stranded linear DNA (130−375 kb) and consists of 1−2 lateral bodies on either side of the virus core (biconcave). Poxviruses proliferate in the infected cytoplasm. Viral genome contains about 185 ORFs, which guide the synthesis of more than 200 viral proteins. Mature virus is released in budding form.

9.10.4.2 Transcription

A defining characteristic of the virus is their ability to carry out both transcription and DNA replication in the cytoplasm rather than the nucleus of their host cells. They do this by encoding all the necessary enzymes and factors rather than using those in the nucleus of the infected cell. They do, however, rely on their host for the cellular machinery of translation and for the precursor metabolites for all the processes of the Central Dogma. Transcription of the poxvirus early genes begins as soon as the viral core is released in the cytoplasm of an infected cell.

9.10.4.3 Replication

Early studies of poxvirus replication indicated that concatemers were formed as part of the process, leading to the notion that genome, whose unique conformation might permit it to open into a single stranded circular form, was copied by a form of rolling circle replication. Sequence analysis of the concatemers showed that the unit genomes were not linked "head to tail" as rolling circle replication would produce, however, but instead were "head to head" and "tail to tail".

9.10.4.4 Maturation

Poxvirus have very complex structures that include several membrane layers. These membranes appear to be derived from the sides of the Golgi complex by a process that does not involve budding. Virion maybe released by cell lysis or by exocytosis through the cytoplasmic membrane.

9.10.4.5 Sources

The source of infection of poxvirus are infected humans or animals, mainly through inhalation of air-borne variola virus, usually droplets expressed from the oral, nasal or mucosa of an infected person. Human poxvirus infections include smallpox, human monkeypox and molluscum contagiosum.

1) Smallpox was a potent infectious disease caused by smallpox virus (variola virus) and has been widely prevalent around the world. Smallpox virus infection, which was mainly spread through the respiratory tract and direct contact, causing high fever, blisters or pustules on the face and whole body and has a high case fatality rate. Some patients with healed scabs have obvious de-pigmented scarring on the face and other parts. In 1977, the Global Smallpox eradication program was launched by the World Health Organization (WHO) and by 1980 it was declared to be eradicated. Variola has 1 serotype, which made eradication possible. At present, attention is being paid to the non-immune community of the population by means of planned immunization, which can lead to stop the variola from becoming a potential biological weapon. It is diagnosed by finding Guarnieri bodies (intracytoplasmic inclusions) in infected cells.

2) The humanmonkeypox has similar clinical manifestations as that of smallpox, although it is often milder. It is characterized by high fever, muscle pains, swollen lymph nodes and systemic blisters and pustules, accompanied by bleeding tendency with a mortality rate of about 11%. The virus is mainly spread due to contact with wild animals (Prairie dogs, etc.) or animal bites or close contact with an infected person. The earliest cases were seen in Africa Zaire, but in recent years few cases in the United States and other places have also been recorded.

3) Cowpox is a mild skin blister-like change caused by cowpox virus. It is caused by close contact with milking workers, generally without serious systemic infection. The vaccinia virus is cross-immunogenic with VACV and is used primarily for the planned immunization of smallpox. Vaccination usually causes mild skin reactions only at the site of vaccination, but may cause severe progressive vaccinia, post-vaccine encephalitis and dilatation in susceptible populations who are immunocompromised and other diseases. Currently, vaccinia virus is widely used as a model for studying the gene regulation of poxvirus or as a carrier for expressing foreign proteins.

4) Molluscum contagiosum is caused by the Molluscum contagiosum virus (MCV) that results in small, raised, pink lesions with a depression in the center. Mainly transmitted through direct contact, fomites or contaminated objects. Human is its only host for infection, more common seen in children. The virus can also be transmitted through sexual contact, causing genital wart molluscum. Soft warts can subside on their own, leaving no scar. It is diagnosed when eosinophilic cytoplasmic inclusion bodies are found in the infec-

ted cells.

Immunization: Immunization by vaccinia virus can prevent smallpox, human monkeypox, although at present it is only used for high-risk groups' inoculation. Generally it is not used during large-scale vaccination as the impenetrable capsid doesn't allow further studies. Injecting vaccinia immunoglobulin (VIG) can get a good passive immune effect. Vaccinia vaccination is recommended for laboratory workers who directly handle cultures or animal infected with:

- Non-highly attenuated vaccinia virus strains.
- Recombinant vaccinia virus from non-highly attenuated vaccinia virus strains.
- Other orthopox virus that can infect humans.

9.10.5 Rabies Virus

The Rabies virus is an enveloped virus with a single stranded RNA genome classified under family*Rhabdoviridae*, genus *Lyssavirus* (Lyssa, meaning rage, a synonym for rabies). Rabies virus is a neurotropic virus that causes rabies in humans and animals. Rabies has been recognized since ancient times as a disease transmitted to humans and animals by the bite of 'mad dogs'. The name rabies comes from the Latin word 'rabidus' meaning 'mad'. The disease in human beings is called 'hydrophobia' because the patient exhibits fear of water, being incapable of drinking though subject to intolerable thirst(Figure 9-21).

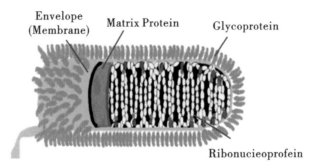

Figure 9-21　Bullet shaped structure of Rabies Virus

Rabies virus is bullet shaped, 180 nm×75 nm in size, with one end rounded and the other end planar or concave. The lipoprotein envelope carries knob-like spikes, composed of glycoprotein G, which is important in pathogenesis, virulence and immunity. Glycoprotein G mediates the binding of the virus to acetylcholine receptors in neural tissues, induces hemagglutination inhibiting (HI) and neutralizing antibodies. Moreover, purified Glycoprotein may act as a safe and effective subunit vaccine.

Spikes do not cover the planar end of thevirion and may be released from the envelope by treatment with lipid solvents or detergents, beneath the envelope is the membrane or matrix (M) protein layer which may be invaginated at the planar end and projects outwards from the planar end of some virions forming a bleb. The core of the virion consists of helically arranged ribonucleoprotein (RNP). The genome is an unsegmented, linear, negative sense RNA. Also present in the nucleocapsid are RNA-dependent RNA transcriptase and some structural proteins. The genetic information is packaged as a RNP complex in which RNA is tightly bound by the viral nucleoprotein. The genome of the virus encodes five genes whose order is highly conserved. These genes code for nucleoprotein (N), phosphoprotein (P), matrix protein (M), glycoprotein (G) and the viral RNA polymerase (L).

The complete genome sequences range from 11,615 to 11,966 nucleotide in length. All transcription and replication events take place in the cytoplasm inside a specialized "virus factory", theNegri body

(named after Adelchi Negri). These are $2-10$ μm in diameter, intracytoplasmic, basophilic inclusion bodies typical for a rabies infection and thus used in definite diagnosis of cases by making histopathological brain impression smears stained by Seller's technique (basic fuchsin and methylene blue in methanol).

Rabies transmission can occur through the saliva of animals during their bite and the virus present in the saliva of animal is deposited in the wound. Rarely, infection may also occur following non-bite exposures such as licks or aerosols or transplantation of cornea or other virus infected tissues. The virus then appears to multiply in muscles, connective tissues or nerve at the site of deposition for 2 to 3 days. It then penetrates the nerve endings and travels passively in theaxoplasm towards the spinal cord and brain, at a speed of 3mm per hour. The infection spreads centripetally from the axon to the neural bodies and progressively up the spinal cord through the synapses of the neurons. The virus then ascends rapidly to the brain, multiplies and spreads centrifugally along the nerve trunks to various parts of the body including the salivary glands, where it multiplies again and shed through saliva.

Rabies disease in human beings is called "hydrophobia" because the patient exhibits fear of water, being incapable of drinking though subject to intolerable thirst. Rabies in animals is not called hydrophobia because they do not have this peculiar feature. In humans the incubation period is usually from $1-3$ months, though it may be as short as 7 days or as long as three years. The incubation period is usually short in persons infected through bite on face or head and long in those bitten on the legs. The course of he disease in humans is classified into four stages-prodromal stage, acute encephalitis phase, coma and death. The onset is marked by prodromal symptoms such as fever, headache, malaise, fatigue and anorexia. An early symptom is often a neuritic pain or paresthesia and fasciculation at the site of virus entry. Apprehension, anxiety, agitation, irritability, nervousness, insomnia or depression characterize the prodromal phase which usually lasts $2-4$ days. Excessive libido, priapism and spontaneous ejection may occur rarely. Acute neurological phase usually begins with hyperactivity, with bouts of bizzare behavior, agitation or seizures appearing between apparently normal periods. The pathognomonic feature is difficulty in drinking, together with intense thirst. Patients may be able to swallow dry solids but not liquids. Attempts to drink bring on painful spasms of the pharynx and larynx producing chocking or gagging that patients develop a dread of even sight or sound of water. Generalized convulsions follow. Death usually occurs within $1-6$ days due to respiratory arrest during convulsions.

Rabies virus, like manyrhabdoviruses, has an extremely wide host range. All animals are susceptible to rabies infection, though differences in susceptibility exists between species. Cattle, cats and foxes are highly susceptible, whereas shunks, opposums and fowl are relatively resistant. Humans and dogs are intermediately susceptible, whereas pups are more susceptible than adult dogs.

In the wild it has been found infecting many mammalian species, while in the laboratory it has been found that birds can be infected, as well as cell cultures from mammals, birds, reptiles and insects. The method most commonly used for diagnosis is the demonstration of rabies virus antigens by immunofluorescence. The specimens tested are corneal smears and skin biopsy or salivaantemortem and brain postmortem. Direct immunofluorescence is done using anti-rabies serum tagged with fluorescein isothiocyanate. The vaccination that can be administered at the time of animal bite is neural vaccine. These are suspensions of nervous tissues of animals infected with the fixed rabies virus. The earliest was Pasteur's cord vaccine prepared by drying over caustic potash, for varying periods, pieces of infected rabbit spinal cord. It has to be given in 3 doses and patient is to be observed for another 10 days.

Chapter 10

Mycology

10.1　Superficial Mycoses

Superficial mycoses are a kind of diseases which caused by some fungi after their invasion into the superficial keratinized tissues such as the epidermis of our skin, hairs or beard, etc. It includes pityriasis versicolor, tinea nigra and piedra, etc.

10.1.1　Pityriasis Versicolor

Pityriasis versicolor is caused by the infection of *Malassezia*. It was named by its discrete, serpentine, hyper or hypopigmented maculae on the skin of the chest, upper back, arms or abdomen. The lesions(Figure 10-1) are chronic and occur as macular patches of discolored skin that may enlarge and coalesce, but scaling, inflammation and irritation are minimal. Indeed, the common affliction is largely a cosmetic problem. There were some short, coarse and branching nonseptate hyphae and groups of yeast-like cells observed in the specimens from the lesion in microscopic detection. Because *Malasseizia furfur* is lipophilic, some olive oils were added into the media to satisfy *Malasseizia furfur* growth. The colonies are usually yeast type colonies. The inducing factors are high gas temperature and sweat, so pityriasis versicoloro ccurs mostly in summer. In the prevention of pityriasis versicolor, good personal hygiene is the most important such as changing and washing clothes in time, the disinfection of clothes, etc. Some creams of antifungal agents are often used in the treatment of pityriasis versicolor in clinic such as clotrimazole, ketoconazole, etc.

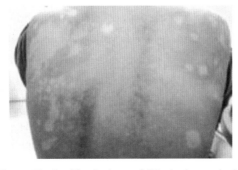

Figure 10-1　The lesions of Pityriasis versicolor

10.1.2 Tinea Nigra

Tinea nigra(or tinea nigra palmaris) occurring mainly in the tropics is a superficial phaeohyphomycosis caused by the dematiaceous fungus *Hottaea(Exophiala) werneckii*, the main pathogens of Tinea nigra in Europe and America and *Microsporum mansonii*, the main pathogens of tinea nigra in Asia and Africa. These two fungi may be free-living in nature and human can be infected by contact with them. This disease occurs more often in young women and is a chronic and asymptomatic infection. The lesions appear as a dark (brown to black) discoloration, often on the palm. At first the lesions appear as light brown spots and then spread all around. Some fuse together. The skin in lesions is smooth and appears as dark color. Occasionally, there is a slight keratinization of the lesion, with a slight keratinized dander edge and a darker color. *Microsporum mansonii* are often in the lesions in the neck and chest and *Hottaea(Exophiala) werneckii* often in the palm. Microscopic examination of skin scrapings from the periphery of the lesion will reveal branched, brown irregular septate hyphae and budding yeast-like cells with melaninized cell walls for *Hottaea(Exophiala) werneckii* and brown slim septate hyphae with no branches and some round or oval microconidia on the side and the top of hyphae for *Microsporum mansonii*. Tinea nigra will respond to treatment with imidazole creams, keratolytic solutions, etc.

10.1.3 Piedra

Piedra is also called as nodular trichomycosis. It is a kind of fungal infection disease of the hair and beard. Black piedra is a nodular infection of the hair shaft caused by *Piedraia hortai*. White piedra, due to infection of *Trichosporon* species, presents as larger, softer, yellowish nodules on the hairs. Axillary, pubic, beard and scalp hair may be infected. There are some dark brown, branching septate hyphae and ascuses within 4–8 spindle ascospores in the nodules of black piedra and some light green hypae around the hair shaft which separate into several oval or rectangle-shaped spores in the nodules of white piedra. Treatments for both of them are to remove the hair and the application of a topical antifungal agent.

10.2 Cutaneous Mycoses

Cutaneous mycoses are a kind of fungal infection diseases in which just the superficial kerantinized tissue(skin, hair and nails) is infected by corresponding fungi. The most important pathogens of these are the dermatophytes which can be identified from each other usually by the properties of their colonies and their spores, a group of about 40 species that belong to 3 genera: *Epidermophyton*, *Trichophyton* and *Microsporum*.

10.2.1 Biological Characterization of Dermatophytes

Epidermophyton, *Trichophyton* and *Microsporum* all belong to imperfect fungi. There is just one specie of *Epidermophyton-Epidermophyton floccosum* which is pathogenic to humans and can infect skin and nails, but not hair, resulting in tinea corporis, tinea pedis, tinea manus, tinea cruris and tinea unguium, etc. The optimum temperature of *Epidermophyton floccosum* in Sabouraud's agar is room temperature or 28 ℃. After cultivation, it produces a waxy colony at first and lastly a powdery colony. While the color of the colony changes from white to yellowish green. There are some rod-shaped macroconidia which are smooth thin-walled, 3–5 cells and formed in groups of two or three and no microconidium (Figure 10–2). The hypha is septate mycelium and fine. Occasionally a racquet, nodular or spiral hyphae can be seen.

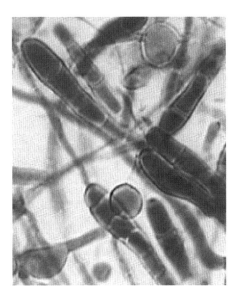

Figure 10-2   *Epidermophyton flocco-sum*(400×)

There are twenty more species in *Trichophyton* and thirteen being pathogenic to humans which can infect skin, hairs and nails. After being cultivated in Sabouraud's agar, the colonial appearance of *Trichophyton* varies between different species. Colonies of *Trichophyton mentagrophytes* may be velvety to granular; Both types display abundant grape-like clusters of spherical microconidia on terminal branches. Coiled or spiral hyphae are commonly found in primary isolates. The typical colony of *Trichophyton rubrum* has a white, velvety surface and a deep red, nondiffusible pigment when viewed from the reverse side of the colony. The microconidia are small and piriform (pear-shaped). *Trichophyton tonsurans* produces a flat, powdery to velvety colony on the obverse surface that becomes reddish-brown on reverse; The microconidia are mostly elongate.

Members in *Microsporum* are mostly pathogenic and can infect only hair and skin. The common pathogenic ones include *Microsporum ferrugineum*, *Microsporum canis* and *Microsporum gypsseum*, etc. *Microsporum* species tend to produce distinctive multicellular macroconidia with echinulate walls. Both types of conidia are borne singly in these genera. *Microsporum canis* forms a colony with a white cottony surface and a deep yellow color on reverse; the thick-walled, 8-to 15-celled macroconidia frequently have curved or hooked tips. *Microsporum gypseum* produces a tan, powdery colony and abundant thin-walled, 4-to 6-celled macroconidia.

10.2.2   Pathogenesis and Immunity of Dermatophytes

Dermatophytes are mainly found in soil, animal and human body or on the surface of animal or human skin or the appendages of skin such as hair and nails. Dermatophytes infect the hosts after trauma and contact. There is evidence that host susceptibility may be enhanced by moistuer, warmth, specific skin chemistry, composition of sebum and perspiration, youth, heavy exposure and genetic predisposition. When dermatophytes grow and reproduce in infected tissue, lesions and inflammation can be caused by mechanical stimulation and metabolic products of fungi. Many patients who develop chronic, noninflammatory dermatophyte infections have poor cell-mediated immune responses to dermatophyte antigen. These patients often are atopic and have immediated-type hypersensitivity and elevated IgE concentrations. In the normal host, immunity to dermatophytosis varies in duration and degree depending on the host, the site and the species of fungus causing the infection.

10.2.3 Clinical Findings

Dermatophyte infections of skin and the appendages are usually called as tinea because of the raised circular lesions. A dermatophyte can result in a variety of tinea and a tinea may be caused by several dermatophytes. Table 10-1 lists different tineas and their pathogens.

Table 10-1　Dermatophytosis of the skin and the common fungus in its skin lesions

Dermatophytosis	E. floccosum	M. canis	T. mentagrophytes	T. rubrum	T. tonsurans
Tinea corporis		+	+	+	+
Tinea unguium	+		+		
Tinea cruris	+		+	+	
Tinea capitis		+	+		+
Tinea barbae			+	+	
Tinea pedis	+		+	+	

"+" means positive, margin means negative

10.2.3.1　Tinea Capitis

Tinea capitis(Figure 10-3) is the infection of the scalp and hair caused by dermatophytes. It includes favus, microsporosis capitis, trichophytosis capitis, kerion.

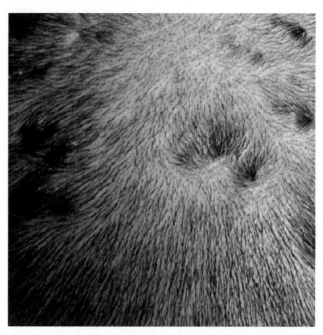

Figure 10-3　The lesions of Tinea capitis

(1) Favus

Favus is the infection of scalp and hair caused by *Trichophyton schoenleinli*. It is the most serious one of tinea capitis. After the infection of the head, it begins to form a pinpointed, light yellowish-red dot under epidermis and then develop into light yellow scabs which are higher on the edge and vary from each other in size. In the scabs, there are a large number of pathogenic fungi and one to several hairs which is rough and dull, being easily broken and shed. Favus patients companied by kerion are rare.

(2) Microsporosis Capitis

Microsporosis capitis is fungal infection of scalp and the peripheral of hair root. A variety of members in *Microsporum* and *Trichophyton* are responsible for the forming of microsporosis capitis. The main ones are *Microsporum canis* and *Microsporum ferrugineum*. Microsporosis capitis occurs often in children and teenagers, seldomly in infants and adults. The incidence is higher in boys than in girls. This disease can be self-healing after adulthood. The reason may be that the pH value of adult scalp is not suitable for the growth of pathogenic fungi. In the early, the rash of microsporosis capitis appeared as dandruff, small red papules with some hairs growing out from it. And then papules developed into spherical or oval white patch. The hairs were weakened and easily broken. The hairs in lesions show a greenish to silvery fluorescence examined under Wood's light. Zoophilic species result in more obvious inflammation than anthropophilic species and even resulting in kerion.

(3) Trichophytosis Capitis

Trichophytosis capitis is the fungal infection of scalp and hair caused by anthropophilic *Trichophyton*, the most important being *Trichophyton violaceum* and *Trichophyton tosurans*. It occurs usually in children at first. It would be a chronic disease from the childhood to adulthood if being untreated. Adults can be infected by contact with the pathogens. The incidence in men is similar to that in women. At first the lesions appear as small papules and dander spots with slightly itching feeling. The lesions are usually scattered all over and it is easily to be ignored. With the development of the disease, the lesions will become larger gradually. Different from microsporosis capitis, the pathogens of trichophytosis capitis produce spores within the hair shaft(endothrix) and no fluorescence in Woodlight.

(4) Kerion

Kerion can be caused by many dermatophytes, especially those zoophilic fungi because they can induce a severe hypersensitivity reaction. It is usually characterized by pyogenic infection of the hair follicle. The hairs in the lesion are easily to be removed, forming permanent hair loss. After healing, scars can be left.

10.2.3.2 Tinea Corporis

Tinea corporis is the fungal infection of the skin except hands, feet and perineum. Almost all dermatophytes can cause tinea corporis, but only a few of them in which *Trichophyton rubrum* is the absolute dominant strain in the global are the pathogens of tinea corporis in clinic. The incidence of tinea corporis may be influenced by climatic conditions, patient's age and immunity and sanitary conditions, etc. Tinea corporis is either primary infection or secondary infection of other tinea. After pathogenic fungi entered the epidermis, they colonized in the cuticle with keratin as nutrients and resulted in mild inflammatory response. The typical syndrome of tinea corporis is that some red papules or small blisters appear at first, followed by the forming of dandruff and then spreading around to form circular lesions with clear edge. With the spreading of the lesion's edge, the state of skin in the centre come back to the common gradually. The appearance of lesions varies from different pathogens.

10.2.3.3 Tinea Cruris

Tinea cruris is actually a kind of tinea corporis. It is listed out alone just because of its especial lesion location(the inner of thigh, perineum and hip) and special notices in treatment. *Trichophyton rubrum* and *Trichophyton mentagrohytes* are the main pathogens of tinea cruris. The clinical manifestation is similar to tinea corporis.

10.2.3.4 Tinea Manus

Tinea manus is the fungal infection of hands' skin. Same as tinea cruris and tinea pedis, the main pathogens of tinea manus are also *Trichophyton rubrum* and *Trichophyton mentagrohytes*. Compared to tinea pedis, the incidence of tinea manus is lower and tinea manus occurs often in one side with fewer complications. There are more mistakes in diagnosis of tinea manus than tinea pedis because of its atypical lesions and unsatisfying laboratory diagnosis-low positive rate of detection. The main clinical manifestations include blisters, papules, dandruff, itching, eczema like changes, etc. There are four clinical types: blister type, dandruff type, keratinized thickening type and erosion type.

10.2.3.5 Tinea Pedis

Tinea pedis is a kind of chronic fungal infection of feet skin. The incidence of tinea pedis is the highest in all tineas. The primary lesions often occur between the toes. The main clinical manifestations are blisters, dandruff and itching, etc. Sometimes, it can also cause the complications such as erysipelas, cellulitis and lymphangitis, etc. There are five clinical typesof tinea pedis: blister type, papule dandruff type, impregnated erosion type, excessive keratinization type and mixed type.

10.2.3.6 Tinea Unguium(Onychomycosis)

Tinea unguium(Onychomycosis)may follow prolonged tinea pedis. Almost all fungi can invade nails. Dermatophytes, yeasts and molds are the main pathogens of tinea unguium. With fungal hyphal invasion, the nails become yellow, brittle and thickened. One or more of feet or hands may be involved. There are five types in clinic: superficial white onychomycosis, distal lateral subungual onychomycosis, proximal subungual onychomycosis, endoonyx onychomycosis and total dystrophic onychomycosis.

10.2.4 Laboratory Diagnosis

Scrapings from the lesions in the skin or nails and hairs involved in lesions are usually used as examination specimens. The specimen will be mixed with a 10% solution of potassium hydroxide preparation and place it under a coverslip. After observation under microscope, the discovery of fungal hyphae and spores can preliminarily make sure of dermatophytes infection. Cultivation of specimens in Sabouraud's agar will be necessary for further identification of fungal species. The properties of colony and the morphological properties of hyphae and spores are helpful to the identification of fungal genera and species.

10.2.5 Treatment

Therapy consists of thorough removal of infected and dead epithelial structures which can avoid further damage and help antifungal agents play their roles better and application of a topical antifungal chemical or antibiotic. To prevent reinfection, the area should be kept dry and sources of infection, such as an infected pet or shared bathing facilities, should be avoided. The treatment of dermatophytoses includes topical and oral administration. Griseofulvin and itraconazole are effective for most of them. For tinea unguium, besides surgical removal of the nail, months of oral itraconazole or terbinafine treatment is necessary.

10.3 Subcutaneous Mycoses

Sporothrix and dematiaceous fungi normally resided in soil or on vegetation are the main two which can cause subcutaneous mycoses. They enter the skin or subcutaneous tissue by traumatic inoculation with contaminated material. In general, they usually grow and reproduce in area of implantation and result in local lesions. But with the development of disease, they can also expand slowly via blood flow or lymph circulation and result in systemic infection and life-threatening disease.

10.3.1   Sporotrichosis

Sporothrix schenckii is the main pathogen of sporotrichosis. *Sporothrix schenckii* is a kind of dimorphic fungus. It appears as molds in nature and yeast-type in the host. It is a kind of saprophytic fungus found in water, soil and plants. They enter the host usually by the trauma resulted from plants' thorns. Besides, they can also come from some rodents. The lesion appears as a slight nodular lump in the trauma at first. And the lump develop into a ulcer, forming a chronic granulomatous infection gradually. The draining lymphatics and lymph nodes can be involved. Besides specific clinical manifestation, the culture of pus or tissue specimens is necessary to the diagnosis. After gram stain, there were some spindle, oval gram positive cells most located in neutrophils or large monocytes. They can also be identified by fluorescent antibody staining. After 3−5 days cultivation in Sabouraud's agar, white colony can be observed. With further cultivation, the color of colony turns into brown gradually and black at last. In microscopic examination of the culture, filamentous fungi with septate hyphae may be seen and there are many pear-shaped or oval microconidia in groups on both sides of mycelium (Figure 10−4). Being free from trauma and good treatment of the wound are effective preventive methods. Cutaneous and lymphatic sporotrichosis can be treated with oral potassium iodide or itraconazole. And the deep infection can be treated with amphotericin B.

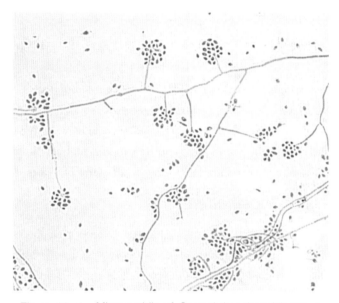

Figure 10−4   Microconidia of *Sporothrix schenckii*(400×)

10.3.2   chromomycosis

Chromomycosis is a variety of disease caused by the pathogenic fungi in dematiaceous fungi. These fungi most are saprophytes and commonly reside in soil and plants. The main pathogenic ones include *Cladosporium corrionii*, *Fonsecaea pedrosoi* and *Phialophora verrucosa*, etc. They usually enter the hosts by wounds. Infection occurs in the exposed parts of skin such as face and limbs, characterized by the changes of skin color of the lesion. They can also invade deep tissue or organs, appeared as chronic infection process. When the body's immunity is low, it can invade the central nervous system and cause infection in the brain. In the infected skin there are some papules appeared at first. And the papules enlarge gradually into nodules. With further development of the nodules, they fuse together appearing as wart-shaped or papilloma-shaped and dark red or black. Because of reoccurence and development of lesions, the lymph circulation would be influenced and it resulted in elephantiasis in limbs. Under direct microscopic examination, brown branching septate hyphae can be seen. On the side or the top of braches, conidiophore can be formed and there are some brown spherical or oval conidia on them. Its dendrite-shaped, sword-apex-shaped and vase-shaped conidia are the important basis for the identification of this fungus. Being free from trauma and good treatment of the wound are important in prevention. Surgical excision with wide margins is the therapy of choice for small lesions. Chemotherapy with flucytosine or itraconazole may be efficacious for larger lesions.

10.3.3　Mycetoma

Mycetoma appears as a localized abscess, usually on the feet, but is not limited to the lower extremity. The abscess discharge pus, serum and blood through sinuses (sinus means "abnormal channel" here). The infection can spread to the underlying bone and results in crippling deformities. The pathogens are various soil fungi. Most common are *Madurella grisea* and *Exophiala jeanselmei*. Mycetomas appear similar to the lesion of chromomycosis, but the defining characteristic of mycetoma is the presence of colored granules, composed of compacted hyphae, in the exudate. The color of the granules (black, white, red or yellow) is characteristic of the causative organism and, therefore, useful in identifying the particular pathogen. There is no effective chemotherapy for fungal mycetoma. Treatment is usually surgical excision.

10.4　Endemic Mycoses

Fungi which can cause endemic mycoses include *Histoplasma capsulatum*, *Coccidiodes immitis*, *Blastomyces dermatitidis* and *Paracoccidioides brasiliensis*. In recent years, it has been proved that *Penicillium marneffei* can cause extensive, disseminated infection (more commonly in AIDS patients) in Southeast Asia. They are all dimorphic fungus. In nature or 25-30 ℃ experimental condition, they exist in the form of molds. And in tissue or 37 ℃ culture condition, they exist in the form of yeasts.

10.4.1　*Histoplasma Capsulatum*

Histoplasma capsulatum is a dimorphic soil saprophyte that causes histoplasmosis. *Histoplasma capsulatum* enters the host mainly by respiratory inhale of fungal spores. At first it infects oral macrophages and cause local granulomas. Most of *Histoplasma capsulatum* infections are inapparent infection and just a few can result in histoplasmosis (pulmonary chronic infectons and systemic disseminated infections). Histoplasmosis are more common in the old men or immunocompromised patients. Direct smear examination, the culture of fungi and histopathological examination are helpful for the diagnosis. Under microscope, yeast-like cells may be seen. After 6-8 weeks' cultivation under 25-30 ℃ in Sabouraud's agar, white or light yellow colony may be observed. The hyphae are septate hypha. Most fungi have specific gear-shaped macroconidia. Besides mycological examination, serological examination can also be used in the diagnosis. ELISA and radioimmunoassay can be used in the detection of polysaccharide antigens. Compliment fixation and immunodiffusion can be used in the detection of antibody. The method of serological diagnosis is rapid, but it is important to take notice of cross reactions. Histoplasmin skin test is commonly used in epidemiological investigations. Ketoconazole is commonly used in the treatment and the patients with severe illness can choose amphotericin B.

10.4.2　*Coccidioides Immites*

The life cycle of *Coccidioides immites* consists of hyphae, arthrospores and spheres. In nature or common media, *Coccidioides immites* produce septate hyphae and arthrospores. In tissue or some special media, arthrospores develop into sphere filled with endospores. Coccidioides immites usually reside in soil. Human can be infected by inhalation of spores. The initial stage is mainly pulmonary infection and the properties of pathology are characterized by acute, subacute or chronic granulomatous reactions accompanied by various fibrosis. For most of us, primary pulmonary infection can be cured by a therapy without anti-fungal agents. But for immunocompromised patients, fungi can spread to the extrapulmonary tissue and cause diseases of extrapulmonry tissue. At the same time, there may be complications such as pulmonary nodules, hollows and purulent pneumothorax, etc. In the direct smear examination of tissue specimens under microscope, the detection of the endospore-filled sphere can make sure of the diagnosis. The patients can be treated with amphotericin B and ketoconazole.

10.4.3   *Blastomyces Dermatitides* and *Paracoccidioides Brasiliensis*

Blastomyces dermatitides and *Paracoccidioides brasiliensis* both are the thermally dimorphic fungal agents of blastomycosis and paracoccidioidomycosis (South American blastomycosis), which are confined to endemic regions of Central and South America. They both infect the hosts by pulmonary inhalation.

For *Paracoccidioides brasiliensis* infection, over 95% patients are men. After a period of dormancy that may last for decades, the pulmonary granulomas may become active, leading to chronic, progressive pulmonary disease or dissemination. According to the clinical manifestations, the paracoccidioidomycosis can be classified into the skin mucosa paracoccidioidomycosis and paracoccidioidomycosis of viscera. In skin mucosa type, the pathogens enter by oral mucosa or skin. The lesions occur initially in the gingival, upper palate and tongue, etc. Skin lesions usually come from the spreading of mucosal lesions or from the blood spreading or from the burst of superficial lymph nodes, forming ulcer. The lesions are often in the face and more commonly in the nose or around the mouth. For viscera type, primary infections are mostly in the lung. Patients may appear as hypodynamia, high fever, chest pain, dyspnea and cough, etc. If pulmonary infection is secondary infection of other lesions, the clinical symptoms of lung may be very mild. The lesions of digestive tract infection are mostly in ileocecum. The intestines may have extensive ulcers accompanied by abdominal pain, nausea, vomiting, hepatosplenomegaly and enlarged lymph nodes, etc. The pathogens can disseminate and result in systemic infection. Laboratory diagnosis includes direct microscopic examination and culture. *Paracoccidioides brasiliensis* appears as yeast-type colony cultivated at 37 ℃ and filamentous colony at 25 ℃. Large, multiply budding yeast cells in tissue specimen can be helpful for the diagnosis. Ketoconazole and amphotericin B can be used in treatment.

Blastomyces dermatitidis grows as a mold in culture, producing hyaline, branching septate hyphae and conidia. But at 37 ℃ or in the host, It converts to a large, singly budding yeast cell. *Blastomyces dermatitidis* causes blastomycosis, a chronic infection with granulomatous and pyogenic lesions that is initiated in the lungs, whence dissemination may occur to any organs but preferentially to the skin and bones. Blastomycosis occurs mainly in North America. Laboratory Diagnosis mainly depends on direct smear microscopic examination and culture. Besides of these, serological tests can be also used in diagnosis. But they are not as useful as they are in the case of other endemic mycoses. Ketoconazole and amphotericin B can be used in treatment.

10.4.4   *Penicillium Marneffei*

Penicillium marneffei is the only dimorphic fungus in *Penicillium* genus. It is a common opportunistic pathogen that causes secondary infections of AIDS, advanced malignancies or other severe immunocompromised patients. The disease caused by the fungus is known as *penicillium marneffei*. After cultivation at 25 ℃, it appears as filamentous fungus. There are branching septate hyphae. The mycelia end in a broom-shaped structure made up of some conidiophores and conidium chains (at the terminal of conidiophore). Being cultivated at 37 ℃, there are some spherical, oval or long yeast cells accompanied by a few short hyphae (septa in parts of them). The infection may be cause by pulmonary inhalation of spore. The initial symptoms are mostly fever and weight loss, which can be accompanied by different degrees of respiratory symptoms (cough, chest pain, etc.), digestive system damage (hepatosplenomegaly), rashes, etc. Direct smear examination, culture of fungi, serological diagnosis and histopathological examination are helpful for the diagnosis. Early diagnosis and early use of sensitive antifungal agents are key to reducing mortality. The drugs currently used for treatment are mainly amphotericin B, azoles and echinocandins.

10.5 Opportunistic Mycoses and Mycotoxin

Currently, in addition to known dermatophytes and some pathogenic dimorphic fungi, there are a number of fungi that are symbiotic with humans or that have been found in nature, which can cause opportunistic infections. The most common opportunistic pathogens are *Candida*, *Aspergillus*, *Cryptococcus* and *Mucor*, etc. In addition, the toxins produced by some fungi can cause some very serious diseases, which seriously threaten human life and health.

10.5.1 Candidiasis

Candidiasis is a series of diseases caused by *Candida albicans* and related yeasts. In the yeast genus candida, *Candida albicans* is the most common pathogen. It can cause acute or chronic inflammation of skin, mucosa and viscera.

Candida albicans

Candida albicans is widely distributed in soil, air, plant surface, animal body surface and the cavity that communicates with the outside and is a member of normal flora of human body. All kinds of candidiasis can be caused when the hosts are in a condition of dysbacteriosis or low immunity.

(1) Biological Characterization

Candida albicans is spherical or oval, budding yeast cell (3 – 6 micrometers in diameter). In Gram's stain, it is gram positive. In tissue, it is easier for them to form blastospores and pseudohyphae (Figure 10 – 5). On nutritionally deficient media *Candida albicans* produces large, spherical chlamydospores derived from the thin-walled, spherical or pear-shaped cell on the top of pseudohypha or between the pseudohyphae. It grows very well in common agar, blood agar and Sabouraud's agar. At 37 ℃, it can form a gray white or cream-colored typical yeast-like colony.

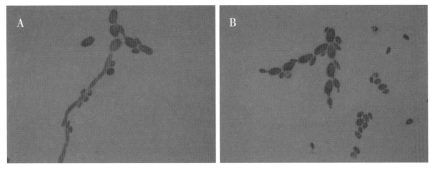

Figure 10-5   *Candida albicans*(1000×,gram stain)

A. pseudohypha of *Candida albicans*

B. blastospore of *Candida albicans*

(2) Pathogenesis and Symptomatology

As a member of human normal flora, *Candida albicans* can be beneficial for us. When the body is in dysbacteriosis or in a low immunity condition, it can invade a variety of tissue and organs, resulting in candidiasis. In the process of infection, fungal virulent factors such as some adhesins and enzymes and the transformation of phenotype (yeast-type and filamentous fungus) can play important roles in the forming of lesions.

Cutaneous candidiasis often occur in somewhere warm, wet and wrinkled such as armpit, groin, crissum, perineum and finger, etc. Mucosal infection is characterized by thrush (Figure 10-6) oral erosion, vulvitis and vaginitis, among which thrush is the most common. Visceral Candidiasis includes Candida pneumonia, bronchitis, enteritis, cystitis, etc. *Candida albicans* can also cause septicemia which has become one of the common pathogen of septicemia. Beside these, it can also spread to central nervous system, resulting in meningitis, meningoencephalitis and brain abscess, etc.

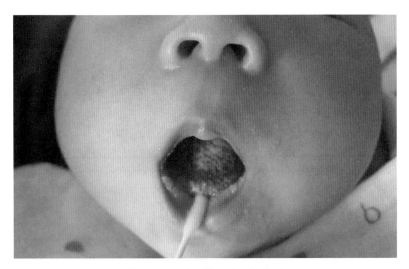

Figure 10-6   Thrush of infant

(3) Laboratory Diagnosis

Sputum, exudate from cutaneous lesions, cerebrospinal fluid, blood, urine and tissue biopsies all can be used as the specimen for laboratory identification. Blastospore and pseudohyphae in direct smear microscopic examination, the specific colony in the culture, the result of germ tube and Chlamydospore production test are important basis of the diagnosis. Appropriate interpretation of positive culture is necessary for the diagnosis because candida species are members of the normal flora. At present, serological diagnosis of candidiasis has limitations of specificity or sensitivity.

(4) Treatment

Both oral and vaginal infections are treated topically with nystatin or clotrimazole. Depending on the severity and extent of a candidal infection, treatment with an azole drug, such as ketoconazole, fluconazole and itraconazole, may be given orally or intravenously. Amphotericin B alone or in combination with flucytosine is used in systemic infection. Echinocandins, such as caspofungin, micafungin and anidulafungin are active against *Aspergillus* and most *Candida*, including those species resistant to azoles.

10.5.2 Cryptococcosis

Cryptococcosis is caused by the yeast *Cryptococcus neoformans*, which is found worldwide, often in soil containing bird (especially pigeon) droppings. Therefore, most are an exogenous infection.

10.5.2.1 Biological Characterization

Cryptococcus neoformans has a characteristic polysaccharide capsule around the budding yeast cell, which is observable on a background of India ink (Figure 10−7). In blood agar or Sabouraud's media, it can produce a whitish mucoid colony in several days. After a longer cultivation, the color of colony may become orange gradually and deep brown at last. Capsule polysaccharides which can be used in serological diagnosis are important antigens of *Cryptococcus neoformans*. There are A, B, C and D this four serotypes and A and D serotype are more common in clinic.

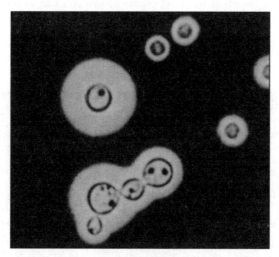

Figure 10−7 *Cryptococcus neoformans* in ink
(400×)

10.5.2.2 Pathogenesis and Symptomatology

Capsule polysaccharides are the important pathogenic material of *Cryptococcus neoformans*. The most form of crytococcosis is a mild, subclinical lung infection caused by inhalation of the yeast cells. *Cryptococcus neoformans* is also a member of human normal flora, it can cause endogenous infection when immunity is weakened. In immunocompromised patients, the infection often disseminates to the brain and meninges, with fatal consequences. However, about 20% of patients with cryptococcal meningitis have no immunologic defect. In AIDS patients, cryptococcosis is the second most common fungal infection(after candidiasis) and is potentially the most serious.

10.5.2.3　Laboratory Diagnosis

Cerebrospinal fluid, tissue, exudates, sputum, blood and urine all can be used as specimen which can be selected depending upon disease types and the stage of disease. Cerebrospinal fluid and urine is centrifuged before microscopic examination and culture which is a better choice for diagnosis. A positive capsule stain on cerebrospinal fluid can give a quick diagnosis of cryptococcal meningitis, but false negatives are common. In the culture, specific yeast type colony is beneficial for identification. In serological identification, ELISA and latex agglutination test can be used to detect its specific capsule polysaccharide antigens.

10.5.2.4　Treatment

Amphotericin B, itraconazole and flucytosine can be used in the treatment of cryptococcosis, the precise treatment regimen depending on the stage of disease, site of infection and whether the patient has AIDS.

10.5.3　Aspergillosis

Aspergillosis is caused by several species of the genus *Aspergillus* – *Aspergillus fumigatus*, *Aspergillus flavus* and *Aspergillus niger*, etc. And in them, *Aspergillus fumigatus* is the most common one. *Aspergillus* is one of the most widely distributed fungi. It has characteristic conidial head structure. They are rarely pathogenic in the normal host, while they can cause disease in immunosuppressed individuals and patients treated with broad-spectrum antibiotics.

10.5.3.1　Biological Characterization

The hyphae of *Aspergillus* species are septate mycelia. In the terminal of its aerial hyphae, it bears characteristic conidial head structure: long conidiophores with terminal vesicles on which phialides produce basipetal chains of conidia. They can be identified according to morphologic differences in the these structure, including the size, shape, texture and color of the conidia. It can grow very well in Sabouraud's agar in 37–45 ℃, producing shiny colonies(initially white in color) which become filamentous colony gradually.

10.5.3.2　Pathogenesis and Symptomatology

Primary infection of *Aspergillus* is ususally caused by inhalation of a large number pathogens, resulting in acute pneumonia. If skin is infected, it will result in primary cutaneous aspergillosis. In immunosuppressed patients, *Aspergillus* can disseminate into a variety of extrapulmonary tissue or organs, resulting in systemic aspergillosis. It can also cause allergic disease (allergic bronchopulmonary aspergillosis) because of inhalation of *Aspergillus* spores in a large number. Some *Aspergillus* can produce some toxins which can induce tumor in human or animals.

10.5.3.3　Laboratory Diagnosis

Sputum, other respiratory tract specimens and lung biopsy tissue can be used for microscopic examination and culture. It can be identified according to the properties of its colony and conidia. Besides, serological detection of soluble antigens (ELISA, latex agglutination test and convective immunoelectrophoresis, etc.)can be used in diagnosis.

10.5.3.4　Treatment

Treatment of aspergillosis is typically by amphotericin B and surgical removal of fungal masses or infected tissue. Itraconazole has been proved to be effective for *Aspergillus* osteomyelitis. Besides of application of antifungal agents, cytokine immunotherapy are necessary for the treatment of allergic aspergillosis.

10.5.4 Mucormycosis

Mucormycosis is an opportunistc mycosis caused by a number of molds classified in the order *Mucorales of the class Zygomycetes*. These fungi are widespread in nature. They are thermotolerant saprophytes with rectangle-shaped branching septate hyphae. Its asexual spore is sporangiosporeand its sexual spore is zygospore.

Mucormycosis is a unusual but lethal fungal infection. It occurs rarely in the normal host and more commonly in patients with diabetes mellitus leukemias, lymohoma, corticosteroid treatment, severe burns, immunodeficiencies and other debilitating diseases, etc. The pathogens enter the host by respiratory inhalation, digestive tract or any breaks in skin and mucosa, resulting in thrombosis, tissue ischemia and necrosis. Mucormycosis can occur in a variety of tissue and organ. Usually mucormycosis occur in the nose or ears at first, resulting in necrotizing inflammation and granuloma. And then it spreads to the brain and results in meningitis. It can also spread to the lungs, the gastrointestinal tract, etc. Sputum and tissue specimen can be used in direct smear examination and culture for the identification. The typical therapy includes the application of amphotericin B and surgical removal of lesions.

10.5.5 Mycotoxin

Besides fungal infectious diseases, some fungi can produce lots of toxins, resulting in food poisoning, malformation or tumor.

The production of toxin is influenced by many factors. Fungi are more likely to grow and produce toxins in natural medium than in artificial synthetic medium. Water, temperature and humidity are the main conditions affecting fungal growth and the production of fungal toxin. After many times artificial cultivation, the strong virulent stain can be transformed into weak virulent strain.

The fungal toxin can be classified according to their chemical structure, their target organ or the name of fungi which produce it. The chemical structure classification is now seldom mentioned because it is lack of specificity and its chemical structure is not closely related with its toxicity. Aflatoxin, ergot and mushroom toxin are important fungal toxin in medicine.

Aflatoxin is the secondary metabolites of *Aspergillus flavus* and some other *Aspergillus*. Aflatoxin is extremely toxic and carcinogenic. All aflatoxins contain the structures of difuran ring and coumarin. Aflatoxin mainly pollutes grains or oil and their products, such as peanut, edible oil, corn, etc. It causes diseases by eating polluted food, including acute poisoning, chronic poisoning or cancer. At present, the metabolites of aflatoxin in the body is considered to be related to the occurring of cancer.

Ergot is the metabolites of *Claviceps purpurea*-a kind of fungus which parasites in rye and wheat. It can cause ergotism after eating polluted food of ergot. Small doses of ergot can be used for treatment of clinical disorders, such as control of childbirth bleeding, drug abortion, migraines and hypotension, etc.

Mushroom toxin exist mainly in all kinds of amanita. It can result in a dose-related disease called mycetismus. They can cause severe or fatal damage to the liver and kidney.

Chapter 11

Microbe Growth Control

Controlling microbe growth can prevent infections and food spoilage. Sterilization is the progress of removing or destroying microbe on objects. Disinfection is the process of reducing or inhibiting microbial growth on nonliving surfaces. Antisepsis is the process of reducing or inhibiting microorganisms on living tissues. There are agents that can affect the growth of microbes, for example, heat or antimicrobial chemicals usually kill bacteria at a constant rate and certain chemical agents damage the plasma membrane of bacteria by altering its permeability. Some microbe control agents damage cellular proteins by breaking hydrogen bonds. Other agents interfere with DNA and RNA replication and protein synthesis of bacteria.

The scientific control of microbial growth began only about 100 years ago. Pasteur's work on microorganisms led scientists to believe that microbes were a possible cause of disease. In the mid-1,800 s, the Hungarian Physician Ignaz Semmelweis and English physician Joseph Lister used this thinking to develop some of the first microbial control practices for medical procedures. These practices included hand washing with microbe killing chloride of lime and use of the techniques of aseptic surgery to prevent microbial contamination of surgical wounds. Until that time, hospital-acquired infections or nosocomial infections, were the cause of death in at least 10% of surgical cases and deaths of delivering mothers were as high as 25% : Ignorance of microbes was such that, during the American Civil War, a surgeon might have cleaned his scalpel on his boot sole between incisions.

11.1 Definitions of Frequently Used Terms

Terminology is especially important when the control of microorganisms is discussed because words such as disinfectant and antiseptic often are used loosely. The situation is even more confusing because a particular treatment can either inhibit growth or kill, depending on the conditions.

Sterilization is the process by which all living cells, spores and acellular entities are either destroyed or removed from an object or habitat. A sterile object is totally free of viable microorganisms, spores and other infectious agents. When sterilization is achieved by a chemical agent, the chemical is called a sterilant. Incontrast, disinfection is the killing, inhibition or removal of microorganisms that may cause disease; disinfection is the substantial reduction of the total microbial population and the destruction of potential pathogens. Disinfectants are agents, usually chemical, used to carry out disinfection and normally used only on inanimate objects. A disinfectant does not necessarily sterilize an object because viable spores and a few microorganisms may remain. Sanitization is closely related to disinfection. In sanitization, the microbial population is reduced to levels that are considered safe by public health standards. The inanimate object is usually cleaned as well as partially disinfected. For example, sanitizers are used to clean eating utensils in restaurants.

Antisepsis is the prevention of infection or sepsis and is accomplished with antiseptics. These are chemical agents applied to tissue to prevent infection by killing or inhibiting pathogen growth; they also reduce the total microbial population. Because they must not destroy too much host tissue, antiseptics are generally not as toxic as disinfectants. Chemotherapy is the use of chemical agents to kill or inhibit the growth of microorganisms within host tissue.

A suffix can be employed to denote the type of antimicrobial Agent. Substances that kill organisms often have the suffix-*cide*; a germicide kills pathogens but not necessarily endospores. A disinfectant or antiseptic can be particularly effective against a specific group, in whichcase it may be called a bactericide, fungicide orviricide. Other chemicals do no kill but rather prevent growth. If these agents are removed, growth will resume. Their names end in-static (Greek *statikos*, causing to stand or stopping)-for example, bacteriostatic and fungistatic.

11. 2　Influences of Environmental Factors on Microbial Growth

The presence of organic matter often inhibits the action of chemical antimicrobial. In hospitals, the presence of organic matter in blood, vomit or feces influences the selection of disinfectants. Microbes in surface biofilms, are difficult for biocides to reach effectively. Because their activity is due to temperature dependent chemical reactions, disinfectants work somewhat better under warm conditions. Directions on disinfectant containers frequently specify the use of a warm solution.

The nature of the suspending medium is also a factor in heart treatment. Fats and proteins are especially protective and a medium rich in these substance protects microbes, which will then have a higher survival rate. Heat is also measurably more effective under acidic conditions. As we have seen, microorganisms must be able to respond to variations in nutrient levels. Microorganisms also are greatly affected by the chemical and physical nature of their surroundings. An understanding of environmental influences aids in the control of microbial growth and the study of the ecological distribution of microorganisms. The adaptation of some microorganisms to extreme and inhospitable environments are truly remarkable. Microbes are present virtually everywhere on Earth. Many habitats in which microbes thrive would kill most other organisms. Bacteria such as *Bacillus infernus* are able to live over 2. 4 kilometers below Earth's surface, without oxygen and at temperatures above 60 ℃. Other microbes live in acidic hot springs, at great ocean depths or in lakes. Microorganisms that grow in such harsh conditions are called extremophiles.

In this section, we briefly review the effects of the most important environmental factors on microbial growth. Major emphasis is given to solutes and water activity, pH, temperature, oxygen level, pressure and radiation. It is important to note that for most environment factors, a range of levels supports growth of a microbe. For example, a microbe might exhibit optimum growth at pH 7 but grows, though not optimally, at pH values down to pH 6 and up to pH 8. Furthermore outside this range, the microbe might cease reproducing but remain viable for some time. Clearly, each microbe must have evolved adaptations that allow it to adjust its physiology within its preferred range and it may also have adaptations that protect it in environments outside this range. These adaptations also discussed in this section.

11.2.1   Solutes and Water Activity

Because a selectively permeable plasma membrane separates microorganisms from their environment, they can be affected by changes in the osmotic concentration of their surroundings. If a microorganism is placed in a hypotonic solution, water will enter the cell and cause it to burst unless something is done to prevent the influx or inhibit plasma membrane expansion. Conversely if it is placed in a hypertonic solution, water will flow out of the cell. In microbes that have cell walls, the membrane shrinks away from the cell wall—a process called plasmolysis. Dehydration of the cell in hypertonic environments may damage the cell membrane and cause the cell to become metabolically inactive.

Clearly it is important that microbes be able to respond to changes in the osmotic concentrations of their environment. Microbes in hypotonic environments can reduce the osmotic concentration of their cytoplasm. For example, some procaryotes have mechanosensitive (MS) channels in their plasma membrane. In a hypotonic environment, the membrane stretches due to an increase in hydrostatic pressure and cellular swelling. MS channels then open and allow solutes to leave. Thus, MS channels act as escape valves to protect cells from bursting. Because many protists do not have a cell wall, they must use contractile vacuoles to expel excess water. Many microorganisms, whether in hypotonic or hypertonic environments, keep the osmotic concentration of their cytoplasm somewhat above that of the habitat by the use of compatible solutes, so that the plasma membrane is always pressed firmly against their cell wall. Compatible solutes are solutes that do not interfere with metabolism and growth when at high intracellular concentration in a hypertonic environment through the synthesis or uptake of choline, betaine, proline, glutamic, acid and other amino acids; elevated levels of potassium ions may also be used. Polyols and amino acids are ideal compatible solutes because they normally do not disrupt enzyme structure and function.

Some microbes are adapted 10 extreme hypertonic environments. Halophiles grow optimally in the presence of NaCl or other salts at a concentration above about 0.2 M. Extreme halophiles have adapted so completely to hypertonic, saline conditions that they require high levels of sodium chloride to grow-concentrations between about 2M and saturation. The archaeon *Halobacterium* can be isolated from the Dead Sea, the Great Salt Lake in Utah and other aquatic habitats with salt concentrations approaching saturation. *Halobacterium* and other extremely halophilic procaryotes accumulate enormous quantities of potassium in order to remain hypertonic to their environment; the internal potassium concentration may reach 4 to 7M. Furthermore, their enzymes, ribosomes and transport proteins require high potassium levels for stability and activity. In addition, the plasma membrane and cell wall of *Halobacterium* are stabilized by high concentrations of sodium ion. If the sodium concentration decreases too much, the wall and plasma membrane disintegrate. Extreme halophiles have successfully adapted to environmental conditions that would destroy most organisms. In the process, they have become so specialized that they have lost ecological flexibility and can prosper only in a few extreme habitats.

Because the osmotic concentration of a habitat has such profound effects on microorganisms, it is useful to express quantitatively the degree of water availability. Microbiologists generally use water activity (a_w) for this purpose. The water activity of a solution is 1/100 the relative humidity of the solution. It is also equivalent to the ratio of the solution's vapor pressure to that of pure water.

The Water activity of a solution or solid can be determined by sealing it in a chamber and measuring the relative humidity after the system has come to equilibrium. Suppose after a sample is treated in this way, the air above it is 95% saturated-that is, the air contains 95% of the moisture it would have when equilibrated at the same temperature with a sample of pure water. The relative humidity would be 95% and the sample's water activity, 0.95. Water activity is inversely related to osmotic pressure; if a solution has high osmotic pressure, its a_w is low.

Microorganisms differ greatly in their ability to adapt to habitats with low water activity. A microorganism must expend extra effort to grow in a habitat with a low aw value because it must maintain a high internal solute concentration to retain water. Some microorganisms can do this and are osmotolerant; they grow over wide ranges of water activity. For example, Staphylococcus aureus is halotolerant, can be cultured in media containing sodium chloride concentration up to about 3M and is well adapted for growth on the skin. The yeast *Saccharomyces rouxii* grows in sugar solutions with aw values as low as 0.6. The photosynthetic protist *Dunaliella viridis* tolerates sodium chloride concentrations from 1.7 M to a saturated solution. Some microbes are true xerophiles. That is, they grow best at low a_w. However, most microorganisms only grow well at water activities around 0.98 or higher. This is why drying food or adding large quantities of salt and sugar effectively prevents food spoilage.

11.2.2 Temperature

Microorganisms are particularly susceptible to external temperatures because they cannot regulate their internal temperature. An important factor influencing the effect of temperature on growth is the temperature sensitivity of enzyme-catalyzed reactions. Each enzyme has a temperature at which it functions optimally. At some temperature below the optimum, it cease to be catalysis increases to that observed for the optimal temperature. The velocity of the reaction roughly doubles for every 10 ℃ rise in temperature. When all enzymes, in a microbe are considered together, as the rate of each reaction increases, metabolism as a whole becomes more active and the microorganism grows faster. However, beyond a certain point, further increase actually slow growth and sufficiently high temperature are lethal. Hightemperatures denature enzymes, transport carriers and other proteins. Temperature also has a significant effect on microbial membranes. At very low temperatures, membranes solidify. At high temperatures, the lipid bilayer simply melts and disintegrates. Thus when organisms are above their optimum temperatures are very low, function is affected but not necessarily cell chemical composition and structure.

Because of these opposing temperature influences, microbial growth has a characteristic temperature dependence with distinct cardinal temperatures-minimum, optimum and maximum growth temperatures. Although the shape of temperature dependence curves varies, the temperature optimumis always closer to the maximum than to the minimum. The cardinal temperatures are not rigidly fixed. Instead they depend to some extent on other environmental factors such as pH and available nutrients. For example, *Crithidia fasciculate*, a flagellated protist living in the gut of mosquitoes, grows in a simple medium at 22 to 27 ℃. However, it cannot be cultured at 33 to 34 ℃ without the addition of extra metals, amino acids, vitamins and lipids.

The cardinal temperatures vary greatly among microorganisms. Optima usually range from 0 ℃ to 75 ℃, whereas microbial growth occurs at temperatures extending from less than-20 ℃ to over 120 ℃. Some archaea even grow at 121 ℃, the temperature normally used in autoclaves. A major factor determining growth range seems to be water. Even at the most extreme temperatures, microorganisms need liquid water to grow. The growth temperature range for a particular microorganism usually spans about 30 degrees. Some species have a small range; others, such as *Enterococcus faecalis*, grow over a wide range of temperatures. The major microbial groups differ from one another regarding their maximum growth temperature. The upper limit for protists is around 50 ℃. Some fungi grow at temperatures as high as 55 to 60 ℃. Procaryotes can grow at much higher temperatures than eucaryotes. It has been suggested that eucaryotes are not able manufacture stable and functional organellar membranes at temperatures above 60 ℃. The photosynthetic apparatus also appears to be relatively unstable because photosynthetic organisms are not found growing at very high temperatures.

Psychrophiles grow well at 0 ℃ or lower; the maximum is around 15 ℃. They are readily isolated from Arctic and tat for psychrophiles because 90% of ocean water is 5 ℃ or colder. The psychrophilic protist *Chlamydomonasnivalis* can actually turn a snowfield or glacier pink with its bright red spores. Psychrophiles are widespread among bacterial taxa and are found in such genera as *Pseudomonas*, *Vibriio*, *Alcaligenes*, *Bacillus*, *Photobacterium*, and *Shewanella*. A psychrophilic archaeon, *Methanogenium*, has been isolated from Ace Lake in Antarctica. Psychrophilic microorganisms have adapted to their environment in several ways. Their machinery function well at low temperatures. The cell membranes of psychrophilic microorganisms have high levels of unsaturated fatty acids and remain semifluid when cold. Indeed, many psychrophiles begin to leak cellular constituents at temperature higher than 20 ℃ because of cell membrane disruption.

Psychrotrophs grow at 0 to 7 ℃ even though they have optima between 20 and 30 ℃ and maxima at about 35 ℃. Psychrotrophic bacteria and fungi are major cause of refrigerated food spoilage.

Mesophiles are microorganisms with growth optima around 20 to 45 ℃. They often have a temperature minimum of 15 to 20 ℃ and their maximum is about 45 ℃ or lower. Most microorganisms probably fall within this category. Almost all human pathogens are mesophiles, as might be expected because the humanbody is a fairly constant 37 ℃.

Thermophiles grow at temperatures between 55 and 85 ℃. Their growth minimum is usually around 45 ℃ and they often have optima between 55 and 65 ℃. The vast majority are procaryotes, although a few photosynthetic protists and fungi are thermophilic. These organisms flourish in many habitats including composts, self-heating hay stacks, hot waterlines and hot springs.

Hyperthermophiles have growth optima between 85 ℃ and about 113 ℃. They usually do not grow well below 55 ℃. *Pyrococcus abyssi* and *Pyrodictium* occultum are examples of marine hyperthermophiles found in hotareas of the seafloor.

Thermophiles and hyperthermophiles differ from mesophiles in many ways. They have heat-stable enzymes and protein synthesis systems that function properly at high temperatures. These proteins are stable for a variety of reasons. Heat-stable proteins have highly organized hydrophobic interiors and more hydrogen and other noncovalent bonds. Larger quantities of amino acids such as proline also make polypeptide chains less flexible and more heat stable. In addition, the proteins are stabilized and aided in folding by proteins called chaperone proteins. Evidence exists that histone like proteins stabilize the DNA of thermophilic bacteria. The membrane lipids of thermophiles and hyperthermophiles are also quite stable. They tend to be more saturated, more branched and of higher molecular weight. This increases themelting points of membrane lipids. Archaeal thermophileshave membrane lipids with ether linkages, which protect the lipids from hydrolysis at high temperatures. Sometimes archaeal lipids actually span the membrane to form a rigid, stable monolayer.

11.2.3   pH

pH is a measure of the relative acidity of a solution of a solution and is defined as the negative logarithm of the hydrogen ion concentration. The pH scale extends from pH0 to pH14 and each pH unit represents a tenfold change in hydrogen ion concentration. Microbial habitats vary widely in pH-from pH 0 to 2 at the acidic end to 2 at the acidic end to alkaline lakes and soil with pH values between 9 and 10.

Each species has a definite pH growth range and pH growth optimum. Acidophiles have their growth optimum between pH 0 and 5.5; neutrophiles, between pH 5.5 and 8.0; and alkalophiles, between pH 8.0 and 11.5. Extreme alkalophiels have growth optima at pH10 or higher. In general, different microbial groups have characteristic pH preferences. Most bacteria and protists are neutrophiles. Most fungi prefer more acidic surroundings, about pH 4 to 6; photosynthetic protists also seem to favor slight acidity. Many archaea are acidophiles. For example, the archaeon *Sulfolobusacidocaldarius*is acommon inhabitant of acidic hot springs; it grows well from pH1to 3 and at high temperature. The archaea *Ferroplasma acidarmanus* and *Pcrophilus oshimae* can actually grow very close to pH 0. Alkalophiles are distributed among all three domains of life. They include bacteria belonging to the genera *Bacillus*, *Micrococcus*, *Pseudomonas* and *Streptomyces*; yeasts and filamentous fungi; and numerous archaea.

Although microorganisms often grow over wide ranges of pH and far from their optima, there are limits to their tolerance. When the external pH is low, the concentration of H^+ is greater outside than inside and HT will move into the cytoplasm and lower the cytoplasmic pH. Drastic variations in cytoplasmic pH can harm microorganisms by disrupting the plasma membrane or inhibiting the activity of enzymes and membrane transport proteins. Most procaryotes die if the internal pH drops much below 5.0 to 5.5. Changes in the external pH also might alter the ionization of nutrient molecules and thus reduce their availability to the organism.

Microorganisms respond to external pH changes using mechanisms that maintain a neutral cytoplasmic pH. Several mechanisms for adjusting to small changes in external pH have been proposed. Neutrophiles appear to exchange potassium for protons using an antiport transport system. Internal buffering also may contribute to pH homeostasis. However, if the external pH becomes too acidic, other mechanisms come into play. When the pH drops below about 5.5 to 6.0, *Salmonella enterica serovar* Typhimurium and E. coli synthesize an array of new proteinsas part of what has been calledtheir acidic tolerance response. A proton-translocating ATPase enzyme contributes to this protective response, either by making more ATP or by pumping protons out of the cell. If theexternal pH decreases to 4.5 or lower, acid shock proteins andheat shock proteins are synthesized. These prevent the denaturation of proteins and aidin the refolding of denaturedconditions.

What about microbes that live at pH extremes? Extremealkalophiles such as *Bacillusalcalophilus* maintain their internal pH close toneutrality by exchanging internal sodium ions for external protons. Acidophiles use a variety of measures to maintain a neutral interhal pH.

These include the transport of cations into the cell, thus decreasing the movement of H^+ into the cell; proton tansporters that pump H^+out if they get in; and highly impermeablecell membranes.

11.2.4 Oxygen

The importance of oxygen to the growth of an organism correlates with its metabolism-in particular, with the processes it uses to conserve the energy supplied by its energy source. Almost all energy metabolic processes involve the movement of electrons through a series of membrane-bound electron carriers called the electron transport chain. For chemotrophs, an externally supplied terminal electron acceptor is critical to the functioning of the ETC. The nature of the terminal electron acceptor is related to an organism's oxygen requirement.

An organism able to grow in the presence of atmospheric O_2 is an aerobe, whereas one that can grow in its absence is anaerobes. Almost all multicellular organisms are completely dependent on atmospheric O_2 for growth-that is, they are obligate aerobes. Oxygen serves as the terminal electron acceptor for the ETC in the metabolic process called aerobic respiration. In addition, aerobic eucaryotes employ O_2 in the synthesis of sterols and unsaturated fatty acids. Microaerophiles such as Campylobacter are damaged by the normal atmospheric level of O_2 and require O_2 levels in the range of 2 to 10% for growth. Facultative anaerobes do not require O_2 for growth but grow better in its presence. In the presence of oxygen, they use O_2 as the terminal electron acceptor during aerobic respiration. Aerotolerant anaerobes such as *Enterococcus faecalis* simply ignore O_2 and grow equally well whether it is present or not; chemotrophic aerotolerant anaerobes are often described as having strictly fermentative metabolism. In contrast, strict or obligate anaerobes are usually killed in the presence of O_2. Strict anaerobes cannot generate energy through aerobic respiration and employ other metabolic strategies such as fermentation or anaerobic respiration, neither of which require O_2. The nature of bacterial O_2 responses can be readily determined by growing the bacteria in culture tubes filled with a solid culture medium or a medium such as thioglycollate broth, which contains a reducing agent to lower O_2 levels.

A microbial group may show more than one type of relationship to O_2. All five types are found among the procaryotes and protists. Fungi are normally aerobic, but a number of species-particularly among the yeasts-are facultative anaerobes. Photosynthetic protists are usually obligate anaerobes are killed by O_2, they may be recovered from habitats that appear to be oxic. In such as cases they associate with facultative anaerobes that use up the available O_2 and thus make the growth of strict anaerobes possible. For example, the strict anaerobe *Bacteroides gingivalis* lives in the mouth where it grows in the anoxic crevices around the teeth. Clearly the ability to grow in both oxic and anoxic environments provides considerable flexibility and is an ecological advantage.

The different relationships with O_2 are due to several factors, including the inactivation of proteins and the effect of toxic O_2 derivatives. Enzymes can be inactivated when sensitive groups such as sulfhydryls are oxidized. A notable example is the nitrogen-fixation enzyme nitrogen fixation enzyme nitrogenase, which is very oxygen sensitive. Toxic O_2 derivatives are formed when proteins such as flavoproteins promote oxygen reduction. The reduction products are superoxide radical, hydrogen peroxide and hydroxyl radical.

These products are extremely toxic because they oxidize and rapidly destroy cellular constituents. A microorganism must be able to protect itself against such oxygen products or it will be killed. Indeed, neutrophils and macrophages, two important immune system cells, use these toxic oxygen products to destroy invading pathogens.

Many microorganisms possess enzymes that protect against toxic O_2 products. Obligate aerobes and facultative anaerobes usually contain the enzymes superoxide dismutase and catalase, which catalyze the destruction of superoxide radical and hydrogen peroxide, respectively. Peroxidase also can be used to destroy hydrogen peroxide. Aerotolerant microorganisms may lack catalase but usually have superoxide dismutase. The aerotolerant bacterium *Lactobacillus plantarum* uses manganous ions instead of superoxide dismutase to destroy the superoxide radical. All strict anaerobes lack both enzymes or have them in very low concentrations and therefore cannot tolerate O_2. However, some microaerophilic bacteria and anaerobic archaea protect themselves from the toxic effects of O_2 with the enzymes superoxide reductase and peroxidase. Superoxide reductase reduces superoxide to H_2O_2 without producing O_2. The H_2O_2 is then converted to water by peroxidase.

Because aerobes need O_2 and anaerobes are killed by it, radically different approaches must be used when they are cultured. When large volumes of aerobic microorganisms are cultured, either they must be shaken to aerate the culture medium or sterile air must be pumped through the culture vessel. Precisely the opposite problem arises with anaerobes-all O_2 must be excluded. This is accomplished in several ways. Special anaerobic media containing reducing agents such as thioglycollate or cysteine may be used. The medium is boiled during preparation to dissolve its components and drive off oxygen. The reducing agents eliminate any residual dissolved O_2 in the medium so that anaerobes can grow beneath its surface. Oxygen also may be eliminated by removing air with a vacuum pump and flushing out residual O_2 with nitrogen gas. Often CO_2 as well as nitrogen is added to the chamber since many anaerobes require a small amount of CO_2 for best growth.

11.2.5　Pressure

Organisms that spend their lives on land or the surface of water are always subjected to a pressure of atmosphere and are never affected significantly by pressure. It is thought that high hydrostatic pressure affects membrane fluidity and membrane-associated unction. Yet many procaryotes live in the deep sea where the hydrostatic pressure can reach 600 to 1,000 atm and the temperature is about 2 to 3 ℃. Many of these procaryotes are barotolerant: increased pressure adversely affects them but not as much as it does nontolerant microbes. Some procaryotes are truly barophilic-they grow more rapidly at high pressures. A barophile recovered from the Mariana trench near the Philippines grows only at pressures between about 400 to 500 atm when incubated at 2 ℃. Barophiles may play an important role in nutrient recycling in the deep sea. Thus far, they have been found among several bacterial genera. Some archaea are thermobarophiles.

11.3　The Pattern of Microbial Death

A microbial population is not killed instantly when exposed to a lethal agent. Population death is generally exponential-that is, the population will be reduced by the same fraction at constant intervals. If the logarithm of the population number remaining is plotted against the time of exposure of the microorganism to the agent, a straight-line plot will result. When the population has been greatly reduced, the rate of killing may slow due to the survival of a more resistant strain of the microorganism. It is essential to have aprecise measure of anagent's killing efficiency. One such measure is the decimal reduction time (D) or D value. The decimal reduction time is the time required to kill 90% of the microorganisms or spores in a sample under specified conditions. For example, in a semilogarithmic plot of the population remaining versus the time of heating, the D value is the time required for the line to drop by one log cycle or tenfold. The D value is usually written with a subscript to indicate the temperature for which it applies.

To study the effectiveness of a lethal agent, one must be able to decide when microorganisms are dead, which may present some challenges. A microbial cell is often defined as dead if it does not grow and reproduce when inoculated into culture medium that would normally support its growth. In like manner, an inactive virus cannot infect a suitable host. This definition has flaws, however. It has been demonstrate that when bacteria are exposed to certain conditions, they can remain alive but are temporarily unable to reproduce. When in this state, they are referred to as viable but nonculturable. In conventional tests to demonstrate killing by an antimicrobial agent, VBNC bacteria would be thought to be dead. This is a serious problem because after a period of recovery, the bacteria may regain their ability tore produce and cause infection.

11.4   Actions of Microbial Control Agents

11.4.1   Alteration of Membrane Permeability

A microorganism's plasma membrane, located just inside the cell wall, is the target of many microbial control agents. This membrane actively regulates the passage of nutrients into the cell and the elimination of wastes from the cells. Damage to the lipids or proteins of the plasma membrane by antimicrobial agents cause cellular contents to leak into the surrounding medium and inferences with the growth of the cell.

11.4.2   Damage to Proteins and Nucleic Acids

Bacteria are sometimes thought of as "little bags of enzymes". Enzymes, which are primarily protein, are vital to all the cellular activities. Recall that the functional properties of proteins are the result of their three-dimensional shape. This shape is maintained by chemical bonds that link adjoining portions of the amino acid chain as it folds back and forth upon itself. Some at those bonds are hydrogen bonds, which are susceptible to breakage by heat or certain chemical; breakage results in denaturation of the protein. Covalent bonds, which are stronger, are also subject to attack. For example, disulfide bridges, which play an important role in protein structure by joining amino acid with exposed sulfhydryl groups, can be broken by certain chemicals or sufficient heat.

The nucleic acids DNA and RNA are the carrier of the cell's genetic information. Damage to these nucleic acids by heat, radiation or chemicals is frequently lethal to the cell; the cell can no longer replicate, nor can it carry our normal metabolic functions such as the synthesis of enzymes.

11.5   Conditions Influencing the Effectiveness of Antimicrobial Agents

Destruction of microorganisms and inhibition of microbial growth are not simple matters because the efficiency of an antimicrobial agent is affected by at least six factors.

11.5.1   Population Size

Because an equal fraction of a microbial population is killed during each interval, a larger population requires a longer time to die than a smaller one.

11.5.2   Population Composition

The effectiveness of an agent varies greatly with the nature of the organisms being treated because microorganisms differ markedly insusceptibility. Bacterial spores are much more resistant to most antimicrobial agents than are vegetative forms and younger cells are usually more readily destroyed than mature organisms. Some species are able to withstand adverse conditions better than others. For instance, *Mycobacterium tuberculosis*, which causes tuberculosis, is much more resistant to antimicrobial agents than most other bacteria.

11.5.3　Concentration or Intensity of an Antimicrobial Agent

Often, but not always, the more concentrated a chemical agent or intense a physical agent, the more rapidly microorganisms are destroyed. However, agent effectiveness usually is not directly related to concentrationor intensity. Over a short range, a small increase in concentration leads to an exponential rise in effectiveness; beyond a certain point, increases may not raise the killing rate much at all. Sometimes an agent is more effectiveat lower concentrations. For example, 70% ethanol is this more bacteriocidal than 95% ethanol because the activity of ethanol is enhanced by the presence of, water.

11.5.4　Duration of Exposure

Chemical antimicrobials often require extended exposure for more-resistant microbes or endospores to be affected. In heat treatments, a longer exposure can compensate for a lower temperature, a phenomenon of particular importance to pasteurization of dairy products. The longer a population is exposed to a microbicidal agent, the more organisms are killed. To achieve sterilization, exposure should be long enough to reduce the probability of survival to 10^{-6} or less.

11.5.5　Local Environment

The population to be controlled isnot isolated but surrounded by environmental factors that may either offer protection or aid in its destruction. For example, because heat kills more readily at an acidic pH, acidic foods and beverages such as fruits and tomatoes are easier to pasteurize than more alkaline foods such as milk. A second important environmental factor is organic matter, which can protect microorganisms against physical and chemical disinfecting agents. Biofilms are a good example. The organic matter in a biofilm protects the biofilm's microorganisms. Furthermore, it has been clearly documented that bacteria in biofilms are alteredphysiologically and this makes them less susceptible to many antimicrobial agents. Because of the impact of organic matter, it may be necessary to clean objects, especially medical and dental equipment, before they are disinfected or sterilized.

Chapter 12

Physical and Chemical Agents for Microbe Control

Moist heat kills bacteria by degrading nucleic acids, denaturing enzymes and other proteins and disrupting cell membranes. Although treatment with boiling water for 10 minutes kills vegetative forms, autoclave at 121 ℃ and 15 pounds of pressure must be used to destroy endospores. Glassware and other heat-stable items may be sterilized by dry heat at 160 to 170 ℃ for 2 to 3 hours. Microorganisms can be efficiently removed by filtration with either depth filters or membrane filters. Biological safety cabinets with high-efficiency particulate filters sterilized air by filtration. Chemical agents usually act as disinfectants because they cannot readily destroy bacterial spores. The effectiveness of disinfectants depends on their concentration, duration of treatment, temperature and presence of organic material. Phenolics and alcohols are popular disinfectants that act by denaturing proteins and disrupting cell membranes. Halogenskill by oxidizing cellular constituents; cell proteins may also be iodinated. Iodine applied as a tincture or iodophor. Chlorine may be added to water as a gas, hypochlorite or an organic chlorine derivative. Heavy metals tend to be bacteriostatic agents. They are employed in specialized situations such as the use of silver nitrate in the eyes of newborn infants and copper sulfate in lakes and pools. Cationic detergents are often used as disinfectants and antiseptics; they disrupt membranes and denature proteins. Aldehydes such as formaldehyde and glutaraldehyde can sterilize as well as disinfect because they kill spores. Ethylene oxide gas penetrates plastic wrapping material and destroys all life forms by reacting with proteins. It is used to sterilize packaged, heat-sensitive materials. Vaporized hydrogen peroxide is used to decontaminate enclosed spaces. The vaporized hydrogen peroxide is a mist that can be circulated throughout the space. The peroxide and its oxy-radical by products are toxic to most microorganisms.

Over the last century, scientists have continued to develop a variety of physical methods and chemical agents to control microbial growth. Although most microorganisms are beneficial, some microbial activities have undesirable consequences such as food spoilage and disease. Therefore it is essential to be able to kill a wide variety of microorganisms or inhibit their growth to minimize their destructive effects. The goal is twofold: ①to destroy pathogens and prevent their transmission. ②to reduce or eliminate microorganisms responsible for the contamination of water, food and other substances. Thus this chapter focuses on the control of microorganisms by physical, chemical and biological agents.

12.1 Physical Methods of Microbial Control

Drying and salting were probably among the earliest techniques. When selecting methods of microbial control, consideration must be given to effects on things besides the microbes. For example, certain vitamins or antibiotics in a solution might be inactivated by heat. Many laboratory or hospital materials, such as rubber and latex tubing, are damaged by repeated heating. There are also economic considerations.

Heat and other physical agents are normally used to control microbial growth and sterilize objects, as can be seen form the continual operation of the autoclave in every microbiology laboratory. The most frequently employed physical agents are heat, filtration and radiation.

12.1.1　Heat

A visit to any supermarket will demonstrate that heat-preserved canned goods represent one of the most common methods of food preservation. Laboratory media and glassware and hospital instruments, are also usually sterilized by heat. Heat appears to kill microorganisms by denaturing their enzymes the resultant changes to the three-dimensional shapes of these proteins inactivate them.

Heat resistance varies among different microbes; these differences can be expressed through some concepts. Thermal death point is the lowest temperature at which all the microorganisms in a liquid suspension will be killed in 10 minutes. Another factor to be considered in sterilization is the length of time required. This is expressed as thermal death time, the minimal length of time for all bacteria in a liquid culture to be killed at a given temperature. Decimal reduction time is a third concept related to bacterial heat resistance. DRT is the time, in which 90% of a population of bacteria at a given temperature will be killed.

12.1.1.1　Moist Heat

Moist heat readily destroys viruses, bacteria and fungi. Moist heat kills by degrading nucleic acids and denaturing enzymes and other essential proteins. It also disrupts cell membranes. Exposure to boiling water for 10 minutes is sufficient to destroy vegetative cells and eukaryotic spores.

These high temperatures are most commonly achieved by steam under pressure in an autoclave. Autoclaving is the preferred method of sterilization, unless the material to be sterilized can be damaged by heat or moisture. Sterilization in an autoclave is most effective when the organisms are either contacted by the steam directly or are contained in a small volume of aqueous liquid. Under these conditions, steam at 8 pressure of about 15 psi (121 ℃) will kill all organisms and their endospores in about 15 minutes.

Some materials cannot withstand the high temperature of the autoclave and spore contamination precludes the use of other methods to sterilize them. For these materials, a process of intermittent sterilization, also known astyndallizationis used. The process also uses steam (30–60 minutes) to destroy vegetative bacteria. However, steam exposure is repeated for a total of three times with 23 to 24 hour incubations between steam exposures. The incubations permit remaining spores to germinate into heat-sensitive vegetative cells that are then destroyed upon subsequent steam exposures.

12.1.1.2　Dry Heat

Many objects are best sterilized in the absence of water by dry heat sterilization. Dry heat kills by oxidation effects. One of the simplest methods of dry heat sterilization is direct flaming. You will use this procedure many times in the microbiology laboratory when you sterilize inoculating loops. To effectively sterilize the inoculating loop, you heat the wire to a red glow. A similar principle is used in incineration, an effective way to sterilize and dispose of contaminated paper cups, bags and dressings.

Another form of dry heat sterilization is hot-air sterilization. Generally, a temperature of about 170 ℃ maintained for nearly 2 hours ensures sterilization. The longer period and higher temperature are required because the heat in water is more readily transferred to a cool body than is the heat in air. For example, imagine the different effects of immersing your hand in boiling water at 100 ℃ and of holding it in a hot-air oven at the same temperature for the same amount of time.

12.1.1.3   Pasteurization

Louis Pasteur found a practical method of preventing the spoilage of beer and wine called pasteurization. Pasteur used mild heating, which was sufficient to kill the organisms that caused the particular spoilage problem without seriously damaging the taste of the product. The same principle was later applied to milk to produce what we now call pasteurized milk the intent of pasteurization of milk was to eliminate pathogenic microbes. It also lowers microbial numbers which prolongs milk's good quality under refrigeration. Many relatively heat-resistant bacteria survive pasteurization, but these are unlikely to cause disease or cause refrigerated milk to spoil. Products other than milk, such as ice cream, yogurt and beer, all have their own pasteurization times and temperatures, which often differ considerably.

In the classic pasteurization treatment of milk, the milk was exposed to a temperature of about 63 ℃ for 30 minutes. Most milk pasteurization today uses higher temperatures, at least 72 ℃, but for only 15 seconds. This treatment, known as high-temperature short-time pasteurization, is applied as the milk flows continuously past a heat exchanger.

Milk can also be sterilized-something quite different from pasteurization-by ultra-high-temperature (UHT) treatments so that it can be stored without refrigeration. To avoid giving the milk a cooked taste, a UHT system is used in which the liquid milk never touches a surface hotter than the milk itself while being heated by steam. The milk falls in a thin film through a chamber of superheated steam and reaches 140 ℃ in less than a second. It is held for 3 seconds in a holding tube and then cooled in a vacuum chamber, where the steam flashes off. With this process, in less than 5 seconds the milk temperature rises from 74 ℃ to 140 ℃ and drops back to 74 ℃.

12.1.2   Filtration

Filtration is the passage of a liquid or gas through a screen like material with pores small enough to retain microorganisms. A vacuum is created in the receiving flask; air pressure then forces the liquid through the filter. Filtration is an excellent way to reduce the microbial population in solutions of heat-sensitive material and sometimes it can be used to sterilize solutions. Rather than directly destroying contaminating microorganisms, the filter simply removes them.

12.1.2.1   Depth Filters

Depth filters consist of fibrous or granular materials that have been bonded into a thick layer filled with twisting channels of small diameter. The solution containing microorganisms is sucked through this layer under vacuum and microbial cells are removed by physical screening or entrapment and by adsorption to the surface of the filter material. Depth filters are made of diatomaceous earth, unglazed porcelain, asbestos or other similar materials.

12.1.2.2   Membrane Filters

Membrane filters have replaced depth filters for many purposes. These circular filers are porous membranes, a little over 0.1 mm thick, made of cellulose acetate, cellulose nitrate, polycarbonate, polyvinylidene fluoride or other synthetic materials. Although a wide variety of pore sizes are available, membranes with pores about 0.2 μm in diameter are used to remove most vegetative cells, but not viruses, from solutions ranging in volume from less than 1 ml to many liters. The membranes are held in special holders and are often preceded by depth filters made of glass fibers to remove larger particles that might clog the membrane filter. The solution is pulled or forced through the filter with a vacuum or with pressure from a syringe, peristaltic pump or nitrogen gas and collected in previously sterilized containers. Membrane filters remove microorganisms by screening them out much as a sieve separates large sand particles from small ones. These filters are used to sterilize pharmaceuticals, ophthalmic solutions, culture media, oils, antibiotics and other heat-sensitive solutions.

12.1.2.3 Air Filtration

Air also can be sterilized by filtration. Two common examples are N-95 disposable masks used in hospitals and labs and cotton plugs on culture vessels that let air in but keep microorganisms out. N-95 masks exclude 95% of particles that are larger than 0.3 μm. Other important examples are laminar flow biological safety cabinets, which employ high-efficiency particulate air (HEPA) filters to remove 99.97% of particles 0.3 μm or larger. Laminar flow biological safety cabinets or hoods force air through HEPA filters, then project a vertical curtain of sterile air across the cabinet opening. This protects a worker from microorganisms being handled within the cabinet and prevents contamination of the room.

12.1.3 Radiation

Radiation has various effects on cell, depending on its wavelength, intensity and duration. Radiation that kills microorganisms is of two types: ionizing and nonionizing.

12.1.3.1 Ionizing

Ionizing radiation-gamma rays, X-rays, of high-energy electron beams—has a wavelength shorter than that of nonionizing radiation, less than about 1 nm. Therefore, it carries much more energy. Gamma rays are emitted by certain radioactive elements such as cobalt and electron beams are produced by accelerating electrons to high energies in special machines. X rays, which are produced by machines in a manner similar to the production of electron beams, are similar in nature to gamma rays. Gamma rays penetrate deeply but may require hours to sterilize large masses; high-energy electron beams have much lower penetrating power but usually require only a few seconds of exposure. The principal effect of ionizing radiation is the ionization of water, which forms highly reactive hydroxyl radicals. These radicals react with organic cellular components, especially DNA.

12.1.3.2 Nonionizing

Nonionizing radiation has wavelength longer than that of ionizing radiation, usually greater than about 1 nm.

Ultraviolet (UV) radiation causes thiamine-thiamine dimerization of the microbial DNA, preventing polymerase-mediated replication and transcription. However, UV does not penetrate glass, dirt films, water and other substances very effectively. Because of this disadvantage, UV radiation is used as a sterilizing agent only in a few specific situations. UV light damages the DNA of exposed cells by causing bonds to form between adjacent pyrimidine bases, usually thymines, in DNA chains. These thymine dimers inhibit correct replication of the DNA during reproduction of the cell. The UV wavelengths most effective for killing microorganisms are about 260 nm; these wavelengths are specifically absorbed by cellular DNA. UV radiation is also used to control microbes in the air. A major disadvantage of UV light as a disinfectant is that the radiation is not very penetrating. Another potential problem is that UV light can damage human eyes and prolonged exposure can cause burns and skin cancer in humans.

The shorter wavelengths—those most effective against bacteria—are screened out by the ozone layer of the atmosphere. The antimicrobial effect of sunlight is due almost entirely to the formation of singlet oxygen in the cytoplasm. Many pigments produced by bacteria provide protection from sunlight.

Microwaves do have much direct effect on microorganisms and bacteria can readily be isolated from the interior of recently operated microwave ovens. Moisture containing foods are heated by microwave action and the heat will kill most vegetative pathogens.

12.1.4   Low Temperatures

The effect of low temperatures on microorganism depends on the microbe and the intensity of the application. For example, at temperatures of ordinary refrigerators, the metabolic rate of most microbes is so reduced that they cannot reproduce or synthesize toxins. In other words ordinary refrigeration has a bacteriostatic effect. Yet psychrotrophs do grow slowly at refrigerator temperatures and will alter the appearance and taste of foods after a time. For example, a single microbe reproducing only three times a day would reach a population of more than 2 million within a week. Pathogenic bacteria generally will not grow at refrigerator temperatures, but for at least one important exception.

12.1.5   High Pressure

High pressure applied to liquid suspensions is transferred instantly and evenly throughout the sample. If the pressure is high enough, the molecular structures of proteins and carbohydrates are altered, resulting in the rapid inactivation of vegetative bacterial cells. Endospores are relatively resistant to high pressure.

12.1.6   Desiccation

In the absence of water, a condition that is known as desiccation, microorganisms cannot grow or reproduce but can remain viable for years. Then, when water is made available to them, they can resume their growth and division. This ability is used in the laboratory when microbes are preserved by lyophilization or freeze-drying, a process described. Certain foods are also freeze-dried. The resistance of vegetative cells to desiccation varies with the species and the organism's environment.

12.1.7   Osmotic Pressure

The use of high concentrations of salts and sugars to preserve food is based on the effects of osmotic pressure. High concentrations of these substances create a hypertonic environment that causes water to leave the microbial cell. This process resembles preservation by desiccation, in that both methods deny the cell the moisture it needs for growth. The principle of osmotic pressure is used in the preservation of foods. For example, concentrated salt solutions are used to cure meats and thick sugar solutions are used to preserve fruits.

12.2   Chemical Agents of Microbial Control

Chemical agents are used to control the growth of microbes on both living tissue and inanimate objects. Unfortunately, few chemical agents achieve sterility. Most of them merely reduce microbial populations to safe levels or remove vegetative forms of pathogens from objects. A common problem in disinfection is the selection of an agent. No single disinfectant is appropriate for all circumstances.

12.2.1   Evaluating a Disinfectant

There is a need to evaluate the effectiveness of disinfectants and antiseptics. For many years the standard test was the phenol coefficient test, which compared the activity of a given disinfectant with that of phenol. However, the current standard is the American Official Analytical Chemist'suse-dilution test.

Thedisk-diffusion method is used in teaching laboratories to evaluate the efficacy of a chemical agent. A disk of filter paper is soaked with a chemical and placed on an agar plate that has been previously inoculated and incubated with the test organism. After incubation and incubated with the test organism. After incubation, if the chemical is effective, a clear zone representing inhibition of growth can be seen around the disk.

12.2.2   Chemical Agents

12.2.2.1   Phenol and Phenolics

Lister was the first to usephenol to control surgical infections in the operating room. Its use had been suggested by its effectiveness in controlling odor in sewage. It is often used in throat lozenges for its local anesthetic effect but has little antimicrobial effect at the low concentrations used. At concentrations above 1%, however, phenol has a significant antibacterial effect.

Derivatives of phenol, called phenolics, contain a molecule of phenol that has been chemically altered to reduce its irritating qualities or increase its antibacterial activity in combination with a soap or detergent. Phenolics exert antimicrobial activity by injuring lipid-containing plasma membranes, which results in leakage of cellular contents.

12.2.2.2   Bisphenols

Bisphenols are derivatives of phenol that contain two phenolic groups connected by a bridge. One bisphenol, hexachlorophene, is an ingredient of a prescription lotion, used for surgical and hospital microbial control procedures. Another widely used bisphenol is triclosan, an ingredient in antibacterial soaps.

12.2.2.3   Biguanides

Chlorhexidine is a member of the biguanide group with a broad spectrum of activity. It is frequently used for microbial control on skin and mucous membranes. Combined with a detergent or alcohol, chlorhexidine is also used for surgical hand scrubs and preoperative skin preparation in patients.

12.2.2.4   Alcohols

Alcohols are among the most widely used disinfectants and antiseptics. They are bactericidal and fungicidal but not sporicidal; some lipid-containing viruses are also destroyed. The two most popular alcohol germicides are ethanol and isopropanol, usual used in about 70% to 80% concentration. They act by denaturing proteins and possibly by dissolving membrane lipids. A 10−15 minute soaking is sufficient to disinfect small instruments.

12.2.2.5   Halogens

The halogens, particularly iodine and chlorine, are effective antimicrobial agents, both alone and as constituents of inorganic or organic compounds. Iodine is one of the oldest and most effective antiseptics. It is effective against all kinds of bacteria, many endospores, various fungi and some viruses. Iodine impairs protein synthesis and alters cell membranes, apparently by forming complexes with amino acids and unsaturated fatty acids.

Iodophoris a combination of iodine and an organic molecule, from which the iodine is released slowly. Iodophors have the antimicrobial activity of iodine, but they do not stain and are less irritating. Povidone is a surface-active iodophor that improves he wetting action and serves as a reservoir of free iodine. Iodine are used mainly for skin disinfection and wound treatment. To treat water, iodine tablets are added or the water can be passed through iodine-treat resin filters.

Chlorine is the usual disinfectant for municipal water supplies and swimming pools and is also employed in the dairy and food industries. It may be applied as chlorine gas (Cl_2), sodium hypochlorite or calcium hypochlorite, all of which yield hypochlorous acid. The result is oxidation of cellular materials and destruction of vegetative bacteria and fungi. Chlorine is also an excellent disinfectant for individual use because it is effective, inexpensive and easy to employ. Small quantities of drinking water can be disinfected with halazone tabreleases chloride when added to water and disinfects it in about a half hour.

12.2.2.6 Surface-active Agents

Surface-active agents or surfactants, can decrease surface tension among molecules of a liquid.

Soap has little value as an antiseptic, but it does have an important function in the mechanical removal of microbes through scrubbing. Soap breaks the only film into tiny droplets, a process called emulsification and the water and soap together lift up the emulsified oil and debris and float them away as the lather is washed off.

Acid-anionic surface-active sanitizers are very important in the cleaning of dairy utensils and equipment. Their sanitizing ability is related to the negatively charged portion of the molecule, which reacts with the plasma membrane. These sanitizers, which act on a wide spectrum of microbes, including troublesome thermoduric bacteria, are nontoxic, noncorrosive and fast acting.

The most widely used surface-active agents are the cationic deter gents, especially the quaternary ammonium compounds (quats). Their cleansing ability is related to the positively charged portion-the cation-of the molecule. Quaternary ammonium compounds are strongly bactericidal against gram-positive bacteria and less active against gram-negative bacteria. Quats are also fungicidal, amoebicidal and virucidal against enveloped viruses. They do not kill endospores or mycobacteria. Their chemical mode of action is unknown, but they probably affect the plasma membrane. They change the cell's permeability and cause the loss of essential cytoplasmic constituents, such as potassium.

12.2.2.7 Heavy Metal

For many years the ions of heavy metals such as mercury, silver, arsenic, zinc and copper were used as germicides. These have now been superseded by other less toxic and more effective germicides. There are a few exceptions. In some hospitals, a 1% solution of silver nitrate is added to the eyes of infants to prevent ophthalmic gonorrhea. Silver sulfadiazine is used on burns. Copper sulfate is an effective algicide in lakes and swimming pools. Heavy metals combine with proteins, often with their sulfhydryl groups and inactivate them. They may also precipitate cell proteins.

Inorganic mercury compounds, such as mercuric chloride, have a long history of use as disinfectants. They have a very broad spectrum of activity; their effect is primarily bacteriostatic. However, their use is now limited because of their toxicity, corrosiveness and ineffectiveness in organic matter.

Copper in the form of copper sulfate or other copper, containing additives is used chiefly to destroy green algae that grow in reservoirs, stock ponds, swimming pools and fish tanks. If the water does not contain excessive organic matter, copper compounds are effective in concentrations of one part per million of water. To prevent mildew, copper compounds such as copper 8-hydroxyquinoline are sometimes included in paint.

Zinc can be seen on weathered roofs of buildings down-slope from galvanized fittings. Copper and zinc treated shingles are available. Zinc chloride is a common ingredient in mouthwashes and zinc oxide is probably the most widely used antifungal agent in paints, mainly because it is often part of the pigment formulation.

12.2.2.8　Chemical Preservatives

Chemical preservatives are frequently added to foods to retard spoilage. Sulfur dioxide (SO_2) has long been used as a disinfectant, especially in wine-making. Sodium nitrate and sodium nitrite are added to many meat products. The active ingredient is sodium nitrite, which certain bacteria in the meats can also produce from sodium nitrate. These bacteria use nitrate as a substitute for oxygen under anaerobic conditions. The nitrite has two main functions: to preserve the pleasing red color of the meat by reacting with blood components in the meat and to prevent the germination and growth of any botulism endospores that might be present. Nitrite selectively inhibits certain iron-containing enzymes of Clostridium botulinum.

12.2.2.9　Aldehydes

Both of the commonly used aldehydes, formaldehyde and glutaraldehyde, are highly reactive molecules that combine with nucleic acids and proteins and inactivate them, probably by cross-linking and alkylating molecules. They are sporicidal and can be used as chemical sterilants. Formaldehyde is usually dissolved in water or alcohol before use. A 2% buffered solution of glutaraldehyde is an effective disinfectant. It is less irritating than formaldehyde and is used to disinfect hospital and laboratory equipment. Glutaraldehyde usually disinfects objects within about 10 minutes but may require as long as 12 hours to destroy all spores.

12.2.2.10　Gaseous Chemosterilizers

Ethylene oxide is both microbicidal and sporicidal. It is a very strong alkylating agent that kills by reacting with functional groups of DNA and proteins to block replication and enzymatic activity. It is a particularly effective sterilizing agent because it rapidly penetrates packing materials, even plastic wraps.

Betapropiolactone is occasionally employed as a sterilizing gas. In the liquid form it has been used to sterilize vaccines and sera.

Vaporized hydrogen peroxidecan be used to decontaminate biological safety cabinets, operating rooms and other large facilities. These systems introduce vaporized hydrogen peroxide into the enclosure for some time, depending on the size of the enclosure and the materials within. Hydrogen peroxide and its oxy radical byproducts are toxic and kill a wide variety of microorganisms. During the course of the decontamination process, it breaks down to water and oxygen, both of which are harmless. Other advantages of these systems are that they can be used at a wide range of temperatures and they do not damage most materials.

12.2.2.11　Peroxygens

Peroxygens exert antimicrobial activity by oxidizing cellular components of the treated microbes. Examples are ozone, hydrogen peroxide and peracetic acid.

Ozoneis a highly reactive form of oxygen that is generated by passing oxygen through high-voltage electrical discharges. It is responsible for the air's rather fresh odor after a lightning storm, in the vicinity of electrical sparking or around an ultraviolet light. Ozone is often used to supplement chlorine in the disinfection of water because it helps neutralize tastes and odors. Although ozone is a more effective killing agent, its residual activity is difficult to maintain in water and it is more expensive than chlorine.

Hydrogen peroxide is found in many household medicine cabinets and in hospital supply rooms. It is not a good antiseptic for open wounds; in fact, it may slow wound healing. It is quickly broken down to water and gaseous oxygen by the action of the enzyme catalase, which is present in human cells. However, hydrogen peroxide does effectively disinfect inanimate objects, an application in which it is even sporicidal, especially at elevated temperatures. On a nonliving surface, the normally protective enzymes of aerobic bacteria and facultative anaerobes are overwhelmed by the high concentrations of peroxide used.

Oxidizing agentsare useful for irrigating deep wounds, where the oxygen released makes an environment that inhibits the growth of anaerobic bacteria.

Benzoyl peroxide is another compound useful for treating wounds infected by anaerobic pathogens, but it is probably more familiar as the main ingredient in over-the-counter medications for acne, which is caused by a type of anaerobic bacterium infecting hair follicles.

Peracetic acid is one of the most effective liquid chemical sporicides available and is considered a sterilant. It is generally effective on endospores and viruses within 30 minutes and kills vegetative bacteria and fungi in less than 5 minutes.

12.3   Antimicrobial Drugs

When the body's normal defenses cannot prevent or overcome a disease, it is often treated with chemotherapy. we focus on antimicrobial drugs, the class of chemotherapeutic agents used to treat infectious diseases. Antimicrobial drugs act by interfering with the growth of microorganisms. Unlike disinfectants, however, they must often act within the host. Therefore, their effects on the cells and tissues of the host are important. The ideal antimicrobial drug kills the harmful microorganism without damaging the host; this is the principle of selective toxicity.

Antibiotics were one of the most important discoveries for modern medicine. Within the memory of many people, an abdominal wound or a ruptured appendix represented nearly certain death from infection. There was little that medicine could do to treat diseases such as typhoid fever, tuberculosis and so-called blood poisoning in which bacteria proliferated uncontrolled in the bloodstream. The use of antimicrobials such as penicillin and sulfanilamide in the treatment of some infections resulted in rapid cures that seemed almost miraculous at the time.

12.3.1   The History of Chemotherapy

The birth of modern chemotherapy is credited to the efforts of Paul Ehrlich in Germany during the early part of the twentieth century. While attempting to stain bacteria without staining the surrounding tissue, he speculated about some "magic bullet" that would selectively find and destroy pathogens but not harm the host. This idea provided the basis for chemotherapy, a term he coined.

In 1928, Alexander FIeming observed that the growth of the bacterium Staphylococcus aureus was inhibited in the area surrounding the colony of a mold that had contaminated a Petri plate. The mold was identified as *Penicillium notatum* and its active compound, which was isolated a short time later, was named penicillin. Similar inhibitory reactions between colonies on solid media are commonly observed in microbiology and the mechanism of inhibition is called antibiosis. From this word comes the term antibiotic, a substance produced by microorganisms that in small amounts inhibits another microorganism. Therefore, the wholly synthetic sulfa drugs, for example, technically are not antibiotics. However, this distinction is often ignored in practice.

In 1940, a group of scientists at Oxford University headed by Howard Florey and Ernst Chain succeeded in the first clinical trials of penicillin. Under war time conditions in the United Kingdom, research into the development and large scale production of penicillin was not possible and this work was transferred to the United States. The original culture of *Penicillium chrysogenum* was not a very efficient producer of the antibiotic. It was soon replaced by a more prolific strain. This valuable organism was first isolated from a moldy cantaloupe bought at a market in Peoria, Illinois.

Antibiotics are actually rather easy to discover, but few are of medical or commercial value. Some are used commercially other than for treating disease—for example, as a supplement in animal feed. Many antibiotics are toxic to humans or lack any advantage over antibiotics already in use.

More than half of our antibiotics are produced by species of streptomyces, filamentous bacteria that commonly inhabit soil. A few antibiotics are produced by endospore-forming bacteria such as Bacillus and others are produced by molds, mostly of the genera Penicillium and Cephalosporium. One study screened 400,000 microbial cultures that yielded only three useful drugs. It is especially interesting to note that practically all antibiotic-producing microbes have some sort of sporulation process.

12.3.2   The Spectrum of Antimicrobial Activity

It is comparatively easy to find or develop drugs that are effective against prokaryotic cells and that do not affect the eukaryotic cells of humans. These two cell types differ substantially in many ways, such as in the presence or absence of cell walls, the fine structure of their ribosomes and details of their metabolism. Thus, selective toxicity has numerous targets. The problem is more difficult when the pathogen is a eukaryotic cell, such as a fungus, protozoan or helminth. At the cellular level, these organisms resemble the human cell much more closely than a bacterial cell does. We will see that our arsenal against these types of pathogens is much more limited than our arsenal of antibacterial drugs. Viral infections are particularly difficult to treat because the pathogen is within the human host's cells and the genetic information of the virus is directing the human cell to make viruses rather than to synthesize normal cellular materials.

Some drugs have a narrow spectrum of microbial activity or range of different microbial types they affect. Penicillin G, for example, affects gram-positive bacteria but very few gram-negative bacteria. Antibiotics that affect a broad range of gram-positive or gram-negative bacteria are therefore called broad-spectrum antibiotics.

A primary factor involved in the selective toxicity of antibacterial action lies in the lipopolysaccharide outer layer of gram-negative bacteria and the porins that form water-filled channels across this layer. Drugs that pass through the porin channels must be relatively small and preferably hydrophilic. Drugs that are lipophilic or especially large do not enter gram-negative bacteria readily.

Because the identity of the pathogen is not always immediately known, a broad-spectrum drug would seem to have an advantage in treating a disease by saving valuable time. The disadvantage is that many normal microbiota of the host are destroyed by broad-spectrum drugs. The normal microbiota ordinarily compete with and check the growth of pathogens or other microbes. If certain organisms in the normal microbiota are not destroyed by the antibiotic and their competitors are destroyed, the survivors may flourish and become opportunistic pathogens. An example that sometimes occurs is overgrowth by the yeastlike fungus Candida albicans, which is not sensitive to bacterial antibiotics. This overgrowth is called a superinfection, a term that is also applied to growth of a target pathogen that has developed resistance to the antibiotic. In this situation, such an antibiotic-resistant train replaces the original sensitive strain and the infection continues.

12.3.3   The Action of Antimicrobial Drugs

Antimicrobial dugs are either bactericidal or bacteriostatic. In bacteriostasis, the host's own defenses, such as phagocytosis and antibody production, usually destroy the microorganisms.

12.3.3.1 The Inhibition of Cell Wall Synthesis

The cell wall of a bacterium consists of a macromolecular network called peptidoglycan. Peptidoglycan is found only in bacterial cell walls. Penicillin and certain other antibiotics prevent the synthesis of intact peptidoglycan; consequently, the cell wall is greatly weakened and the cell undergoes lysis. Because penicillin targets the synthesis process, only actively growing cells are affected by these antibiotics-and, because human cells do not have peptidoglycan cell walls, penicillin has very little toxicity for host cells.

12.3.3.2 The Inhibition of Protein Synthesis

Because protein synthesis is a common feature of all cells, whether prokaryotic or eukaryotic, it would seem an unlikely target for selective toxicity. One notable difference between prokaryotes and eukaryotes, however, is the structure of their ribosomes. Eukaryotic cells have 80S ribosomes; prokaryotic cells have 70S ribosomes. The difference in ribosomal structure accounts for the selective toxicity of antibiotics that affect protein synthesis. However, mitochondria also contain 70S ribosomes similar to those of bacteria. Antibiotics targeting the 70S ribosomes can therefore have adverse effects on the cells of the host. Among the antibiotics that interfere with protein synthesis are chloramphenicol, erythromycin, streptomycin and the tetracyclines.

Reacting with the 50S portion of the 70S prokaryotic ribosome, chloramphenicol inhibits the formation of peptide bonds in the growing polypeptide chain. Most drugs that inhibit protein synthesis have a broad spectrum of activity; erythromycin is an exception. Because it does not penetrate the gram-negative cell wall, it affects mostly gram-positive bacteria.

Some other antibiotics react with the 30S portion of the 70S prokaryotic ribosome. The tetracyclines interfere with the attachment of the tRNA carrying the amino acids to the ribosome, preventing the addition of amino acids to the growing polypeptide chain. Tetracyclines do not interfere with mammalian ribosomes because they do not penetrate very well into intact mammalian cells. However, at least small amounts are able to enter the host cell, as is apparent from the fact that the intracellular pathogenic rickettsias and chlamydias are sensitive to tetracyclines. The selective toxicity of the drug in this case is due to a greater sensitivity of the bacteria at the ribosomal level.

Aminoglycoside antibiotics, such as streptomycin and gentamicin, interfere with the initial steps of protein synthesis by changing the shape of the 30S portion of the 70S prokaryotic ribosome. This interference causes the genetic code on the mRNA to be read incorrectly.

12.3.3.3 Injury to the Plasma Membrane

Certain antibiotics, especially polypeptide antibiotics, bring about changes in the permeability of the plasma membrane; these changes result in the loss of important metabolites from the microbial cell. For example, polymyxin B causes disruption of the plasma membrane by attaching to the phospholipids of the membrane.

Some antifungal drugs, such as amphotericin B, miconazole and ketoconazole, are effective against a considerable range of fungal diseases. Such drugs combine with sterols in the fungal plasma membrane to disrupt the membrane. Because bacterial plasma membranes generally lack sterols, these antibiotics do not act on bacteria. However, the plasma membranes of animal cells do contain sterols and amphotericin B and ketoconazole can be toxic to the host. Fortunately, animal cell membranes have mostly cholesterol and fungal cells have mostly ergosterol, against which the drug is most effective, so that the balance of the toxicity is tilted against the fungus.

12.3.3.4 The Inhibition of Nucleic Acid Synthesis

A number of antibiotics interfere with the processes of DNA replication and transcription in microorganisms. Some drugs with this mode of action have an extremely limited usefulness because they interfere with mammalian DNA and RNA as well. Others, such as rifampin and the quinolones, are more widely used in chemotherapy because they are more selectively toxic.

12.3.3.5 Inhibiting the Synthesis of Essential Metabolites

A particular enzymatic activity of a microorganism can be competitively inhibited by a substance that closely resembles the normal substrate for the enzyme. An example of competitive inhibition is the relationship between the antimetabolite sulfanilamide and para-aminobenzoic acid (PABA). In many microorganisms, PABA is the substrate for an enzymatic reaction leading to the synthesis of folic acid, a vitamin that functions as a coenzyme for the synthesis of the purine and pyrimidine bases of nucleic acids and many amino acids. In the presence of sulfanilamide, the enzyme that normally converts PABA to folic acid combines with the drug instead of with PABA. This combination prevents folic acid synthesis and stops the growth of the microorganism. Because humans do not produce folic acid from PABA, sulfanilamide exhibits selective toxicity-it affect microorganisms that synthesize their own folic acid but does not harm the human host. Other chemotherapeutic agents that act as antimetabolites are the sulfones and trimethoprim.

12.3.4 Introduction of Commonly Used Antimicrobial Drugs

12.3.4.1 Antibacterial Antibiotics

(1) Inhibitors of Cell Wall Synthesis

1) Penicillin: The term penicillin refers to a group of over 50 chemically related antibiotics. All penicillins have a common core structure containing a β-lactam ring called the nucleus. Penicillin molecules are differentiated by the chemical side chains attached to their nuclei. Penicillins can be produced either naturally or semisynthetically. Penicillins prevent the cross-linking of the peptidoglycans, which interferes with the final stages of the construction of the cell wall.

2) Natural penicillins: Penicillin extracted from cultures of the mold Penicillium exists in several closely related forms. These are the so-called natural penicillins. The prototype compound of all the penicillins is penicillin G. It has a narrow but useful spectrum of activity and is often the drug of choice against most staphylococci, streptococci and several spirochetes. When injected intramuscularly, penicillin G is rapidly excreted from the body in 3 to 6 hours. When taken orally, the acidity of the digestive fluids in the stomach diminishes its concentration. Procaine penicillin, a combination of the drugs procaine and penicillin G, is retained at detectable concentrations for up to 24 hours; concentration peaks at about 4 hours. Still longer retention times can be achieved with benzathine penicillin, a combination of benzathine and penicillin G. Although retention times of as long as 4 months can be obtained, the concentration of the drug is so low that the organisms must be very sensitive to it. Penicillin V, which is stable in stomach acids and can be taken orally and penicillin G are the natural penicillins most often used.

Natural penicillins have some disadvantages. Chief among them are their narrow spectrum of activity and their susceptibility to penicillinases. Penicillinases are enzymes produced by many bacteria, especially Staphylococcus species, that cleave the β-lactam ring of the penicillin molecule. Because of this characteristic, penicillinases are sometimes called β-lactamases.

3) Semisynthetic penicllins: A large number of semisynthetic penicillins have been developed in attempts to overcome the disadvantages of natural penicillins. Scientists develop these penicillins in either of two ways. First, they can interrupt synthesis of the molecule by Penicillium and obtain only the common penicillin nucleus for use. Second, they can remove the side chains from the completed natural molecules and then chemically add other side chains that make them more resistant to penicillinase or the scientists

can give them an extended spectrum. Thus the term semisynthetic：part of the penicillin is produced by the mold and part is added synthetically.

4）Penicillinase-resistant penicillins：The first semisynthetic penicillin designed to evade the action of penicillinases was methicllin. Eventually, so many strains of staphylococci developed resistance to methicillin that the abbreviation MRSA made its appearance. Resistance became so prevalent that methicillin has been discontinued in the United States. Replacement antibiotics similar to methicillin, such as oxacillin and nafcillin, have been developed.

5）Extended-Spectrum penicillins：To overcome the problem of the narrow spectrum of activity of natural penicillins, broader-spectrum semisynthetic penicillins have been developed. These new penicillins are effective against many gram-negative bacteria as well as gram-positive ones, although they are not resistant to penicillinases. The first such penicillins were the aminopenicillins, such as ampicillin and amoxicillin. When bacterial resistance to these became more common, the carboxypenicillins were developed. Members of this group, such as carbenicillin and ticarcillin, have even greater activity against gram-negative bacteria and have the special advantage of activity against Pseudomonas aeruginosa.

Among the more recent additions to the penicillin family are the ureidopenicillins, such as mezlocillin and azlocillin. These broader-spectrum penicillins are modifications of the structure of ampicillin. The search for even more effective modifications of penicillin continues.

6）Penicillins plus β-lactamase inhibitors：A different approach to the proliferation of penicillinase is to combine penicillins with potassium clavulanate, a product of a streptomycete. Potassium clavulanate is a noncompetitive inhibitor of penicillinase with essentially no antimicrobial activity of its own. It has been combined with some new broader-spectrum penicillins, such as amoxicillin.

7）Carbapenems：The carbapenems are a class of β-lactam antibiotics that substitute a carbon atom for a sulfuratom and add a double bond to the penicillin nucleus. These antibiotics, which inhibit cell wall synthesis, have an extremely broad spectrum of activity. Representative of the group is Primaxin, a combination of imipenem and cilastin. The cilastin has no antimicrobial activity but prevents degradation of the combination in the kidneys. Tests have demonstrated that Primaxin is active against 98% of all organisms isolated from hospital patients.

8）Monobactams：Another method of avoiding the effects of penicillinase is shown by aztreonam, which is the first member of a new class of antibiotics. It is a synthetic antibiotic that has only a single ring rather than the conventional β-lactam double ring and is therefore known as a monobactam. Aztreonam's spectrum of activity is remarkable for a penicillin-related compound-this antibiotic, which has unusually low toxicity, affects only certain gram-negative bacteria, including pseudomonads and *E. coli*.

9）Cephalosporins：In structure, the nuclei of cephalosporins resemble those of penicillin. Cephalosporins inhibit cell wall synthesis in essentially the same way as do penicillins. However cephalosporins differ from penicillin in that they are resistant to penicillinases and are effective against more gram-negative organisms than the natural penicillins. However, the cephalosporins are susceptible to a separate group of β-lactamases.

The number of second, third and even fourth generation cephalosporins has proliferated in recent years；there are now more than 70 versions. Each generation tends to be more effective against gram-negatives and has a broader spectrum of activity than the previous generation. A first-generation cephalosporin is cephalothin；a representative second generation is cefamondole. Oral administration is preferred by patients and several newer cephalosporins allow this. Cefpodoxime and cefixime are two cephalosporins that have been approved for oral administration.

10) Bacitracin: Bacitracin is a polypeptide antibiotic effective primarily against gram-positive bacteria, such as staphylococci and treptococci. Bacitracin inhibits the synthesis of cell walls at an earlier stage than penicillins and cephalosporins. It interferes with the synthesis of the linear strands of the peptidoglycans. Its use is restricted to topical application for superficial infections.

11) Vancomycin: Vancomycin is one of a small group of glycopeptide antibiotics derived from a species of Streptomyces found in the jungles of Borneo. Originally, toxicity of vancomycin was a serious problem, but improved purification procedures in its manufacture have largely corrected this. Although it has a very narrow spectrum of activity, which is based on inhibition of cell wall synthesis, vancomycin has been extremely important in addressing the problem of MRSA. Vancomycin has been considered the last line of antibiotic defense for treatment of Staphylococcus aureus infections that are resistant to other antibiotics. The widespread use of vancomycin to treat MRSA has led to the selection of vancomycin-resistant enterococci. These are opportunistic, gram-positive pathogens that are particularly troublesome in hospital settings. This appearance of vancomycin-resistant pathogens, leaving almost no effective alternative, is considered a medical emergency.

12) Antimycobacterial antibiotics: The cell wall of members of the genus Mycobacterium differs from the cell wall of most other bacteria. It incorporates mycolic acids that are a factor in their staining properties, causing them to stain as acid-fast. The genus includes important pathogens, such as those that cause leprosy and tuberculosis.

Isoniazid (INH) is a very effective synthetic antimicrobial drug against Mycobacterium tuberculosis. The primary effect of INH is to inhibit the synthesis of mycolic acids, which are components of cell walls only of the mycobacteria. It has little effect on nonmycobacteria. When used to treat tuberculosis, INH is usually administered simultaneously with other drugs, such as rifampinor ethambutol. This minimizes development of drug resistance. Because the tubercle bacillus is usually found only within macrophages or walled off in tissue, any antitubercular drug must be able to penetrate into such sites.

Ethambutol is effective only against mycobacteria. The drug apparently inhibits incorporation of mycolic acid into the cell wall. It is a comparatively weak antitubercular drug; its principal use is as the secondary drug to avoid resistance problems.

(2) Inhibitors of Proteinsynthesis

1) Chlora mphenicol: Chloramphenicol is a broad-spectrum antibiotic with serious toxicity problems. Because of its relatively simple structure, it is less expensive for the pharmaceutical industry to synthesize it chemically than to isolate it from Streptomyces. Because it is relatively inexpensive, chloramphenicol is often used where low cost is essential. Its relatively small molecular size promotes its diffusion into areas of the body that are normally inaccessible to many other drugs. However, chloramphenicol has serious adverse effects; most important is the suppression of bone marrow activity. This suppression affects the formation of blood cells. In about 1 in 40,000 users, the drug appears to cause aplastic anemia, a potentially fatal condition; the normalrate for this condition is only about 1 in 500,000 individuals. Physicians are advised not to use the drug for trivial conditions or ones for which suitable alternatives are available.

2) Aminoglycosides: Aminoglycosides are a group of antibiotics in which aminosugars are linked by glycoside bonds. They were among the first antibiotics to have significant activity against gram-negative bacteria. Probably the best-known aminoglycoside is streptomycin, which was discovered in 1944. Streptomycin is still used as an alternative drug in the treatment of tuberculosis, but rapid development of resistance and serious toxic effects have diminished itsusefulness.

Aminoglycosides are bactericidal and inhibit protein synthesis. They can affect hearing by causing permanent damage to the auditory nerve and damage to the kidneys has also been reported. Because of his, their use has been declining. Neomycin is present in many nonprescription topical preparations. Gentamicin is especially useful against Pseucdomonas infections. Pseudomonads are a major problem for persons suffering from cystic fibrosis. The aminoglycoside tobramycin is administered in an aerosol to aid in the control of infections that occur in patients with cystic fibrosis.

3)Tetracyclines：Tetracyclines are a group of closely related broad-spectrum antibiotics produced by *Streptomyces* spp. Tetracyclines inhibit protein synthesis. They not only are effective against gram-positive and gram-negative bacteria but also penetrate body tissues well and are especially valuable against the intracellular rickettsias and chlamydias. Three of the more commonly used tetracyclines areoxytetracycline,chlortetracycline and tetracycline itself. Some semisynthetic tetracyclines,such as doxycycline and minocycline, are available. They have the advantage of longer retention in the body.

Tetracyclines are used to treat many urinary tract infections,mycoplasmal pneumonia and chlamydial and rickettsial infections. They are also frequently used as alternative drugs for such diseases as syphilis and gonorrhea. Tetracyclines often suppress the normal intestinal microbiota because of their broad spectrum, causing gastrointestinal upsets and often leading to superinfections,particularly by the fungus Candida albicans. They are not advised for children,who might experience a brownish discoloration of the teeth or for pregnant women,in whom they might cause liver damage. Tetracyclines are among the most common antibiotics added to animal feeds,where their use results in significantly faster weight gain；however,some human health problems can also result.

4)Macrolides：Macrolides are a group of antibiotics named for the presence of a macrocyclic lactone ring. The best-known macrolide in clinical use is erythromycin. Its mode of action is the inhibition of protein synthesis. However,erythromycin is not able to penetrate the cell walls of most gram-negative bacilli. Its spectrum of activity is therefore similar to that of penicillin G and it is a frequent alternative drug to penicillin. Because it can be administered orally,an orange-flavored preparation of erythromycin is a frequent penicillin substitute for the treatment of streptococcal and staphylococcal infections in children. Erythromycin is the drug of choice for the treatment of legionellosis,my coplasmal pneumonia and several other infections.

Other macrolides now available include azithromycin and clarithromycin. Compared to erythromycin, they have a broader antimicrobial spectrum and penetrate tissues better. This is especially important in the treatment of conditions caused by intracellular bacteria such as Chlamydia,a frequent cause of sexually transmitted infection.

A new generation of semisynthetic macrolides,the ketolides,is being developed to cope with increasing resistance to other macrolides. The prototype of this generation is telithromycin.

5)Streptogramins：We mentioned previously that the appearance of vancomycin-resistant pathogens constitutes a serious medical problem. One answer may be a unique group of antibiotics,the streptogramins. The first of these drugs to be released,Synercid,is a combination of two cyclic peptides,quinupristin and dalfopristin,which are distantly related to the macrolides. They block protein synthesis by attaching to the 50S potion of the ribosome,as do other antibiotics such as chloramphenicol. Synercid,however,acts at uniquely different points on the ribosome. Dalfopristin blocks an early step in protein synthesis and quinupristin blocks a later step. The combination causes incomplete peptide chains to be released and is synergistic in its action. Synercid is effective against a broad range of gram-positive bacteria that are resistant to other antibiotics. This makes Synercid especially valuable,even though it is expensive and has a high incidence of adverse side effects.

6)Oxazolidinones   The oxazolidinones are another new class of antibiotics developed in response to vancomycin resistance. When the FDA approved this class of antibiotic in 2001, it represented the first new class of antibiotics approved in 25 years. Like several other antibiotics that inhibit protein synthesis, oxazolidinone antibiotics act on the ribosome. However, they are unique in their target, binding to the 50S ribosomal subunit close to the point where it interfaces with the 30S subunit. These drugs are totally synthetic, which may make resistance slower to develop. Like vancomycin, they have no usefulness against gram-negative bacteria, but they are active against certain enterococci that are not sensitive to Synercid. One member of this antibiotic group is linezolid, used mainly to combat MRSA.

(3) Injury to the Plasmsa Membrane

Polymyxin B is a bactericidal antibiotic effective against gram-negative bacteria. For many years, it was one of very few drugs against infections by gram-negative used Pseudomonas. The mode of action of polymyxin B is to injure plasma membranes. Polymyxin B is seldom used today except in the topical treatment of superficial infections. Both bacitracin and polymyxin B are available in nonprescription antiseptic ointments, in which they are usually combined with neomycin, a broad-spectrum aminoglycoside. In a rare exception to the rule, these antibiotics do not require a prescription. Many of the antimicrobial peptides discussed on page 605 target the synthesis of the plasma membrane.

(4) Inhibitors of Nucleicacid Synthesis

1) Rifamycins: The best known derivative of the rifamycin family of antibiotics is rifampin. These drugs are structurally related to the macrolides and inhibit the synthesis of mRNA. By far the most important use of rifampin is against mycobacteria in the treatment of tuberculosis and leprosy. A valuable characteristic of rifampin is its ability TO penetrate tissues and reach therapeutic levels in cerebrospinal fluid and abscesses. This characteristic is probably an important factor in its antitubercular activity, because the tuberculosis pathogen is usually located inside issues or macrophages. An unusual side effect of rifampin is the appearance of orange-red urine, feces, saliva, sweat and event ears.

2) Quinolones and fluoroquinolones: In the early 1960s, the synthetic drug nalidixic acid was developed-the first of the quinolone group of antimicrobials. It exerted a unique bactericidal effect by selectively inhibiting an enzyme needed for the replication of DNA. Although nalidixic acid found only limited, it led to the development in the 1980s of a prolific group of synthetic quinolones, the fluoroquinolones. The most widely used fluoroquinolones are norfloxacin and ciprofloxacin. The latter is better known under its trade name of Cipro and gained widespread publicity for its use against anthrax infections. Although they are relatively safe for adults, fluoroquinolones adversely affect the development of cartilage and their use is limited among children, adolescents and pregnant women.

A third generation of fluoroquinolones includes moaxi-floxacin and gatifloxacin. These have a broader antimicrobial spectrum, especially against gram-positives and can be taken orally. Gatifloxacin is also available in a liquid formulation for treatment of eye infections.

(5) Competitive Inhibitors of the Synthesisof Essentialmetabolites

Sulfonamides: As noted earlier, sulfonamides or sulfa drugs, we are the first synthetic antimicrobial drugs used to treat among microbial diseases. Antibiotics have diminished the importance of sulfa drugs in chemotherapy, but they continue to be used to treat certain urinary tract infections and have other specialized uses, as in the combination drug silver sulfadiazine, used to control infections in burn patients. Sulfonamides are bacteriostatic; as mentioned, their action is due to their structural similarity to para-aminobenzoic acid (PABA).

Probably the most widely used sulfa drug today is a combination of trimethoprim and sulfamethoxazole. This combination is an excellent example of drug synergism. When used in combination, only 10% of the concentration is needed, compared to when each drug issued alone. The combination also has a broader spectrum of action and greatly reduces the emergence of resistant strains.

12.3.4.2   Antifungal Drugs

Eukaryotes, such as fungi, use the same mechanisms to synthesis proteins and nucleic acids as higher animals. Therefore it is more difficult to find a point of selective toxicity in eukaryotes than in prokaryotes. Moreover, fungal infections are becoming more frequent because of their role as opportunistic infections in immunosuppressed individuals, especially those with AIDS.

(1) Agents Affecting Fungal Sterols

Many antifungal drugs target the sterols in the plasma membrane. In fungal membranes, the principal sterol is ergosterol; in animal membranes, cholesterol. When the biosynthesis of ergosterol in a fungal membrane is interrupted, the membrane becomes excessively permeable, killing the cell. Inhibition of ergosterol biosynthesis is the which basis for the selective toxicity of many antifungals, which include members of the polyene, azole and allylamine Groups.

1) Polyenes: Amphotericim B is the most commonly used member of the antifungal polyene antibiotics. For many years amphotericin B, produced by Streptomyces species of soil bacteria, has been a mainstay of clinical treatment for systemic fungal diseases such as histoplasmosis, coccidioidomycosis and blastomycosis. The drug's toxicicy particularly to the kidneys, is a strongly limiting factor in these uses. Administering the drug encapsulated in lipids (liposomes) appears to minimize toxicity.

2) Azoles: Some of the most widely used antifungal drugs are represented among the azole antibiotics. Before they made their appearance, the only drugs available for systemic fungal infect ions were amphotericin B and flucytocine. The first azoles were imidazoles, such as clotrimazole and miconazole, which are now sold without a prescription for topical application for treatment of cutaneous mycoses, such as athlete's foot and vaginal yeast infections. An important addition to this group was ketocomazole, which has an unusually broad spectrum of activity among fungi. Ketoconazole, taken orally, is often used as a less toxic alternative to amphotericin B for many systemic fungal infections, although occasional liver damage has been reported. Ketoconazole topical ointments are used to treat dermatomycoses. A promising new broad spectrum antifungal, voriconazole, is expected to replace amphotericin B for treatment of many systemic antifungal infections. It has a special advantage in treatment of aspergillosis of the central nervous system because it is able to penetrate the blood-brain barrier.

The use of ketoconazole diminished sharply upon the introduction of the triazole antibiotics. Drugs of this group, such as flucomazole and itraconzole, are less toxic and have other advantages as well. Unlike ketoconazole, they are very water soluble, which makes their administration for systemic infections easier and more effective.

3) Allylamines: The allylamines represent a recently developed class of antifungals that inhibit the biosynthesis of ergosterols in a manner that is functionally distinct. Terbinafine and naftifine, examples of this group, are when resistance to azole-type antifungals arises.

(2) Agents Affecting Fungal Cell Walls

The fungal cell wall contains compounds that are unique to these organisms. A primary target for selective toxicity among these compounds is B-glucan. Inhibition of the biosynthesis of this glucan results in an incomplete cell wall and results in lysis of the fungal cell. The first of a new class of antifungal drugs is the echinocandins, which inhibit the biosynthesis of glucans. A member of thee chinocandin group, caspofungin is now available commercially. This new antifungal agent is expected to become especially valuable for combating systemic Aspergillus infections in persons whose immune system is compromised. It is also effective against important fungi such as *Candida* spp. and *Pneumocystis jiroveci*, which causes a pneumonia often seen in AIDS patients.

(3) Agents Inhibiting Nucleic Acids

Flucytosine, an analog of the pyrimidine cytosine, interferes with the biosynthesis of RNA and therefore protein synthesis. The selective toxicity lies in the ability of theflucytocine into 5-fluorouracil, fungal cell to convert which is incorporated into RNA and eventually disrupts protein synthesis. Mammalian cells lack the enzyme to make this conversion of the drug. Flucytosine has a narrow spectrum of activity and toxicity to the kidneys and bone further limit its use.

(4) Other Antifungal Drugs

Griseofulvin is an antibiotic produced by a species of Penicllium. It has the interesting property of being active against superficial dermatophytic fungal infections of the hair and nails, even though its route of administration is oral. The drug apparently binds selectively to the keratin found in the skin, hair follicles, is primarily to block and nails. Its modeof action microtubules assembly, which interferes with mitosis and thereby inhibits fungal reproduction.

Tolnaftate is a common alternative to miconazole as a topical agent for the treatment of athlete's foot. Its mechanism of action is not known. Undecylenic acid is a fatty acid that has antifungal activity against athlete's foot, although it is not as effective as effective as tolnaftate or the imidazoles.

Pentamidine isethionate is used in the treatment of Pneumocystis pneumonia. The drug's mode of action is unknown, but it appears to bind DNA.

12.3.4.3 Antiviral Drugs

In developed parts of the world, it is estimated that at least 60% of infectious illnesses are caused by viruses and about 15% by bacteria. Every year, at least 90% of the U. S population suffers from a viral disease. Yet relatively few antiviral drugs have been approved in the United States and they are effective against only an extremely limited group of diseases. Many of the recently developed antiviral drugs are directed against HIV, the pathogen responsible for the pandemic of AIDS. Therefore, as a practical matter the discussion of antivirals is often separated into agents that are directed at chemotherapy of HIV and those with more general applications.

Because viruses replicate within the host's cells, very often using the genetic and metabolic mechanisms of the host's own cells, it is relatively difficult to target the virus without damaging the host's cellular machinery. Many of the antivirals in use today are analogs of components of viral DNA or RNA. However as more becomes known about the reproduction of viruses, more targets suggest themselves for antiviral action.

(1) Nucleoside and Nucleotide Analogs

Several important antiviral drugs are analogs of nucleosides and nucleotides. Among the nucleoside analogs, acyclovir is the one more widely used. While best known for treating genital herpes, it is generally useful for most herpesvirus infections, especially in immunosuppressed individuals. The antiviral drugs famiciclovir, which can be taken orally and ganciclovir are derivatives of acyclovir and have a similar mode of action. Ribavirin resembles the nucleoside guanine and accelerates the already high mutation rate of RNA viruses until the accumulation error reaches a crisis point, killing the virus. The nucleoside analog, lamivrudine, is used to treat hepatitis B. More recently, a nucleotide analog adefovir dipivoxil has been introduced for patients resistant to the nucleoside lamivudine. A nucleosideanalog, cidofovir, is presently used for treatment of cytomegalovirus infections of the eye, but this drug is especially interesting because it shows promise as a possible treatment of smallpox.

Antiertrovirals: The need for effective chemotherapy of HIV infections has led to the development of a relatively numerous group of antiviral drugs. HIV is an RNA virus and its reproduction depends on the enzyme reverse transcriptase, which controls the synthesis of RNA from DNA. Analogs of nucleotides or nucleosides are often a basis for drugs to block this essential step. In fact, the term antiretroviral currently implies that HIV infection. A well-known example of a nucleotide analog is zidovdine. Currently, the only nucleotide reverse transriptase inhibitor is tenofovir. Only recently approved, it is often used when other regimens have filed.

Not all drugs that inhibit reverse transcriptase are nucleoside or nucleotide analogs. For example, several non-nucleoside agents, such as nevirapine, block RNA synthesis by other mechanisms.

(2) Other Enzyme Inhibitors

Another approach to the control of HIV infections is to inhibit the enzymes that control the last stage of viral reproduction. When the host cell (at the direction of the infecting HIV) makes a new virus, it must begin by cutting up large proteins with protease enzymes. The resulting fragments are used to assemble new viruses. Analogs of amino acid sequences in the large proteins can serve as inhibitors of these proteases by competitively interfering with their ac tivity. The protease inhibitors atazanavir, indinavir and saquinavir have proved especially effective when combined with inhibitors of reverse transcriptase. Other enzymatic targets of HIV are the enzymes, integrases, that integrate the viral DNA into the host's DNA, forming a provirus—by integrase inhibitors. Entry of HIV into the cell by fusion can be blocked by fusion inhibitors such as envuvirtide—which, however, is dauntingly expensive.

(3) Interferon

Cells infected by a virus often produce iterferon, which inhibits further spread of the infection. Interferons are classified as cytokines. Alpha-interferon is currently a drug of choice for viral hepatitis infections. The production of interferons can be stimulated by a recently introduced antiviral, imiquimod. This drug is often prescribed to treat genital warts caused by a herpesvirus.

12.3.4.4 Antiprotozoan and Antihelminthic Drugs

For hundreds of years, quinine from the Peruvian cinchona tree was the only drug known to be effective for the treatment of a parasitic infection. It was first introduced into Europe in the early 1600 s and was known as "Jesuit's powder". There are now many antiprotozoan and antihelminthic drugs, although many of them are still considered experimental. This does not preclude their use, however, by qualified physicians. The CDC provides several of them on request when they are not available commercially.

(1) Antiprotozoan Drugs

Quinine is still used to control the protozoan disease malaria, but synthetic derivatives, such as chloroquine, have largely replaced it. For preventing malaria in areas where the disease has developed resistance to chloroquine, the new drug mefloquine is recommended, although serious psychiatric side effects have been reported. Quinacrine is the drug of choice for treating the protozoan disease giardiasis. Diiodohydroxyquin is an important drug prescribed for several intestinal amoebic diseases, but its dosage must be carefully controlled to avoid optic nerve damage. Its mode of action is unknown.

Metronidazole is one of the most widely used antiprotozoan drugs. It is unique in that it acts not only against parasitic protozoa but also against obligately anaerobic bacteria. For example, as an antiprotozoan agent, it is the drug of choice for vaginitis caused by Trichomonas vaginalis. It is also used in the treatment of giardiasis and amoebic dysentery. The mode of action is to interfere with anaerobic metabolism, which incidentally these protozoans share with certain obligately anaerobic bacteria Clostridium.

Tinidazole, a drug similar to metronidazole are cently been approved for use in the United States—although it has long been used elsewhere under the trade name of Fasigyn. It is effective in the treatment of giardiasis, amebiasis and trichomoniasis. Another new antiprotozoan agent and the first to be approved for the chemotheraphy of diarrhea caused by Cryptosporidium hominis, is nitazoxanide. It is active in treatment of giardiasis and amebiasis. Interestingly, it is also effective in treating several helminthic diseases, as well as having activity against some anaerobic bacteria.

(2) Anithelminthic Drugs

With the increased popularity of sushi, a Japanese specialty often made with raw fish, the CDC began to notice an increased incidence of tapeworm infections. To estimate the incidence, the CDC documents requests for niclosamide, which is the usual first choice in treatment. The drug is effective because it inhibits ATP production under aerobic conditions. Praziquantel is about equally effective for the treatment of tapeworms; it kills worms by altering the permeability of their plasma membranes. Praziquantel has a broad spectrum of activity and is highly recommended for treating several fluke-caused diseases, especially schistosomiasis. It causes the helminths to undergo muscular spasms and apparently makes them susceptible to attack by the immune system. Apparently, its action exposes surface antigens, which antibodies can then reach.

Mebendazole and albendazole are broad-spectrum antihelminthics that have few side effects and have become the drugs of choice for treatment of many intestinal helminthic infections. The mode of action of both drugs is to inhibit the formation of microtubules in the cytoplasm, which interferes with the absorption of nutrients by the parasite. These drugs are also widely used in the livestock industry; for veterinary applications they are relatively more effective in ruminant animals.

Ivermectin is a drug with a wide range of applications. It is known to be produced by only one species of organism, Sreptomyces avermectinius, which was isolated from the soil near a Japanese golf course. It is effective against many nematodes and several mites, ticks and insects. Its primary use has been in the livestock industry as a broad-spectrum antihelminthic. Its exact mode of action is uncertain, but the final result is paralysis and death of the helminth without effectingmammalian hosts.

12.3.5   Tests to Guide Chemotherapy

Different microbial species and strains have different degrees of susceptibility to different chemotherapeutic agents. Moreover, the susceptibility of a microorganism can change with time, even during therapy with a specific drug. Thus, a physician must know the sensitivities of the pathogen before treatment can be started. However, physicians often cannot wait for sensitivity tests and must begin treatment based on their "best guess" estimation of the most likely pathogen causing the illness.

Several tests can be used to indicate which chemotherapeutic agent is most likely to combat a specific pathogen. However, if the organisms have been identified—for example, Pseudomonas aeruginosa, beta-hemolytic streptococci or gonococci-certain drugs can be selected without only specific testing for susceptibility. Tests are necessary when susceptibility is not predictable or when antibiotic resistance problems develop.

12.3.5.1   The Diffusion Methods

Probably the most widely used, although not necessarily the best, method of testing is the disk-diffusion method, also known as the Kirby-Bauer test. A Petri plate containing an agar medium is inoculated uniformly over its entire surface with a standardized amount of a test organism. Next, filter paper disks impregnated with known concentrations of chemotherapeutic agents are placed on the solidified agar surface. During incubation, the chemotherapeutic agents diffuse from the disks into the agar. The farther the agent diffuses from the disk, the lower its concentration. If the chemotherapeutic agent is effective, a zone of inhibition forms around the disk after a standardized incubation. The diameter of the zone can be measured; in general, the larger the zone, the more sensitive the microbe is to the antibiotic. The zone diameter is compared to a standard table for that drug and concentration and the organism is reported as sensitive, intermediate or resistant. For a drug with poor solubility, however, the zone of inhibition indicating that the microbe is sensitive will usually be smaller than for another drug that is more soluble and has diffused more widely. Results obtained by the disk-diffusion method are often inadequate for many clinical purposes. However, the test is simple and inexpensive and is most often used when more sophisticated laboratory facilities are not available.

A more advanced diffusion method, the E test, enables a lab technician to estimate the minimal inhibitory concentration (MIC), the lowest antibiotic concentration that prevents visible bacterial growth. A plastic-coated strip contains gradient of antibiotic conentrations and the MIC can be read from a scale printed on the strip.

12.3.5.2　Broth Dilution Test

A weakness of the diffusion method is that it does not determine whether a drug is bactericidal and not just bacteriostatic. A broth dilution test is often useful in determining the minimal bactericidal concentration of an antimicrobial drug. The MIC is determined by making a sequence of decreasing concentrations of the drug in a broth, which is then inoculated with the test bacteria. The wells that do not show growth can be cultured in broth or on agar plates free of the drug. If growth occurs in this broth, the drug was not bactericidal and the MBC can be determined. Determining the MIC and MBC is important because it avoids the excessive or erroneous use of expensive antibiotics and minimizes the chance of toxic reactions that larger-than-necessary doses might cause.

Dilution tests are often highly automated. The drugs are purchased already diluted into broth in wells formed in a plastic tray. A suspension of the test organism is prepared and inoculated into all the wells simultaneously by a special inoculating device. After incubation, the turbidity may be read visually, although clinical laboratories with high workloads may read the trays with special scanners that enter the data into a computer that provides a printout of the MIC.

Other tests are also useful for the clinician; a determination of the microbe's ability to produce β-lactamase is one example. One popular, rapid method makes use of a cephalosporin that changes color when its β-lactam ring is opened. In addition, a measurement of the serum concentration of an antimicrobial is especially important when toxic drugs are used. These assays tend to vary with the drug and may not always be suitable for smaller laboratories.

12.3.6　The Effectiveness of Chemotherapeutic Agents

12.3.6.1　Drug Resistance

Variations on these mechanisms also occur. For example, a microbe could become resistant to trimethoprim by synthesizing very large amounts of the enzyme against which the drug is targeted. Conversely, polyene antibiotics can become less effective when resistant organisms produce smaller amounts of the sterols against which the drug is effective. Of particular concern is the possibility that susceptible normal populations.

Hereditary drug resistance is often carried by plasmids or by small segments of DNA called transposons that can jump from one piece of DNA to another. Some plasmids, including those called resistance factors, can be transferred between bacterial cells in a population and between different but closely related bacterial populations. R factors often contain genes for resistance to several antibiotics.

Antibiotics have been a much misused product, nowhere more so than in the less developed areas of the world. Well-trained personnel are scarce, especially in rural areas, which is perhaps one reason why antibiotics can almost universally be purchased without prescription in these countries. In much of the world, antibiotics are sold to treat headaches and for other inappropriate uses. Even when the use of antibiotics is appropriate, dose regimens are usually shorter than needed to eradicate the infection. This encourages the survival of resistant strains of bacteria. Outdated, adulterated and counterfeit even antibiotics are common.

The developed world is also contributing to the rise of antibiotic resistance. The CDC estimates that in the United States, 30% of antibiotic prescriptions for ear infections, 100% of prescriptions for the common cold and 50% of prescriptions for sore throats were unnecessary or not appropriate to treat the probable pathogen. At least half of the more than 100,000 tons of antibiotics consumed in the United States each year are not used to treat disease but are used in animal feeds to promote growth-a practice that many feel should be curtailed. Patients also contribute to survival of antibiotic-resistant microbes when they fail to finish the full regimen of the prescription or use leftover antibiotics.

Strains of bacteria that are resistant to antibiotics are particularly common among hospital workers, where antibiotics are in constant use. Many hospitals have special monitoring committees to review the use of antibiotics for effectiveness and cost.

12.3.6.2 Antibiotic Safety

In our discussions of antibiotic, we have occasionally mentioned side effects. These may be potentially serious, such as liver or kidney damage or hearing impairment. Administration of almost any drug involves an assessment of risks against benefits; this is called the therapeutic index. Sometimes, the use of another drug can cause toxic effects that do not occur when the drug is taken alone. One drug may also neutralize the intended effects of the other. For example, a few antibiotics have been reported to neutralize the effectiveness of contraceptive pills. Also, some individuals may have hypersensitivity reactions for example, to penicillins.

12.3.6.3 Effects of Combinations of Drugs

The chemotherapeutic effect of two drugs given simultaneously is sometimes greater than the effect of either given alone. This phenomenon, called synergism, was introduced earlier. For example, in the treatment of bacterial endocarditis, penicillin and streptomycin are much more effective when taken together than when either drug is taken alone. Damage to bacterial cell walls by penicillin makes it easier for streptomycin to enter.

Other combinations of drugs can show antagonism. For example, the simultaneous use of penicillin and tetracycline is often less effective than when either drug is used alone. By stopping the growth of the bacteria, the bacteriostatic drug tetracycline interferes with the action of penicillin, which requires bacterial growth.

Chapter 13

Principles of Control Infection

13.1 Immunoprophylaxis of Microorganism Infection

An important contribution of microbiology to medicine has been immunization, which is only one of the most effective measures that may be used for the control of infectious diseases. An animal or human may acquire immunity to a disease in several ways. ①The individual may acquire an infection and then develop the immunity. This is natural active immunity because the immunization was a natural outcome of infection in the infected individual producing the immune response. ②The individual may be exposed to an antigen to induce formation of antibodies, a type of immunity known as artificial active immunity because the individual produced the antibodies. This process is commonly known as vaccination, properly termed immunization. ③Alternatively, the individual may receive injections of an antiserum derived from another individual who has previously infected and formed antibodies against the disease. This is called artificial passive immunity because the individual receiving the antibodies played no active part in the antibody-producing process. ④Finally, natural passive immunity also occurs. For several months after birth, newborns have mater IgG antibodies in their blood. These antibodies, acquired across the protection while the immune system of the new-born is maturing. By systematic active immunization, therefore, many developed countries have virtually eliminated 'vaccine preventable diseases' (VPD) such as diphteria, pertussis, tetanus, measles, mumps, rubella and poliomyelitis. The global eradication of smallpox, of course, has been the crowning glory of immunization.

Immunoprophylaxis may be in the form of ①routine immunization, which forms part of basic health care; or ②immunization of individuals or selected groups exposed to risk of specific infections.

13.1.1 Routine Immunization

Routine immunization schedules have been developed for different countries and modified from time to time, based on the prevalence of infectious diseases. their public health importance availability of suitable vaccines, their cost benefit factors and logistics. In China, the Expanded Programme on Immunization (EPI) and the Universal Immunization Programme (UIP) have been able to afford protection for much of the target population against VPDS.

Immunization with three doses of OPV has not been consistently effective in China and other developing countries, with high rates of seroconversion failures. This is sought to be met through the strategy of mop up rounds by giving OPV to all the children in an area on the same day, expecting natural spread of the vaccine virus among the children to reinforce immunization. These rounds are preferably held during October to April, as the polio season in China is from May to October, with a peak in July-August.

Different countries employ different immunization schedules depending on their priorities.

13.1.2 Active Immunization

Immunization is the most effective method to provide individual and community protection against many epidemic diseases. Immunization can be active, with stimulation of the body's immune mechanisms through administration of a vaccine or toxin or passive, through administration of plasma or globulin containing preformed antibody to the agent desired. Active immunization mimics an infection and can mount an immune response to control the second infection. The common types of vaccine list as following.

13.1.2.1 Vaccines

Protection against pathogenic microorganisms requires the generation of effective immune mechanisms. Thus, vaccines must be capable of targeting the immune system appropriately i. e. cellular and/or humoral mechanisms. The available vaccines and their indications are showed in Table 13-1.

Table 13-1　Bacterial vaccines for active immunization

Disease	Products	Type of antigen
Anthrax	*Bacillus anthracis*	Partially purified proteins
Cholera	*Vibrio cholerae*	Killed organisms
Diphtheria	*Corynebacteriumdiphtheriae*	Toxoid
Haemophilusinfluenzae infections	Polysaccharide capsule conjugated with protein	Polysaccharide protein conjuagate
Lyme disease	*Borreliaburgdorferi*	Recombinant outer surface protein A
Meningitis	*Haemophilusinfluenzae*	Capsular polysaccharide conjugated to carrier protein, e. g. diphtheria toxoid
Plague	*Yersinia pestis*	Killed organisms
Pneumonia	*Streptococcus pneunomiae*	Capsular polysaccharide
Q fever	*Coxiellaburnetii*	Killed organisms
Tetanus	*Clostridium tetani*	Toxoid
Tuberculosis	*Mycobacterium bovis* (BCG)	Live organisms
Tularemia	*Franciisellatularensis*	Live organisms
Typhoid fever	*Salmonella typhi*	
Typhus	*Rickettsia prowazekii*	Killed organisms
Whooping cough	*Bordetella pertussis*	Killed organisms or acellular (purified proteins)

Continue to Table 13-1

Disease	Products	Type of antigen
Diphtheria	DTP(diphtheria, tetanus, pertussis)	Killed bacteria. also an "acellular" vaccine containing two or more antigens but not the whole cell
Tetanus	DTaP(diphtheria, tetanus)	
Pertussis		
Hepatitis A	Hepatitis A	Live
Hepatitis B	Hepatitis B	Genetic engineering
Influenza	Influenza A and B	Killed
Measles	Measles	Live
Mumps	Mumps	Live
Poliovirus	Poliovirus	Live/Killed
Japanese encephalitis	Japanese encephalitis	Live/Killed
Rabies	Rabies	Killed
Rubella	Rubella	Live
Hemorrhagic fever	Hemorrhagic fever	Killed

(1) Attenuated Live Vaccines

Attenuated vaccines consist of organisms that have been attenuated by growth in unfavorable conditions, forcing them to mutate their genes; mutants that have lost virulence but retain antigenicity are repeatedly selected. The approach is to use suspensions of living organisms that are reduced in their virulence (attenuated) but still immunogenic. Nowadays, mutation is usually 'site-directed'by recombinant DNA technology. Such organism, which are essentially new strains, can sometimes regain virulence by back-mutation and can also cause severe disease in immunocompromised individuals. On the other hand they often induce stronger and better localized immunity, do not often require adjuvants or booster injections. Moreover, the immunity induced is usually more appropriate for protection against the pathogenic strain of the organism, e. g. Th1 vs Th2 responses. The example of attenuated bacteria vaccine is mumps measles and rubella vaccines (now combined), the live-virus polio vaccine and yellow fever vaccine.

(2) Inactivated Vaccines

Inactivated vaccines use microbes that have been killed by a chemical such as formalin, acetone or phenol. If the disease is not mediated by a single toxin, inactivated vaccine may be possible to stimulate the production of protective antibodies. This is done as a routine with vaccines against pertussis (whooping cough), typhoid and influenza. There is also an inactivated polio vaccine.

(3) Subunit Vaccine

Subunit vaccines(acellular vaccine) contain only those antigenic fragments of a microorganism that stimulate a maximum immune response without causing side effects. Subunit vaccines that are produced by genetic engineering techniques, meaning that other microbes are programmed to produce the desired antigenic fraction, are called recombinant vaccines. For example, the vaccine against the hepatitis B virus consists of a portion of the viral protein coat that is produced by genetically engineered yeast.

(4) Conjugated Vaccine

Conjugated vaccines have been developed in recent years to deal with the poor immune response of children to vaccines based on capsular polysaccharides. The polysaccharides are combined with proteins such as diphtheria toxoid thereby making them much more powerful antigens; this approach has led to the very successful vaccine for *Haemophilusinfluenzae* type B, which gives significant protection even at 2 months.

(5) Peptide Vaccine

A related approach is to attach short, chemically synthesized peptides (usually<20 amino acids) that correspond to known epitopes from an infectious organism onto a carrier to create peptide vaccines. These strategies are based on the concept that isolated carbohydrate or polypeptide epitopes can act as haptens to induce antibodies, whichi may then recognize the same epitopes in the native pathogen, though usually with lower affinity. For this approach to succeed, however, the vaccine must incorporate both B-and T-cell epitopes alone induce little or no immunologic memory. Moreover, T-cell epitopes must be carefully chosen to ensure that they can be recognized, presented and responded by all members of the population at risk.

(6) Recombinant Vaccine

Advances in molecular bacteriology have provided the immunologist with many new targets for vaccine development. Scientist have identified the components of the immune system that are protective for many infectious agents. Using molecular genetics, selective recombinant proteins of defined epitopes can be prepared that protect the host. This approach overcomes the problem of disease complications which might occur with modified live vaccines. If the host is inoculated with the defined peptide, they develop responses to the epitope and do not have to worry about resulting disease from vaccination with a modified live vaccine.

(7) DNA Vaccine

Bacterial plasmids containing cloned DNA are injected intramuscularly into a host animal and the DNA is transcribed and translated to produce an immunogenic protein and this triggers an immune response. These plasmids are called DNA vaccines or nucleic acid vaccines. Experiments with animals show that plasmids of "naked" DNA injected into muscle results in the production of the protein encoded in the DNA. These proteins persist and stimulate an immune response.

DNA vaccines provide considerable advantages over many conventional immunization protocols. For example, since only a single foreign gene is injected, there is no chance of infection as there might be with an attenuated vaccine. Second, antigens and even single antigenic determinants can be used in a vaccine to target the immune response to a particular cell component such as a tumor-specific antigen. Finally, this is the only method known in which immunization with a single bioengineered antigen elicits a Tc response, in addition to the antibody response.

A problem with this type of vaccine is that the DNA remains effective only until it is degraded. Indications are that RNA, which could replicate in the recipient, might be a more effective agent.

13.1.2.2　Toxoids

Toxoids were the first acellular vaccines, which are purified exotoxins that have been inactivated by chemicals or heat. If the signs and symptoms of a disease can be attributed essentially to the effects of a single toxin, the toxoid can provide the key to successful active immunization against the disease. Immunization against diphtheria is indicated for every child and given in three doses at 2,4 and 6 months of age, thereafter. Tetanus toxoid of *Clostridium tetani* is given to everyone both early in life and later as boosters for protection against tetanus.

13.1.2.3　Adjuvants

The response to an immunogen can often be enhanced if it is administered as a mixture with substances called adjuvants. Adjuvants function in one or more of the following ways: ①by prolonging retention of the immunogen; ②by increasing the effective size of the immunogen and so promoting phagocytosis and presentation by macrophages;③by stimulating the influx of macrophages or other immune cell types to the injection site;④by promoting local cytokine production and other immunologic activities of such immune cells.

A number of adjuvants have been used in experimental animals, the most potent being complete Freund's adjuvant(CFA), a water-in-oil emulsion containing killed mycobacteria. The only adjuvants approved for clinical use are aluminum salts-fine particles of aluminum phosphate or hydroxide onto which the immunogen is adsorbed. These widely used adjuvants increase the stability and effective particle size of an immunogen and also promote release of certain cytokines, such as interleukin-1.

13.1.3 Passive Immunization-homologous and Heterologous Sera

Artificial passive immunization is used in clinical practice when it is considered necessary to protect a patient at short notice and for a limited period. Therefore, passive immunization is a kind of antibody transfusion. Antibodies which may be antitoxic, antibacterial or antiviral produced by human or animal donors are injected to give temporary protection. Human preparations are referred to as homologous and are much less likely to give rise to the adverse reactions, occasionally associated with the injection of animal (heterologous) sera. Although homologous antisera do not confer durable protection, an additional advantage of them is that their effect may persist for 3−6 months, whereas the protection afforded by a heterologous serum is likely to last only for a few weeks.

(1)Pooled Immunoglobulins

Human normal immunoglobulin (HNIG) is available in the China and elsewhere for the short-term prophylaxis of hepatitis A in contacts or travellers who intend to visit countries where hepatitis A is common because protective levels of antibody to a range of diseases are present in pooled normal human serum. HNIG can also protect an immunocompromised child temporarily against measles if given promptly after contact with a case. Nevertheless, HNIG does not give reliable post-exposure protection against mumps or rubella. Specific immunoglobulins. Preparations of specific immunoglobulins, gamma globulin containing high titers of specific antibodies, are available in the China for passive immunization against tetanus human tetanus immunoglobulin(HTIG), Hepatitis B(HBIG), rabies (HRIG) varicella-zoster(ZIG) and vaccinia (AVIG).

(2)Animal Sera and Antitoxins

These preparations are used only when human globulin is not available, because they carry a much higher risk of anaphylactic reactions. They are usually prepared from hyperimmunized horse or rabbits.

No antiserum of animal origin should be given without carefully inquiring about prior exposure or allergic response to any product of the specific animal source. Whenever a foreign antiserum is administered, a syringe containing aqueous epinephrine, 1 : 1,000, should be available. If allergy(to foreign antiserum) is suspected by history or shown by skin testing and no alternative to serum therapy is possible, desensitization may be attempted. Passive immunotherapy or immunoprophylaxis should always be administered as soon as possible after exposure to the offending agent. Immune antisera and globulin are always given intramuscularly unless otherwise noted. always question carefully and test for hypersensitivity before administering animal sera.

The various materials available for passive immunization, of both human and animal origin, are detailed in Table 13−2.

Table 13-2 Material available for passive immunization

Disease	Products	Source of antiserum
Black widows spider bite	Antivenin widow spider	Horse
Botulism	ABE polyvalent antitoxin	Horse
Diphtheria	Diphtheria antitoxin	Horse
Gas gangrene	Polyvalent antitoxin	Horse
Snakebite	Antivenin coral snake, Antivenin rattlesnake, Copperhead and moccasin	Horse
Tetanus	Tetanus immune globulin	Immune human, horse

13.2 Therapy of Microorganism Infection

13.2.1 Antibacterial Therapy

Infections are so common in general practice that it is not practical for every patient to be fully investigated a rational choice of antimicrobial agent made on the results. Because clinically effective antimicrobial agents are all designed to exhibit selective toxicity toward the parasite rather than the host, many patients who make the effort to see a doctor expect drug treatment. There are three main points in the diagram of choice of antibiotics which is applicable to many common conditions: ①Patients may be categorized on clinical grounds into those with mild moderate or severe infection and also into those who were previously healthy or have underlying disease which may affect their response to therapy; ②The microorganisms causing many common clinical syndromes have predictable antibiotic sensitivities allowing a rational choice to be made; ③The results of laboratory tests may lead to modification or withdrawal of chemotherapy.

13.2.1.1 Antibacterial Mechanism of Drugs

(1) Inhibit Bacterial Cell Wall Synthesis

Since most bacteria possess a rigid cell wall that is lacking in mammalian cells, this structure is a prime target for agents that exhibit selective toxicity, the ability to inhibit or destroy the microbe without harming the host. However, the bacterial cell wall can also prevent access of agents that would otherwise be effective. Thus, the complex outer envelope of Gram-negative bacteria is impermeable to large hydrophilic molecules, which may be prevented from reaching an otherwise susceptible target. Inhibitors of bacterial cell wall synthesis act on the formation of the peptidoglycan layer. Bacteria that lack peptidoglycan, such as mycoplasmas, are resistant to these agents.

(2) Inhibit Bacterialprotein Synthesis

Bacterial ribosomes are sufficiently different from those of mammalian cells to allow selective inhibition of protein synthesis. Most of these agents are true antibiotics (or derivatives thereof) produced by *Streptomyces* species or other soil organisms.

(3) Inhibitnucleic Acid Synthesis

Nucleic acids are ubiquitous in living cells and it is perhaps surprising that a number of important antibacterial agents act directly or indirectly on DNA or RNA synthesis.

13.2.1.2　Antibacterial Agents

The principal types of antibacterial agent are listed in Table 13-3. Because there are so many of them it is convenient to group them according to their site of action.

Table 13-3　Antibacterial agents in clinical use

Agent	Site action	Usual activity[a] against					
		Staphylococci	Streptococci	Enterobacteria	Pseudomonas aeruginosa	Mycobacterium tuberculosis	Anaerobes
Penicillins	Cell wall	(+)	+	v	v	−	+[b]
Cephalosporins	Cell wall	+	+	+	v	−	+[b]
Otherβ-lactam agents	Cell wall	v	v	+	v	−	v
Glycopeptides	Cell wall	+	+	−	−	−	+[c]
Tetracyclines	Ribosome	(+)	(+)	(+)	−	−	(+)
Chloramphenicol	Ribosome	+	+	+	−	−	−
Aminoglycosides	Ribosome	+	−	+	v	v	−
Macrolides	Ribosome	+	+	−	−	−	+
Lincosamides	Ribosome	+	+	−	−	−	+
Fusidic acid	Ribosome	+	+	−	−	+	+
Rifamycins	RNA synthesis	+	+	+	−	+	+
Sulphonamides	Folate metabolism	(+)	(+)	(+)	−	−	−
Diaminopyrimldines	Folate metabolism	+	+	(+)	−	−	−
Quinolones	DNA synthesis	v	v	+	v	v	−
Nitrofurans	DNA synthesis	−	−	+	−	−	+
Nitroimidazoles	DNA synthesis	−	−	−	−	−	+

v, variable activity among different agents of the group.

[a] Usual spectrum of intrinsic activity; parentheses indicate that resistance is common. bPoor

[b] Poor activity against anaerobes of the Bacteroidesfragilis group.

[c] Poor activity against most Gram-negative anaerobes.

13.2.2 Antiviral Therapy

13.2.2.1 Antiviral Mechanism of Drugs

(1) Inhibit Attachment

Attachment to a cell receptor is virus-specific event. Antibody can bind to extracellular virus and prevent this attachment. However, although therapy with antibody is useful in prophylaxis, it has beem minimally effective in treatment.

(2) Inhibit Penetration and Uncoating

Rimantadine differs from amantadine by the substitution of a methyl group for a hydrogen ion. These two amines inhibit several early steps in viral replication, including viral uncoating. They are extremely selective, with activity against only influenza A. In addition, they are effective in preventing influenza but are less useful in treatment of this viral infection due in part to the brief period of viral replication. And influenza A strains resistant to these agents may appear rapidly in patients treated for clinical illness. Such strain can spread to patients receiving the drug prophylatically and can impair its efficacy as a preventive.

(3) Inhibit Fusion

Fuzeon is a large peptide that blocks the virus and cellular membrane fusion step involved in entry of HIV-1 into cells.

(4) Inhibit Biological Synthesis

At present, most antiviral agents are nucleoside analogs that are active against virus specific nucleic acid polymerases or transcriptases and have much less activity against analogous host enzymes. Some of these agents serve as nucleic acid chain terminators after incorporation into nucleic acids.

(5) Inhibit Assembly

The protease inhibitors are the newest agents that inhibit HIV. These agents block the action of the viral-encoded enzyme protease, which cleaves polyproteins to produce structural proteins. Inhibition of this enzyme leads to blockage of viral assembly and release. The protease inhibitors are potent suppressors of HIV replication in vitro and in vivo, particularly when combined with other antiretroviral agents.

13.2.2.2 Antiviral Drugs

In developed parts of the world, it is estimated that nearly 60% of infectious diseases are caused by viruses. Yet relatively few antiviral drugs have found a place in the prophylaxis or treatment of viral infections (Table 13-4). Most of those presently available are nucleoside analogues, which are phosphorylated within cells and inhibit DNA replication.

Table 13-4　Antiviral agents in clinical use

Compound	Mode of action	Indication
Acyclovir[a]	Nucleosideanalogue	Herpes simplex
Amantadine (and rimantadine)	Viral uncoating and assembly	Influenza A
Dideoxynucleosides	Nucleoside analogues	HIV
Foscarnet	Inhibition of polymerase	Cytomegalovirus retinitis
Ganciclovir	Nucleoside analogue	Cytomegalovirus

Continue to Table 13-4

Compound	Mode of action	Indication
Idoxuridine (and trifluridine)	Nucleoside analogue	Herpes simplex(topical)
Interferon-α	Immunomodulator	Hepatitis B and C
Penciclovir[a]	Nucleosiode analogue	Herpes simplex
Ritonavir	Protease	HIV
Saquinavir	inhibitor	HIV
Tribavirin[b]	Nucleoside analogue	Respiratory syncytial virus
Zidovudine	Nucleoside analogue	HIV

HIV, human immunodeficiency virus.

[a] Available in pro-drug formulations.

[b] Also known as ribavirin.

Targets for antiviral drugs are various points in viral replication, involving attachment, penetration, uncoating, RNA-directed DNA synthesis(reverse transcription) and assembly and release of the intact virion. In some cases, antivirals selectively inhibit DNA polymerase. Inhibitors of this enzyme take advantage of the fact that the synthesis of viral nucleic acids is more rapidly than that of the cell, so there is relatively greater inhibition of viral than cellular DNA.

The most widely used antiviral agent, acyclovir(acyclovir) and the related penciclovir, are phosphorylated by a thymidine kinase produced by the herpes simplex virus. Since the drugs are activated only in cells infected with the virus, they exhibit true selective toxicity. Valaciclovir and famciclovir are oral pro-drug formulations of acyclovir and penciclovir, respectively. Granciclovir, which exhibit preferential activity against cytomegalovirus is phosphorylated by cellular enzymes and is much more toxic. Another nucleoside analogue, tribavirin(ribavirin), has no useful antiherpes activity, but is used in the treatment of respiratory syncytial virus infection and Lassa fever.

Interferons, naturally occurring antiviral compounds are produced by mammalican cells in response to viral infection. Recombinant DNA techniques now allow relatively inexpensive large-amounts of interferons by bacteria and yeasts. Interferons are used to treat chronic active hepatitis B and C infections, although its efficacy is often transient. Topical interferon application is beneficial in the treatment of human papilloma virus infections. Unfortunately, interferons have been ineffective in treating many viral infections and cause symptomatic systemic toxicity, (e. g. , fever, malaise), partly because of their effect on host cell protein synthesis.

The acquired immune deficiency syndrome (AIDS) pandemic has generated an enormous interest in potential antiviral agents. Several nucleoside analogues, including zidovudine (azidothymidine) and the dideoxynucleosides, didanosine (dideoxyinosine), zalcitsbine (deoxycytidine), stavudine (didehydrodeoxythymidine) and lamivudine(deoxythiacytidine) are now in use. A number of other compounds, including some HIV protease inhibitors, which act at a later stage in the viral cycle by interfering with the cleavage of essential polyprotein precursors, are showing promise. Saquinavir and ritonavir are examples of such compounds that are in limited chinical use, principally in combination with zidovudine or zalcitabine.

13.2.3 Antifungal Therapy

Although fungi cause a wide variety of infections, relatively few drugs are available for treatment, especially for the systemic therapy of serious mycoses, because they use the same mechanisms to synthesize proteins and nucleic acids as humans. Superficial fungal infections of the skin and mucous membranes are very common and can often be treated with topical agents including polyenes, such as nystatin or azole derivatives. More effective is griseofulvin, given orally, sometimes over long periods, for dermatophyte infection of the nail; the new allylamineterbinafine, seems to be at least as effective in these conditions, since these agents are deposited in newly formed keratin. Systematic fungal disease is relatively rare in the China, except in patients who are immunosuppressed or otherwise compromised. There are few effective antifungal agents that can be used systemically and some have considerable toxicity. Serious systemic disease, such as systemic candidosis, cryptococcal infections and aspergillosis, is often treated parenterally with the polyene, amphotericin B, which is extremely toxic. Flucytosine is also active against yeasts and has been used in combination with amphotericin B. Amphotericin B is toxic and treatment has to be carefully monitored to obtain the most satisfactory clinical results. The pyrimidine analogue 5-fiuorocytosine is also active against many yeasts and has been used in combination with amphotericin B.

Azole derivatives also exhibit the broadest spectrum of activity, embracing yeasts, filamentous fungi and dimorphic fungi and are being used more widely in the treatment of systemic fungal disease because of their relative lack of toxicity, although resistance may be a problem.

The characteristics of currently used antifungal agents are summarized in Table 13−5. Most act by interfering with the integrity of the fungal cell membrane, either by binding to membrane sterols (polyenes) or by preventing the synthesis of ergosterol (azoles and allylamines).

Table 13−5 Antifungal agents in clinical use

Agent	Mechanism of action	Mechanism of resistance	Route	Clinical use
Polyenes				
Nystatin	Membrane disruption	Sterol modification	Topical	Most fungi
Amphotericin B	Membrane disruption		Intravenous	Most fungi
Azoles				
Ketoconazole	Demethylase block of ergosterol synthesis	Active efflux, demethylasealteration oroverproduction[a]	Oral	*Candida*, *Cryptolcoccus*, dimorphic fungi[b]
Fluconazole	Demethylase block of ergosterol synthesis	Active efflux, demethylasealteration oroverproduction[a]	Oral, intravenous	*Candida*, *Cryptolcoccus*, dimorphic fungi
Itraconazole	Demethylase block of ergosterol synthesis	Active efflux, demethylasealteration oroverproduction[a]	Oral, intravenous	*Candida*, *Cryptolcoccus*, dimorphic fungi, invasive molds (*Aspergillus*)
Clotrimazole	Demethylase block of ergosterol synthesis	Unknown[c]	Topical	*Candida*, some yeasts

Continue to Table 13–5

Agent	Mechanism of action	Mechanism of resistance	Route	Clinical use
Miconazole	Demethylase block of ergosterol synthesis	Unknown[c]	Topical	*Candida*, some other ergosterol yeasts
Voriconazole	Demethylase block of ergosterol synthesis	Unknown[c]	Oral, intravenous	*Candida*, some yeasts and molds
Allyamines				
Terbinafine	Squalene accumulation	Active efflux	Oral	Dermatophytes, combined with azoles for*Candida*,*Aspergillus*
Naftifine	Squalene accumulation	Unknown	Topical	Dermatophytes
Flucytosine	RNA and DNA modifying	Permease or*Cryptococcus*, enzymes[d]absent or decreased	Oral	*Candida*and synthesis resistance emerges in monotherapy
Echinocandins				
Caspofungin	Block of glucan synthesis	Unknown	Intravenous	*Aspergillus*, *Candida*
Griseofulvin	Microtubule disruption	Unknown	Oral	Dermatophytes
Potassium Iodide	Unknown	Unknown	Oral	*Sporothrix-schenckii*
Tolnaftate	Unknown	Unknown	Oral	Dermatophytes

a Most work is fluconazole and Candida,other azoles are to be assumed similar.

b Generall less absorbed and less active than fluconazole or itraconazole.

c Probably similar to other azoles,but resistance to the concentrations in topical preparations may differ.

d Cytosine deaminase and uracil phosphoribosyltransferase (the enzyme that forms 5-fluorodoxyuridine from 5-flucytosine).

Chapter 14

Biosafety

Clinical personnel can be exposed to potential hazards when collecting, delivering and analyzing the patient specimen. The infection easily occurs especially among microbiological laboratory staffs, because the infectious agent may be present in the diagnostic specimen and reproduced during the stages of culture identification.

Recent researches showed that poor laboratory techniques and accident occurrence can make relevant personnel expose to hazards and cause laboratory acquired infections. Reasonable laboratory design, appropriate safety facilities, establishment of standardized operating procedures, training of qualified personnel and perfect management can minimize the exposure to hazards that can cause laboratory acquired infections.

The biosafety is responsible for the development and oversight of programs to ensure the safe handling, use, transport and disposal of biological materials. Biosafety activities include registration, review, monitoring and training for research involving infectious agents and recombinant DNA molecules; consultation and training regarding occupational exposure to bloodborne pathogens distribution, collection and destruction of sharps disposal containers; treatment and incineration of pathological waste; selection, proper use and maintenance of biosafety cabinets; and emergency response to incidents involving biological materials.

Biosafety of laboratory is defined by the knowledge, technology and operation procedures for the protection of research staff and community population against laboratory accidents and bio-terrorism attack. In China, the standards of building construction, equipment and operation procedures are established according to the international rules.

14.1 Classification of Pathogenic Microorganisms

In China, microorganisms are divided into four groups according to their communicability and hazards affecting the safety of individuals or population:

Group 1: A pathogen that usually causes serious human or animal disease or a certain microorganism that has not yet been discovered or announced to be eliminated in China, such as alastrim virus, Xinjiang hemorrhagic fever virus (XHF), Ebola virus, yellow fever virus (YFV), smallpox virus, nipah virus (NiV), monkey pox virus, marburg virus, etc.

Group 2:A pathogen that usually causes serious human or animal disease and that can be readily transmitted from one individual to another, directly or indirectly, such as human immunodeficiency virus (HIV), High pathogenic avian influenza virus (HPAIV), foot-and-mouth disease virus (FMDV), Japanese encephalitis virus (JEV), Newcastle disease virus (NDV), poliovirus, rabies virus (RV), SARS coronavirus, etc.

Group 3:A pathogen that can cause human or animal disease but is unlikely to be a serious hazard to laboratory workers, community, livestock or environment. Laboratory exposures rarely cause serious infection and effective treatment and preventive measures are available and the risk of spread of infection is limited, such as A B C D E hepatitis viruses, measles virus, parainfluenza virus, rotavirus, rubella virus, etc.

Group 4 (no or low individual and community risk):A microorganism that is unlikely to cause human or animal disease, such as guinea pig herpesvirus, hamster leukemia virus, mouse leukemia virus, etc.

14.2　Microbiological Risk Assessment

The backbone of the practice of biosafety is risk assessment. While there are many tools available to assist in the assessment of risk for a given procedure or experiment, the most important component is professional judgment.

One of the most helpful tools available for performing a microbiological risk assessment is the listing of risk groups for microbiological agents. However, simple reference to the risk grouping for a particular agent is insufficient in the conduct of a risk assessment. Other factors that should be considered, as appropriate, include

1) Pathogenicity of the agent and infectious dose

2) Potential outcome of exposure

3) Natural route of infection

4) Other routes of infection, resulting from laboratory manipulations (parenteral, airborne, ingestion)

5) Stability of the agent in the environment

6) Concentration of the agent and volume of concentrated material to be manipulated

7) Presence of a suitable host (human or animal)

8) Information available from animal studies and reports of laboratory-acquired infections or clinical reports

9) Laboratory activity planned (sonication, aerosolization, centrifugation, etc.)

10) Any genetic manipulation of the organism that may extend the host range of the agent or alter the agent's sensitivity to known, effective treatment regimens

11) Local availability of effective prophylaxis or therapeutic interventions.

Risk assessments should be performed by the individuals most familiar with the specific characteristics of the organisms being considered for use, the equipment and procedures to be employed, animal models that may be used and the containment equipment and facilities available.

On the basis of the information ascertained during the risk assessment, a biosafety level can be assigned to the planned work, appropriate personal protective equipment selected and standard operating procedures (SOPs) incorporating other safety interventions developed to ensure the safest possible conduct of the work. The laboratory director or principal investigator is responsible for ensuring that adequate and timely risk assessments are performed and for working closely with the institution's safety committee and biosafety personnel to ensure that appropriate equipment and facilities are available to support the work being considered. Once performed, risk assessments should be reviewed routinely and revised when necessary, taking into consideration the acquisition of new data having a bearing on the degree of risk and other relevant new information from the scientific literature.

14.3 Biosafety Levels

The primary risk criteria used to define biosafety levels are infectivity, severity of disease, transmissibility and the nature of the work being conducted. Biosafety levels of laboratory range from the lowest biosafety level 1 (BSL-1) to the highest at level 4 (BSL-4).

Biosafety level 1 (BSL-1) belongs to basic laboratory. It is applicable to basic teaching and research laboratory. Biosafety level 1 is appropriate for agents that are not known to cause disease in normal, healthy humans or opportunistic pathogens that may cause infection in the young, the aged and immunodeficient or immunosuppressed individuals. BSL-1 laboratories are not necessarily separated from the general traffic patterns in the building. Work is typically conducted on open bench tops using standard microbiological practices. Special containment equipment or facility design isnot required, but may be used as determined by appropriate risk assessment.

Biosafety level 2 (BSL-2) belongs to basic laboratory. It is applicable to diagnostic and research laboratory. BSL-2 is suitable for work involving agents that pose moderate hazards to personnel and the environment. It differs from BSL-1 in that: ①laboratory personnel have specific training in handling pathogenic agents and are supervised by scientists competent in handling infectious agents and associated procedures; ②access to the laboratory is restricted when work is being conducted; ③all procedures in which infectious aerosols or splashes may be created are conducted in BSCs or other physical containment equipment. Due to the potential infectiousness of clinical specimens, laboratory standard operating procedures should be strictly followed when accepting, handlingand testing the specimens, so as to clearly identify the risk of infection of various clinical specimens.

Biosafety level 3 (BSL-3) belongs to containment laboratory. It is applicable to specific diagnostic and research laboratory in which work is done with indigenous or exotic agents with a potential for respiratory transmission and which may cause serious and potentially lethal infection. Laboratory personnel must receive specific training in handling pathogenic and potentially lethal agents and must be supervised by scientists competent in handling infectious agents and associated procedures.

Biosafety level 4 belongs to the maximum containment laboratory. It is applicable for work with dangerous and exotic agents that pose a high individual risk of aerosol-transmitted laboratory infections and life-threatening disease that is frequently fatal, for which there are no vaccines or treatments or a related agent with unknown risk of transmission. Laboratory staff must have specific and thorough training in handling extremely hazardous infectious agents. Laboratory staff must understand the primary and secondary containment functions of standard and special practices, containment equipment and laboratory design characteristics. All laboratory staff and supervisors must be competent in handling agents and procedures requiring BSL-4 containment. The laboratory supervisor in accordance with institutional policies controls access to the laboratory.

14.4 Laboratory Equipment

Appropriate laboratory design, use of suitable laboratory equipment and standard operating procedures can minimize the risk of staffs infection. Basic safety equipments of laboratory include biological safety cabinets(BSCs) and personal protective equipment.

14.4.1   Biological Safety Cabinets

Biological safety cabinets are designed to protect the operator, the laboratory environment and work materials from exposure to infectious aerosols and splashes that may be generated when manipulating materials containing infectious agents, such as primary cultures, stocks and diagnostic specimens. Biosafety cabinets are classified into three levels by a variety of design and performance factors. These include air velocity, air recirculation proportion, contaminated plenum pressure and exhaust function.

14.4.1.1   Class Ⅰ Biological Safety Cabinet

The Class Ⅰ BSC was the first recognized BSC and, because of its simple design, is still in wide use throughout the world. It protects the operator and the environment from exposure to biohazards, it does not prevent samples being handled in the cabinet from coming into contact with airborne contaminants that may be present in room air. Room air is drawn in through the front opening at a minimum velocity of 0.38 m/s, it passes over the work surface and is discharged from the cabinet through the exhaust duct. The directional flow of air whisks aerosol particles that may be generated on the work surface away from the laboratory worker and into the exhaust duct. The front opening allows the operator's arms to reach the work surface inside the cabinet while he or she observes the work surface through a glass window. The window can also be fully raised to provide access to the work surface for cleaning or other purposes. The air from the cabinet is exhausted through a HEPA filter:①into the laboratory and then to the outside of the building through the building exhaust;②to the outside through the building exhaust;③directly to the outside. The HEPA filter may be located in the exhaust plenum of the BSC or in the building exhaust. Some Class Ⅰ BSCs are equipped with an integral exhaust fan, whereas others rely on the exhaust fan in the building exhaust system.

14.4.1.2   Class Ⅱ Biological Safety Cabinets

As the use of cell and tissue cultures for the propagation of viruses and other purposes grew, it was no longer considered satisfactory for unsterilized room air to pass over the work surface. The Class Ⅱ BSC was designed not only to provide personnel protection but also to protect work surface materials from contaminated room air. Class Ⅱ BSCs, of which there are four types (A1, A2, B1 and B2), differ from Class Ⅰ BSCs by allowing only air from a HEPA-filtered (sterile) supply to flow over the work surface. The Class Ⅱ BSC can be used for personnel working with infectious agentscausing moderate or high individual risk, low community risk. Class Ⅱ BSCs can be used for personnel working with infectious agents causing high individual and community risk when positive-pressure suits are used.

14.4.1.3   Class Ⅲ Biological Safety Cabinet

This type provides the highest level of personnel protection and is used forpersonnel working with infectious agents causing high individual and community risk. All penetrations are sealed "gas tight". Supply air is HEPA-filtered and exhaust air passes through two HEPA filters. Airflow is maintained by a dedicated exhaust system exterior to the cabinet, which keeps the cabinet interior under negative pressure (about 124.5 Pa). Access to the work surface is by means of heavy duty rubber gloves, which are attached to ports in the cabinet. The Class Ⅲ BSC should have an attached pass-through box that can be sterilized and is equipped with a HEPA-filtered exhaust. The Class Ⅲ cabinet may be connected to a double-door autoclave used to decontaminate all materials entering or exiting the cabinet. Several glove boxes can be joined together to extend the work surface. Class Ⅲ BSCs are suitable for work in Biosafety Level 3 and 4 laboratories.

14.4.2　Personal Protective Equipment

Personal protective equipment and clothing may act as a barrier to minimize the risk of exposure to aerosols, splashes and accidental inoculation. The clothing and equipment selected is dependent on the risk assessment and the nature of the work performed.

Personal protective equipment and clothing may act as a barrier to minimize the risk of exposure to aerosols, splashes and accidental inoculation. The clothing and equipment selected is dependent on the nature of the work performed.

14.4.2.1　Protective Clothing

Laboratory coats should preferably be fully buttoned. However, long-sleeved, back-opening gowns or coveralls give better protection than laboratory coats and are preferred in microbiology laboratories and when working at the biological safety cabinet. Aprons may be worn over laboratory coats or gowns where necessary to give further protection against spillage of chemicals or biological materials such as blood or culture fluids. Laundering services should be provided at/near the facility.

Laboratory coats, gowns, coveralls or aprons should not be worn outside the laboratory areas. Dispose of protective clothing appropriately. Contaminated clothing must be changed and deposited in marked anti-leakage bag to transport.

14.4.2.2　Eye and Face Protection

The choice of equipment to protect the eyes and face from splashes and impacting objects will depend on the activity performed. Prescription or plain eye glasses can be manufactured with special frames that allow lenses to be placed in frame from the front, using shatterproof material either curved or fitted with side shields (safety glasses). Safety spectacles do not provide for adequate splash protection even when side shields are worn with them. Goggles for splash and impact protection should be worn over normal prescription eye glasses and contact lenses (which do not provide protection against biological or chemical hazards). Face shields (visors) are made of shatterproof plastic, fit over the face and are held in place by head straps or caps.

Goggles, safety spectacles or face shields should not be worn outside the laboratory areas.

14.4.2.3　Respirators

Respiratory protection may be used when carrying out high-hazard procedures (e. g. cleaning up a spill of infectious material). The choice of respirator will depend on the type of hazard. Respirators are available with interchangeable filters for protection against gases, vapours, particulates and microorganisms. It is imperative that the filter is fitted in the correct type of respirator. To achieve optimal protection, respirators should be individually fitted to the operator's face and tested. Fully self-contained respirators with an integral air supply provide full protection. Advice should be sought from a suitably qualified person, e. g. an occupational hygienist, for selection of the correct respirator. Surgical type masks are designed solely for patient protection and do not provide respiratory protection to workers. Some single-use disposable respirators have been designed for protection against exposures to biological agents.

Respirators should not be worn outside the laboratory areas.

14.4.2.4　Gloves

Contamination of hands may occur when laboratory procedures are performed. Hands are also vulnerable to "sharps" injuries. Disposable microbiologically approved latex, vinyl or nitrile surgical-type gloves are used widely for general laboratory work and for handling infectious agents and blood and body fluids. Reusable gloves may also be used but attention must be given to their correct washing, removal, cleaning and disinfection.

Gloves should be removed and hands thoroughly washed after handling infectious materials, working in a biological safety cabinet and before leaving the laboratory. Used disposable gloves should be discarded with infected laboratory wastes.

Allergic reactions such as dermatitis and immediate hypersensitivity have been reported in laboratory and other workers wearing latex gloves, particularly those with powder. Alternatives to powdered latex gloves should be available.

Stainless steel mesh gloves should be worn when there is a potential exposure to sharp instruments e. g. during postmortem examinations. Such gloves protect against slicing motion but do not protect against puncture injury.

Gloves should not be worn outside the laboratory areas.

Before leaving the laboratory, personal protective equipment and clothing should be removed and hands should be washed.

Table 14-1 summarizes some personal protective equipment used in laboratories and the protection afforded.

Table 14-1   **Personal protective equipment**

Equipment	Hazard corrected	Safety features
Laboratory coats, Gowns, coveralls	Contamination of clothing	· Back opening · Cover street clothing
Plastic aprons	Contamination of clothing	· Waterproof
Footwear	Impact and splash	· Closed-toe
Goggles	Impact and splash	· Impact-resistant lenses (must be optically correct or worn over corrective eye glasses) · Side shields
Safety spectacles	Impact	· Impact-resistant lenses (must be optically correct) · Side shields
Face shields	Impact and splash	· Shield entire face · Easily removable in case of accident
Respirators	Inhalation of aerosols	· Designs available include single-use disposable; full-face or half-face air purifying; full-face or hooded powered air purifying (PAPR); and supplied air respirators
Gloves	Direct contact with microorganisms	· Disposable microbiologically approved latex, vinyl or nitrile · Hand protection
	Cuts	· Mesh

14.4.2.5 Safety Check List of Personal Protection

1) Is protective clothing of approved design and fabric provided for all staff for normal work, e. g. , gowns, coveralls, aprons, gloves?

2) Is additional protective clothing provided for work with hazardous chemicals and radioactive and carcinogenic substances, e. g. , rubber aprons and gloves for chemicals and for dealing with spillages; heat-resistant gloves for unloading autoclaves and ovens?

3) Are safety glasses, goggles and shields (visors) provided?

4) Are there eye-wash stations?

5) Are there emergency showers (drench facilities)?

6) Is radiation protection in accordance with national and international standards, including provision of dosimeters?

7) Are respirators available, regularly cleaned, disinfected, inspected and stored in a clean and sanitary condition?

8) Are appropriate filters provided for the correct types of respirators, e. g. , HEPA filters for microorganisms, appropriate filters for gases or particulates?

9) Are respirators fit-tested?

14.5 Biosecurity and Bioterrorism

Microbiology laboratories should protect personnel against exposure to biological agents and reduce environmental hazards. It is also necessary to protect laboratory and laboratory materials to prevent intentional actions leading to human or environmental hazards.

14.5.1 Laboratory Biosecurity

Laboratory biosecurity refers to institutional and personal security measures designed to prevent the loss, theft, misuse, diversion or intentional release of pathogens and toxins. Biosecurity precautions should become a routine part of laboratory work. Effective and standard biosafety practices are the very foundation of laboratory biosecurity activities.

Laboratory biosecurity measures should be based on a comprehensive programme of accountability for pathogens and toxins that includes an updated inventory with storage location, identification of personnel with access, description of use, documentation of internal and external transfers within and between facilities and any inactivation and/or disposal of the materials. Likewise, an institutional laboratory biosecurity protocol should be established for identifying, reporting, investigating and remediating breaches in laboratory biosecurity, including discrepancies in inventory results. The involvement and roles and responsibilities of public health and security authorities in the event of a security infraction must be clearly defined.

Laboratory biosecurity training, distinct from laboratory biosafety training, should be provided to all personnel. Such training should help personnel understand the need for protection of such materials and the rationale for the specific biosecurity measures and should include a review of relevant national standards and institution-specific procedures. Procedures describing the security roles and responsibilities of personnel in the event of a security infraction should also be presented during training.

The professional and ethical suitability for working with dangerous pathogens of all personnel who have regular authorized access to sensitive materials is also central to effective laboratory biosecurity activities.

14.5.2   Bioterrorism Precaution

The bioterrorism is one kind of activity using microorganisms such as bacteria and virus with strong pathogenicity to attack the human, which brings severe damage to the social public and the environment

14.5.2.1   Bioterrorism Threat Graduation

According to CDC classification of USA is the biological terror threat is divided into three levels, namely A level (the biggest harm), B level (medium harm) and C level (the lowest harm). The several pathogens can be used as the A level biowarfare agent, such as *B anthrax*, *Y pestis*, *Francisellatularensis* type A, Hemorrhagic fever virus (Ebola virus, Marburg virusand epidemic hemorrhagic fever virus), Smallpoxvirus and T2 mycotoxin which is produced by the fungus of *Fusarium*.

14.5.2.2   The Dissemination Way of Biowarfareagent

The pathogen used in the biological terrorism is often made into tiny particles, so it is easily disseminated in the aerosol form in the air. The human may be infected through the respiratory tract and the skin. Another way is to use the medium insects, such as the mosquito, fly, cockroach, louse, flea and rodents carried pathogens to infect human through the digestive tract, skin and respiratory tract by biting the people or polluting the environment.

14.5.2.3   Precaution

To research the related pathogen and develop effective vaccine and medicine are major methods. The vaccine antitoxin and antibiotic can be in advanced development to cure the patients and control disease.

14.6   Biosafety Techniques

In this section, we introduce the common laboratory techniques and accident handling in order to avoid or reduce the laboratory-acquired infections as possible.

14.6.1   Laboratory Techniques

There are biosafety-related problems in the process of collection, transport and manipulation of specimens. Therefore, the standard practices and procedures should be studied and followed strictly.

14.6.1.1   Handling of Infectious or Potentially Infectious Materials

(1) Transport of Specimens

To avoid accidental leakage or spillage, secondary containers, such as boxes, should be used, fitted with racks so that the specimen containers remain upright. The secondary containers may be of metal or plastic, should be autoclavable or resistant to the action of chemical disinfectants and the seal should preferably have a gasket. They should be regularly decontaminated.

(2) Freeze-dryers of Infectious Materials

Ampoules of infectious materials should be opened in biological safety cabinets to avoid microbe dispersal and contamination. First decontaminate the outer surface of the ampoule. Make a file mark on the tube near to the middle of the cotton or cellulose plug, if present. Hold the ampoule in alcohol-soaked cotton to protect hands before breaking it at a file scratch. Remove the top gently and treat as contaminated material. If the plug is still above the contents of the ampoule, remove it with sterile forceps. Add liquid for resuspension slowly to the ampoule to avoid frothing.

Ampoules containing infectious materials should never be immersed in liquid nitrogen because cracked or imperfectly sealed ampoules may break or explode on removal. If very low temperatures are required, ampoules should be stored only in the gaseous phase above the liquid nitrogen. Otherwise, infectious materials should be stored in mechanical deep-freeze cabinets or on dry ice. Laboratory workers should wear eye and hand protection when removing ampoules from cold storage.

(3) Separation of Serum

Only properly trained staff should be employed for this work. Gloves and eye and mucous membrane protection should be worn. Splashes and aerosols can only be avoided or minimized by good laboratory technique. Blood and serum should be pipetted carefully, not poured. Pipetting by mouth must be forbidden. After use, pipettes should be completely submerged in suitable disinfectant. They should remain in the disinfectant for the appropriate time before disposal or washing and sterilization for reuse. Discarded specimen tubes containing blood clots, etc. (with caps replaced) should be placed in suitable leakproof containers for autoclaving and/or incineration. Suitable disinfectants should be available for clean-up of splashes and spillages.

(4) Prions

As complete inactivation of prions is difficult to achieve, it is important to stress the use of disposable instruments whenever possible and to use a disposable protective covering for the work surface of the biological safety cabinet. The main precaution to be taken is to avoid ingestion of contaminated materials or puncture of the laboratory worker's skin. All manipulations must be conducted in biological safety cabinets. Bench waste, including disposable gloves, gowns and aprons, should be autoclaved using a porous load steam sterilizer at 134–137 ℃ for a single cycle of 18 min or six successive cycles of 3 min each, followed by incineration.

14.6.1.2 Use of Common Instruments

Common instruments used in the microbiological laboratory include microbiological transfer loops, pipettes, safety cabinets, centrifuges, etc.

(1) Transfer Loops

In order to avoid the premature shedding of their loads, microbiological transfer loops should have a diameter of 2–3 mm and be completely closed. The shanks should be not more than 6 cm in length to minimize vibration. The risk of spatter of infectious material in an open Bunsen burner flame should be avoided by using an enclosed electric microincinerator to sterilize transfer loops. Disposable transfer loops, which do not need to be resterilized, are preferable.

(2) Pipettes

All pipettes should have cotton plugs to reduce contamination of pipetting devices. A pipetting aid must always be used. Pipetting by mouth must be prohibited. Air should never be blown through a liquid containing infectious agents. To avoid dispersion of infectious material dropped from a pipette, an absorbent material should be placed on the working surface; this should be disposed of as infectious waste after use.

(3) Centrifuges

Centrifuges should be placed at such a level that workers can see into the bowl to place trunnions and buckets correctly. The buckets must be loaded, equilibrated, sealed and opened in a biological safety cabinet. Buckets, rotors and centrifuge bowls should be decontaminated after each use. The interior of the centrifuge bowl should be inspected daily for staining or soiling at the level of the rotor. If staining or soiling are evident then the centrifugation protocols should be re-evaluated.

(4) Biological Safety Cabinets

The cabinet must not be used unless it is working properly. The cabinet will not protect the operator from spillage, breakage or poor technique. All work must be carried out in the middle or rear part of the working surface and be visible through the viewing panel. The glass viewing panel must not be opened when the cabinet is in use. Air grills must not be blocked with notes, pipettes or other materials, as this will disrupt the airflow causing potential contamination of the material and exposure of the operator. Bunsen burners must not be used in the cabinet. The heat produced will distort the airflow and may damage the filters. An electric microincinerator is permissible but sterile disposable transfer loops are better. The cabinet fan should be run for at least 5 min before beginning work and after completion of work in the cabinet. The operator should not disturb the airflow by repeated removal and reintroduction of his or her arms. Paperwork should never be placed inside biological safety cabinets.

(5) Others

When in use, homogenizers, shakers and sonicators should be covered by a strong transparent plastic casing. This should be disinfected after use. Where possible, these machines should be operated, under their plastic covers, in a biological safety cabinet.

14.6.1.3　Standard Precautions with Blood and other Body Fluids, Tissues and Excreta

Standard precautions are designed to reduce the risk of transmission of microorganisms from both recognized and unrecognized sources of infection.

(1) Prevention of Specimen Leakage

To avoid accidental leakage or spillage, secondary containers, such as boxes, should be used, fitted with racks so that the specimen containers remain upright.

(2) Protection of Personal Safety and Hand Hygiene at Work

Gloves and eye and mucous membrane protection should be worn.

(3) Allocation of Biological Safety Cabinet

The known or unknown infectious specimens or microbes should be treated in the biological safety cabinet.

(4) Handling Precautions

Pipetting by mouth must be prohibited. A pipetting aid must always be used. Standard precautions should be followed when using syringes and needles to avoid sharp injury.

(5) Sterilization

The contaminated surface of the biological safety cabinet should be wiped using an appropriate disinfectant after work is completed and at the end of the day. The laboratory coats, gowns, coveralls or aprons should not be worn outside the laboratory areas. Laboratory workers should wash their hands before leaving the laboratory. Contaminated, reusable materials should be decontaminated and then washed. Contaminated instruments should be decontaminated and then repaired or discarded.

14.6.2　Emergency Procedures for Microbiological Laboratories

14.6.2.1　Puncture Wounds, Cuts and Abrasions

The affected individual should remove protective clothing, wash the hands and any affected area, apply an appropriate skin disinfectant and seek medical attention as necessary.

14.6.2.2　Ingestion of Potentially Infectious Material

Protective clothing should be removed and medical attention sought. Identification of the material ingested and circumstances of the incident should be reported and appropriate and complete medical records kept.

14.6.2.3 Potentially Infectious Aerosol Release

All persons should immediately vacate the affected area and any exposed persons should be referred for medical advice. No one should enter the room for an appropriate amount of time, to allow aerosols to be carried away and heavier particles to settle. If the laboratory does not have a central air exhaust system, entrance should be delayed (e. g. for 24 h).

14.6.2.4 Broken Containers and Spilled Infectious Substances

Broken containers contaminated with infectious substances and spilled infectious substances should be covered with a cloth or paper towels. Disinfectant should then be poured over these and left for the appropriate amount of time. The cloth or paper towels and the broken material can then be cleared away; glass fragments should be handled with forceps. The contaminated area should then be swabbed with disinfectant. If dustpans are used to clear away the broken material, they should be autoclaved or placed in an effective disinfectant. Cloths, paper towels and swabs used for cleaning up should be placed in a contaminated-waste container. Gloves should be worn for all these procedures. If laboratory forms or other printed or written matter are contaminated, the information should be copied onto another form and the original discarded into the contaminated-waste container.

14.6.2.5 Breakage of Centrifuges

If a breakage occurs or is suspected while the machine is running, the motor should be switched off and the machine left closed (e. g. for 30 min) to allow settling. If a breakage is discovered after the machine has stopped, the lid should be replaced immediately and left closed (e. g. for 30 min). Strong (e. g. thick rubber) gloves, covered if necessary with suitable disposable gloves, should be worn for all subsequent operations. Forceps or cotton held in the forceps, should be used to retrieve glass debris. All broken tubes, glass fragments, buckets, trunnions and the rotor should be placed in a noncorrosive disinfectant known to be active against the organisms concerned (see Chapter 14). Unbroken, capped tubes may be placed in disinfectant in a separate container and recovered.

14.6.3 Treatment of Infectious Waste

Infectious waste refers to discarded infectious or potentially infectious substances. The principle of treatment is to discard these substances after decontamination or transport after proper packaging and treat them in other places, so as not to cause potential harm to the participants. Decontamination methods include autoclaving (first choice), incineration, etc.

Sharps such as glass fragments and injection needles should be placed in a puncture-proof container and treated according to the above principles.

14.6.4 Transport of Infectious Substances

Transport of infectious and potentially infectious materials is subject to strict national and international regulations. These regulations describe the proper use of packaging materials, as well as other shipping requirements.

Laboratory personnel must ship infectious substances according to applicable transport regulations. Compliance with the rules will reduce the likelihood that packages will be damaged and leak, reduce the exposures resulting in possible infections and improve the efficiency of package delivery.

The triple packaging system, the choice for the transport of infectious and potentially infectious substances, consists of three layers: the primary receptacle, the secondary packaging and the outer packaging. The primary receptacle containing the specimen must be watertight, leakproof and appropriately labelled as to content. A second watertight, leakproof packaging is used to enclose and protect the primary receptacle. The third layer protects the secondary packaging from physical damage while in transit. Requirements for the transport of highly hazardous substances are more stringent, which can be found in the relevant regulations.

Appendix I

Bacterial classification

1 革兰氏阳性球菌（*Gram-positive Coccus*）

Abiotrophia［乏养（球）菌属］

　A. *adiacens*（毗邻乏养菌）

　A. *balaenopterae*（鲸乏菌）

　A. *defective*（软弱乏养菌）

　A. *elegans*（苛求乏养菌）

　A. *pare-adiacens*（副毗邻乏养菌）

Aerococcus（气球菌属）

　A. *christensenii*（克氏气球菌）

　A. *homari*（虾气球菌）

　A. *sanguinicola*（住血气球菌）

　A. *suis*（肉猪气单胞菌）

　A. *urinae*（尿道气球菌）

　A. *urinaeequi*（马尿气球菌）

　A. *urinaehominis*（人尿气球菌）

　A. *vitidans*（绿色气球菌）

Alloiococcus（异球菌属）

　A. *otiti s*（耳炎异球菌）

Dermacoccus（皮球菌属）

　D. *abyssi*（深渊皮球菌）

　D. *harathri*（深海坑皮球菌）

　D. *nishinomiyaensis*（西宫皮球菌）

　D. *Profundi*（深海皮球菌）

Dolosicoccus（狡诈球菌属）

　D. *paucivorans*（窄食狡诈球菌）

　D. *olosigranulum*（蒙球菌属）

　D. *pigrum*（惰性蒙球菌）

Enterococcus（肠球菌属）

    E. aquimarinus（海水肠球菌）

    E. caccae（粪便肠球菌）

    E. columbae（鸽肠球菌）

    E. dispar（殊异肠球菌）

    E. faecium（屎肠球菌）

    E. gilvus（浅黄肠球菌）

    E. hirae（拉氏肠球菌）

    E. malodoratus（病臭肠球菌）

    E. porcinus（猪肠球菌）

    E. silesiacus（西里西亚肠球菌）

Eremococcus（孤立球菌属）

    E. coleocola（居阴道孤立球菌）

Facklamia（法肯莱姆菌属）

    F. hominis（人法肯莱姆菌）

    F. ignava（懒惰法肯莱姆菌）

    F. languida（活法肯莱姆菌）

    F. miroungae（象海豹法肯莱姆菌）

    F. sourekii（索尔克法肯莱姆菌）

    F. tabacinasalis（鼻烟法肯莱姆菌）

Gemella（孪生球菌属）

    G. haemolysans（溶血孪生球菌）

    G. morbillorum（麻疹孪生球菌）

    G. bergeri（伯杰氏孪生球菌）

    G. cuniculi（兔孪生球菌）

    G. palaticanis（狗龈孪生球菌）

    G. sanguinis（血孪生球菌）

Globicatella（圆短链菌属）

    G. sanguis（血圆短链菌）

    G. sulfidifaciens（产硫化物圆短链菌）

    G. ranulicatella（小链球菌属）

    G. adiacens（毗邻小链球菌）

    G. balaenopterae（鲸小链球菌）

    G. elegans（苛求小链球菌）

Helcococcus（创伤球菌属）

    H. kaunzii（孔兹创伤球菌）

    H. ovis（绵羊创伤球菌）

    H. sueciensis（瑞士创伤球菌）

Ignavigranum（惰球菌属）

    I. ruoffiae（劳夫惰性菌）

Kocuria［柯克（球）菌属］

    K. aegyptica（埃及柯克菌）

    K. carniphila（喜肉柯克菌）

    K. erythromyxa（红黏液柯克菌）

    K. flava（黄色柯克菌）

    K. halotolerans（耐盐柯克菌）

    K. kristinae（克氏柯克菌）

    K. marina（海洋柯克菌）

    K. polaris（极地柯克菌）

    K. rosea（玫瑰色柯克菌）

    K. varians（变异柯克菌）

Kytococcus（皮肤球菌属）

    K. aerolatus（气生皮肤球菌）

    K. schroeteri（锡伦特皮肤球菌）

    K. sedentarius（栖息皮肤球菌）

Lactococcus（乳球菌属）

    L. acidipiscis（酸鱼乳杆菌）

    L. brevis（短乳杆菌）

    L. cacaonum（可可豆乳杆菌）

    L. compost（堆肥乳杆菌）

    L. dextrinicus（糊精乳杆菌）

    L. equi（马乳杆菌）

    L. farraginis（香肠乳杆菌）

    L. gasseri（家氏乳杆菌）

    L. halotolerans（耐盐乳杆菌）

    L. parabuchneri（类布氏乳杆菌）

Leuconostoc（明串珠菌属）

    L. amelibiosum（酵母促生明串珠菌）

    L. carnosum（肉明串珠菌）

    L. durionis（榴莲明串珠菌）

    L. ficulneum（无花果明串珠菌）

    L. gelidum（冷明串珠菌）

    L. inhae（仁荷明串珠菌）

    L. kimchii（泡菜明串珠菌）

    L. mesenteroides（肠膜明串珠菌）

    L. palmae（棕榈明串珠菌）

    L. pseudoficulneum（假无花果明串珠菌）

Luteococcus（黄球菌属）

    L. japonicus（日本黄球菌）

    L. peritonei（腹膜黄球菌）

    L. sanguinis（血黄球菌）

Macrococcus（大球菌属）

    M. bovicus（牛大球菌）

    M. brunensis（布尔诺大球菌）

    M. carouselicus（赛马大球菌）

    M. caseolyticus（溶酪大球菌）

    M. eqipercius（马珀西大球菌）

    M. hajekii（哈氏大球菌）

    M. lamae（美洲驼大球菌）

Micrococcus（微球菌属）

    M. agilis（活泼微球菌）

    M. endophyticus（植物内微球菌）

    M. flavus（黄色微球菌）

    M. luteus（藤黄微球菌）

    M. terreus（土地微球菌）

    M. yunnanensis（云南微球菌）

    M. lactis（乳微球菌）

    M. lylae（里拉微球菌）

    M. roseus（玫瑰色微球菌）

    M. varians（变异微球菌）

Nesterenkonia［纳斯特连柯（球）菌属］

    N. alba（白色纳斯特连柯菌）

    N. aethiopica（埃塞俄比亚纳斯特连柯菌）

    N. flava（黄色纳斯特连柯菌）

    N. halobia（喜盐纳斯特连柯菌）

    N. halophila（嗜盐纳斯特连柯菌）

    N. jeotgal（盐渍海鲜纳斯特连柯菌）

    N. lacusekhoensis（回音湖纳斯特连柯菌）

    N. lutea（浅黄纳斯特连柯菌）

    N. sandarakina（橙色纳斯特连柯菌）

    N. xinjiangensis（新疆纳斯特连柯菌）

Peptococcus（消化球菌属）

    P. niger（黑色消化球菌）

Peptoniphilus（亲胨菌属）

    P. asaccharolyticus（不解糖亲胨菌）

    P. gorbachii（戈巴赫氏亲胨菌）

    P. harei（哈氏亲胨菌）

    P. indolicus（产吲哚亲胨菌）

    P. ivorii（爱氏亲胨菌）

    P. lacrimalis（人泪亲胨菌）

    P. methioninivorans（食甲硫氨酸亲胨菌）

    P. olsenii（奥尔森亲胨菌）

    P. stomatis（口腔亲胨菌）

Peptostreptococcus（消化链球菌属）

　　P. anaerobius（厌氧消化链球菌）

　　P. barnesae（巴尔涅斯消化链球菌）

　　P. harei［海（哈）氏消化链球菌］

　　P. indolicus（吲哚消化链球菌）

　　P. ivorii（艾弗消化链球菌）

　　P. lacrimalis（人眼消化链球菌）

　　P. magnus（大消化链球菌）

　　P. octavius（第八消化链球菌）

　　P. stomatis（口腔消化链球菌）

　　P. tetradius（四联消化链球菌）

Planococcus（动性球菌属）

　　P. antarcticus（南极动性球菌）

　　P. citreus（柠檬色动性球菌）

　　P. donghaensis（东海动性球菌）

　　P. kocurii（科氏动性球菌）

　　P. maitriensis（麦特瑞动性球菌）

　　P. maritimus（滨海动性球菌）

　　P. plakortidis（海绵动性球菌）

　　P. rifietoensis（动性球菌）

　　P. salinarum（盐场动性球菌）

　　P. stackebrandtii（斯托克布兰的特氏动性球菌）

Rhodococcus（红球菌属）

　　R. aichiensis（爱知红球菌）

　　R. artemisiae（艾蒿红球菌）

　　R. bronchialis（支气管红球菌）

　　R. chubuensis（楚布红球菌）

　　R. equi（马红球菌）

　　R. globerulus（圆红球菌）

　　R. jostii（宙斯红球菌）

　　R. kyotonensis（京都红球菌）

　　R. maris（海红球菌）

　　R. opacus（混浊红球菌）

Sarcina（八叠球菌属）

　　S. maxima（最大八叠球菌）

　　S. ventriculi（胃八叠球菌）

Staphylococcus（葡萄球菌属）

　　S. agnetis（阿格尼丝葡萄球菌）

　　S. aureus（金黄色葡萄球菌）

　　S. capitis（头状葡萄球菌）

　　S. carnosus（肉葡萄球菌）

　　S. cohnii（孔氏葡萄球菌）

S. *delphini*(海豚葡萄球菌)

S. *equorum*(马葡萄球菌)

S. *hominis*(人葡萄球菌)

S. *lentus*(缓慢葡萄球菌)

S. *xylosus*(木糖葡萄球菌)

Streptococcus(链球菌属)

S. *equi*(马链球菌)

S. *iniae*(海豚链球菌)

S. *pyogenes*(化脓链球菌)

S. *ferus*(野生链球菌)

S. *mitior*(温和链球菌)

S. *rattus*(鼠链球菌)

S. *avium*(鸟链球菌)

S. *lactis*(乳链球菌)

S. *hansenii*(汉氏链球菌)

S. *adjacens*(毗邻链球菌)

Vagococcus(游球菌属)

V. *acidifermentans*(发酵产酸游球菌)

V. *carniphilus*(喜肉游球菌)

V. *elongates*(长形游球菌)

V. *fessus*(乏活游球菌)

V. *fluvialis*(河流游球菌)

V. *lutrae*(水獭游球菌)

V. *penaei*(对虾游球菌)

V. *salmoninarum*(鲑鱼游球菌)

2 *Gram positive aerobic spore-bearing bacilli*(革兰氏阳性需氧芽孢杆菌)

Alicyclobacillus(脂环酸芽孢杆菌属)

A. *acidiphilus*(嗜酸脂环酸芽孢杆菌)

A. *aeris*(金属矿脂环酸芽孢杆菌)

A. *contaminans*(污染脂环酸芽孢杆菌)

A. *fastidiosus*(脆弱脂环酸芽孢杆菌)

A. *herbarius*(草脂环酸芽孢杆菌)

A. *hesperidum*(神话环酸芽孢杆菌)

A. *pohliae*(苔脂环酸芽孢杆菌)

A. *pomorum*(水果脂环酸芽孢杆菌)

A. *sacchari*(糖脂环酸芽孢杆菌)

A. *tolerans*(耐受环酸芽孢杆菌)

Ammoniphilus(嗜氨菌属)

A. *oxalaticus*(草酸嗜氨菌)

A. *oxalivorans*(食草酸嗜氨菌)

Aneurinibacillus（解硫胺芽孢杆菌属）

　　A. aneurinolyticus（解硫胺解硫胺芽孢杆菌）

　　A. danicus（丹拜解硫胺芽孢杆菌）

　　A. migulanus（米氏解硫胺芽孢杆菌）

　　A. themoaerophilus（嗜热氧解硫胺芽孢杆菌）

Bacillus（芽孢杆菌属）

　　B. alvei（蜂房芽孢杆菌）

　　B. badius（粟褐芽孢杆菌）

　　B. cereus（蜡样芽孢杆菌）

　　B. firmus（坚强芽孢杆菌）

　　B. insolitus（异常芽孢杆菌）

　　B. larvae（幼虫芽孢杆菌）

　　B. marinus（海洋芽孢杆菌）

　　B. polymyxa（多黏芽孢杆菌）

　　B. pumilus（短小芽孢杆菌）

　　B. subtillis（枯草芽孢杆菌）

Brevibacillus（短芽孢杆菌属）

　　B. agri（土壤短芽孢杆菌）

　　B. brevis（短短芽孢杆菌）

　　B. centrosporus（中孢短芽孢杆菌）

　　B. choshinensis（桥石短芽孢杆菌）

　　B. fluminis（河短芽孢杆菌）

　　B. formosus（美丽短芽孢杆菌）

　　B. invocatus（未邀短芽孢杆菌）

　　B. panacihumi（人参园土短芽孢杆菌）

　　B. reuszeri（罗尹氏短芽孢杆菌）

　　B. thermoruber（热红短芽孢杆菌）

Geobacillus（土壤芽孢杆菌属）

　　G. debilis（弱土壤芽孢杆菌）

　　G. gargensis（加尔加土壤芽孢杆菌）

　　G. haustophilus（嗜热土壤芽孢杆菌）

　　G. jurassicus（侏罗纪土壤芽孢杆菌）

　　G. kaustophilus（嗜热土壤芽孢杆菌）

　　G. lituanicus（立陶宛土壤芽孢杆菌）

　　G. pallidus（苍白土壤芽孢杆菌）

　　G. tepidamans（温生土壤芽孢杆菌）

　　G. uzenensis（乌津土壤芽孢杆菌）

　　G. vulcani（瓦尔肯土壤芽孢杆菌）

Gracilibacillus（柔芽孢杆菌属）

　　G. boraciitolerans（耐硼柔芽孢杆菌）

　　G. diposauri（荒漠鼹鼠柔芽孢杆菌）

　　G. halolerans（耐盐柔芽孢杆菌）

G. halophilus（嗜盐柔芽孢杆菌）

G. kekensis（凯凯盐湖柔芽孢杆菌）

G. lacisalsi（盐湖柔芽孢杆菌）

G. orientalis（东方柔芽孢杆菌）

G. saliphilus（喜盐柔芽孢杆菌）

G. thailandensis（泰国柔芽孢杆菌）

G. ureilyticus（解脲柔芽孢杆菌）

Paenibacillus（类芽孢杆菌属）

P. aestuarii（湿地类芽孢杆菌）

P. alvei（蜂房类芽孢杆菌）

P. borealis（北方类芽孢杆菌）

P. cineris（火山土类芽孢杆菌）

P. durum（坚韧类芽孢杆菌）

P. elgii（生科类芽孢杆菌）

P. filicis（蕨类类芽孢杆菌）

P. gordonae（戈氏类芽孢杆菌）

P. lactis（乳类芽孢杆菌）

P. pabuli（饲料类芽孢杆菌）

Salibacillus（盐芽孢杆菌属）

S. marismortui（死海盐芽孢杆菌）

S. salexigens（需盐盐芽孢杆菌）

Virgibacillus（枝芽孢杆菌属）

V. arctics（北极枝芽孢杆菌）

V. carmonensis（卡莫那枝芽孢杆菌）

V. campisalis（盐场枝芽孢杆菌）

V. dokdonensis（全罗北道枝芽孢杆菌）

V. halophilus（嗜盐枝芽孢杆菌）

V. kekensis（柯柯盐湖枝芽孢杆菌）

V. necropolis（墓地枝芽孢杆菌）

V. olivae（橄榄废水枝芽孢杆菌）

V. salarium（盐枝芽孢杆菌）

V. soli（土壤枝芽孢杆菌）

3　*aerobic Gram-Positive Rods*［革兰氏阳性杆菌（需氧的）］

Agromyces（壤霉菌属）

A. allii（壤霉菌）

A. striae（珧壤霉菌）

A. aurantiacus（金色壤霉菌）

A. brachium［细枝（末梢）壤霉菌］

A. cerinus（蜜黄壤霉菌）

A. flavus（黄壤霉菌）

A. mucosus（岩藻糖壤霉菌）

A. hip puratus(酸盐壤霉菌)

A. humanus(地壤霉菌)

A. italicus(大利壤霉菌)

Arthrobacter(节杆菌属)

A. agii(活泼节杆菌)

A. albius(发白节杆菌)

A. albus(白色节杆菌)

A. alkali philus(喜碱节杆菌)

A. alpinus(高山节杆菌)

A. antarcticus(南极节杆菌)

A. ardlevensis(阿德雷岛节杆菌)

A. laoensis[阿里莱特(乳研联)节杆菌]

A. arron venets(黑蓝节杆菌)

A. aurescens(金黄节杆菌)

Aureobacterium(金杆菌属)

A. barkeri(巴氏金杆菌)

A. flavescens(浅黄金杆菌)

A. liquefaciens(液化金杆菌)

A. saperda(天牛金杆菌)

A. terregens(需土金杆菌)

A. testacean(砖红色金杆菌)

A, arabinogalactanolyticum(解阿拉伯糖半乳聚糖金杆菌)

A. estro 扩 maicer(酯香金杆菌)

A. ieraranolwtieun(解角质素金杆菌)

A. Trichet vieth(解单端霉毒系金菌)

Brevibacterium(短杆菌属)

B. casei(乳酪短杆菌)

B. epidermidis(表皮短杆菌)

B. frigoritolerans(耐寒短杆菌)

B. halotoler(耐盐短杆菌)

B. iodine(紫色短杆菌)

B. linens(扩展短杆菌)

B. acet vlicun(乙酰短杆菌)

B. ru/ascend(微红短杆菌)

B. album(白色短杆菌)

B. antiqua(代短杆菌)

Caseobacter(酪杆菌属)

C. polymorphus(多形酪杆菌)

Clavibacter(棍状杆菌属)

C. uranium(伊朗棍状杆菌)

C. michiganensis(密执安棍状杆菌)

C. ratha yi(拉氏棍状杆菌)

  C. toxicus（中毒棍状杆菌）

  C. tritici（小麦棍状杆菌）

  C. xyli（棉花棍状杆菌）

Cryptobacterium（隐杆菌属）

  C. curtum（短隐杆菌）

Curtobacterium（短小杆菌属）

  C. ammomulgenes（广氨短小秆菌）

  C. citreum（柠檬色短小杆菌）

  C. flaccum faciens（萎蔫短小杆菌）

  C. ginsengisoli（人参土短小杆菌）

  C. herbart（草短小杆菌）

  C. luteum（藤黄短小杆菌）

  C. pusillum（极小短小杆菌）

Gordona（戈登菌属）

  G. alkanivorans（噬烷烃戈登菌）

  G. amicalis（友谊戈登菌）

  G. arai（新井戈登菌）

  G. bronchialis（支气管戈登菌）

  G. holesterolivorans（噬胆固醇戈登菌）

  G. defruit（污水戈登菌）

  G. desul/ ricans（脱硫戈登菌）

  G. e//usa（扩散戈登菌）

  G. hankookensis（韩国戈登菌）

  G. hirsuta［粗糙（蓬发）戈登菌］

Leucobacter（明杆菌属）

  L. prolatus（气生明杆菌）

  L. albus（白色明杆菌）

  L. alluvia（冲积土明杆菌）

  L. rudicollis（干丘明杆菌）

  L. celer（速明杆菌）

  L. chironomid（摇蚊明杆菌）

  L. chromiireducens（铬还原明杆菌）

  L. chromiiresistens（铬抵抗明杆菌）

  L. denitrificans（脱硝明杆菌）

  L. albidus（显白明杆菌）

Microbacterium（微杆菌属）

  M. aerolatum（空气微杆菌）

  M. agaric（松茸微杆菌）

  M. aoyamense（青山微杆菌）

  M. aquimaris（海水微杆菌）

  M. bore（树状微杆菌）

  M. arthros phaerae（千足虫微杆菌）

M. aurantiacum(橙色微杆菌)

M. aur"Ldm(金黄微杆菌))

M. awajiense(淡路岛微杆菌)

M. azadirachtae(印楝微杆菌)

Mycobacterium(分枝杆菌属)

M. avium(鸟分枝杆菌)

M. bohemium(波希米亚分枝杆菌)

M. botniense(帕特省分枝杆菌)

M. bovis(牛型分枝杆菌)

M. celatum(秘密分枝杆菌)

M. chimaera(嵌合体分枝杆菌)

M. cookii(库氏分枝杆菌)

M. doricum(安科纳分枝杆菌)

M. europaeum(欧洲分枝杆菌)

Nocardia(诺卡菌属)

N. abscessus(脓肿诺卡菌)

N. acidovorans(嗜酸诺卡菌)

N. africana(非洲诺卡菌)

N. alba(白色诺卡菌)

N. altamirensis(阿尔塔米拉诺卡菌)

N. anamensis(天美诺卡菌)

N. amarae(沟诺卡菌)

N. anaemia(贫血诺卡菌)

N. gobonis(青叶诺卡菌)

N. arom(花落诺卡菌)

Rathayibacter(拉思菌属)

R. caries(薹草拉思菌)

R. festucae(紫羊茅拉思菌)

R. ratha vi(拉思拉思菌)

R. tritici(小麦拉思菌)

R. iranicus(伊朗拉思菌)

R. tories(中毒拉思菌)

Rhodococcus(红球菌属)

R. chloro phenolics(氯酚红球菌)

R. chubuens(楚布红球菌)

R. chubutensis(楚布红球菌)

R. coprophilous(嗜粪红球菌)

R. corallinus(珊瑚红球菌)

R. equi(马红球菌)

R. erythropolis(红城红球菌)

R. fascians[束(聚集)红球菌]

R. glomerulus(圆红球菌)

R. gordonia（戈登红球菌）

Streptomyces（链霉菌属）

    S. antibioticus（抗生链霉菌）

    S. biverticillatus（双重轮丝链霉菌）

    S. albicans（白蓝链霉菌）

    S. thermophilus（嗜热链霉菌）

    S. chromatidis（色直丝链霉菌）

    S. pestis（疫霉链霉菌）

    S. roseus（玫瑰英链霉菌）

    S. flavus（黄色链霉菌）

    S. globisporus（球孢链霉菌）

    S. erythreus（红霉素链霉菌）

    S. splendens（华美链霉菌）

Terrabacter（地杆菌属）

    T. aeriphilus（喜空气地杆菌）

    T. aerolatus（气携地杆菌）

    T. carboxydivorans（食一氧化碳地杆菌）

    T. ginsenosidimutans（人参苷转化地杆菌）

    T. lapitti（小石头地杆菌）

    T. terrae（土地地杆菌）

    T. erigena（地生地杆菌）

    T. tumescent（肿胀地杆菌）

Tsukamurella（冢村菌属）

    T. paurometabolun（稍变冢村菌）

    T. carbox ydivorans（食一氧化碳冢村菌）

    T. inchonensis（仁川冢村菌）

    T. pseudo puma（假泡沫冢村菌）

    T. pulmonis（肺冢村菌）

    T. soli（土壤冢村菌）

    T. spongia（海绵冢村菌）

    T. spume（泡沫冢村菌）

    T. strandjordae（斯特朗冢村菌）

Turicella（苏黎世菌属）

    T. otitidis（耳炎苏黎世菌）

4 *Gram-positive Rods of facultative anaerobic and akinesis*［革兰氏阳性杆菌（兼性厌氧,无动力）］

Weissella（魏斯菌属）

    W. beninensis（贝宁魏斯菌）

    W. ceti（鲸鱼魏斯菌）

    W. cibaria（食物魏斯菌）

    W. fabaria（可可豆魏斯菌）

W. ghanensis(加纳魏斯菌)

W. hellenica(希腊魏斯菌)

W. kandern(坎氏魏斯菌)

W. kimchii(渍菜魏斯菌)

W. koreensis(韩国魏斯菌)

W. soli(土地魏斯菌)

5 *Gram-positive Rods of facultative anaerobic, rodlike and aerobic*[革兰氏阳性杆菌(棒状,需氧和兼性厌氧的)]

Actinobaculum(放杆菌属)

A. massiliense(马赛放杆菌)

A. schaalii(斯氏放杆菌)

A. suis(猪放杆菌)

A. urinale(脲放杆菌)

Actinomyces(放线菌属)

A. bernardine(伯纳德放线菌)

A. bovis(牛型放线菌)

A. bowdenii(伯氏放线菌)

A. canis(犬放线菌)

A. catuli(小狗放线菌)

A. coleocanis(犬阴道放线菌)

A. dentalis(牙齿放线菌)

A. denticolens(齿垢放线菌)

A. europaeus(欧洲放线菌)

A. funke(芬克放线菌)

Arachnia(蛛网菌属)

A. propionica(丙酸蛛网菌)

Arcanobacterium(隐秘杆菌属)

A. a bortisuls(猪流产隐秘杆菌)

A. bernardine(伯氏隐秘杆菌)

A. bialowiezense(比亚罗维茨)

A. bonas(欧洲野牛)

A. haemolyticum(溶血隐秘杆菌)

A. hi p pocoleae(马阴道隐秘杆菌)

A. phocae(海豹隐秘杆菌)

A. pluranimalium(多动物隐秘杆菌)

A. pyogenes(化脓隐秘杆菌)

Carnobacterium(肉杆菌属)

C. alter funditum(副深层肉杆菌)

C. divergens(差异肉杆菌)

C. funditum(深层肉杆菌)

C. gallinarum(鸡肉杆菌)

C. inhibins（抑制肉杆菌）

C. jeotgali（酵海鲜肉杆菌）

C. maltaromaticun（麦香肉杆菌）

C. mobile（动力肉杆菌）

C. piscicola（居栖鱼肉杆菌）

C. pleistocene（更新世肉杆菌）

Cellulomonas（纤维单胞菌属）

C. biazotea（双氮纤维单胞菌）

C. cellose（纤维纤维单胞菌）

C. chitinilvtica（解几丁纤维单胞菌）

C. com post（堆肥纤维单胞菌）

C. denverensis（丹佛纤维单胞菌）

C. fermentans（发酵纤维单胞菌）

C. flavigena（产黄纤维单胞菌）

C. fimi（粪肥纤维单胞菌）

C. gelida（冷纤维单胞菌）

C. hominis（人纤维单胞菌）

Corynebacterium（棒状杆菌属）

C. accolens（依赖棒状杆菌）

C. fermentans（非发酵棒状杆菌）

C. ammoniagenes（产氨棒状杆菌）

C. amycolatum（无枝菌酸棒状杆菌）

C. aquilae（鹰棒状杆菌）

C. argentorate（斯特拉斯堡棒状杆菌）

C. typicum（非典型棒状杆菌）

C. aurtmucosun（黏黄棒状杆菌）

C. auris（耳棒状杆菌）

C. nuristanis（犬耳棒状杆菌）

Dermabacter（皮肤杆菌属）

D. hominis（人皮肤杆菌）

Dermatophilus（嗜皮菌属）

D. abyssi（深渊皮球菌）

D. marathi（深海坑皮球菌）

D. nishinomiya（西宫皮球菌）

D. pro/undi（深海皮球菌）

Erysipelothrix（丹毒丝菌属）

E. inopinata（意外丹毒丝菌）

E. rhusio patriae（猪红斑丹毒丝菌）

E. tonsillaris（扁桃体丹毒丝菌）

Facklamia（法肯莱姆菌属）

F. hominis（人法肯莱姆菌）

F. Agnano(懒惰法肯莱母菌)

F,languida(活法肯莱姆菌)

F. mirounga(象海豹法肯莱姆菌)

F. bourkii(索尔克法肯莱姆菌)

F. tabacinasalis(鼻烟法肯莱姆菌)

Gardnerella(加德纳菌属)

G. vaginalis(阴道加德那菌)

Globicatella(圆短链菌属)

G. sanguis(血圆短链菌)

G. sulfidifaciens(产硫化物圆短链菌)

Lactobacillus(乳杆菌属)

L. acidi piscis(酸鱼乳杆菌)

L. acidophilus(嗜酸乳杆菌)

L. agilis(敏捷乳杆菌)

L,algidus(冷乳杆菌)

L. alimentarius(食品乳杆菌)

L. amylolyticus(解淀粉乳杆菌)

L. amylophilus(嗜淀粉乳杆菌)

L. amylotrophicus(食淀粉乳杆菌)

L. amylovorus(解淀粉乳杆菌)

L. aquarius(水生乳杆菌)

Leifsonia(利夫森菌属)

L. antarctica(南极利夫森菌)

L. aquatica(水生利夫森菌)

L. aurea(金黄色利夫森菌)

L. bigeumensis(飞禽岛利夫森菌)

L. cynodontis(狗牙根利夫森菌)

L. ginseng(人参利夫森菌)

L. kafniensis(卡夫里冰川利夫森菌)

L. kribbensis(韩生科院利夫森菌)

L. pinderiensis(平达里冰川利夫森菌)

L. poae(早熟禾草利夫森菌)

Listeria(李斯特菌属)

L. innocua(无害李斯特菌)

L. ivanovi(依氏李斯特菌)

L. ivanoviisubsp. anova(依氏李斯特菌依氏亚种)

L. ivanoviisubsp. londongensis(依氏李斯特菌伦顿亚种)

L. marthin(马斯李斯特菌)

L. monocytogenes(单核细胞增生李斯特菌)

L. rocourtiae(罗考尔特李斯特菌)

L. seeligeri(斯氏李斯特菌)

L. welshimeri(韦尔希默李斯特菌)

Luteococcus(黄球菌属)

  L. japonicus(日本黄球菌)

  L. peritonei(腹膜黄球菌)

  L. sanguinis(血黄球菌)

Oerskovia(厄氏菌属)

  O. enterophila(嗜肠厄氏菌)

  O. genesis(耶纳厄氏菌)

  O. paurometabolic(稍变厄氏菌)

  O. turbata(颤动厄氏菌)

  O. xanthinol utica(解黄嘌呤厄氏菌)

Paralactobacillus(副乳杆菌属)

  P. selangorensis(雪兰省副乳杆菌)

Rothia(罗氏菌属)

  R. dentocariosa(龋齿罗氏菌)

  R. aeria(空气罗氏菌)

  R. amarae(污沟罗氏菌)

  R. dentocariosa(龋齿罗氏菌)

  R. mucilaginosa(黏滑罗氏菌)

Sanguibacter(血杆菌属)

  S. antarcticus(南极血杆菌)

  S. inulinase(菊糖血杆菌)

  S. keddie(科氏血杆菌)

  S. marinus(海生血杆菌)

  S. solih(壤血杆菌)

  S. suarez(苏氏血杆菌)

6   *Gram-positive Rods of anaerobism*[革兰氏阳性杆菌(厌氧的)]

Atopobium(陌生菌属)

  A. fossor(挖蚀陌生菌)

  A. minutum(小陌生菌)

  A. parvulum(极小陌生菌)

  A. rimae(裂陌生菌)

  A. vaginae(阴道陌生菌)

Bifidobacterium(双歧杆菌属)

  B. angulatum(有角双歧杆菌)

  B. animalis(动物双歧杆菌)

  B. bifidum(两叉双歧杆菌)

  B. bou(牛双歧杆菌)

  B. catenulata(链状双歧杆菌)

  B. denticolens(居齿双歧杆菌)

  B. dentium(齿双歧杆菌)

　　　　B. gallicum（高卢双歧杆菌）

　　　　B. infantis（婴儿双歧杆菌）

　　　　B. longum（长双歧杆菌）

　Brucella（布鲁氏菌属）

　　　　B. abortus（流产布鲁氏菌）

　　　　B. canis（犬布鲁氏菌）

　　　　B. ceti［海洋大动物（鲸）布鲁氏菌］

　　　　B. inopinata（意外布鲁氏菌）

　　　　B. melitensis（马耳他布鲁氏菌）

　　　　B. microf（田鼠布鲁氏菌）

　　　　B. neotomae（森林鼠布鲁氏菌）

　　　　B. ovis（羊布鲁氏菌）

　　　　B. pinnipedialis（海豹布鲁氏菌）

　　　　B. suis（猪布鲁氏菌）

　Clostridium（梭菌属）

　　　　C. abson（不同梭菌）

　　　　C. aciduric（尿酸梭菌）

　　　　C. algidicarnis（冷肉梭菌）

　　　　C. amygdalina（苦杏仁味梭菌）

　　　　C. barkeri（巴克梭菌）

　　　　C. botulinum（肉毒梭菌）

　　　　C. cadaveris（尸毒梭菌）

　　　　C. carnis（肉梭菌）

　　　　C. celatum（隐藏梭菌）

　　　　C. cellobioparu（产纤维二糖梭菌）

　Cryptobacterium（隐杆菌属）

　　　　C. curtum（短隐杆菌）

　Dorea（杜尔菌属）

　　　　D. formicigenerans（产甲酸杜尔菌）

　　　　D. longicatena（长链杜尔菌）

　Eggerthella（埃格菌属）

　　　　E. hongkongensis（香港埃格菌）

　　　　E. lenta（迟缓埃格菌）

　　　　E. sinensis（中国埃格菌）

　Eubacterium［真（优）杆菌属］

　　　　E. aerofaciens（产气真杆菌）

　　　　E. aggregans（聚集真杆菌）

　　　　E. barkeri（巴克真杆菌）

　　　　E. biforme（两形真杆菌）

　　　　E. branchy（短真杆菌）

　　　　E. cellulosolvens（溶纤维真杆菌）

E. contorting(扭曲真杆菌)

E. cylindroid(柱状真杆菌)

E. dolicum(长链真杆菌)

E. aligns(挑剔真杆菌)

Holdemania(霍尔德曼菌属)

H. filiformis(线型霍尔德曼菌)

Mobiluncus(动弯杆菌属)

M. curtus(柯氏动弯杆菌)

M. curtisii subsp. curtisii(柯氏动弯杆菌柯氏亚种)

M. curtisii subsp. holmes(柯氏动弯杆菌霍氏亚种)

M. mulieris(羞愧动弯杆菌)

Mogibacterium(难养杆菌属)

M. diversum(多样难养杆菌)

M. neglectum[(易)忽视难养杆菌]

M. pumilum(微菌落难养杆菌)

M. timidun(怯生难养杆菌)

M. vescum(弱生难养杆菌)

Parascardovia(副斯加都伟菌属)

P. denticolens(居齿副斯加都伟菌)

Propionibacterium(丙酸杆菌属)

P. acidifaciens(产酸丙酸杆菌)

P. acidipropionici(丙酸丙酸杆菌)

P. acnes(痤疮丙酸杆菌)

P. avidum(贪婪丙酸杆菌)

P. cyclohexanicum(环己酸丙酸菌)

P. freudenreichii(费氏丙酸杆菌)

P. granulosum(颗粒丙酸杆菌)

P. innocuum(无害丙酸杆菌)

P. jensenii(詹氏丙酸杆菌)

P. thoenii(特氏丙酸杆菌)

Propionimicrobium(产丙酸菌属)

P. lymphophilum(嗜淋巴产丙酸菌)

Pseudoramibacter(假枝杆菌属)

P. alactolyticus(不解乳假肢杆菌)

Scardovia(斯加都伟菌属)

S. inopinata(异形斯加都伟菌)

S. wiggsiae(威格斯斯加都伟菌)

Shuttleworthia(舒特勒沃斯菌属)

S. satelles(卫星舒特勒沃斯菌)

Slackia(斯莱克菌属)

S. exigua(乏生斯莱克菌)

S. faecicanis(狗粪斯莱克菌)

S. heliotrinireducens(还原天芥菜碱斯莱克菌)

S. isoflavoniconvertens(异黄酮转化斯莱克菌)

S. piriformis(梨形斯莱克菌)

Turicibacter(苏黎世杆菌属)

T. sanguinis(血苏黎氏杆菌)

7　*Gram-negative Coccus*(革兰氏阴性球菌)

Anaeroglobus(厌氧球菌属)

A. hydrogenalis(氢厌氧球菌)

A. lactolyticus(解乳厌氧球菌)

A. murdochii(默多克氏厌氧球菌)

A. octavius(第八厌氧球菌)

A. prevotii(普氏厌氧球菌)

A. tetradius(四联厌氧球菌)

A. vaginalis(阴道厌氧球菌)

Neisseria(奈瑟菌属)

N. animalis(动物奈瑟菌)

N. denitrificans(脱硝奈瑟菌)

N. flava(黄色奈瑟菌)

N. gonorrhoeae(淋病奈瑟菌)

N. lactamica(乳糖奈瑟菌)

N. macacae(猕猴奈瑟菌)

N. meningitids(脑膜炎奈瑟菌)

N. perflava(深黄奈瑟菌)

N. sicca(干燥奈瑟菌)

N. weaveri(韦弗氏奈瑟菌)

Veillonella(韦荣球菌属)

V. alcalescens subsp. *alcalescens*(产碱韦荣球菌产碱亚种)

V. alcalescens subsp. *Ratti*(产碱韦荣球菌大鼠亚种)

V. atypica(非典型韦荣球菌)

V. caviae(豚鼠韦荣球菌)

V. criceti(仓鼠韦荣球菌)

V. magna(大韦荣球菌)

V. parvula(小韦荣球菌)

V. ratti(鼠韦荣球菌)

V. rogosae(罗格斯韦荣球菌)

Victivallis(食谷菌属)

V. vadensis(瓦赫宁根食谷菌)

8 *Gram-negative bacilli of obligate aerobic and pole hair*[革兰氏阴性杆菌(专性需氧,极毛)]

Acidovorax(食酸菌属)

A. delafieldii(德氏食酸菌)

A. facilis(敏捷食酸菌)

A. temperans(中泛食酸菌)

Allorhizobium(别根瘤菌属)

A. undicola(居水别根瘤菌)

Alteromonas(异单胞菌属、交替单胞菌属)

A. addita(加入异单胞菌)

A. atlantica(大西洋异单胞菌)

A. citrea(柠檬异单胞菌)

A. colwelliana(科氏异单胞菌)

A. communis(普遍异单胞菌)

A. espejiana(埃氏异单胞菌)

A. marina(海异单胞菌)

A. rubra(红色异单胞菌)

A. tagae(塔加氏异单胞菌)

A. vaga(漫游异单胞菌)

Balneatrix(浴者菌属、巴氏丝菌属)

B. alpica(阿尔卑斯浴者菌)

Bradyrhizobium(慢生根瘤菌属)

B. betae(甜菜慢生根瘤菌)

B. canariense(卡那里岛慢生根瘤菌)

B. cytisi(金雀儿慢生根瘤菌)

B. denitrificans(脱硝慢生根瘤菌)

B. elkanii(埃尔肯氏慢生根瘤菌)

B. japonicum(大豆慢生根瘤菌)

B. lablabi(扁豆慢生根瘤菌)

B. liaoningense(辽宁慢生根瘤菌)

B. pachyrhizi(豆薯慢生根瘤菌)

B. yuanmingense(圆明园慢生根瘤菌)

Brevundimonas(短波毛单胞菌属)

B. alba(白色短波毛单胞菌)

B. bacteroides(杆状短波毛单胞菌)

B. bullata(泡状短波毛单胞菌)

B. diminuta(缺陷短波毛单胞菌)

B. intermedia(中间短波毛单胞菌)

B. kwangchunensis(光春短波毛单胞菌)

B. lenta(黏性短波毛单胞菌)

B. nasdae(航天短波毛单胞菌)

B. poindexterae(波氏短波毛单胞菌)

B. terrae(土壤短波毛单胞菌)

Burkholderia(伯克菌属、伯克霍尔德菌属)

B. acidipaludis(酸性沼泽伯克菌)

B. anthina(花园伯克菌)

B. bannensis(版纳伯克菌)

B. caledonica(苏格兰伯克菌)

B. caribensis(加勒比伯克菌)

B. diffusa(广布伯克菌)

B. ferrariae(铁矿伯克菌)

B. glathei(格氏伯克菌)

B. lata(普通伯克菌)

B. mimosarum(含羞草伯克菌)

Chryseomonas(华丽单胞菌属、华丽金色单胞菌属)

C. antarcticun(南极华丽杆菌)

C. anthropi(人体华丽杆菌)

C. bovis(牛华丽杆菌)

C. caeni(污泥华丽杆菌)

C. daecheongense(大清湖华丽杆菌)

C. elymi(野生黑麦华丽杆菌)

C. flavum(黄色华丽杆菌)

C. gambrini(干布里那斯华丽杆菌)

C. jeonii(杰氏华丽杆菌)

C. lathyri(山黛豆华丽杆菌)

Comamonas(丛毛单胞菌属)

C. acidovorans(食酸丛毛单胞菌)

C. aquatica(水生丛毛单胞菌)

C. badia(栗色丛毛单胞菌)

C. composti(堆肥丛毛单胞菌)

C. denitrificans(脱硝丛毛单胞菌)

C. granuli(颗粒丛毛单胞菌)

C. nitrativorans(含硝丛毛单胞菌)

C. ondototermitis(白蚁丛毛单胞菌)

C. terrigena(土生丛毛单胞菌)

C. zonglianii(宗濂丛毛单胞菌)

Delftia(代尔夫特菌属)

D. acidovorans(食酸代尔夫特菌)

D. lacustris(湖代尔夫特菌)

D. tsuruhatensis(清臣代尔夫特菌)

Flavimonas(黄素单胞菌属)

F. oryzihabitans(栖稻黄素单胞菌)

Hydrogenophaga（嗜氢菌属）

   H. bisanensis（釜山噬氢菌）

   H. caeni（污泥噬氢菌）

   H. defluvii（污水噬氢菌）

   H. flava（黄色噬氢菌）

   H. intermedia（中间噬氢菌）

   H. palleronii（帕氏噬氢菌）

   H. pseudoflava（类黄噬氢菌）

   H. taenionspiralis（螺纹噬氢菌）

Massilia（马赛菌属）

   M. aerilata（气生马赛菌）

   M. albidiflava（黄白马赛菌）

   M. brevitalea（短杆马赛菌）

   M. consociata（联系马赛菌）

   M. dura（硬马赛菌）

   M. flava（黄色马赛菌）

   M. jejuensis（济州马赛菌）

   M. niabensis（农技院马赛菌）

   M. oculi（眼马赛菌）

   M. plicata（绕叠马赛菌）

Mesorhizobium（中间根瘤菌属）

   M. albiziae（山槐中间根瘤菌）

   M. alhagi（骆驼刺中间根瘤菌）

   M. caraganae（锦鸡儿中间根瘤菌）

   M. chacoense（查科中间根瘤菌）

   M. ciceri（鹰嘴豆中间根瘤菌）

   M. gobiense（戈壁中间根瘤菌）

   M. loti（百脉中间根瘤菌）

   M. mediterraneum（地中海中间根瘤菌）

   M. metallidurans（抗金属中间根瘤菌）

   M. opportunistum（机会中间根瘤菌）

Pandoraea（潘多拉菌属）

   P. apista（奸诈潘多拉菌）

   P. faecigallinarum（母鸡粪潘多拉菌）

   P. nortmbergensis（纽伦堡潘多拉菌）

   P. oxalativorans（食草酸潘多拉菌）

   P. pnomenusa（驻肺潘多拉菌）

   P. pulmonicola（居肺潘多拉菌）

   P. sputorum（痰潘多拉菌）

   P. thiooxydans（硫氧化潘多拉菌）

   P. vervacti（休耕地潘多拉菌）

Pseudoalteromonas（假交替单胞菌属、假异单胞菌属）

  P. aliena（另种假交替单胞菌）

  P. atlantica（大西洋假交替单胞菌）

  P. bynsanensis（边山假交替单胞菌）

  P. carrageenovora（嗜角叉菜假交替单胞菌）

  P. distincta（明显假交替单胞菌）

  P. elyakovii（艾氏假交替单胞菌）

  P. flavipulchra（金色假交替单胞菌）

  P. haloplanktis（游海假交替单胞菌）

  P. issachenkonii（伊萨臣柯假交替单胞菌）

  P. marina（海假交替单胞菌）

Pseudomonas（假单胞菌属）

  P. aeruginosa（铜绿假单胞菌）

  P. alcaliphila（嗜碱假单胞菌）

  P. amygdali（扁桃假单胞菌）

  P. borbori（污水假单胞菌）

  P. brenneri（布伦那假单胞菌）

  P. cannabina（大麻假单胞菌）

  P. delafieldii（德氏假单胞菌）

  P. facilis（敏捷假单胞菌）

  P. japonica（日本假单胞菌）

  P. kilonensis（基尔假单胞菌）

Rhizobium（根瘤菌属）

  R. aggregatum（成团根瘤菌）

  R. borbori（污泥根瘤菌）

  R. ciceri（鹰嘴豆根瘤菌）

  R. daejeonense（大田根瘤菌）

  R. etli（菜豆根瘤菌）

  R. galegae（山羊豆根瘤菌）

  R. herbae（草药根瘤菌）

  R. japonicum（大豆根瘤菌）

  R. lupini（羽扇豆根瘤菌）

  R. mongolense（内蒙古根瘤菌）

Roseomonas（玫瑰单胞菌属）

  R. aerilata（气生玫瑰单胞菌）

  R. cervicalis（宫颈玫瑰单胞菌）

  R. fauriae（费氏玫瑰单胞菌）

  R. lacus（湖玫瑰单胞菌）

  R. mucosa（黏液玫瑰单胞菌）

  R. pecuniae（硬币玫瑰单胞菌）

  R. rosea（玫瑰色玫瑰单胞菌）

  R. stagni（池塘玫瑰单胞菌）

R. terrae(土壤玫瑰单胞菌)

R. vinacea(葡萄酒色玫瑰单胞菌)

Sinorhizobium(中华根瘤菌属)

S. fredii(费氏中华根瘤菌)

S. meliloti(苜蓿中华根瘤菌)

S. saheli(萨赫勒中华根瘤菌)

S. teranga(适宜中华根瘤菌)

S. xinjiangensis(新疆中华根瘤菌)

S. arboris(树中华根瘤菌)

S. morelense(莫雷洛斯中华根瘤菌)

Sphingomonas(鞘氨醇单胞菌属)

S. abaci(台鞘氨醇单胞菌)

S. aerolata(粘连鞘氨醇单胞菌)

S. cloacae(阴沟鞘氨醇单胞菌)

S. dokdonensis(独岛鞘氨醇单胞菌)

S. faeni(干草鞘氨醇单胞菌)

S. ginsenosidimutans(人参苷转化鞘氨醇单胞菌)

S. insulae(岛鞘氨醇单胞菌)

S. japonica(日本鞘氨醇单胞菌)

S. mucosissima(极黏鞘氨醇单胞菌)

S. natatoria(泳池鞘氨醇单胞菌)

S. pruni(桃鞘氨醇单胞菌)

Spirillum(螺菌属)

S. volutans(迂回螺菌)

S. winogradskyi(维诺格拉德斯基氏螺菌)

S. minus(减少螺菌)

S. pulli(雏鸡螺菌)

Stenotrophomonas(寡养单胞菌属、寡食单胞菌属)

S. acidaminiphila(喜氨酸寡养单胞菌)

S. africana(非洲寡养单胞菌)

S. chelatiphaga(食螯合剂寡养单胞菌)

S. daejeonensis(大田寡养单胞菌)

S. dokdonensis(独岛寡养单胞菌)

S. humi(土寡养单胞菌)

S. koreensis(韩国寡养单胞菌)

S. pavanii(帕文寡养单胞菌)

S. rhizophila(嗜根寡养单胞菌)

S. terrae(土壤寡养单胞菌)

Telluria(土地菌属)

T. chitinolytica(解几丁土地菌)

T. mixta(混毛土地菌)

Vogesella（沃格菌属）

    V. indigofera（产靛沃格菌）

    V. lacus（湖沃格菌）

    V. mureinivorans（食胞壁质沃格菌）

    V. perlucida（透明沃格菌）

Xanthomonas（黄单胞菌属）

    X. albilineans（白纹黄单胞菌）

    X. ampelina（葡萄酒黄单胞菌）

    X. bromi（雀麦草黄单胞菌）

    X. campestris（野油菜黄单胞菌）

    X. codiaei（巴豆黄单胞菌）

    X. fragariae（草莓黄单胞菌）

    X. hortorum（花园黄单胞菌）

    X. hyacinthi（风信子黄单胞菌）

    X. melonis（甜瓜黄单胞菌）

    X. oryzae（水稻黄单胞菌）

Zavarzinia（扎瓦菌属）

    Z. compransoris（餐伴扎瓦菌）

Zoogloea（动胶菌属）

    Z. caeni（污泥动胶菌）

    Z. oryzae（稻动胶菌）

    Z. remigera（生枝动胶菌）

    Z. resiniphila（嗜树脂动胶菌）

9 *Gram-negative bacilli of obligate aerobic and peritrichal*［革兰氏阴性杆菌（专性需氧，周毛）］

Achromobacter（无色杆菌属）

    A. denitrificans（反硝无色杆菌）

    A. insoletus（稀有无色杆菌）

    A. piechaudii（皮氏无色杆菌）

    A. ruhlandii（卢氏无色杆菌）

    A. spanius（少见无色杆菌）

    A. xylosoxidans（木糖氧化无色杆菌）

    A. xylosoxidans subsp. *denitrificans*（木糖氧化无色杆菌反硝化亚种）

    A. xylosoxidans subsp. *xylosoxidans*（木糖氧化无色杆菌木糖氧化亚种）

Agrobacterium（土壤杆菌属）

    A. atlanticum（大西洋土壤杆菌）

    A. ferrugineum（锈色土壤杆菌）

    A. gelatinovorum（食明胶土壤杆菌）

    A. meteori（梅氏土壤杆菌）

    A. radiobacter（放射形土壤杆菌）

A. rhizogenes（发根土壤杆菌）

A. stellulatum（星斑土壤杆菌）

A. tumefaciens（根癌土壤杆菌）

A. vitis（葡萄土壤杆菌）

Alcaligenes（产碱菌属）

A. denitrificans（反硝化产碱菌）

A. faecalis（粪产碱菌）

A. aestus（海潮产碱菌）

A. cupidus（渴望产碱菌）

A. eutrophus（真养产碱菌）

A. latus（广泛产碱菌）

A. pacificus（太平洋产碱菌）

A. venustus（优美产碱菌）

A. aquatilis（水产碱菌）

A. piechaudii（皮氏产碱菌）

Azorhizobium（固氮根瘤菌属）

A. caulinodans（茎瘤固氮根瘤菌）

A. doebereinerae（多氏固氮根瘤菌）

Ochrobactrum（苍白杆菌属）

O. anthropi（人苍白杆菌）

O. ciceri（鹰嘴豆苍白杆菌）

O. gallinifaecis（鸡粪苍白杆菌）

O. haematophilum（中间苍白杆菌）

O. lupini（白羽扇豆苍白杆菌）

O. oryzae（稻苍白杆菌）

O. pectoris（牲畜苍白杆菌）

O. thiophenivorans（噻吩苍白杆菌）

O. rhizophaerae（根围苍白杆菌）

O. tritici（小麦苍白杆菌）

Variovorax（贪噬菌属）

V. boronicumulans（集硼贪噬菌）

V. dokdonensis（独岛贪噬菌）

V. ginsengisoli（人参土贪噬菌）

V. paradoxus（争论贪噬菌）

V. soli（土贪噬菌）

Wautersia（沃特菌属）

W. basilensis（巴塞尔沃特菌）

W. campinensis（坎皮纳沃特菌）

W. eutropha（真养沃特菌）

W. gilardii（吉氏沃特菌）

W. metallidurans（耐金属沃特菌）

W. numazuensis（沼津沃特菌）

W. oxalatica(草酸盐沃特菌)

W. paucula(罕有沃特菌)

W. respiraculi(呼吸道沃特菌)

W. taiwanensis(台湾沃特菌)

10　*Gram-negative bacilli of obligate aerobic and akinesis*[革兰氏阴性杆菌(专性需氧,无动力)]

Acinetobacer(不动杆菌属)

A. *baumannii*(鲍氏不动杆菌)

A. *baylyi*(拜尔利不动杆菌)

A. *brisouii*(布雷索不动杆菌)

A. *calcoaceticus*(乙酸钙不动杆菌)

A. *gerneri*(格尔纳不动杆菌)

A. *haemolyticus*(溶血不动杆菌)

A. *johnsonii*(约氏不动杆菌)

A. *lwoffi*(鲁氏不动杆菌)

A. *parvus*(小不动杆菌)

A. *rudis*(粗初不动杆菌)

Bergeyella(伯杰菌属)

B. *zoohelum*(动物伤口伯杰菌)

Branhamella(布兰汉菌属)

B. *catarrhalis*(卡他布兰汉菌)

B. *caviae*(豚鼠布兰汉菌)

B. *cuniculi*(兔布兰汉菌)

B. *ovis*(绵羊布兰汉菌)

Brucella(布鲁氏菌属)

B. *abortus*(流产布鲁氏菌)

B. *canis*(犬布鲁氏菌)

B. *ceti*(海洋大动物布鲁氏菌)

B. *inopinala*(意外布鲁氏菌)

B. *melitensis*(马耳他布鲁氏菌)

B. *microti*(田鼠布鲁氏菌)

B. *neotomae*(森林鼠布鲁氏菌)

B. *ovis*(羊布鲁氏菌)

B. *pinnipedialis*(海豹布鲁氏菌)

B. *suis*(猪布鲁氏菌)

Calymmatobacterium(鞘杆菌属)

C. *granulomatis*(肉芽肿鞘杆菌)

Chryseobacterium(华丽杆菌属、华丽金黄杆菌属)

C. *anthropi*(人体华丽杆菌)

C. *aquaticum*(水华丽杆菌)

C. bovis（牛华丽杆菌）

C. caeni（污泥华丽杆菌）

C. daecheongense（大清湖华丽杆菌）

C. elymi（野生黑麦华丽杆菌）

C. flavum（黄色华丽杆菌）

C. gambrini（干布里那斯华丽杆菌）

C. luteum（橙色华丽杆菌）

C. miricola（居米尔空间站华丽杆菌）

Empedobacter（稳杆菌属）

E. brevis（稳杆菌）

Flavobacterium（黄杆菌属）

F. acidificum（酸化黄杆菌）

F. acidurans（耐酸黄杆菌）

F. breve（短黄杆菌）

F. cheniae（陈氏黄杆菌）

F. defluvii（污泥黄杆菌）

F. esteraromaticum（酯香黄杆菌）

F. ferrugineum（锈色黄杆菌）

F. phragmitis（芦苇黄杆菌）

F. rivuli（小河黄杆菌）

F. saliperosum（怕盐黄杆菌）

Francisella（弗朗西丝菌属）

F. halioticida（杀鲍鱼弗朗西丝菌）

F. hispaniensis（西班牙弗朗西丝菌）

F. noatunensis（海岸弗朗西丝菌）

F. novicida（新凶手弗朗西丝菌）

F. philomiragia（蜃楼弗朗西丝菌）

F. piscicida（杀鱼弗朗西丝菌）

F. tularensis（土拉热弗朗西丝菌）

Moraxella（莫拉菌属）

M. atlantae（亚特兰大莫拉菌）

M. boeveri（鲍氏莫拉菌）

M. bovis（牛莫拉菌）

M. canis（狗莫拉菌）

M. lacunata（腔隙莫拉菌）

M. nonliquefaciens（非液化莫拉菌）

M. oblonga（伸长莫拉菌）

M. pluranimalium（多动物莫拉菌）

M. saccharolytica（解糖莫拉菌）

M. urethralis（尿道莫拉菌）

Myroides（类香菌属）

M. marinus（海洋类香菌）

M. odoratimimus（拟气味类香菌）

M. odoratus（气味类香菌）

M. pelagicus（海类香菌）

M. phaeus（棕色类香菌）

M. profoundi（深海类香菌）

Oligella（寡源菌属）

O. ureolytica（解尿寡源菌）

O. urethralis（尿道寡源菌）

Paracoccus（副球菌属）

P. alcaliphilus（时间副球菌）

P. caeni（污泥副球菌）

P. denitrifyicans（脱硝副球菌）

P. fistulariae（管鱼副球菌）

P. isoporae（珊瑚副球菌）

P. kocurii（科氏副球菌）

P. marcusii（马氏副球菌）

P. methylutens（甲基副球菌）

P. niistensis（国立多科院）

P. solventlvorans（食溶剂副球菌）

Pedobacter（土杆菌属）

P. aquatilis（水生土杆菌）

P. caeni（污水土杆菌）

P. duraquae（硬水土杆菌）

P. ginsengisoli（人参土杆菌）

P. hartonius（哈茨山土杆菌）

P. insulae（岛土杆菌）

P. lentus（慢生土杆菌）

P. metabolipauper（迟代谢土杆菌）

P. rhizophaerae（根围土杆菌）

P. saltan（滑动土杆菌）

Pelistega（居鸽菌属）

P. europaeaa（欧洲居鸽菌）

Psychrobacter（冷杆菌属）

P. aestuarii（潮间带冷杆菌）

P. celer（速生冷杆菌）

P. faecalis（粪冷杆菌）

P. fozii（弗兹冷杆菌）

P. glacincola（冰栖冷杆菌）

P. immobilis（不动冷杆菌）

P. jeotgali（盐渍海鲜冷杆菌）

P. luti（污泥冷杆菌）

P. marincola（海居冷杆菌）

  P. namhaensis（南海冷杆菌）

Psychroflexus（冷弯菌属）

  P. gondwanense（关德瓦那冷弯菌）

  P. salinarum（盐场冷弯菌）

  P. sediminis（沉淀冷弯菌）

  P. torques（弯曲冷弯菌）

  P. tropicus（热带冷弯菌）

Sphingobacterium（鞘氨醇杆菌属）

  S. anhuiense（安徽鞘氨醇杆菌）

  S. bambusae（竹鞘氨醇杆菌）

  S. canadense（加拿大鞘氨醇杆菌）

  S. daejeonense（大田鞘氨醇杆菌）

  S. faecium（屎鞘氨醇杆菌）

  S. heparinum（肝素鞘氨醇杆菌）

  S. mizutae（水谷氏鞘氨醇杆菌）

  S. piscium（鱼鞘氨醇杆菌）

  S. shayense（沙雅氨醇杆菌）

  S. wenxiniae（文新鞘氨醇杆菌）

Weeksella（威克菌属）

  W. virosa（黏液威克菌）

  W. zoohelcum（动物溃疡威克菌）

11　*gram-negative bacillus, obligate aerobic, indefinite Flagella*［革兰氏阴性杆菌（专性需氧，鞭毛不定）］

Advenella（颇陌菌属）

  A. incenata（禁食颇陌菌）

  A. kashmirensis（克什米尔颇陌菌）

  A. mimigardefordensis（明斯特颇陌菌）

Afipia（军院菌属、阿菲波菌属）

  A. birgiae（贝格军院菌）

  A. broomeae（布鲁姆军院菌）

  A. clevelandensis（克里夫兰军院菌）

  A. felis（猫军院菌）

  A. massiliensis（马赛军院菌）

Bordetella（鲍特菌属）

  B. ansorpii（亚洲监网鲍特菌）

  B. avium（鸟鲍特菌）

  B. bronchiseptica（支气管败血鲍特菌）

  B. hinzii（欣茨鲍特菌）

  B. holmesii（霍姆鲍特菌）

  B. parapertussis（副百日咳鲍特菌）

B. pertussis（百日咳鲍特菌）

B. petrii（哌替鲍特菌）

B. trematum（伤口鲍特菌）

Janthinobacterium（紫色杆菌属）

J. agaricidamnosum（蘑软腐紫色杆菌）

J. lividum（暗蓝紫色杆菌）

Kerstersia（凯斯特菌属）

K. gyiorum（肢体凯斯特菌）

Legionella（军团菌属）

L. anisa（茴香军团菌）

L. beliardensis（蒙贝利亚尔军团菌）

L. cherrii（彻里军团菌）

L. dresdensis（德雷斯顿军团菌）

L. erythra（红色军团菌）

L. fallonii（法龙军团菌）

L. geestiana（吉士厅军团菌）

L. hackeliae（哈克军团菌）

L. impletisoli（土注军团菌）

L. lansingensis（兰辛军团菌）

Novosphingobium（新鞘氨醇菌属）

N. acidiphilum（嗜酸新鞘氨醇菌）

N. capsulatum（荚膜新鞘氨醇菌）

N. hassiacum（黑森新鞘氨醇菌）

N. indicum（印度新鞘氨醇菌）

N. lentum（慢新鞘氨醇菌）

N. mathurense（马图拉新鞘氨醇菌）

N. naphthalenivorans（食萘新鞘氨醇菌）

N. panipatense（帕尼帕特新鞘氨醇菌）

N. resinovorans（食树脂新鞘氨醇菌）

N. rosa（玫瑰新鞘氨醇菌）

Ralstonia（罗尔斯顿菌属）

R. basilensis（巴塞尔罗尔斯顿菌）

R. campinensis（坎皮纳罗尔斯顿菌）

R. eutropha（真养罗尔斯顿菌）

R. gilardii（吉氏罗尔斯顿菌）

R. metallidurans（耐金属罗尔斯顿菌）

R. oxalateica（草酸盐罗尔斯顿菌）

R. paucula（罕见罗尔斯顿菌）

R. respiraculi（呼吸罗尔斯顿菌）

R. solanacearum（青枯罗尔斯顿菌）

R. syzygii（蒲桃罗尔斯顿菌）

Sphingobium（鞘氨醇菌属）

　　S. abikonense（我孙子鞘氨醇菌）

　　S. amiense（阿见鞘氨醇菌）

　　S. chinhatense（金赫德鞘氨醇菌）

　　S. faniae（范氏鞘氨醇菌）

　　S. herbicidovorans（嗜除草剂鞘氨醇菌）

　　S. indicum（印度鞘氨醇菌）

　　S. japanicum（日本鞘氨醇菌）

　　S. lactosutens（乳糖同化鞘氨醇菌）

　　S. olei（油鞘氨醇菌）

　　S. qiquonii（其国鞘氨醇菌）

Sphingopyxis（鞘氨醇盒菌属）

　　S. alaskensis（阿拉斯加鞘氨醇盒菌）

　　S. baekryungensis（白翔岛鞘氨醇盒菌）

　　S. chilensis（智利鞘氨醇盒菌）

　　S. flavimaris（黄海鞘氨醇盒菌）

　　S. ginsengisoli（人参土鞘氨醇盒菌）

　　S. litoris（海岸鞘氨醇盒菌）

　　S. marina（海洋鞘氨醇盒菌）

　　S. soli（土壤鞘氨醇盒菌）

　　S. taejonensis（大田鞘氨醇盒菌）

　　S. witflariensis（威兹拉鞘氨醇盒菌）

12　*gram-negative bacillus*, *facultative anaerobic*, Pseudomonos or lateral setae, purpurin［革兰氏阴性杆菌（兼性厌氧，极毛或侧毛，紫色素）］

Chromobacterium（色杆菌属）

　　C. aquaticum（水生色杆菌）

　　C. fluviatile（河流色杆菌）

　　C. haemolyticus（溶血色杆菌）

　　C. lividum（蓝黑色杆菌）

　　C. piscinae（池塘色杆菌）

　　C. pseudoviolaceum（假紫色色杆菌）

　　C. subtsugae（铁衫土色杆菌）

　　C. violaccum（紫色色杆菌）

Iodobacter（紫杆菌属、碘杆菌属）

　　I. fluviatile（河生紫杆菌）

13　*gram-negative bacillus*, *microaerophilic or anaerobic*［革兰氏阴性杆菌（微需氧或厌氧）］

Peltstega（居鸽菌属）

　　P. europaeaa（欧洲居鸽菌）

Sutterella(萨特氏菌属)

    S. parvirubra(小红萨特氏菌)

    S. stercoricans(狗粪萨顿氏菌)

    S. wadsworthensis(沃兹沃思萨特氏菌)

14 *gram-negative bacillus, aerobic and facultative anaerobic, unpowered* [革兰氏阴性杆菌（需氧和兼性需氧，无动力）]

Actinobacillus(放线杆菌属)

    A. anseriformium(鹅放线杆菌)

    A. capsulatus(荚膜放线杆菌)

    A. delphinicola(居海豚放线杆菌)

    A. euuli(马驹放线杆菌)

    A. hominis(人放线杆菌)

    A. indolicus(吲哚放线杆菌)

    A. minor(小放线杆菌)

    A. pleuropneumoniae(胸膜肺炎放线杆菌)

    A. rossii(罗氏放线杆菌)

    A. scotiae(苏格兰放线杆菌)

Alishewanella(别施万菌属)

    A. aestuarii(河口别施万菌)

    A. agri(田野别施万菌)

    A. fetalis(胎儿别施万菌)

    A. jeotgali(发酵海鲜别施万菌)

Cardiobacterium(心杆菌属)

    C. hominis(人心杆菌)

    C. valvarum(瓣膜心杆菌)

Coenonia(联系菌属)

    C. anatina(鸭联系菌)

Dichelobacter(偶蹄杆菌属)

    D. nodosus(节拟杆菌)

Eikenella(艾肯菌属)

    E. corrodens(啮蚀艾肯菌)

Gallibacterium(鸡杆菌属)

    G. anatis(鸭鸡杆菌)

    G. melopsittaci(鹦鹉鸡杆菌)

    G. salpingitidis(卵管炎鸡杆菌)

    G. trehalosifermentans(酵海藻糖鸡杆菌)

Haemophilus(嗜血杆菌属)

    H. actinomycetemcomitans(伴放线菌嗜血菌)

Kingella(金氏菌属)

    K. denitrificans(脱硝金氏菌)

K. *kingae*(金氏金氏菌)

K. *indologenes*(产吲哚金氏菌)

K. *orale*(口腔金氏菌)

K. *potus*(蜜熊金氏菌)

Mannheimia(曼海姆菌属)

M. *caviae*(豚鼠苷曼海姆菌)

M. *glucosida*(葡糖苷曼海姆菌)

M. *granulomatis*(肉芽肿曼海姆菌)

M. *haemolytica*(溶血曼海姆菌)

M. *ruminalis*(反刍曼海姆菌)

M. *varigena*(异源曼海姆菌)

Ornithobacterium(鸟杆菌属)

O. *rhinotracheale*(鼻气管鸟杆菌)

Pasteurella(巴斯德菌属)

P. *aerogenes*(产气巴斯德菌)

P. *bettyae*(贝特巴斯德菌)

P. *cabalii*(马巴斯德菌)

P. *dagmatis*(咬啮马巴斯德菌)

P. *granulomatis*(肉芽肿巴斯德菌)

P. *haemolytica*(溶血巴斯德菌)

P. *langaaensis*(郎氏巴斯德菌)

P. *mairii*(麦氏巴斯德菌)

P. *penetrans*(侵入巴斯德菌)

P. *stomatis*(咽喉巴斯德菌)

Riemerella(里默尔菌属)

R. *anatipestifer*(鸭病里默尔菌)

R. *columbina*(鸽里默尔菌)

Suttonella[苏同(萨顿)菌属]

S. *indologenes*(产吲哚萨顿菌)

S. *ornithocala*(居鸟萨顿菌)

15 *gram-negative campylobacter, microaerophilic, powered*[革兰氏阴性弯曲杆菌(微嗜氧,有动力)]

Arcobacter(弓形菌属)

A. *butzleri*(巴策尔弓形菌)

A. *cibarius*(食物弓形菌)

A. *defluvii*(污泥弓形菌)

A. *ellisii*(埃利斯弓形菌)

A. *halophilus*(嗜盐弓形菌)

A. *marinus*(海洋弓形菌)

A. *mytili*(贻贝弓形菌)

A. nitrofigilis（硝化弓形菌）

A. skirrowii（斯氏弓形菌）

A. thereius（动物弓形菌）

Campylobacter（弯曲菌属）

C. avium（鸟弯曲菌）

C. butzleri（巴策尔弯曲菌）

C. canadensis（加拿大弯曲菌）

C. coli（结肠弯曲菌）

C. concisus（简洁弯曲菌）

C. curvus（弯弯曲菌）

C. fetus（胎儿弯曲菌）

C. lari（海豚弯曲菌）

C. rectus（直肠弯曲菌）

C. sputorum（唾液弯曲菌）

Helicobacter（螺杆菌属）

H. acinonychis（猎豹螺杆菌）

H. anseris（鹅螺杆菌）

H. aurati（金仓鼠螺杆菌）

H. bilis（胆汁螺杆菌）

H. bizzozeronii（毕氏螺杆菌）

H. brantae（加拿大鹅螺杆菌）

H. canadensis（加拿大螺杆菌）

H. canis（犬螺杆菌）

H. cetorum（海豚螺杆菌）

H. felis（猫螺杆菌）

16   *gram-negative bacillus*, *Enterobacteriaceae*［革兰氏阴性杆菌（肠杆菌科）］

Brenneria（布伦那菌属）

B. alni（桤木布伦那菌）

B. nigrifluens（流黑布伦那菌）

B. paradisiaca（类百合布伦那菌）

B. quercina（栎布伦那菌）

B. rubrifaciens（生红布伦那菌）

B. salicis（柳布伦那菌）

Budvicia（布戴维采菌属）

B. aquatica（水生布戴维采菌）

Buttiauxella（布丘菌属）

B. agrestis（乡间布丘菌）

B. brennerae（布伦那布丘菌）

B. ferragutiae（费氏布丘菌）

B. gaviniae（加文布丘菌）

    B. izardii(伊泽布丘菌)

    B. noackiae(诺亚克布丘菌)

    B. warmboldiae(沃氏布丘菌)

Cedecea(西蒂西菌属)

    C. davisae(戴维西蒂西菌)

    C. lapagei(拉帕西蒂西菌)

    C. neteri(奈特西蒂西菌)

Citrobacter(柠檬酸杆菌属)

    C. braakii(布拉克柠檬酸杆菌)

    C. diversus(异型柠檬酸杆菌)

    C. farmeri(法默柠檬酸杆菌)

    C. freundii(弗劳地柠檬酸杆菌)

    C. gillenii(吉伦柠檬酸杆菌)

    C. koseri(科泽柠檬酸杆菌)

    C. malonatica(丙二酸盐柠檬酸杆菌)

    C. rodentium(啮齿柠檬酸杆菌)

    C. sedlakii(塞德拉克柠檬酸杆菌)

    C. youngae(杨氏柠檬酸杆菌)

Edwardsiella(爱德华菌属)

    E. hoshinae(保科爱德华菌)

    E. intaluri(鲶鱼爱德华菌)

    E. tarda(迟钝爱德华菌)

Enterobacter(肠杆菌属)

    E. aerogenes(产气肠杆菌)

    E. agglomerans(聚团肠杆菌)

    E. arachidis(花生肠杆菌)

    E. cloacae(阴沟肠杆菌)

    E. cowanii(科恩肠杆菌)

    E. dissolvens(溶解肠杆菌)

    E. gergoviae(格高肠杆菌)

    E. intermedius(中间肠杆菌)

    E. kobei[神户(科比)肠杆菌]

    E. mori(桑肠杆菌)

Erwinia(欧文菌属)

    E. alni(桤木欧文菌)

    E. amylovora(解淀粉欧文菌)

    E. ananas(菠萝欧文菌)

    E. oleae(油橄榄欧文菌)

    E. papayae(木瓜欧文菌)

    E. persicinus(桃色欧文菌)

    E. quercina(栎欧文菌)

    E. salicis(柳欧文菌)

    E. toletana(托莱多欧文菌)

    E. typographi(树皮甲虫欧文菌)

Escherichia(埃希菌属)

    E. albertii(阿勃特氏埃希菌)

    E. blattae(蟑螂埃希菌)

    E. coli(大肠埃希菌)

    E. fergusenii(弗格森氏埃希菌)

    E. hermanii(赫曼氏埃希菌)

    E. vulneris(伤口埃希菌)

Ewingella[尤因(欧文)菌属]

    E. americana(美国尤因氏菌)

H. afnia(哈夫尼亚菌属)

    H. afnia alvei(蜂房哈夫尼亚菌)

    H. paralvei(类蜂房哈夫尼亚菌)

Klebsiella(克雷伯菌属)

    K. granulomatis(肉芽肿克雷伯菌)

    K. ornithinolytica(解鸟氨酸克雷伯菌)

    K. pneumoniae subsp. pneumoniae(肺炎克雷伯菌肺炎亚种)

    K. pneumoniae subsp. azaenae(肺炎克雷伯菌臭鼻亚种)

    K. pneumoniae subsp. rhinoscleromatis(肺炎克雷伯菌鼻硬结亚种)

    K. oxytoca(催产克雷伯菌)

    K. planticola(植生克雷伯菌)

    K. singaporensis(新加坡克雷伯菌)

    K. terrigena(土生克雷伯菌)

    K. variicola[多栖(变栖)克雷伯菌]

Kluyvera(克雷瓦菌属)

    K. aegyptica(埃及克雷瓦菌)

    K. ascorbata(抗坏血酸克雷瓦菌)

    K. carniphila(喜肉克雷瓦菌)

    K. cochleae(蜗牛克雷瓦菌)

    K. cryocrescens(栖冷克雷瓦菌)

    K. georgiana(佐治亚克雷瓦菌)

    K. himachalensis(喜马偕尔拜雷瓦菌)

Koserella(科泽菌属)

    K. trabulsii(特拉伯氏科泽菌)

Leclercia(勒克菌属)

    L. adecarboxylata(非脱羧勒克菌)

Leminorella(勒米诺菌属)

    L. grimontii(格氏勒米诺菌)

    L. richardii(理氏勒米诺菌)

Moellerella（米勒菌属）

　　M. wisconsensis（威斯康星米勒菌）

Morganella（摩根氏菌属）

　　M. morganella subsp. morganella（摩根氏摩根氏菌摩根氏菌亚种）

　　M. morganella subsp. sibonii（摩根氏摩根氏菌塞氏亚种）

　　M. psychrotolerans（耐冷摩根氏菌）

Obesumbacterium（肥杆菌属）

　　O. proteus（变形肥杆菌）

Pantoea（泛菌属）

　　P. agglomerans（成团泛菌）

　　P. allii（洋葱泛菌）

　　P. ananatis（菠萝泛菌）

　　P. antyophila（喜花泛菌）

　　P. breneri（布伦纳氏泛菌）

　　P. calida（温热泛菌）

　　P. citrea（柠檬泛菌）

　　P. deleyi（迪莱氏泛菌）

　　P. dispersa（分散泛菌）

　　P. eucrina（易鉴泛菌）

Pectobacterium（果胶杆菌属）

　　P. atrosepticum（黑腐果胶杆菌）

　　P. betavasculorum（纤维束果胶杆菌）

　　P. carnegieana（大仙人掌果胶杆菌）

　　P. cacticidum（灭仙人掌果胶杆菌）

　　P. chrysanthemi（菊果胶杆菌）

　　P. cypripedii（勺兰果胶杆菌）

　　P. rhapontici（大黄果胶杆菌）

　　P. wasabiae（山蒿菜果胶杆菌）

　　P. carotovorum subsp. carotovorum（胡萝卜软腐果胶杆菌胡萝卜软腐亚种）

　　P. . carotovorum subsp. atrosepticum（胡萝卜软腐果胶杆菌黑腐亚种）

Photorhabdus（光杆菌属）

　　P. asymbiotica（非共生光杆菌）

　　P. asymbiotica subsp. asymbiotica（非共生光杆菌非共生亚种）

　　P. asymbiotica subsp. australis（非共生光杆菌南部亚种）

　　P. damsela（美人鱼光杆菌）

　　P. luminescens（发光光杆菌）

　　P. luminescens subsp. akhurstii（发光光杆菌阿氏亚种）

　　P. luminescens subsp. kayaii［发光光杆菌克氏（凯氏）亚种］

　　P. luminescens subsp. laumondii（发光光杆菌劳氏亚种）

　　P. luminescens subsp. luminescens（发光光杆菌发光亚种）

　　P. luminescens subsp. thracensis（发光光杆菌色雷斯光杆菌）

Pragia(布拉格菌属)

    P. fontium(泉水布拉格菌)

Proteus(变形杆菌属)

    P. hauseri(豪氏变形杆菌)

    P. inconstans[不稳定(无恒)变形杆菌]

    P. mirabilis(奇异变形杆菌)

    P. myxofaciens(产黏变形杆菌)

    P. vulgaris(普通变形杆菌)

Providencia(普罗非登斯菌属)

    P. alcalifaciens(产碱普罗非登斯菌)

    P. burhodogranariea(大红仓普罗非登斯菌)

    P. friedericiana(弗里德普罗非登斯菌)

    P. heimbachae[海氏(亨巴赫)普罗非登斯菌]

    P. rettgeri(雷氏普罗非登斯菌)

    P. rustigianii[拉氏(鲁氏)普罗非登斯菌]

    P. sneebia(斯尼大学普罗非登斯菌)

    P. stuartii(斯氏普罗非登斯菌)

    P. vermicola(居线虫普罗非登斯菌)

Rahnella(兰恩菌属)

    R. aquatilis(水生兰恩菌)

Raoultella(劳特菌属)

    R. ornithinolytica(解鸟氨酸劳特菌)

    R. planticola(植生劳特菌)

    R. terrigena(土生劳特菌)

Salmonella(沙门菌属)

    S. choleraesuis(猪霍乱沙门菌)

    S. enteritidis(肠炎沙门菌)

    S. gallinarum(鸡沙门菌)

    S. hirschfeldii(希氏沙门菌)(副伤寒 C)

    S. paratyphi-A(甲型副伤寒沙门菌)

    S. schottmuelleri(薛氏沙门菌)(副伤寒 B)

    S. typhi(伤寒沙门菌)

    S. typhimurium(鼠伤寒沙门菌)

    S. sailamae(萨拉姆沙门菌)

    S. azizonae(亚利桑那沙门菌)

Serratia(沙雷菌属)

    S. entomophila(嗜虫沙雷菌)

    S. facaria(无花果沙雷菌)

    S. glossinae(采采蝇沙雷菌)

    S. grimesii[葛氏(格氏)沙雷菌]

    S. liquefaciens(液化沙雷菌)

*S. marcescen*s（黏质沙雷菌）

S. marcescens subsp. Sakuensis（黏质沙雷菌长野亚种）

S. nematodiphila（嗜线虫沙雷菌）

S. odorifera（气味沙雷菌）

S. plymuthia（蒲城沙雷菌）

Shigella（志贺菌属）

S. boydii（鲍氏志贺菌）

S. dysenteriate（痢疾志贺菌）

S. flexneri（福氏志贺菌）

S. sonnei（宋内氏志贺菌）

Tatumella（塔特姆菌属）

T. citrea（柠檬塔特姆菌）

T. . mobirosea（凤梨病塔特姆菌）

T. punctata（斑点塔特姆菌）

T. ptyseos（痰塔特姆菌）

T. terreae（土壤塔特姆菌）

Trabulsiella（特拉伯菌属）

T. guamensis（关岛特拉伯菌）

T. odontotermitis（黑翅白蚁特拉伯菌）

Xenorhabdus（致病杆菌属）

X. griffiniae（格里芬致病杆菌）

X. hominickii（霍氏致病杆菌）

X. indica（印度致病杆菌）

X. innexi（因耐公司致病杆菌）

X. japonicus（日本致病杆菌）

X. koppenhoeferi（霍潘菏芬致病杆菌）

X. kozodoii（库氏致病杆菌）

X. luminescens（发光致病杆菌）

X. mauleonii（莫氏致病杆菌）

X. poinarii（波因那致病杆菌）

Yersinia（耶氏菌属）

Y. aldovae（阿氏耶氏菌）

Y. aleksiciae（阿利克西奇耶氏菌）

Y. beicovieri（伯氏耶氏菌）

Y. enterocolitica（小肠结肠炎耶氏菌）

Y. entomophaga（食昆虫耶氏菌）

Y. frederiksenii（弗氏耶氏菌）

Y. intermedia（中间耶氏菌）

Y. kristensenii（克氏耶氏菌）

Y. massiliensis（马赛耶氏菌）

Y. nurmii（纳氏耶氏菌）

Y. pestis（鼠疫耶氏菌）

Yokenella(约克菌属)

    Y. regensburgei(雷金斯堡约克菌)

17   *gram-negative bacillus*, *Vibrionaceae*[革兰氏阴性杆菌(弧菌科)]

Aeromonas(气单胞菌属)

    A. aquariorum(鱼缸气单胞菌)

    A. bestiarum(兽生气单胞菌)

    A. bivalvium(双壳贝气单胞菌)

    A. caviae(豚鼠气单胞菌)

    A. diversa(多样气单胞菌)

    A. encheleia(鳗气单胞菌)

    A. media(间气单胞菌)

    A. rivull(小溪气单胞菌)

    A. simiae(猴气单胞菌)

    A. sobria(温和气单胞菌)

Aliivibrio(别弧菌属)

    A. fischeri(费氏别弧菌)

    A. finisterrensis[菲尼斯泰(地之角)别弧菌]

    A. logi(火神别弧菌)

    A. salmonicida(杀蛙别弧菌)

    A. sifiae(挪威女神别弧菌)

    A. wodanis(渥顿别弧菌)

Enterovibrio(肠弧菌属)

    E. calviensis(卡尔维湾肠弧菌)

    E. coralii(珊瑚肠弧菌)

    E. nigricans(产黑肠弧菌)

    E. norvegicus(挪威肠弧菌)

Listonella(利斯顿菌属)

    L. anguillara(鳗利斯顿菌)

    L. damsela(美人鱼利斯顿菌)

    L. pelagia(海利斯顿菌)

Moritella(默里特菌属)

    M. abyssi(深渊默里特菌)

    M. dasanensis(北极站默里特菌)

    M. japonica(日本默里特菌)

    M. marina(海默里特菌)

    M. profunda(海底默里特菌)

    M. viscose(黏默里特菌)

    M. yayanosii(亚雅诺斯默里特菌)

Photobacterium(发光杆菌属)

    P. angustum(狭小发光杆菌)

P. aphoticum（无冷光发光杆菌）

P. aplysiae（海兔发光杆菌）

P. aquimaris（海水发光杆菌）

P. damsela（美人鱼发光杆菌）

P. fischeri（费氏发光杆菌）

P. frigidiphilus（嗜冷发光杆菌）

P. gaetbulicola（栖滩涂发光杆菌）

P. indicum（印度洋发光杆菌）

P. jeanii（琼氏发光杆菌）

Plesiomonas（邻单胞菌属）

P. shigelloides（类志贺邻单胞菌）

Salinivibrio（嗜盐弧菌属）

S. bovis（牛嗜盐弧菌）

S. costicola［肋生（住肋）嗜盐弧菌］

S. costicola subsp. alscaliphilus（住肋嗜盐弧菌嗜碱亚种）

S. costicola subsp. costicol（住肋嗜盐弧菌住肋亚种）

S. costicola subsp. vallismortis（住肋嗜盐弧菌死谷亚种）

S. proteolyticus（解蛋白嗜盐弧菌）

S. sharmensis（沙姆沙伊赫嗜盐弧菌）

S. siamensis（暹罗嗜盐弧菌）

Shewanella（施万菌属 希瓦菌属）

S. abyssi（深渊施万菌）

S. affinis（邻附施万菌）

S. alga（海藻施万菌）

S. algidipiscicola（居冷鱼施万菌）

S. amazonensis（亚马逊施万菌）

S. aquimarina（海水施万菌）

S. arctica（北极施万菌）

S. atlantica（大西洋施万菌）

S. baltica（波罗的海施万菌）

S. basaltis（玄武岩施万菌）

Vibrio（弧菌属）

V. aerogenes（产气弧菌）

V. aestuarianus（河口弧菌）

V. agarivorans（食琼脂弧菌）

V. albensis（易北河弧菌）

V. alginolyticus（溶藻弧菌）

V. anguillarum（鳗弧菌）

V. angustum（狭窄弧菌）

V. areninigre（黑沙弧菌）

V. atlanticus（大西洋弧菌）

V. atypicus（非典型弧菌）

18 *gram-negative bacillus, obligate anaerobic* [革兰氏阴性杆菌(专性厌氧)]

Alistipes(另枝菌属)

A. *finegoldii*(芬戈尔德另枝菌)

A. *indistinctus*(难辨另枝菌)

A. *onderdonkii*(翁德顿另枝菌)

A. *putredinis*(腐败另枝菌)

A. *shahii*(谢氏另枝菌)

Anaerobiospirillum(厌氧螺菌属)

A. *succiniciproducens*(产琥珀酸厌氧螺菌)

A. *thomasii*(托马斯厌氧螺菌)

Bacteroides[类(拟)杆菌属]

B. *caccae*(粪类杆菌)

B. *distasonis*(吉氏类杆菌)

B. *eggerthii*(埃氏类杆菌)

B. *fragilis*(脆弱类杆菌)

B. *ovatus*(卵形类杆菌)

B. *uniformis*(单形类杆菌)

B. *bivius*(二路类杆菌)

B. *clarus*(光泽类杆菌)

B. *dorei*(多尔类杆菌)

B. *fluxus*(易死类杆菌)

Bilophila(嗜胆菌属)

B. *ilophila wadsworthia*(沃兹沃嗜胆菌)

Capnocytophaga(嗜二氧化碳噬纤维菌属)

C. *canimorsus*(狗咬嗜二氧化碳噬纤维菌)

C. *cynodegmi*(犬咬嗜二氧化碳噬纤维菌)

C. *gingivalis*(牙龈嗜二氧化碳噬纤维菌)

C. *granulosa*(颗粒嗜二氧化碳噬纤维菌)

C. *haemolytica*(溶血嗜二氧化碳噬纤维菌)

C. *leadbetteri*(利德比特嗜二氧化碳噬纤维菌)

C. *ochracea*(黄褐嗜二氧化碳噬纤维菌)

C. *sputigena*(生痰嗜二氧化碳噬纤维菌)

Catonella(卡顿菌属)

C. *morbi*(病害卡顿菌)

Desulfovibrio[脱硫(硫还原)弧菌属]

D. *desulfuricans*(脱硫脱硫弧菌属)

D. *intestinalis*(蚁肠脱硫弧菌属)

D. *piger*(惰性脱硫弧菌属)

D. *termitidis*(白蚁脱硫弧菌属)

Dialister(小杆菌属, 戴阿利斯特菌属)

    D. invisus(不显浊小杆菌)

    D. microaerophilus(微嗜氧小杆菌)

    D. pneumosintes(侵肺小杆菌)

    D. propionicifaciens(产丙酸小杆菌)

    D. succinatiphilus(喜琥珀酸小杆菌)

Dichelobacter(偶蹄杆菌属)

    D. modosus(节偶蹄杆菌)

Fibrobacter(纤杆菌属)

    F. intestinalis(肠纤杆菌)

    F. succinogenes(产琥珀酸纤杆菌)

Fusobacterium(梭杆菌属)

    F. alocis(龈沟梭杆菌)

    F. equinum(马梭杆菌)

    F. mortiferum(死亡梭杆菌)

    F. nucleatum(具核梭杆菌)

    F. perfoetens(极臭梭杆菌)

    F. plautii(普劳特梭杆菌)

    F. russii(鲁斯梭杆菌)

    F. simiae(猴梭杆菌)

    F. sulci(沟迹梭杆菌)

    F. varium(变形梭杆菌)

Hallella(霍尔菌属)

    H. allella seregens(需血清霍尔菌)

Johnsonella(约翰逊菌属)

    J. ignava(无力约翰逊菌)

Megamonas(巨单胞菌属)

    M. funiformis(线状巨单胞菌)

    M. hypermegas(趋巨巨单胞菌)

    M. rupellensis(拉罗歇尔巨单胞菌)

Mitesuokella(光岗菌属)

    M. dentalis(牙光岗菌)

    M. jalaludinii(贾拉路光岗菌)

    M. multiacidus(多酸光岗菌)

Oribaculum(口杆菌属)

    O. cantoniae(卡特口杆菌)

Oxalobacter(草酸杆菌属)

    O. formigenes(产甲酸草酸杆菌)

    O. vibrioformis(弧形草酸杆菌)

Porphyromonas(卟啉单胞菌属)

    P. asaccharolytica(不解糖卟啉单胞菌)

    P. bennonis[辨野(板东)卟啉单胞菌]

    P. cangingivalis(犬齿龈液卟啉单胞菌)

    P. cansulci(犬口腔卟啉单胞菌)

    P. circumdentaria(牙周卟啉单胞菌)

    P. endodontails(牙髓卟啉单胞菌)

    P. gingivalis(牙龈卟啉单胞菌)

    P. gulae(兽口卟啉单胞菌)

    P. levii[列氏(利氏)卟啉单胞菌]

    P. macacae(猕猴卟啉单胞菌)

Prevotella(普雷沃菌属)

    P. albensis[阿尔巴(苏格兰)普雷沃菌]

    P. amnii(羊水普雷沃菌)

    P. aurantiaca(橙色普雷沃菌)

    P. baroniae(巴隆氏普雷沃菌)

    P. bergensis(卑尔根普雷沃菌)

    P. bivia(双路普雷沃菌)

    P. brevis(短普雷沃菌)

    P. buccae(颊普雷沃菌)

    P. buccalis(口颊普雷沃菌)

    P. fusca(深色普雷沃菌)

Rikenella(立肯菌属)

    R. microfusis(小锤立肯菌)

Ruminobacter(瘤胃杆菌属)

    R. amylophilus(嗜淀粉瘤胃杆菌)

    R. ruminicola(栖瘤胃瘤胃杆菌)

    R. succinogenes(产琥珀酸瘤胃杆菌)

Schwartzia(施瓦茨氏菌属)

    S. succinivorans(嗜琥珀酸施瓦茨氏菌)

Sebaldella(塞巴鲁德菌属)

    S. termitidis(白蚁塞巴鲁德菌)

Selenomonas(月形单胞菌属)

    S. acidaminovorans(嗜氨酸月形单胞菌)

    S. artemidis(蛛形月形单胞菌)

    S. bovis(牛月形单胞菌)

    S. dianae(月神月形单胞菌)

    S. flueggei(福氏月形单胞菌)

    S. infelix(不幸月形单胞菌)

    S. lacticifex(产乳酸月形单胞菌)

    S. lipolytica(解脂月形单胞菌)

S. noxia(有害月形单胞菌)

S. sputigena(生痰月形单胞菌)

Tannerella(坦娜菌属)

T. forsythensis(福赛斯坦娜菌)

Tissierella[泰氏(替策)菌属]

T. cereatinini(肌酐泰氏菌)

T. creatinophila(喜肌酸泰氏菌)

T. praeacuta(前瑞泰氏菌)

Wolinella(沃林菌属)

W. curva(弯曲沃林菌)

W. recta(直肠沃林菌)

W. succinogenes(产琥珀酸沃林菌)

19 *Other prokaryotes*(其他原核细胞微生物)

Bartonella(巴尔通体属)

B. alsatica(阿尔萨斯巴尔通体)

B. bovis(牛巴尔通体)

B. caprecoli(狍巴尔通体)

B. doshiae(多斯巴尔通体)

B. elizabethae(伊丽莎白巴尔通体)

B. grahamii(格雷厄姆氏巴尔通体)

B. henselae(亨氏巴尔通体)

B. japonica(日本巴尔通体)

B. silvatica(森林巴尔通体)

B. talpae(鼹巴尔通体)

Borrelia(疏螺旋体属)

B. anserina(鹅疏螺旋体)

B. brasiliensis(巴西疏螺旋体)

B. caucasica(高加索疏螺旋体)

B. dugesii(杜氏疏螺旋体,扁虱疏螺旋体)

B. graingeri(格氏疏螺旋体)

B. harveyii(哈氏疏螺旋体)

B. tillae(蒂氏疏螺旋体)

B. afzelii(阿氏疏螺旋体)

B. bissettii(比氏疏螺旋体)

B. garinii(加林疏螺旋体)

Brachyspira(短螺旋菌属)

B. aalborgi(奥尔堡短螺旋菌)

B. alvinipulli[雏鸡(鸡腹泻)短螺旋菌]

B. hyodysenteriae(猪痢疾短螺旋菌)

B. innocens(无害短螺旋菌)

B. murdochii(莫多克短螺旋菌)

B. intermedia(中间短螺旋菌)

B. pilosicoli(多毛短螺旋菌)

Brevinema(短螺旋体属)

B. andersonii(安得森短螺旋体)

Chlamydia(衣原体属)

C. muridarum[小鼠(鼠类)衣原体]

C. suis(猪衣原体)

C. trachmatis(沙眼衣原体)

Chlamydophila(亲衣原体属)

C. abortus(流产亲衣原体)

C. caviae(豚鼠亲衣原体)

C. felis(猫亲衣原体)

C. pecorum[畜(羊)群亲衣原体]

C. pneumoniae(肺炎支原体)

C. psittaci(鹦鹉热亲衣原体)

Coxiella(考克斯体属)

C. burneii(贝氏考克斯体)

Ehrlichia(埃里希体属)

E. canis(犬埃里希体)

E. chaffeensis(查氏埃里希体)

E. equi(马埃里希体)

E. ewingii(尤因氏埃里希体)

E. muris(小鼠埃里希体)

E. phagocytophila(嗜噬胞埃里希体)

E. ristinii(里氏埃里希体)

E. ruminantium(反刍类埃里希体)

E. sennetsu(腺热埃里希体)

Leptospira(钩端螺旋体属)

L. alexanderi(亚历山大钩端螺旋体)

L. biflexa(双曲钩端螺旋体)

L. broomii(布鲁姆钩端螺旋体)

L. fainei(费恩钩端螺旋体)

L. interrogans(问号钩端螺旋体)

L. kirschneri(基氏钩端螺旋体)

L. kmetyi(柯氏钩端螺旋体)

L. meyeri(迈氏钩端螺旋体)

L. parva(弱小钩端螺旋体)

L. weilii(韦氏钩端螺旋体)

Mycoplasma(支原体属)

M. adleri(艾德勒支原体)

M. auris（山羊支原体）

M. anatis（鸭支原体）

M. bovis（牛支原体）

M. arthritidis（关节炎支原体）

M. buccale（颊支原体）

M. canis（犬支原体）

M. citelli（地鼠支原体）

M. coccoides（球形支原体）

M. dispar（殊异支原体）

Orientia（东方次体属）

O. rientia tsutsugamushi（恙虫病东方次体）

Rickettsia（立克次体属）

R. prowazekii（普氏立克次体）

R. canadensis（加拿大立克次体）

R. akari（螨立克次体）

R. australis（南方立克次体）

R. conorii（康氏立克次体）

R. parkeri（帕氏立克次体）

R. montana（蒙大拿立克次体）

R. rickettsii（立氏立克次体）

R. aficae（非洲立克次体）

R. tamurae（田村立克次体）

Serpulina（小蛇菌属）

S. alvinipulli（鸡腹泻小蛇菌）

S. murdochii（默多克小蛇菌）

S. intermedia（中间小蛇菌）

S. pilosicoli（多毛小蛇菌）

S. innocens（无害小蛇菌）

S. hyodysenteriae（猪痢疾小蛇菌）

Treponema（密螺旋体属）

T. amylovorum（食淀粉密螺旋体）

T. azotonutricium（偶氮营养密螺旋体）

T. berlinense（柏林密螺旋体）

T. brennaborense（伯兰登堡密螺旋体）

T. bryantii（布氏密螺旋体）

T. carateum（斑点病密螺旋体）

T. denticola（齿垢密螺旋体）

T. innocens（无害密螺旋体）

T. medium（中等密螺旋体）

T. minutum（微细密螺旋体）

Tropheryma（养障菌属）

T. whipplei（惠普尔病养障菌）

Ureaplasma（脲原体属）

U. *canigenitalium*（犬生殖道脲原体）

U. *cati*（猫脲原体）

U. *diversum*（差异脲原体）

U. *felinum*（猫口咽脲原体）

U. *gallorale*（鸡口脲原体）

U. *parvum*（小脲原体）

U. *urealyticum*（解脲脲原体）

Waddlia（华诊原体属）

V. *chondrophila*（嗜线粒体华诊原体）

Appendix II

Clinical Cases

Case 1   Bacterial Pneumonia

A 35-year-old man came to theemergency room because of fever because of fever and pain in his left chest when he coughed. Five days earlier he had developed signs of a viral upper respiratory infection with sore throat, runny nose and increased cough. The day before presentation he developed left lateral chest pain when he coughed or took a deep breath. Twelve hours before coming to the emergency room he was awakened with a severe shaking chill and sweating. Further history taking disclosed that the patient drank moderate to heavy amounts of alcohol and had smoked one package of cigarettes daily for about 17 years. He worked as an automobile repairing man. He had a history of two prior hospitalizations-4 years ago for alcohol withdrawal and 2 years ago for acute bronchitis.

Clinical Features

Temperature was 39 ℃, pulse 130/min and respirations 28/min. Blood pressure was 120/80 mmHg. Physical examination showed a slightly overweight man who was coughing frequently and holding his left chest when he coughed. He produced very little thick rusty-colored sputum. His chest examination showed normal movement of the diaphragm. There was dullness to percussion of the left lateral posterior chest, suggesting consolidation of the lung. Tubular(bronchial) breath sounds were heard in the same area along with dry crepitant sounds (rales), consistent with lung consolidation and viscous mucus in the airway. The remainder of his physical examination was normal.

Laboratory Findings & Imaging

Chest films showed a dense left lower lobe consolidation consistent with bacterial pneumonia. The hematocrit was 45% (normal). The white blood cell count was 16,000/L (markedly elevated) with 80% PMN forms with an absolute PMN count of 12,800/L (markedly elevated), 12% lymphocytes and 8% monocyte. Blood chemistry tests, including electrolytes, were normal. Sputum was thick, yellow to rusty-colored and purulent in appearance. Gram stain of the sputum showed many PMN cells lancet-shaped gram-positive diplococci. Twenty-four hours later, the blood cultures were positive for Streptococcus pneumoniae. Cultures of sputum grew numerous S pneumonia and a few colonies of H influenzae.

Treatment

The initial diagnosis was bacterial pneumonia, possibly pneumococcus. Intra-intestinal aqueous penicillin G therapy was initiated and the patient was infused with parenteral fluid. Within 48 hours, his body temperature was normal and he had a large amount of purulent sputum. Penicillin G lasted 7 days. At 4 weeks after admission, lung consolidation cleared.

Case 2　Peritonitis & Abscesses

An 18-year-old male student was admitted to the hospital because of fever and abdominal pain. He had been well until 3 days prior to admission, when he developed diffuse abdominal pain and vomiting following the evening meal. The pain persisted through the night and was worse the following morning. He was seen in the emergency room, where abdominal tenderness was noted; X-rays of the chest and abdomen were normal; the white blood cell count was 24,000/L; and other laboratory tests, including tests of liver, pancreas and renal function, were normal. The patient returned home, but the abdominal pain and intermittent vomiting persisted and fever to 38 ℃ developed. The patient was admitted to the hospital on the third day of illness. There was no history of use of medication, drug or alcohol abuse, trauma or infection and the family history was negative.

Clinical Features

The temperature and was 38 ℃, the pulse 100/min, respirations 24/min. The blood pressure was 110/70 mmHg. Physical examination showed a normally developed young man who appeared acutely ill and complained of diffuse abdominal pain. The chest and heart examinations were normal. The abdomen was slightly distended. There was diffuse periumbilical and right lower quadrant tenderness to palpation with guarding (muscle rigidity with palpation). There was a suggestion of a right lower quadrant mass. Bowel sounds were influent.

Laboratory Findings & Imaging

The hematocrit was 45% (normal) and the white blood cell count was 20,000/L (markedly elevated) with 90% polymorphonuclear cells (markedly elevated) and 12% lymphocytes. The serum amylase (a test for pancreatitis) was normal. Electrolytes and tests of liver and renal function were normal. X-ray films of the chest and abdomen were normal, though several distended loops of small bowel were seen. CT scan of the abdomen showed a fluid collection in the right lower quadrant with extension into the pelvis.

Treatment

The patient was taken to the operating room. During surgery, a perforated appendix was found, with a large appendix abscess extending into the pelvis. Remove the appendix, collect about 300 mL of odor abscess fluid and place a drainage tube. The patient received gentamicin, ampicillin and metronidazole for 2 weeks. One week after surgery, drainage was performed daily and completely removed. Cultures of abscess fluids showed at least 6 species of bacteria, including E. coli, Bacteroides fragilis, S. aureus and enterococci (normal gastrointestinal flora). The patient recovered uneventfully.

Case 3 Mycobacterium Tuberculosis Infections-Pulmonary Tuberculosis

A 64-year-old man was admitted to the hospital and had a history of 5 months of progressive weakness and a weight loss of 13 kilograms. He also has fever, chills and chronic coughing, producing a pale yellowish sputum and occasionally blood. The patient drank a lot of alcohol and lived in a homestay next door to his frequented tavern. He has smoked a pack of cigarettes every day for the past 45 years. The patient did not have a history of tuberculosis, had no previous history of skin disease, tuberculosis or chest radiographs and had no known history of tuberculosis exposure.

Clinical Features

His temperature was 39 ℃, pulse 110/min, respirations 32/min and blood pressure 120/80 mmHg. He was a slender man. His dentition was poor, but the remainder of his head and neck examination was normal. On chest examination, many crackles were heard over the upper lung fields. The remainder of the physical examination was normal.

Laboratory Findings & Imaging

The hematocrit was 30% (low) and the white blood cell count was 9,600/L. Electrolyte concentrations and other blood tests were normal. The test for HIV-1 antibody was negative. A chest radiograph showed extensive cavitary infiltrates in both upper lobes. A tuberculin skin test was negative, as were skin tests with mumps and candida antigens, indicating anergy. A sputum specimen was obtained immediately and an acid-fast stain was done before the sputum concentration procedure. Numerous acid-fast bacteria were seen on the smear. Culture of the decontaminated and concentrated sputum was positive for acid-fast bacteria after 14 days' incubation; Mycobacterium tuberculosis was identified by molecular probe 2 days later. Susceptibility tests of the organisms showed susceptibility to isoniazid, rifampin, pyrazinamide, ethambutol and streptomycin.

Hospital Course & Treatment

Patients were treated with isoniazid, rifampicin, pyrazinamide and streptomycin for 2 weeks, followed by direct observation of the same drug twice a week for 6 weeks, followed by direct observation of twice-weekly isolation of isoniazid and rifampicin for 16 weeks. Follow-up sputum culture negative tuberculosis. During hospitalization, the patient was placed in isolation and was required to wear a mask at any time. However, medical students and resident physicians are exposed to patients before the masks and isolation are implemented. The resident converted her tuberculin skin test and received 12 months of isoniazid prophylaxis. Trying to track the patient's close contact. A total of 34 tuberculin-positive human tuberculin tests were found to be positive. People aged 35 or under receive one-year isoniazid prophylaxis; those over 35 years of age regularly follow chest X-rays. Two cases of active tuberculosis have also been diagnosed and treated. Mycobacterium tuberculosis isolates from two patients were identical to the target patient isolates by DNA fingerprinting.

Case 4   Anthrax in the United States, 2001-The Index Case in South Florida

On October 2, 2001, a 63-year-old man was admitted to the emergency department of a South Florida medical center because of fever, vomiting and confusion. Four days earlier he had developed fever, myalgia and malaise without specific focal symptoms. The patient had a history of mild heart disease but had otherwise been in good health.

On physical examination, the patient was lethargic and disoriented. His temperature was 39 ℃, blood pressure 150/80 mmHg, pulse 110/min and respirations 18/min. The only other potential abnormality on physical examination was the presence of rhonchi on auscultation of the chest. Rales were not heard. Nuchal rigidity was not present and Kernig and Brudzinski signs were not positive. Multiple blood cultures were obtained. Treatment with intravenous cefotaxime and vancomycin was begun prior to a spinal tap. The hematocrit was 46%, the white blood cell count 9,400/L with 77% polymorphonuclear cells, 15% lymphocytes and 8% monocytes. Blood chemistry tests were normal. The initial chest radiograph (see N Eng JMed 2001;354:1607) showed basilar infiltrates and a widened mediastinum. A spinal tap yielded cloudy CSF with a glucose of 57 mg/dL, a protein of 666 mg/dL and a white cell count of 4,750/L with 81% PMN cells and 19% monocytes. Red blood cells were also present in the CSF. Gram stain of the CSF revealed numerous PMNs and numerous large gram-positive rods, often in chains. A diagnosis of anthrax was considered and high-dose intravenous penicillin G was added to the therapeutic regimen. The medical center laboratory identified Bacilus anthracis 18 hours after the CSF had been cultured. B anthracis was also identified in the blood cultures. On the day of the second hospitalization, the patient developed a generalized seizure. He was intubated and began assisted ventilation. Hypotension and renal failure occur. The patient died on the third hospitalization day. At necropsy, extensive fluid edema is present in the peritoneal cavity. There is lung collapse and lung tissue is not consolidated. There are subpleural and hematoma haemorrhage sites. The mediastinum has thick blood and lymphadenopathy. The heart, liver and spleen are normal. The brain is not checked. The patient served as a photo editor at a large newspaper agency in Palm Beach County, Florida. On July 19, 2001, the patient examined a colleague who described it as suspicious and contained powder. This letter has never been found. Bacillus anthracis was cultured from 20 out of 136 survey-guided environmental samples obtained from October 8 – 10, 2001. Positive cultures included 2 of 21 from the patient's work area. Other positive cultures were obtained from the company's mailrooms, postal and asymptomatic mail operators' offices. These mailers had a positive response to Bacillus anthracis. During the period from October 25 to November 8, 2001, more positive cultures were obtained from other areas of the workplace. It is recommended that more than 1,000 people use antibiotic prophylaxis. The second patient worked at a publishing company and had contact with a large number of work-related e-mails. He developed symptoms on January 1st on January 28 and reported on 4 October that he may have inhaled anthrax. He was admitted to hospital on October 1 and began treatment for antibiotics. The nasal swab B-type anthrax obtained on October 5, 2002 was positive, but the blood, bronchial washing fluid and pleural fluid obtained after the initiation of antibiotic treatment were negative. The two pleural fluid samples were positive for Bacillus anthracis by the polymerase chain reaction. Therefore, this patient is the second inhaled anthrax. He survived and was discharged on October 17, 2001.

Case 5   HIV-1 & AlDS-Disseminated Mycobacterium A Vium Complex(MAC)Infection

A 44-year-old male patient had intermittent fever,sometimes with a history of chills. His frequency of bowel movements increased,there was no candid diarrhea and occasional cramps and abdominal pain occurred. No headache or cough. He has lost about 5 kg of body weight. The rest of his medical history is negative. Ten years before the current disease,the patient's activities made him at risk of contracting HIV. He has never conducted a laboratory test to determine his HIV status.

Clinical Features

His temperature was 38 ℃ ,pulse 90/min,respirations 18/min and blood pressure 110/70 mmHg. He did not appear to be acutely ill. The tip of the spleen was palpable in the left upper abdominal quadrant 3 cm below the ribs(suggesting splenomegaly). Hepatomegaly and lymphadenopathy were not present and there were no neurologic or meningeal signs. The balance of the physical examination was normal.

Laboratory Findings & Imaging

The patient's white count was stable at 3,000/L (below normal). The hematocrit was 29% (below normal). A CD4 T helper-inducer cell count was 75 cells/L (normal,425-1,650/L). The chemistry panel was notable only for the liver enzyme alkaline phosphatase concentration of 210 U/L (normal, 36 – 122 U/L). Further assessment of the cause of the patient's fever revealed normal urinalysis,negative blood cultures and normal chest radiographs. The serum cryptococcal antigen test was negative. Two blood cultures for mycobacteria were obtained. After 10 and 12 days after they were drawn,these became positive. Three days later,the organism was identified as Mycobacterium avium complex (MAC) by a molecular probe. The standard ELISA test for anti-HIV-1 antibodies is the HIV-1 major antigen group,each of the Gag,Pol and Env proteins. Branched DNA analysis measuring HIV-1 RNA was positive at 300,000 copies/ml.

Treatment & Follow-Up

The patient started using the MAC's three-drug regimen:clarithromycin,ethambutol and ciprofloxacin. He noticed that his sense of well-being increased,his fever and sweating decreased significantly and his appetite increased. Concomitantly,patients started receiving highly active antiretroviral therapy (HAART). The drugs used were two nucleoside reverse transcriptase inhibitors,zidovudine (AZT) and lamivudine (3TC) and one protease inhibitor,indinavir. After 4 months of starting antiretroviral therapy,the patient's HIV-1 RNA viral load assay showed no detectable virus levels;the CD4 T cell count was 250 cells/L.

Case 6   Staphylococcus Aureas Infection

While on call on a saturday night in July,you receive a call from the mother of a 15-year-old man who developed the acute onset of nausea,vomiting and diarrhea shortly after returning from an outdoor party that was held at the home of a friend. At the party,picnic lunch of hamburgers,hot dogs,potato salad,baked beans and lemonade was served. The food was served on an outdoor picnic table and the guests were free to eat at any time during the party. None of the food tested spoiled or tainted. His symptoms started abruptly about an hour after he returned home, which was about 4 hours after he had eaten. He currently is unable to keep down anything. He does not have a fever and has not passed any blood in his stool or vomitus. Prior to calling you, your patient's mother spoke with the hostess of the party, who said that she had heard from three other guests who became ill with similar symptoms.

Please answer following questions:

1. Which organism is the most likely cause of this patient's illness? Please interprete the possible pathogenisis.

2. Your patient's mother requests that you call in a prescription for an antibiotic to treat the infection. What is your response?

3. How to develop the microbiological diagnosis for the pathogen?

Case 7　Vibrio Cholerae Infection

A 35-year-old woman had a history of severe diarrhea and vomiting in the emergency room for two days. She began her symptoms shortly after returning from her mission and she brought her church to a rural area in central Africa. She recalled eating shrimp that seemed to be undercooked. Her symptoms suddenly started with watery diarrhea followed by vomiting. She has no fever and denies abdominal pain. At the time of examination, the body temperature was 37.2 ℃, the pulse rate was 115/min and the blood pressure was 80/50 mmHg. Her mucous membranes are dry and her eyes are sunken. When she gently squeezed, her skin was dry and her tent was clean. Her abdomen has an overactive bowel sound, but it is soft and implicated. Her stool was a water sample and her blood test was negative. Whole blood counts show elevated white blood cell counts and elevated hematocrit. The metabolic group showed hypokalemia, low serum bicarbonate and prerenal azotemia. You assess whether this patient is suffering from hypovolemic shock and metabolic acidosis and take appropriate treatment. Please answer following questions:

1. What organism is most likely to be identified on school culture?

2. What is the cause of this patient's diarrhea?

3. What suggestions you could provide for public biosafety?

Case 8　Hepatitis Virus Infection

A 26-year-old woman, who worked in a restaurant as a service, was brought to the outpatient-room with the chief complaint of low-grade fever, nausea and liver pain for 3 weeks. She was pregnant for five months now.

Results of laboratory tests:

Hb 115 g/L (normal:110-160 g/L)

ELISA:HBsAg(+),HBeAg(+);

Alanine aminotransferase (ALT) 200 U/L(normal:0-49 U/L)

Please answer following questions:

1. What's your preliminary impression for this patient?

2. Please describe the different types of Hepatitis Virus and their transmitted routes?

3. According to the basic information of the patient, please offer a good suggestion for her?

Case 9   HIV Infection

Five years ago, a 24-year-old girl developed hepatitis B and is now entering an antenatal clinic late in pregnancy. She was worried because her husband had just told her that he had AIDS.

Please answer following questions:

1. What laboratory tests would you perform for her?

2. If all of the laboratory tests results are bad, please provide a correct suggestion for her?

3. If the girl is HIV positive, what specific cell types are most commonly infected with this virus? What cell surface receptor is the binding site of this virus?

Case 10   Candida Albicans Infection

A 28-year-old woman presents to the office complaining of 2-days of itchy vaginal discharge. One week ago you saw and treated her for a urinary tract infection (UTI) with sulfamethoxazole and trimethoprim (SMX-TMP). She completed her medication as ordered and developed the vaginal discharge shortly thereafter. She denies abdominal pain and her dysuria has resolved. She is not currently taking any medications. On examination, she is comfortable appearing and has normal vital signs. Her general physical examination is normal. A pelvic examination reveals a thick, crud-like, white discharge in her vagina that is adherent to the vaginal sidewalls. There is no cervical discharge or cervical motion tenderness and bimanual examination of the uterus and adnexa is normal.

Please answer following questions:

1. What is the most likely cause of these symptoms?

2. What are the most likely reservoirs of this organism in this patient?

3. How to perform the detection of pathogen in laboratory medicine?

Appendix Ⅲ

Microbiology Webs

一、WHO 总部：http：//www.who.int/

二、中国微生物学会主页：http：//csm.im.ac.cn/index.php

三、中华医学会：http：//www.cma.org.cn/

四、国际传染病学会：http：//www.isid.org

五、美国微生物学会系列杂志：http：//www.journals.asm.org

六、美国微生物学会出版社：http：//www.asmpress.org

七、美国国家医学图书馆：http：//www.nlm.nih.gov

八、美国食品和药品管理局：http：//www.fda.gov

九、中国医药文献数据库：http：//www2.cpi.ac.cn/demo/search_wz.html

十、中国中医药信息网：http：//www.cintcm.ac.cn

十一、中国生物医学文献数据库：http：//www.imicams.ac.cn/cbm/index.asp

十二、中文医学杂志网址

1. JAMA：http：//jama.ama-assn.org/

2. 中华微生物学和免疫学志：http：//www.chininfo.gov.cn/periodical

3. 中华实验和临床学毒杂志：http：//www.chinainfo.gov.cn/periodical

4. 中华医学杂志：http：//www.chinainfo.gov.cn/periodical

5. 病毒学报：http：//www.chinajourmal.net/BDXB.html

6. 中华流行病学杂志：http：//www.chinainfo.gov.cn//periodical

7. 军事医学科学院院刊：http：//www chinainfo gov cnperiodical jsyxkxyyk/index htm

8. 中华传染病学杂志：http：//www.chinainfo.gov.cn/periodical/zhcrbzz/index.htm

9. 中国新药杂志：http：//www.chinfo.gov.cn/periodical/zgxzz/index.htm

10. 中国医学科学院学报 http：//www.chinainfo.gov.cn/periodical/zgyxkxyxb

11. 英国医学杂志中文版：http：//www.chinainfo.gov.cn/periodical/zh-bmj-c/index.htm

12. 中国病毒学：http：//www.chinainfo.gov.cn/periodical/zgbdx/index.htm

13. 北京大学医学报：http：//www.chinainfo.gov.cn/periodical/biykdxxx/index.htm

14. 中国皮肤性病学杂志：202.117.168.22/pifu/index.html

15. 免疫学杂志：http：//www.chinainfo.gov.cn/periodical/myxzz/index.htm

16. 中国抗生素杂志：http：//www.antibiotics-cn.com/anti_front/front_maga/

17. 白求恩医科大学学报：http：//www.chinainfo.gov.cn/periodical/bqeykdxxb/index.htm

18. 中国免疫学杂志：http：//www. chinainfo. gov. cn/periodical/zgyxzz/index. htm

19. 中国药学杂志：http：//www. chinainfo. gov. cn/periodical/zgyxzz/index. htm

20. 第三军医大学学报：http：//www. chinainfo. gov. cn/periodical/dsjydxxb/index. htm

21. 湖北医科大学学报：http：//www. china journal. net. cn

22. 中药研究与信息：http：//www. china-herbs. com. cn/

十三、英文医学杂志网址

1. Sciencehttp：//www. sciencemag. org/

2. Naturehttp：//www. nature. com

http：//www. natureasia. com（自然杂志的中文网址）

3. Proceedings of the National Academy of Scienceshttp：//www. pnas. org/

4. Centers for Disease Control and Preventionhttp：//www. cdc. gov/

5. Emerging Infectious Diseaseshttp：//www. cdc. gov/eid

6. The Microbiology Networkhttp：//microbiol. org/

7. Virology Informationhttp：//virology. science. org/

8. Journal of General Virologyhttp：//vir. sgmjournals. org/

9. All the Virology on theWWW. the full table of contents with links to all the virology websites   http：//www. tulane. edu/-dmsander/garryfavweb. html

10. Institute for Molecular Virology at the University of Wisconsin-Madisonhttp：//www. bocklabs. wisc. edu/welcome. html

11. Harvard medical Schoolhttp：//www. medicine. iu edu/home. html

12. Medicine College of Wisconsinhttp：//www. mcw. edu/

13. Stanford University School of Medicinehttp：//www. mce. stanford. cdu/school/

14. Boston University School of Medicinehttp：//www. bumc. bu. edu/

15. Infectionhttp：//www. urban-vogel. de（go to infection；pdf-format）

16. Cancer Controlhttp：//www. moffitt. usf. edu/ocjournal/

17. Journal of Infectious Diseaseshttp：//www. journals. uchicago. edu/jid/home. html

18. National Center for Biotechnology Informationhttp：//www. ncbi. nlm. nih. gov/

19. Computer Molecular Biology at NIHhttp：//www. molbio. info. mih. gov/molbio/

20. The American Society of Gene Therapyhttp：//www. asgt. org/

21. Nature Biotechnologyhttp：//www. biotech. nature. com/

22. University of Alabama School of Dentistryhttp：//www. dental. uab. edu/

23. Baylor College of Dentistryhttp：//www. tambcd. edu/

24. Harvard School of Dental Medicinehttp：//www. hsdm. med. harvard. edu/

25. Indiana University School of Dentistryhttp：//www. iusd. iupui. edu/

26. New York University College of Dentistry   http：//www. nyu. edu/dental/

27. The Amarican Dental Association http：//www. dental-resources. com/

28. Dental Globe http：//dentalglobe. com/

29. National Cancer Center http：//www. ncc. go. jp/Gopher/

30. National Cancer Institute http：//www. nci. nih. gov/

31. Amarican Cancer Society http：//www. cancer. org/

32. Pharmaceutical Information Network http：//pharminfo. com/

33. Pharmaceutical Manufacturers on the Internet http：//users. erols. com/Ipincock/

34. Cornell Univercity medical college http：//www. med. cornell. edu/

35. Radiology http://radiology. rsnajnls. org/

36. Physiological Genomics http://archneur. ama. -assn. org/

37. Archives of Neurology http://archneur. ama. -assn. org/

38. Center of Epidimiology Research：//www. orau. gov/cer/

39. Bioscience Network http://biochemie. net/

40. BioScience Research Tool http://biochemie. net/links/index. html/

41. Parasitology，Microbiology，Immunolog http://www. Isumc. edu/campus/micr/www. htm

42. The journal of Immunology http://www. jimmunol. orn

43. Immunology Today http://www. elsevier. nl/locate/ito

十四、微生物基因组研究网址

1. http://www. sanger. ac. uk/projects Sanger 中心（结核杆菌、麻风杆菌镰刀状虐原虫、淋病奈瑟菌）

2. http://www. genome. ou. edu Oklahoma 大学（淋病奈瑟菌、化脓链球菌、放线共生放线杆菌、构巢曲霉）

3. http://www. tigr. org/tdb/CMR/gmt/htmls/splashpage. html

4. http://www. pasteur. fr 巴斯德研究所网页

5. http://www. mcs. anl. gov/home/ gaasterl/magpic. html MAGPIE 计划

6. http://www. tigr. org Genomic 研究所（流感嗜血杆菌、生殖器衣原体、幽门螺杆菌）

7. http://www. seqnet. dl. ac. uk//home. html Daresbury 的 SEQNET

8. http://www. ncbi. nlm. gov 生物技术信息国家中心

9. http://www. ai. sri. com/ecocyc/hincyc. html 流感嗜血杆菌基因和代谢

10. http://www. ai. sri. com/ecocyc/ecocyc. html 大肠杆菌基因和代谢

11. http://www. pdb. bnl. gov. 蛋白数据

十五、微生物感染与抗生素耐药网址

1. http://www. asmusa. org/

2. http://www. fda. gov/fdac/features/795 antibio. htm

3. http://www. earss. rivm. nl/

4. http://www. healthsic. tufts. edu/apua/roarhome. htm

5. http://resistanceweb. mfhs. edu/cit/Index. asp

6. http://www. sciam. com/1998/0398issue/0398levy. html

十六、防治结核信息网址

1. http://www. who. int/gtb/

2. http://www. cdc，gov/nchstb/tb/links. htm

3. http://www. niaid. nih. gov/publications/blueprint/toc. htm

4. http://www. niaid. nih. gov/dmid/tb/tb. htm

5. http://www. niaid. nih. gov/dmid/tb/plan. htm

6. http://www. taacf. org/

7. http://www. southernresearch. com

8. http://www. cdc. gov/nchstp/tb/faps/qa. htm

十七、结合杆菌耐药性、应用基因芯片技术检测网址

1. http://www. harc. edu

2. http://www. elsevier. nl

3. http://www. ncbi. nlm. nih. gov

十八、与病毒有关的网址

1. http://www.cdc.gov

2. http://www.mad/cow.org

十九、DNA 疫苗网址

1. http://www.fda.gov/cber

2. http://www.dnavaccine.com

3. http://www.genweb.com

References

[1] KAREN C, CARROLL, TIMOTHY MIETZNER, J, et al. Jawetz Melnick & Adelberg's Medical Microbiology[M]. 27th edition. McGraw-Hill Education, 2015.

[2] PATRICK R MURRAY, KEN S ROSENTHAL, MICHAEL A Pfaller. Medical Microbiology[M]..8th edition, Elsevier, 2015

[3] BROOKS G F, CARROLL K A, BUTEL J S, et al. Medical biology[M]. 26th edition. New York: McGraw-Hill Companies, 2013.

[4] ALEKSHUN M N, LEVY S B. Molecular mechanisms of antibacterial multidrug resistance[J]. Cell, 2007 Mar 23, 128(6):1037-1050.

[5] CROFTS T S, GASPARRINI A J, DANTAS G. Nat Rev Microbiol[J]. Next-generation approaches to understand and combat the antibiotic resistome, 2017, 15(7):422-434.

[6] FURUYA E Y, LOWY F D. Antimicrobial-resistant bacteria in the community setting[J]. Nat Rev Microbiol, 2006, 4(1):36-45.

[7] JESSICA M A, BLAIR, MARK A W, ALISON J B, et al. Molecular mechanisms of antibiotic resistance [J]. Nat Rev Microbiol, 2015, 13(1):42-51.

[8] LEVY S B, MARSHALL B. Antibacterial resistance worldwide: causes, challenges and responses[J]. Nat Med, 2004, 10 (12 Suppl):122-129.

[9] SMITH P A, ROMESBERG F E. Combating bacteria and drug resistance by inhibiting mechanisms of persistence and adaptation[J]. Nat Chem Biol, 2007, 3(9):549-556.

[10] ALEKSHUN M N, LEVY S B. Molecular mechanisms of antibacterial multidrug resistance[J]. Cell, 2007, 128(6):1037-1050.

[11] MURRAY P A, ROSENTHAL K S, KOBAYASHI G S, et al. Medical Microbiology[M].5th ed Mosby, Missouri, USA:2006.

[12] 王丽. 真菌学概述[M].//李明远,徐志凯. 医学微生物学.3 版. 北京:人民卫生出版社,2016:438-450.

[13] 王丽. 真菌学总论[M].//李凡,徐志凯. 医学微生物学.8 版. 北京:人民卫生出版社,2013:327-334.

[14] 邓毛子. 真菌学总论[M].//韩莉. 医学微生物学.2 版. 西安:世界图书出版公司,2014:174-179.

[15] Moselio Schaechter. 真菌和原生生物植物病原体[M].//Moselio Schaechter. 真核微生物. 北京:科学出版社,2012:105-126.

[16] 李若瑜,王端礼. 真菌的形态与分类[M].//温海,李若瑜. 医学真菌学. 北京:人民卫生出版社,2012:1-8.

[17] 王爱平. 抗真菌药物[M].//温海,李若瑜. 医学真菌学. 北京:人民卫生出版社,2012:42-65.

[18] 吕桂霞,吕雪莲,刘维达. 真菌检验[M].//温海,李若瑜. 医学真菌学. 北京:人民卫生出版社,2012:67-83.

[19] 李明远. General Properties of Fungi[M].//汪世平,叶嗣颖. 医学微生物学与寄生虫学. 北京:科学出版社,2006:387-397.

[20] 李明远. General Properties of Fungi[M].//贾文祥. 医学微生物学. 北京:人民卫生出版社,2008:289-294.

[21] 王丽. 主要的病原性真菌[M].//李明远,徐志凯. 医学微生物学. 3 版. 北京:人民卫生出版社,
2016:451-462.

[22] 王丽. 主要病原性真菌[M].//李凡,徐志凯. 医学微生物学. 8 版. 北京:人民卫生出版社,2013:
335-344.

[23] 邓毛子. 主要病原性真菌[M].//韩莉. 医学微生物学. 2 版. 西安:世界图书出版公司,2014:
180-190.

[24] Moselio Schaechter. 人类致病曲霉[M].//Moselio Schaechter. 真核微生物. 北京:科学出版社,
2012:21-24.

[25] 潘炜华,温海. 浅部真菌病[M].//温海,李若瑜. 医学真菌学. 北京:人民卫生出版社,2012:84-
103.

[26] 张浩,冉玉平. 马拉色菌属[M].//温海,李若瑜. 医学真菌学. 北京:人民卫生出版社,2012:104-
115.

[27] 李福秋. 孢子丝菌病[M].//温海,李若瑜. 医学真菌学. 北京:人民卫生出版社,2012:151-160.

[28] 席艳丽. 组织胞浆菌病[M].//温海,李若瑜. 医学真菌学. 北京:人民卫生出版社,2012:174-
181.

[29] 齐显龙,刘斌. 着色真菌病[M].//温海,李若瑜. 医学真菌学. 北京:人民卫生出版社,2012:182-
189.

[30] 李明远. Pathogenic Fungi[M].//汪世平,叶嗣颖. 医学微生物学与寄生虫学. 北京:科学出版社,
2006:398-422.

[31] 李明远. Major Pathogenic Fungi[M].//贾文祥. 医学微生物学. 北京:人民卫生出版社,2008:
295-304.

[32] BECKER K,HEILMANN C,PETERS G. Coagulase-negative staphylococci[J]. Clin Microbiol Rev,
2014(27):870-926.

[33] KRZYSCIAK W,PLUSKWA KK,JURCZAK A,et al. The pathogenicity of the *Streptococcus* genus[J].
European journal of clinical microbiology & infectious diseases:official publication of the European
Society of Clinical Microbiology,2013(32):1361-1376.

[34] ASAM D,SPELLERBERG B. Molecular pathogenicity of *Streptococcus anginosus*[J]. Mol Oral Microbiol,2014(29):145-155.

[35] HAMADA S,KAWABATA S,NAKAGAWA I. Molecular and genomic characterization of pathogenic
traits of group A *Streptococcus pyogenes*[J]. Proc Jpn Acad Ser B Phys Biol Sci,2015(91):539-559.

[36] FISHER K,PHILLIPS C. The ecology,epidemiology and virulence of *Enterococcus*[J]. Microbiology,
2009(155):1749-1757.

[37] GILMORE M S,CLEWELL D B,IKE Y,et al. Enterococci:From Commensals to Leading Causes of
Drug Resistant Infection [Internet][M]. Boston:Massachusetts Eye and Ear Infirmary,2014.

[38] ROUPHAEL N G,STEPHENS D S. Neisseria meningitidis:biology,microbiology and epidemiology
[J]. Methods Mol Biol,2012(799):1-20.

[39] VAN DER POLL T,OPAL S M. Pathogenesis,treatment and prevention of pneumococcal pneumonia
[J]. Lancet,2009(374):1543-1556.

[40] VIRJI M. Pathogenic neisseriae:surface modulation,pathogenesis and infection control[J]. Nature re-
views Microbiology,2009(7):274-286.

[41] GALINSKA E M,ZAGORSKI J. Brucellosis in humans:etiology,diagnostics,clinical forms[J]. Ann
Agric Environ Med,2013(20):233-238.

[42] SPENCER R C. *Bacillus anthracis*[J]. J Clin Pathol,2003(56):182-187.

[43]PERRY R D,FETHERSTON J D. *Yersinia pestis* :etiologic agent of plague[J]. Clin Microbiol Rev, 1997(10):35-66.

[44]BOTTONE E J. *Bacillus cereus*,a volatile human pathogen[J]. Clin Microbiol Rev,2010(23):382- 398.

[45]GIKAS A,KOKKINI S,TSIOUTIS C. Q fever:clinical manifestations and treatment[J]. Expert Rev Anti Infect Ther,2010(8):529-539.

[46]WILSON B A,HO M. *Pasteurella multocida* :from zoonosis to cellular microbiology[J]. Clin Microbiol Rev,2013(26):631-655.

[47]BECK J,NASSAL M. Hepatitis B virus replication[J]. World J Gastroenterol. 2007,13(1):48-64.

[48]FALLAHIAN F,ALAVIAN S M,RASOULINEJAD M. Epidemiology and transmission of hepatitis G virus infection in dialysis patients[J]. Saudi J Kidney Dis Transpl,2010,21(5):831-834.

[49]MOOSAVY S H,DAVOODIAN P,NAZARNEZHAD M A,et al. Epidemiology,transmission,diagnosis and outcome of Hepatitis C virus infection[J]. Electron Physician,2017,9(10):5646-5656.

[50]MUKHERJEE R,BURNS A,RODDEN D,et al. Diagnosis and Management of Hepatitis C Virus Infection[J]. J Lab Autom,2015,20(5):519-538.

[51]BRIESE,THOMAS,PALACIOS,et al. Genetic detection and characterization of Lujo virus,a new hemorrhagic fever-associated arenavirus from Southern Africa[J]. Plos Pathogens,2009(5):5.

[52]DROSTEN C,KüMMERER B M,SCHMITZ H,et al. Molecular diagnostics of viral hemorrhagic fevers [J]. Antiviral Res,2003,57(1-2):61-87.

[53]HAMMON W M,RUDNICK,ADNICK A,et al. Virusesassociated with epidemic hemorrhagic fevers of the Philippines and Thailand[J]. Science,1960(131):1102-1103.

[54]IPPOLITO G,FELDMANN H,LANINI S,et al. Viral hemorrhagic fevers:advancing the level of treatment[J]. BMC Med,2012(10):31.

[55]MATTAR S,GUZMáN C,FIGUEIREDO L T. Diagnosis of hantavirus infection in humans[J]. Expert Rev Anti Infect Ther,2015,13(8):939-946.

[56]TOWNER,JONATHAN S,SEALY,et al. Newly discovered Ebola virus associated with hemorrhagic fever outbreak in Uganda[J]. Plos Pathogens,2008(4):11.

[57]YOSHIMATSU K,ARIKAWA J. Serological diagnosis with recombinant N antigen for hantavirus infection[J]. Virus Res,2014(187):77-83.